Social Gerontology
A Multidisciplinary Perspective

Social Gerontology
A Multidisciplinary Perspective

Nancy R. Hooyman

H. Asuman Kiyak

University of Washington

Allyn and Bacon, Inc.

Boston   London   Sydney   Toronto

Copyright © 1988 by Allyn and Bacon, Inc.
A Division of Simon & Schuster
160 Gould Street
Needham Heights, Massachusetts 02194

Library of Congress Cataloging-in-Publication Data

Hooyman, Nancy.
  Social gerontology.

  Bibliography: p.
  Includes index.
  1. Gerontology. 2. Aging. 3. Aged—United States.
I. Kiyak, H. Asuman, 1951–   . II. Title.
HQ1061.H583   1988   305.2'6   87-26916
ISBN 0-205-11312-5

Cover administrator: Linda Dickinson
Cover designer: Susan Slovinsky
Photo credits: Page 21, Courtesy of V. A. Medical Center, Seattle, WA; page 53, Special Collections Division, University of Washington Libraries; pages 68, 135, 272, and 476, Charles Heib; page 108, George T. Kruse; page 176, Joseph Freeman; pages 206, 303, 326, 358, and 617, Christian Staub; pages 365, 417, 528, 562, and 587, © Isabel Egglin, 1987; page 513, Marianne Gontarz; page 533, Universal Press Syndicate.

Printed in the United States of America
10 9 8 7 6 5 4 3   92 91 90 89

To Joe, for always being there, to Lara,
and to my parents, who have learned the secrets of aging gracefully.

HAK

To Gene, Kevin, and Christopher, for their constant support.
To my father, Hugh Runkle, for his 87-year example.

NRH

Contents

Preface

Aging is a complex and fascinating process, one which we all experience. It is complex because of its many facets—physiological, emotional, cognitive, economic, and interpersonal—that influence our social functioning and well-being. It is a fascinating process because these changes occur differently in each one of us. There is considerable truth to the statement that, as we grow older, we become more unlike each other.

Aging is also a process that has begun to attract the attention of the media, politicians, and the general public, largely because we live in a rapidly aging society. Changes in the numbers and proportion of older people in our population have numerous implications for societal structures, including the family, health care, pension and retirement practices, political processes, community and recreational services, and housing. In addition, these changes are of growing concern because of the problems of poverty, inadequate housing, and chronic disease faced by some elderly, particularly women, ethnic minorities, and the oldest-old. Public officials as well as individuals in the private sector are faced with the challenge of planning for a future in which the segment of the population over age 55 will experience the most rapid growth.

These changes have also meant that most colleges and universities now offer courses in gerontology, or the study of aging. Some of these courses aim to prepare students to work effectively with older people. Most of them seek to enhance students' personal understanding of their own and others' aging. Frequently, students take such a course simply to meet a requirement, discounting the relevance of the aging process to their own lives. Thus, instructors often are faced with the need to help students see the connection between learning about aging and understanding their own behavior, the behavior of their relatives, and oftentimes of their clients.

This book grew out of our experiences in teaching gerontology courses to undergraduate students. In doing so, we have been unable to locate a textbook that conveys the excitement and relevance of understanding the aging process, or one that adequately addresses the biological, psychological, and social aspects of aging. For years, we have been frustrated by the lack of a text that is comprehensive, thorough, and timely in its review of the rapidly growing research on the elderly. As a psychologist and sociologist/social worker, we are committed to developing a text that could be useful to a wide range of disciplines, including nursing, social work, sociology, psychology, health education, and the allied health professions.

The primary focus of this book is social gerontology. As the title implies, however, our goal is to present the diversities of the aging experience and the older population in a multidisciplinary manner. It is our premise that an examination of the social lives of older people requires a basic understanding of the historical, cultural, biological, physiological, psychological, and social contexts of aging. It is important to understand the changes that occur within the aging individual, how these changes influence interactions with social and physical environments, and how the older person is, in turn, affected by such interactions. Throughout this book, the significance of these dynamic interactions between older people and their environments is a unifying theme.

Social gerontology is a growing field with numerous salient areas of research. This book does not purport to cover all these areas, but rather to highlight major research findings that illuminate the processes of aging. Through such factual information, we intend to dispel some of the myths and negative attitudes about aging. We also hope to encourage the reader to pursue this field, both academically and for the personal rewards that come from gaining insight into older people's lives.

This book begins by reviewing major demographic, historical, and cross-cultural changes and their implications for the development of the field of gerontology and, in particular, of social theories of aging. We then turn to the major biological and physiological changes that affect older people's daily functioning, as well as their risk of chronic diseases and consequent utilization of health services. The third section considers psychological changes, particularly in learning and memory, personality, and mental health. Given our emphasis on how such physical and psychological changes affect the social aspects of aging, we consider in depth the social contexts of the family, the community, the economy, living arrangements, and the conditions under which people die. Throughout the book, the differential impact these changes have on women and ethnic minorities are identified, with two chapters focusing specifically on such differences. To highlight the application of research findings to everyday situations, each chapter integrates discussions of both the policy and practice implications of the aging process. We conclude by turning to the larger context of societal myths and stereotypes, social and health policy issues, and future implications for the field.

Given the scope of this book, it has taken several years to complete. We are grateful to the many people who have contributed significantly to its successful fruition. In particular, we thank Lauri Bosworth, Susan Edyvean, Suzanne Metcalf, and Sally Stewart for their tireless efforts in assisting us with library research. Mary Beth Ofstedal, Susan Cellier, Mary Grembowski, Laurie Pollack, Suzanne Condict, Karen Miller, and Gail Nyman-York spent many long hours and weekends at the word processor and copying machine with countless drafts of the manuscript. Ruth Pelz and Sue Davidson have been most valuable in editing the chapters to make them readable for a wide audience. Cathi Soriano and Heather Hovey have provided humor and perspective during some of the most stressful periods. Christian Staub, Joseph Freeman, Charlie Heib, Isabel Egglin, Marianne Gontarz, and George Kruse have enriched the book through their sensitive photographs. Our families, Joe Clark, and Gene, Kevin, and Christopher

Hooyman, have been the mainstay of support, even during weekends and vacations dominated by the ever-present manuscript. Finally, we would like to thank our editor at Allyn and Bacon, Alicia Reilly, for her continued encouragement in completing this book.

Social Gerontology
A Multidisciplinary Perspective

Introduction:
Why Study Aging?

Toward Understanding Aging

From the perspective of youth and middle age, old age seems a remote and, to some, an undesirable period of life. Throughout history, humans have made attempts to prolong youth and to delay aging. The attempts to discover a substance to rejuvenate the body and mind have driven explorers to far corners of the globe, and have inspired alchemists and scientists to search for ways to restore youth and prolong life. Indeed, the discovery of Florida by Ponce de Leon in 1513 was an accident, as he searched for a fountain in Bimini whose waters were rumored to bring back one's youth. The theme of prolonging or restoring youth is evident today in advertisements for skin creams, soaps, vitamins, and certain foods; in the popularity of cosmetic surgery; in books and movies that feature attractive, youthful-looking older characters; and even in medical research and technology that extends life.

All of these concerns point to underlying fears of aging. Many of our concerns and fears arise from misconceptions about what happens to our bodies, our minds, our status in society, and our social lives as we reach our seventies, eighties, and even nineties. They arise, in part, from negative attitudes toward the elderly within our own culture. These attitudes are sometimes identified as manifestations of *ageism,* a term that was coined by Robert Butler, former Director of the National Institute on Aging, to describe stereotypes about old age. As is true for sexism and racism, ageism attributes certain characteristics to all members of a group solely because of a characteristic they share; in this case, their age. In fact, ageism is one prejudice that we are all likely to encounter sooner or later regardless of our gender, ethnic minority status, or sexual preference. A frequent result of ageism is discriminatory behavior against the target group (i.e., older

---

Ponce de Leon's Search for the Fountain of Youth

The quest for gold and other riches attracted many Spanish adventurers to the New World in the fifteenth and sixteenth centuries. Among these was Ponce de Leon, who landed on Puerto Rico in 1508. He heard stories from Indians in the area of a fountain whose waters were believed to rejuvenate older people and restore their youth. This fountain was said to be located on the island of Bimini in the Bahamas. He set forth in 1512 from Puerto Rico in search of this fountain. By then, word of the magic fountain had spread to Europe; both the Spanish court and the Pope encouraged Ponce de Leon in his efforts. Of course, he never did find the fountain of youth, but his search was not futile; he found Florida instead.

From O. Segerberg, *The immortality factor* (New York: E. P. Dutton & Co., 1974).

persons). For example, some aging advocates maintain that hiring younger people for jobs in agencies that serve primarily older people is age discrimination.

To distinguish the realities of aging from the social stereotypes surrounding this process requires an understanding of the "normal" changes that can be expected in the aging body, in mental and emotional functioning, and in social interactions and status. Aging can then be understood as a phase of growth and development—a universal biological phenomenon. Accordingly, the normal processes due to age alone need to be differentiated from pathological changes or disease. As life expectancy increases, as the older proportion of our population grows, and as more of us can look forward to becoming elderly ourselves, concerns and questions about the aging process have attracted widespread public and professional attention.

The Field of Gerontology

The growing interest in understanding the process of aging has given rise to the multidisciplinary field of *gerontology*, the study of the biological, psychological, and social aspects of aging. Gerontologists include researchers and practitioners in such diverse fields as biology, medicine, nursing, dentistry, psychology, sociology, economics, political science, and social work. These individuals are concerned with many aspects of aging, from studying and describing the cellular processes involved, to seeking ways of improving the quality of life for older people. *Geriatrics* is focused on how to prevent or manage the diseases of aging. The field has recently developed as a specialty in medicine, nursing, and dentistry, and is receiving more attention with the increase in the number of older people who have long-term health problems.

Gerontologists view aging in terms of four distinct processes, which will be examined throughout this book.

1. *Chronological aging* is the definition of aging on the basis of a person's years from birth. Thus, a 75-year-old is chronologically older than a 45-year-old. Chronological age is not necessarily related to a person's physical health, mental abilities, or social status.

2. *Biological aging* refers to the physical changes that reduce the efficiency of organ systems, such as the lungs, heart, and circulatory system. A major cause of biological aging is the decline in the number of cell replications as an organism becomes chronologically older. Another factor is the loss of certain types of cells that do not replicate.

3. *Psychological aging* includes the changes that occur in sensory and perceptual processes, mental functioning (e.g., memory, learning, and intelligence), personality, drives, and motives.

4. *Social aging* refers to an individual's changing roles and relationships in the social structure—with family and friends, with the work world, and within organizations such as religious and political groups. As people age chronologically, biologically, and psychologically, their social roles and relationships also alter. The social context, which can vary considerably for different people, determines the meaning of aging for an individual and whether the aging experience will be primarily negative or positive.

Social Gerontology

The purpose of this book is to introduce you to *social gerontology*. This term was first used by Clark Tibbitts in 1954 to describe the area of gerontology that is concerned with the impact of social and sociocultural conditions on the process of aging and with the social consequences of this process. This field has grown as we have recognized the extent to which aging differs across cultures and societies.

Social gerontologists are interested in how the older population and the varieties of aging experiences both affect and are affected by the social structure. Older people are now the fastest growing population segment in the United States, with a growth rate much higher than that for younger age groups. The number of people over age 75 is expected to expand rapidly in the coming decades. This fact has far-reaching social implications for the areas of health care, workplace pension and retirement practices, community facilities, and patterns of government spending. Already, it has led to new specialties in health care—the growth of specialized services such as retirement housing, nursing homes, adult day health programs, and a leisure industry aimed at the older population. Changes in the sociopolitical structure, in turn, affect characteristics of the older population. For example, the widespread availability of secondary and higher education, health promotion programs, and employment-based pensions offer hope that future generations of older people will be better educated, healthier, and economically more secure than the current generation.

Social gerontologists study the impact of changes on both the elderly and our social structures. They also study social attitudes toward aging, and the effects of these attitudes on the older population. For example, as a society, we have tended to undervalue older people and to assume that most elderly are unintelligent, unemployable, nonproductive, senile, and asexual—assumptions not supported by facts. As a result, the activities open to older people, particularly in the areas of employment and leadership in community organizations, have been limited. As Robert Butler has noted, "The tragedy of old age is not that each of us must grow old and die, but that the process of doing so has been made unnecessarily and at times excruciatingly painful, humiliating, debilitating, and isolating" (Butler, 1975, pp. 2–3).

However, since stereotypes of old age are socially constructed, they are capable of undergoing change if society's values alter. Fortunately, such changes are beginning to occur as the public becomes more aware of older people's capabilities and realizes that most elderly are not poor, most do not live in nursing homes, most are not victims of senile dementia, and many are capable of productive employment. With the growth in the number and diversity of older persons, societal myths and stereotypes have been challenged. The public has become increasingly aware of older citizens' strengths and contributions. The result of these actions has been to change the status of older people in our society and the way that other groups view them. Contemporary advertising, for example, is beginning to reflect the changing status of older people, from a group that is viewed as weak, ill, and poor, to one perceived as politically and economically powerful.

As older people have become more politically active and as advocacy groups have emerged in support of seniors' rights, they have influenced not only public perceptions, but also laws that govern Social Security and other age-based policies and programs. Organized groups of elderly have helped to bring changes in retirement and pension policies, housing options, community facilities, health and welfare organizations, continuing education, and other services. Such political and attitudinal changes, which can profoundly transform the condition of older people, are also important issues in the study of social gerontology.

Equally significant in this area of study are the social problems that continue to affect a large percentage of older people. Even though the elderly are financially better off then they were twenty years ago, over 12 percent still fall below our government's official poverty line, with that percentage rising rapidly for women, ethnic minorities, and the oldest of the old. Although less than 5 percent of the elderly are institutionalized, those who are in nursing homes often lack family and other informal supports. Growing percentages of the elderly in the community face chronic diseases that may limit their daily activities. One problem that affects an even larger proportion of the older population is escalating health care costs, with the elderly paying a higher proportion of their income for health care than they have at any time in the past. Therefore, many gerontologists are also concerned with developing policy and practice interventions to address these problems.

What Is Old Age?

Contrary to the messages on birthday cards, aging does not start at age 40 or 65. Even though we are less conscious of age-related changes in earlier stages of our lives, we are all aging from the moment of birth—although the earlier stages are generally referred to as *development* or *maturation,* because the individual develops and matures, both socially and physically, from birth through adolescence. After age 30, additional changes occur that reflect normal declines in all organ systems. This is called *senescence*. Senescence occurs gradually throughout the body, ultimately reducing the viability of different bodily systems and increasing their vulnerability to disease. This is the final stage in the development of an organism.

Our place in the social structure also changes throughout our life span. Every society is age-graded; that is, it assigns different roles, expectations, opportunities, status, and constraints to people of different ages. For example, there are common social expectations about the appropriate age to attend school, begin work, have children, and retire—even though many people deviate from these expectations, and some of these expectations change over time. To call someone a *toddler, child, young adult,* or *old person* is to imply a full range of social characteristics. As we age, we pass through a sequence of defined stages, each with its own social norms and characteristics. In sum, age is a social construct with social meanings and social implications.

The specific effects of age grading, or age stratification, vary across different cultures and historical time periods. A primitive society, for instance, has very different expectations associated with stages of childhood, adolescence, and old age than does our contemporary American culture. Even within our own culture, those who are old today have different experiences of aging than previous or future groups of elderly. The term *cohort* is used to describe groups of people who were born at approximately the same time and therefore share many common experiences. For example, current cohorts of older persons have experienced the Great Depression, the World Wars, and other events that have shaped their lives. Its members include large numbers of immigrants who came to the United States before 1920 and many who have grown up in rural areas. Their average levels of education are lower than later generations. Such factors set today's elderly apart from other cohorts and must be taken into account in any studies of the aging process.

A Diverse Population

Throughout this book, we will refer to the phenomenon of aging and the population of older or elderly people. These terms are based, to some extent, on chronological criteria, but more importantly on individual differences in social, psychological, and biological functioning. In fact, each of us differs somewhat in the way we define old age. You may know an 80-year-old who seems youthful, and a 50-year-old whom you consider elderly. Elderly people also define themselves differently. Some individuals, even in their eighties, do not want to associate with "those old people," whereas others readily join age-based organizations and are proud of the years they have lived. Neugarten (1974) and other researchers have pointed to significant differences between the "young-old" (ages 55 to 75) and the "old-old" (over age 75); more recently, Riley and Riley (1986) have identified the "young-old" (ages 65 to 74), the "old-old" (ages 75 to 85), and the "oldest-old" (over age 85), or, as one of the authors likes to express it, the "frisky, the frail, and the fragile." However, there is diversity even within these divisions.

Older people vary greatly in their health status, their social and work activities, and their family situations. Some are still employed full-time; some are retired. Most are healthy; some are frail, confused, or home-bound. Most still live in a house or apartment; a small percentage are in nursing homes. Some receive large incomes from pensions and investments; many depend primarily on Social Security and have little discretionary income. Most men over age 65 are married, whereas women are more likely to become widowed and live alone as they age. For all these reasons, it is impossible to consider the social aspects of aging without also assessing the impact of individual variables such as physiological changes, health status, psychological well-being, socioeconomic class, and ethnic minority status. It is likewise impossible to define aging only in chronological terms, since chronological age only partially reflects the biological, psychological, and sociological processes that define life stages. Although the terms *elderly* and *older persons* are often used to mean those over 65 years in chronological age, this book is based on the principle that aging is a complex process that involves many different factors and is unique to each individual.

A Model of Dynamic Interaction

As we noted at the outset, this text is primarily concerned with social gerontology, and thus with the relationship between older people and society. These social relationships, in turn, are affected by physiological and psychological changes that occur with age. All these domains—the social, the physical, and the psychological—affect older persons' relationships with their environments, including the social world of family, friends, work colleagues, and neighbors, and physical features such as the layout of their homes, neighborhoods, or communities.

This social environmental perspective (Hendricks and Hendricks, 1981), or person-environment transactional approach (Schwartz, 1974), suggests that the environment is not a static backdrop but changes continually as the older person takes from it what he or she needs, controls what can be manipulated, and adjusts to conditions that cannot be changed. Adaptation thus implies a dual process in which the individual adjusts to some characteristics of the environment (e.g., completing the numerous forms required by Medicare), and brings about changes in others (e.g., attempting to change Social Security laws so that working beyond age 70 does not penalize individuals by reducing their benefits).

ENVIRONMENTAL PRESS

One useful way to view the dynamic interactions between the physical and psychological characteristics of the aging individual with the social and physical environment is Lawton and Nahemow's (1973) model of an individual's competence relative to environmental press. *Environment* in this model, which is shown in Figure 1, may refer to the larger society, the community, the neighborhood, or the home. *Environmental press* refers to the demands that social and physical environments make on the individual to adapt, respond, or change.

The environmental press model can be approached from a variety of disciplinary perspectives. A concept fundamental to social work, for example, is that of person-in-environment and the need to develop practice and policy

FIGURE 1 Diagrammatic Representation of the Behavioral and Affective Outcomes of Person-Environment Transactions

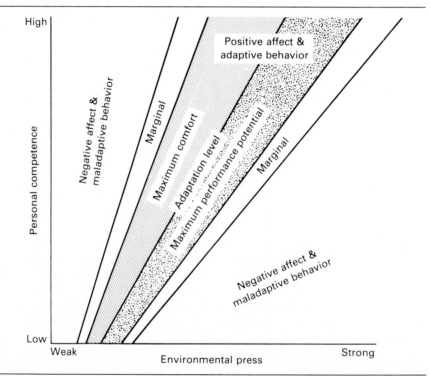

Source: M. P. Lawton and L. Nahemow, Ecology and the aging process. In C. Eisdorfer and M. P. Lawton (Eds.), *Psychology of adult development and aging* (Washington, D.C.: American Psychological Association, 1973), p. 661. Copyright 1973 by the American Psychological Association. Reprinted by permission of the author and publisher.

interventions that achieve a better fit between the person and his or her environment. Health care providers are increasingly aware of the necessity to take account of social environmental factors in their assessments of health problems. Architects and advocates for the disabled are developing ways to make environments more accessible for the elderly with chronic health care problems. Psychologists are interested in how the physical and social environments may be modified to maximize the older person's ability to learn new tasks and perform familiar ones such as driving, taking tests, and self-care. Sociologists study ways that the macro-environment (larger political and economic structures) affects and is affected by an individual's interactions with it. Because the concepts of this model are so basic to understanding the elderly's position in our society and to developing ways to improve the quality of their lives, such environmental interactions will be referred to throughout this text.

The amount of press in an individual's living situation may range from minimal to quite high. For example, very little environmental press is present in an institutional setting where an individual is not responsible for self-care, such as grooming and housekeeping, and has few resources to stimulate the senses or challenge the mind. Other environments can create a great deal of press, for example, a multigenerational household with many members in which the older person plays a pivotal role. Living in a familiar setting with few visitors generates low levels of environmental press. An increase in the number of people sharing the living arrangement or a move to a new home would increase the environmental demands. As the demands change, the individual must adapt to the changes in order to maintain a sense of well-being. Individuals perform at their maximum level when the environmental press slightly exceeds the level at which they adapt. In other words, the environment challenges them to test their limits, but does not overwhelm them. If the level of environmental demand becomes too high, the individual experiences excessive stress or overload. When the environmental press is below the individual's adaptation level, sensory deprivation, boredom, learned helplessness, and dependence on others may result. In either situation—too much or too little environmental press—the person or the environment must change, if the individual's adaptive capacity is to be restored.

Competence is defined by Lawton and Nahemow (1973) as the theoretical upper limit of an individual's abilities to function in the areas of health, social behavior, and cognition. Some of the abilities needed to adapt to environmental press include problem solving and learning, performing on the job, and managing the basic activities of daily living such as dressing, grooming, and cooking (Lawton, 1983). As suggested by the model in Figure 1, the higher a person's competence, the higher the levels of environmental press that can be tolerated. Thus, an older person with multiple physical disabilities and chronic illnesses has reduced physical competence, thereby limiting the level of environmental demands with which the individual can cope.

ENVIRONMENTAL INTERVENTIONS

Most services for older people are oriented toward minimizing environmental demands and increasing supports. These services may focus on changing the physical or social environment, or both. Physical environmental modifications such as ramps and handrails, and community services such as Meals-on-Wheels and escort vans are relatively simple ways to reestablish the older person's level of adaptation and to ease the burdens of daily coping. Such arrangements are undoubtedly essential to the well-being of disabled older people who require supports to enhance their independence. For example, many older people with chronic conditions are able to remain in their own homes because of environmental modifications such as lowered cupboards and countertops, electronic mechanisms that allow them to call for help, and vans equipped for wheelchairs.

A fine line exists, however, between minimizing excessive environmental press and creating an unstimulating or "too easy" environment. Well-intentioned families, for example, may do too much for the older person, assuming responsibility for daily activities, so that their older relative no longer has to exert any effort and may no longer feel he or she is a contributing family member. Likewise, professionals and family members may try to shield the older person from experiencing too many changes. For example, they may presume that an older person is too set in her or his ways to adjust to sharing a residence, thereby denying the person the opportunity to learn about and make an independent decision on home-sharing options. Well-intentioned nursing home staff may not challenge residents to perform such daily tasks as getting out of bed or going to the dining hall. Protective efforts such as these can remove all challenge from the older person's environment, with the result that the person's social, psychological, and physical levels of functioning may decline. Understimulating conditions, then, can be as negative in their effects on the elderly as those in which there is excessive environmental press.

Rather than attempting to minimize or prevent changes, a more appropriate intervention is to introduce positive changes and maximize individual options. Appropriate strategies include both altering environments to be more supportive of the older person's changing needs, and increasing their competence through activities such as counseling, rehabilitation training, health promotion, or social support groups that emphasize reciprocal exchanges. For example, an environment may be made more supportive by placing handrails along steps of the home, putting textured or colored strips along stairs, raising the level of illumination in the home (without producing glare), and installing automatic timers on irons, stoves, ovens, and toasters. Individual competence may be enhanced by encouraging residents of a retirement community to participate in the landscaping and maintenance of the area, to volunteer as teachers' aides in local schools, or to join exercise and peer counseling groups within the retirement complex. Other examples of both environmental and individual interventions to enhance older people's choices are considered throughout this text.

Organization of the Text

This book is divided into five parts. Part I is a general introduction to the field of gerontology and includes a brief history of the field, a discussion of research methods and designs, and a review of several social theories of aging. It also includes information on the demographics (population characteristics) of older people, and a perspective on aging in other historical periods and cultures.

Part II addresses the physiological changes that accompany aging. It begins with a review of normal age-related changes in the body's major organ systems, followed by a description of sensory changes that frequently occur in old age, and their social/environmental effects. It also discusses the diseases that occur most frequently among older people and the factors that influence health care behavior (e.g., when and why older people are likely to seek professional care).

In Part III, we move to the psychological context of aging, including normal and disease-related changes in cognitive functioning (learning, intelligence, and memory), theories of personality development and coping styles, mental health issues of importance to the elderly, and the use of mental health services.

The social issues of aging are explored in Part IV, beginning with the importance of family, friends, and neighbors and how the array of housing arrangements for the elderly affect their social interactions. Issues related to income, employment, and retirement are next explored, followed by a review of changing roles in the community, religious institutions and politics, and topics related to death, dying, and the status of widowhood. The last two chapters of Part IV cover two populations at special risk in old age: ethnic minorities and women.

Part V goes beyond the individual's social context to address the perspective of society as a whole—societal myths and stereotypes about aging and their consequences, and social and health policy issues of importance to the older population.

Each part begins with an introduction to the key issues of aging that are discussed in that section. In order to emphasize the variations in physiological, psychological, social, and societal aspects of aging, vignettes of older people representing these differences are presented.

Why Study Aging?

As you begin this text, you may find it useful to think about your own motivations for learning about older adults and the aging process. Some of you may be in a required course, questioning its relevance, and approaching this text as something you must read to satisfy requirements. Others may have personal reasons for wishing to learn about aging. You may be concerned about your own age-related changes, wondering whether reduced energy or alterations in physical features are inevitable with age. After all, since middle and old age together encompass a longer time span than any other stage of our lives, it is important that we understand and prepare for these years. Perhaps you are looking forward to the freedom made possible by retirement and the "empty nest." Through increased knowledge about the aging process, you may be hoping to make decisions that can enhance your own positive adaptation to aging and old age. Or perhaps you are interested in helping aging relatives, wanting to know what can be done to help them maintain their independence in old age, what housing options exist for them, and how you can improve your caregiving abilities.

Learning about aging not only gives us insight into our own interpersonal relationships, self-esteem, competence, and meaningful activities as we grow older, but it also helps us comprehend the aging process of our parents, grandparents, clients, patients, and friends. It is important to recognize that change and growth take place throughout the life course, and that the concerns of older people are not distinct from those of the young, but represent a continuation of earlier life stages. Such understanding can improve our effectiveness in communicating with relatives, friends, or professionals. In addition, such knowledge can help change any assumptions we may hold about behavior appropriate to various ages. Perhaps some of you wish to work professionally with older people, or are already doing so. You may genuinely enjoy your work, but at the same time be concerned about the social and economic problems facing some elderly and thus feel a responsibility to work to change these negative conditions. As professionals or future professionals working with older people, you are probably eager to learn more about policy and practice options for altering older people's environments to support their independence.

Regardless of your motivations for reading this text, chances are that like most Americans, you have some misconceptions about older people and the aging process. As products of our youth-oriented society, we have all learned negative attitudes about aging, although our own personal experiences with older people may counter many stereotypes and myths. By studying aging and older people, you will not only become more aware of the older population's competence, but also be able to differentiate the normal changes that are associated with the aging process from pathological or disease-related changes. Such an understanding may serve to reduce some of your own fears about aging, as well as positively affect your professional and personal interactions with older people. Our challenge as educators and authors is to present you with the facts and the concepts that will give you a more accurate picture of the experience of aging in American society. We also want to convey to you the excitement and importance of learning about the field of aging. We hope that by the time you have completed this text, you will have acquired information that strengthens positive attitudes toward living and working with older people and toward your own experience of aging.

References

Butler, R. *Why survive? Being old in America.* New York: Harper and Row, 1975.

Hendricks, J., and Hendricks, C. D. *Aging in mass society: Myths and realities.* Cambridge, Mass.: Winthrop, 1981.

Lawton, M. P. Environment and other determinants of well-being in older people. *The Gerontologist,* 1983, *23,* 349–357.

Lawton, M. P., and Nahemow, L. Ecology and the aging process. In C. Eisdorfer and M. P. Lawton (Eds.), *Psychology of adult development and aging.* Washington, D.C.: American Psychological Association, 1973, 619–674.

Neugarten, B. Age groups in American society and the rise of the young-old. In F. Eisele (Ed.), *Political consequences of aging.* The Annals of the American Academy of Political and Social Science, September 1974, *415,* 187–198.

Riley, M. W., and Riley, J. Longevity and social structure: The potential of the added years. In A. Pifer and L. Bronte (Eds.), *Our aging society: Paradox and promise.* New York: W. W. Norton, 1986, 53–77.

Schwartz, A. N. A transactional view of the aging process. In A. N. Schwartz and I. M. Mensh (Eds.), *Professional obligations and approaches to the aged.* Springfield, Ill.: Charles C. Thomas, 1974, 5–29.

Part I

The Field of Social Gerontology

As stated in the Introduction, the study of aging has grown dramatically over the past 100 years. Chapter 1 describes some of the early investigations of aging in both the United States and Europe. The greatest impetus to gerontological research, however, has been the significant growth in the proportion of older persons in the population. The development of major gerontology research centers around the country, the emergence of journals devoted to gerontology, and an increase in research activity all stem from demographic trends that reflect a substantial rise in the older population. Chapter 1 highlights changes in life expectancy, shifts in population pyramids and dependency ratios around the world, and the implications of these changes for social and economic policies. Research methods in gerontology are also described, with particular emphasis on the need to design studies that distinguish age differences from age changes. Research designs that have been developed in an effort to prevent the confounding of age, period, and cohort are presented.

Chapter 2 reviews briefly the role of older persons in a historical context, from prehistoric times to ancient civilizations, through the medieval period, and in colonial times. The effects of modernization on society's views of aging and on older people's roles are presented in a discussion of modernization theory. Other perspectives on the changing roles of older persons are described further in Chapter 2 where cross-cultural differences in older people's status, social participation, and control of resources are reviewed. Understanding these historical and cross-cultural variations can be useful for developing ways to alter contemporary environments to enhance older people's competence.

The focus of Chapter 3 is on social theories of aging. Social scientists have attempted to explain systematically age-related changes in social relationships. Many of these explanations have emerged from basic sociological theories and are not unique to gerontology. These include role theory, age stratification, social exchange, social interaction, and the political economy perspectives. Other theories have been developed as a result of findings from research efforts to define successful aging. These include activity, disengagement, and continuity theories. Although none of these theories fully explains the phenomenon of aging in a manner that accounts for all the variations in older people's behavior, each one contributes to our understanding of the aging experience.

Chapter 1

The Older Population and How It Is Studied

You are undoubtedly aware that more researchers are studying older people and the process of aging now than at any time in the past. Some of the concerns that have motivated this increasing professional interest in the field have probably influenced your own decision to study gerontology. As we noted in the Introduction, the single most important reason is the rapid current growth in the older population. This, in turn, has numerous effects. It influences social and health policies, and marketing and manufacturing decisions, and it has a profound effect on service providers and relatives of older people, on the elderly themselves, and ultimately on all of us as we look forward to longer lives than those normally experienced by past generations.

This chapter examines these population changes, exploring first their effects on the growth of gerontology as a field and then addressing the demographic issues of aging, including: How much has the older population grown, and why? How does this compare to other age groups? What differences can be identified, demographically, with respect to gender, ethnic minority status, and geographic location? And what is the social impact of these statistics? Finally, this chapter turns to the question of how these populations are studied: What are the particular challenges of social gerontological research, and how are they addressed? The net effect of this information is to give you a basic orientation to the field, including how it has developed, what populations are studied, and how.

Development of the Field

Although the scientific study of social gerontology is relatively recent, it has its roots in biological studies of the aging processes and in the psychology of human development. Biologists have long explored the reasons for aging in living organisms. Several key publications and research studies can be identified as milestones in the history of the field.

One of the first textbooks on aging, *The History of Life and Death*, was written in the thirteenth century by Roger Bacon. Focusing on the potential causes of aging, Bacon suggested that life expectancy could be extended if health practices, such as personal and public hygiene, were improved. The first scientist to explain aging as a developmental process, rather than as stagnation or deterioration, was a nineteenth-century Belgian mathematician-statistician named Adolph Quetelet. His interest in age and creative achievement preceded the study of these issues by social scientists by 100 years (Elias, Elias, and Elias, 1977). His training in the field of statistics also led him to consider the problems of *cross-sectional research*; that is, the collection of data on people of different ages at one time, instead of the study of the same person over a period of months or years (*longitudinal research*). These problems will be examined in greater detail in the next section of this chapter.

EARLY COMMUNITY-BASED AND LABORATORY STUDIES

Later in the nineteenth century, Russian scientist S. P. Botkin provided some of the earliest data on the differences between normal and *pathological aging* (i.e., diseases that may speed the process of aging, but are not a normal part of the process), sex differences in atherosclerosis, and the link between alcohol abuse and longevity (Birren and Clayton, 1975). He derived his data from a large community-based study, conducting extensive physiological analyses and comparing these with the social characteristics of nearly 3,000 older residents of St. Petersburg in Russia.

One of the first laboratory studies of aging was undertaken in the 1920s by another Russian physiologist, Ivan Pavlov, and his students. Pavlov is best known for his research with animals, which has provided the foundations for stimulus-response theories of behavior. Recognizing that the ability of older animals to learn and extinguish a response differed from that of younger animals, Pavlov explored the reasons for these differences in the brains of these animals (Birren, 1961). The work of Raymond Pearl and colleagues in the 1920s established the insect species *Drosophila* as an ideal animal model for studying biological aging and longevity. During this era, in 1922, American psychologist G. Stanley Hall published one of the first books on the social psychological aspects of aging in the United States. Titled *Senescence, the Last Half of Life*, it remains a landmark text in gerontology, because it provided the experimental framework for examining changes in cognitive processes and social and personality functions.

HISTORICAL FORCES OF THE LATE NINETEENTH
AND EARLY TWENTIETH CENTURIES

Two important forces led to the expansion of research in social gerontology in the late nineteenth and early twentieth centuries: the growth of the population over age 65 and the emergence of retirement policies in industrial settings. Changes in policies toward the elderly were first evident in many European countries (e.g., West Germany) where social services and health insurance programs were developed specifically for older citizens. In the United States, these changes came somewhat later. At the turn of the century, the focus on economic growth and the immediate problems of establishing workers' rights and child welfare laws took precedence over interest in the welfare of older people. The prevailing belief in this country had been that families should be responsible for their aging members. However, the Great Depression of the 1930s brought to policymakers the stark realization that families struck by unemployment and homelessness could not be responsible for their elders. The older segments of society suffered a disproportionate share of the economic blight of the Depression. New concern for the special needs of the aging population was exemplified by the Social Security system, established in 1935 to help people maintain a minimal level of economic security after retirement. Early work in social gerontology dealt largely with social and economic problems of aging. For example, E. V. Cowdry's *Problems of Aging*, published in 1939, focused on society's treatment of older people and on their particular needs.

FORMAL DEVELOPMENT OF THE FIELD

As society grew more aware of issues facing the older population, the formal study of aging emerged in the 1940s. In 1945, the Gerontological Society was founded, bringing together the small group of researchers and practitioners who were interested in gerontology and geriatrics. Today, this organization numbers its membership between 6,000 and 7,000, and it is the major professional association for people in diverse disciplines who are working in the field of aging. Gerontology became a division of the American Psychological Association in 1945 and, later, of the American Sociological Association.

The *Journal of Gerontology*, which began publishing in 1946, served as the first vehicle for transmitting new knowledge in this growing field. Although it remains a major journal, today numerous others are devoted to the study of aging and to the concerns of those who work with older people, some of which are listed in Table 1–1. An indicator of the knowledge explosion in the field is that the literature on aging published between 1950 and 1960 equalled that of the previous 115 years (Birren and Clayton, 1975). An effort to compile a bibliography of biomedical and social research from 1954 to 1974 produced 50,000 titles (Woodruff, 1975). Today, the burgeoning periodicals in diverse disciplines focused on gerontology have resulted in a proliferation of research publications in this field.

TABLE 1–1 Some Representative Journals Devoted to Gerontology

International Journal of Aging and Human Development
Aging and Society
Experimental Aging Research
Geriatrics
The Gerontologist
Gerodontology
Gerontology and Geriatrics Education
Journal of the American Geriatrics Society
Journal of Gerontology
Journal of Geriatric Nursing
Journal of Geriatric Psychiatry
Journal of Gerontological Social Work
Research on Aging
Psychology and Aging

MAJOR RESEARCH CENTERS FOUNDED

Research in gerontology took on growing significance after these developments, and an interest in the social factors associated with aging grew in the late 1950s and early 1960s. In 1946, a national gerontology research center, headed by Nathan Shock, was established at Baltimore City Hospital by the National Institutes of Health. This federally funded research center undertook to study longitudinally a large group of healthy middle-aged and older men living in the community, by testing them annually, or less often, on numerous physiological parameters. Later, the researchers began tests of cognitive, personality, and social-psychological characteristics of these men. Much later, in 1978, older women were included in their samples. These studies, known as the Baltimore Longitudinal Studies, are still continuing, now under the direction of the National Institute on Aging, founded in 1975. The results of this ongoing research effort continue to provide valuable information about normal age-related changes in physiological and psychological functions.

Concurrently with the Baltimore Longitudinal Studies, several university-based centers were developed to study the aging process and the needs of older

Increased research attention has been directed at physiological functioning among healthy older people.

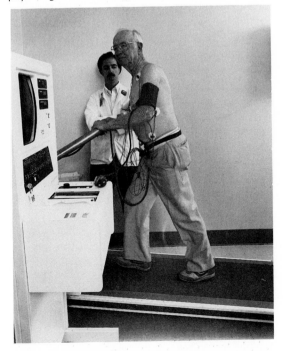

adults. One of the first, the Duke University Center on Aging, focused initially on the mental health of older people but also conducted pioneering research on the social issues of aging. The University of Chicago, under the direction of Robert Havighurst, developed the first research center devoted exclusively to the social aspects of aging. The Kansas City studies of adult development, discussed in Chapter 3, represent the first major social-psychological studies of adult development, and were conducted by researchers from the Chicago center. Research and training centers in aging have since evolved at many other universities, generally stimulated by government sponsorship of gerontological research through the National Institute on Aging (1975), the Center for Studies of the Mental Health of the Aging through the National Institute on Mental Health (1976), and the Administration on Aging (1965).

Growth of the Older Population

As we noted earlier, the most important factor affecting current interest in the field of gerontology is the growing size of the elderly population. In 1900, people over age 65 accounted for approximately 4 percent of the U.S. population—less than one person in 25. By 1985, one in nine Americans, or 11.7 percent of the population, was 65 years or older—a substantial increase. By 2010, because of the maturation of the baby boomers, one in seven Americans will be at least 65 years old (U.S. Senate Special Committee on Aging, 1986).

The growth of the aged population is a worldwide phenomenon. The proportion of people living beyond age 65 is increasing in almost every country, with the greatest increase in the developing nations (World Health Organization, 1982). Many European countries, including Sweden, Norway, Austria, and Great Britain, have a higher proportion of older persons in their populations than does the United States (U.N. Secretariat, 1982).

The most significant increase has been among the so-called "old-old" (Neugarten, 1982), those over age 85. In 1984, of the 28 million persons aged 65 and over in the United States, about 8.8 million were ages 75 to 84, and almost 2.6 million persons were age 85 and over (U.S. Bureau of the Census, 1986a). This 85-plus population has grown more rapidly than any other age group in our country, up 165 percent from 1960 to 1982; it is expected to increase fivefold by the middle of the next century, when it will form 5 percent of the total population and 24 percent of the 65-plus population, as shown in Figure 1–1 (U.S. Senate Special Committee on Aging, 1985). Since World War II, mortality rates in adulthood have declined significantly, resulting in an unprecedented number of people who are reaching advanced old age and are most likely to require health and social services (Rosenwaike, 1985).

FIGURE 1–1 Population 55 Years and Over by Age: 1900–2050

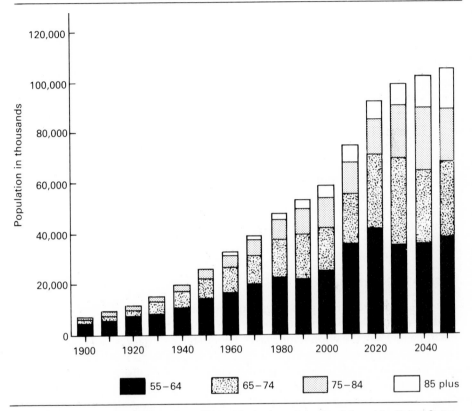

Source: U.S. Census of Population, 1890–1980 and Projections of the Population of the United States: 1983 to 2080, *Current Population Reports,* Series P-25, No. 952, Middle Series.

CHANGES IN LIFE EXPECTANCY

Why have these changes in the aged population occurred? Chiefly because people are living longer. In 1900, the average life expectancy in the United States—the average length of time one could expect to live if one was born that year—was 47 years. At that time, there were approximately 772,000 people between the ages of 75 and 84 in this country, and only 123,000 aged 85 or older. Today, there are almost 2.6 million in this oldest group. The average life expectancy is now much longer. For a child born in 1986, it is 74.9 years. Life expectancy at age 65 was an additional 16.8 years (U.S. Senate Special Committee on Aging, 1986). About four out of five individuals can now expect to reach age 65, at which point there is a better than 50 percent chance of living past age 80 (Kingson, Hirshorn, and Cornman, 1986).

The reasons for these changes have to do with technical advances in medicine. A hundred years ago, adults generally died from acute diseases, with influenza and pneumonia as the principal killers. Few people survived these diseases long enough to need care for chronic conditions. Today, death from acute diseases is rare. Maternal, infant, and early childhood death rates have also declined considerably. The result is a growing number of people who survive to old-old age, often with one or more chronic health care problems.

It is important to distinguish *life expectancy* from *maximum life span*. Whereas life expectancy is a probability estimate based on environmental conditions such as disease and health care, as described above, life span is the maximum number of years a given species could expect to live if environmental hazards were eliminated. As will be described in Chapter 4, there appears to be a maximum biologically determined life span for the cells that comprise an organism, so that even with the elimination of all diseases, we could not expect to live much beyond 120 years.

POPULATION PYRAMIDS

The rise in longevity is partly responsible for an unusually rapid rise in the median age of the U.S. population—from 28 in 1970 to 31.5 years in 1985—meaning that half the population was older and half younger than 31.5 in the latter year. From an historic perspective, a 3.5-year increase in the median age over a 14-year period is a noteworthy demographic event (U.S. Bureau of the Census, 1986a). The other key factors contributing to this rise include a dramatic decline in the birth rate after the mid-1960s, high birth rates in the periods from 1890 to 1915 and just after World War II (these "baby boomers" are now all older than the median), and the large number of immigrants who arrived here before the 1920s.

The baby-boom generation (currently aged 29 to 39), which resulted from increased birth rates after World War II, will dominate the age distribution in the United States well into the next century. In fact, by the early part of the twenty-first century, they will form the "senior boom," and swell the ranks of the 65-plus generation to the point that one in five Americans will be elderly. The projected growth in the older population will raise the median age of the U.S. population from 31 today to 36 by the year 2000 and to age 42 by the year 2050. If current birth rates and immigration levels remain stable, the only age groups to experience significant growth in the next century will be those past age 55 (U.S. Bureau of the Census, 1986a).

One of the most dramatic examples of the changing age distribution of the American population is the shift in the proportion of elderly in relation to the proportion of young persons, as illustrated in Figure 1–2. In 1900, when approximately 4 percent of the population was age 65 and over, young persons aged

FIGURE 1–2 Actual and Projected Change in Distribution of Children and 65-Plus Persons in the Population

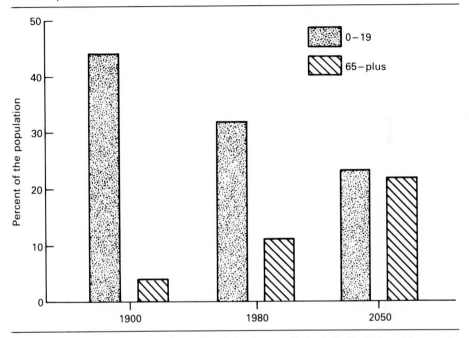

Source: U.S. Bureau of the Census, Current Population Reports, Series P-25, No. 952; and Census of the Population, 1900.

zero to 19 years made up 44 percent of the population. By 1982, reduced birthrates in the 1970s and early 1980s resulted in a decrease of young persons to 32 percent. The U.S. Census Bureau (1986b) predicts that, by the middle of the next century, the proportion of young persons and elderly will be almost equal, with persons zero to 19 years forming 23 percent and the elderly forming 22 percent of the population.

One way of illustrating the changing proportions of young and old persons in the population is the population pyramid. Figure 1–3 contrasts population pyramids for 1910 and 1980. Each horizontal bar in these pyramids represents a ten-year birth cohort (i.e., people born within the same 10-year period). By comparing these bars, we can determine the relative proportion of each birth cohort. As you can see in the first graph, the distribution of the population in 1910 represented a true pyramid, with the smallest proportion aged 60 and older; the largest proportion aged zero to 10. The pyramid has grown more rectangular over the years, as shown in the second graph. This change reflects declines in birth rates in 1930–1940 and 1965–1975, as well as the reduced death rates for older cohorts.

FIGURE 1–3 Population Pyramids for the United States: 1910 vs. 1980

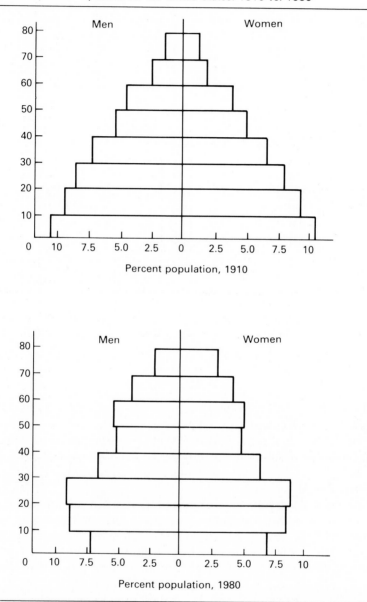

Percent population, 1910

Percent population, 1980

Source: U.S. Bureau of the Census, Projections of the Population of the U.S. *Current Population Reports.* Series P-25, No. 922 (Washington D.C., 1982).

DEPENDENCY RATIOS

An aspect of the changing age distribution in our population that has raised public concern is the so-called *dependency ratio,* or "elderly support ratio" (U.S. Senate Special Committee on Aging, 1986). This ratio has generally been used to indicate the relationship between the proportion of the population that is employed (defined as "productive" members of society) and the proportion that is not in the workforce (and is thus viewed as "dependent"). This rough estimate is obtained by comparing the proportion of the population aged 18 to 64 (the presumed working years) to the proportion under age 18 (yielding the childhood dependency ratio) and over age 65 (yielding the old age dependency ratio). This ratio has increased steadily, such that there appears to be proportionately fewer employed people to support older persons today. In 1910, the ratio was less than .10 (i.e., 10 working people per older person), compared with .18 in 1980 (i.e., five or six employed people per older person). Assuming that the lower birthrate continues, this trend will continue into the early twenty-first century, as the baby-boom cohort reaches old age. Studies using the rough calculation of dependency ratios have concluded that the result will be an increased "burden" on the working age population (Torrey, 1980; Schulz, 1984).

There are problems with such a crude measure, however. It is flawed by the fact that many of the younger and older persons are actually in the workforce and not dependent, while many people of workforce age may not be employed. A number of analysts have criticized the use of dependency ratios that do not take into account the workforce participation rates of different groups; for example, the workforce participation rates of women aged 16 to 59 are expected to increase from 1985 to 2000, while that of men of all ages are projected to decline. When these variations are taken into account, studies have found that although the total dependency ratio increases as the population ages, even in the year 2050 it will remain lower than levels attained in recent decades. Moreover, despite population aging, those under the age of 16 will continue to constitute the largest "dependent" group in future years (Torrey, 1981; Crown, 1985). Therefore, we need to be cautious when we hear policymakers predict "burdens" on the younger population and blame rising costs of public pension programs primarily on the changing dependency ratio.

POPULATION TRENDS BY ETHNIC MINORITY STATUS AND GENDER

In addition to the proportional growth of the older population in general, there are other demographic trends of interest to gerontologists. These include statistics related to the ethnic minority, gender, and geographic distributions of older populations. This section reviews some of these trends, beginning with the demographics of ethnic minorities in the United States.

Today, the ethnic minority populations of our country include a smaller proportion of elderly and a larger proportion of younger adults than the white population. In 1984, approximately 13 percent of whites, but only 8 percent of Blacks, 5 percent of Hispanics, 6 percent of Asian-Americans, and 5 percent of Native Americans were age 65 and over. The difference results primarily from the higher rates of fertility and higher mortality rates among the nonwhite population under age 65 than among the white population under 65 years of age. However, beginning in the early part of the twenty-first century, the proportion of older persons is expected to increase at a higher rate among ethnic minorities than the white population, partly because of the large proportion of children in these groups who, unlike their parents and especially their grandparents, are expected to reach old age (Greene and Siegler, 1984; U.S. Bureau of the Census, 1986a). Differences among the ethnic minority population are further discussed in Chapter 15.

Older women now outnumber older men three to two (Figure 1–4). In 1984, there were 80 men between 65 and 69 years for every 100 women in the same age group. Among those age 85 and over, there were only 40 men for every 100 women. Improvement in life expectancy has been especially dramatic for women. In 1985, life expectancy at birth for women was 78.8 years, whereas for men it was 71.5 years (Kingson, Hirshorn, and Cornman, 1986). This trend of lower mortality and higher life expectancy for women is expected to continue well into the twenty-first century. By the year 2040, life expectancy for women is projected to be 83.1 years, compared to 75.0 years for men (U.S. Senate Special Committee on Aging, 1986).

GEOGRAPHIC DISTRIBUTION

Demographic information on the location of older populations is important for a variety of reasons. For example, the comparison of demographic patterns in different nations and cultures may provide insights into various aspects of the aging process. The differing needs of rural and urban elderly may affect research designs as well as local government policy decisions. Likewise, statistical information on elderly populations state-to-state is necessary in planning for the distribution of federal funds. The following are some of the most salient statistics on the geographic distribution of the elderly today. Their implications will be considered in later chapters, including the impact of these differences on living arrangements, social and health policies, and cross-cultural issues.

Although older adults live in every state and region of the United States, they are not evenly distributed. More live in metropolitan areas; in 1980, 32 percent of the older population lived in central cities, 39 percent in suburbs, and 29 percent in rural areas. Some states have a much higher proportion of residents over age 65 than others; for example, they represent 17.5 percent of the population in Florida

FIGURE 1–4 Men per 100 Women, Selected Ages: 1985

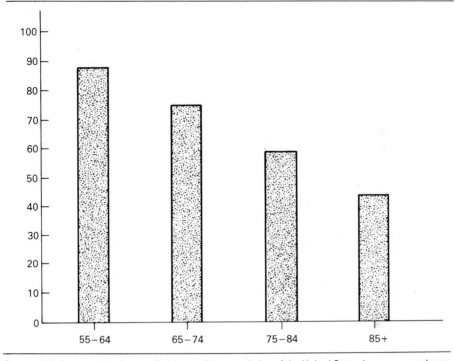

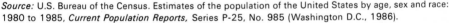

Source: U.S. Bureau of the Census. Estimates of the population of the United States by age, sex and race: 1980 to 1985, *Current Population Reports,* Series P-25, No. 985 (Washington D.C., 1986).

and 14 percent in Arkansas, Iowa, Missouri, Pennsylvania, Rhode Island, and South Dakota—compared to 3 percent of the population in Alaska and 7.6 percent in Utah (U.S. Bureau of the Census, 1986b). These proportions are increasing throughout the country. In some states, such as Florida, migration of retired persons to the state explains the increase, whereas in others, such as Arkansas and South Dakota, migration of younger persons out of the state leaves a greater proportion of older people. Other states may simply reflect the generalized "graying of America." Residential relocation is relatively rare for older people in the United States (23 percent of the older population moved between 1975 and 1980, compared with 48 percent of those under age 65). Such movement tends to be within the same types of environment; that is, people over age 65 generally move from one metropolitan area to another, or from one rural community to another (Longino, 1980). These trends and their implications for adaptation to aging will be described further in Chapter 11.

WORLDWIDE TRENDS

All world regions are experiencing an increase in the absolute and relative size of their older populations. The number of persons aged 65 or older in the world is expected to increase from 259 million in 1980 to 761 million in 2025, a threefold increase. This will result in a world population in which one out of every seven people will be 69 years of age or older by the year 2025 (United Nations Secretariat, 1982; Myers, 1985).

There are substantial differences in the current numbers and expected growth of the older population between industrialized and developing countries. For example, in 1975, 12.3 percent of the population of Europe was age 65 or older; almost 2 percent were 80 years or older. In contrast, Africa and South Asia each counted only 3 percent of their population aged 65 and over. However, the less developed regions of the world expect to show a nearly fivefold increase, from 3.8 percent in 1975, to 17 percent in 2075. An even greater rise in the proportion of the old old (age 80 and beyond) is expected in these countries, from the current 0.5 percent to 3.5 percent in 2075. By the year 2025, only 28 percent of the world's elderly are expected to reside in industrialized nations, while 72 percent will live in developing countries (World Health Organization, 1982). Table 1–2 presents these population trends.

Impact of Demographic Trends

As will be discussed in later parts of this book, the growth of older populations has wide-ranging implications. The impact of demographic changes in the United States is most striking when we look at patterns of federal spending. The growth in numbers and proportions of older people has already placed pressures on our

TABLE 1–2 Proportion of the Population Aged 65 and Older Worldwide: 1950, 1975, and Projections (reported in percent)

	1950	1975	2000	2025	2050	2075
Africa	3.5%	3.1%	3.2%	4.8%	9.3%	16.0%
Latin America	3.4	4.0	4.7	6.9	12.2	17.7
North America	8.1	10.3	12.1	17.0	17.5	17.8
East Asia	4.7	5.5	7.8	13.4	17.1	18.0
South Asia	3.4	3.0	3.7	6.2	12.2	17.0
Europe	8.7	12.3	14.3	17.1	17.7	18.0
Australia/New Zealand	7.5	7.6	8.9	12.5	15.4	17.4
USSR	6.1	8.9	12.0	14.3	16.4	18.0

Source: Adapted from a *Report of United Nations Population Division,* ESA/P/WP.75, August 1981.

health and social service systems. Nearly 29 percent of the U.S. federal budget—$265 billion in 1985—is allocated to programs that primarily benefit the elderly (U.S. Senate Special Committee on Aging, 1986). Social Security accounts for about half this amount, although it is in a different category than other federal expenditures since Social Security taxes are levied separately. In the early 1980s, there was great concern when projections showed that Social Security reserves were inadequate to meet coming needs. More recent studies predict solvency for at least the next 75 years. However, the Medicare program, which now accounts for nearly 7 percent of all federal spending, is less secure. Moreover, as expensive as Medicare has become, it has not adequately protected the elderly from rising health care costs. Even with this federal subsidy, older Americans pay more for their health care today than before Medicare was enacted in 1965. In addition, little help is available—either through public programs or through the private sector—to pay the high costs of long-term care (e.g., nursing homes and other community-based services for people with chronic health problems).

The increase in life expectancy has brought with it a change in expectations about the quality of life in late adulthood. Increasingly in our society, those facing retirement anticipate living 20 to 30 years in relatively good health, with secure and adequate retirement incomes. When these expectations are not met, because of catastrophic medical costs, widowhood, or a retirement income eroded by inflation, the elderly may not be prepared to manage the change in lifestyle. For other segments of the older population, particularly women and ethnic minorities, old age may represent a continuation of a lifetime of poverty or near poverty. Fortunately for most older people, the problems associated with old age, particularly chronic illness and the attendant costs, are forestalled until very old age. As noted, however, the particularly rapid growth of the frail elderly, the majority of whom are women, may severely strain current health and income systems designed to provide resources in old age.

A change among the older male population that is of concern to policymakers is the growth in the number and proportion of older veterans. Of all men age 65 and over, 27 percent were veterans in 1980. By the year 2000, 63 percent will be veterans eligible for health care benefits. However, the proportion of veterans in the 65-plus male population will actually decrease after the turn of the century. Only about 4 percent of aged veterans are projected to be women (U.S. Veterans Administration, 1984).

Another consequence of the increase in life expectancy is a growth in the multigenerational family. More than any other time in history, it is common for middle-aged and older adults to face caregiving responsibilities for older relatives. Approximately 80 percent of these caregivers are women (Brody, 1985). Today, American women can expect to spend more years caring for an aging parent than for a dependent child.

In sum, America is an aging society. The growth in the numbers and proportions of older people, especially the oldest-old, will require that both public and private policies affecting employment, housing and retirement, health care, and social services be modified to meet the needs and expand the opportunities for productivity of those who are living longer. Fundamental issues will have to be resolved about who will receive what societal resources and what will be the roles of the private and public sectors for sharing responsibilities of elder care. The ways in which our society meets these challenges will determine the quality of life available not only to current generations of elderly, but also to those for whom old age seems remote.

How Is Aging Studied?

The previous discussion has introduced the historic growth of gerontology and the demographic trends that underlie the growing importance of this field. Before moving on to an examination of the issues and areas of special concern to social gerontologists, let us first consider the ways in which information about the aging process is gathered. The topic of research methodologies in gerontology may seem an advanced one to introduce so early in a basic text, but in fact, it is essential to understanding the meaning and validity of information presented throughout this book.

The study of aging presents particular conceptual and methodological difficulties. A major one is how research is designed and data interpreted regarding age changes. A point that complicates research in aging and also produces some misleading interpretations of data is how to distinguish *age changes* from *age differences.* This differentiation is necessary if we are to understand the process of aging and the conditions under which age differences occur. If we wish to determine what changes or effects are experienced as an individual moves from middle age to old age and to advanced old age, we must examine the same individual over a period of years, or at least months. In order to understand age changes, longitudinal research is necessary; that is, the repeated measurement of the same person over a specified period of time.

Unfortunately, the time and cost of such studies prevent many researchers from undertaking longitudinal research. Instead, much of the research in this field focuses on age differences, by comparing people of different chronological ages at the same measurement period. These studies, cross-sectional in nature, are the most common ones in gerontology.

The unique problems inherent in how gerontological research is designed and how data are interpreted are evident in the following question: Given that aging in humans is a complex process that proceeds quite differently among different individuals in different geographic, cultural, and historic settings, and that it takes place over a time span as long as 100–120 years, how does one study it? Obviously, scientists cannot follow successive generations—or even a single generation of subjects—throughout their life span. Nor can they be expected to address the entire range of variables that affect aging—including lifestyle, social class, cultural beliefs, public policies, and so on—in a single study.

THE AGE/PERIOD/COHORT PROBLEM

The problem in each case is that of distinguishing *age differences* (ways that one generation differs from another) from *age changes* (ways that people normally change over time). This has been referred to as the "age/period/cohort" problem (Maddox, 1979). (The word *cohort*, you will recall, refers to those people born at roughly the same time. *Period* refers to the effects of the specific historical period involved.) The concept of cohort is an important one in gerontology because historical events differentiate one cohort from another in attitudes and behaviors. Those people in the same cohort are likely to be more similar to each other because of comparable social forces acting on them during a given era (Ryder, 1965; Maddox and Campbell, 1985).

CROSS-SECTIONAL STUDIES

As noted earlier, the most common approach to studying aging is cross-sectional; that is, researchers compare a number of subjects of different ages on the same characteristic. One reason that cross-sectional studies are frequently used is that, compared to other designs, data can be readily gathered. Some examples might include a comparison of the lung capacity of men aged 30 with those who are aged 40, 50, 60, 70, and 80, or a study comparing church attendance by American adults under age 65 with those over age 65. The average differences among different age groups in each study might suggest conclusions about the changes that come with age.

The danger with such cross-sectional studies is that these differences might not be due to the process of aging, but rather to particular cultural and historic conditions that shaped each group of subjects being studied. For example, a higher rate of church attendance among today's elderly than among younger adults might (and indeed probably does) reflect a change in social attitudes during this century toward attending church, as opposed to, say, an increased need for spiritual and religious life as one grows older.

Even in studies of biological factors, such as lung capacity, there may be many intervening variables that threaten the validity of comparative results. In this case, they include the effects of exercise, smoking, and other lifestyle factors, genetic inheritance, and exposure to pollution (this, in turn, might be a product of work environments and social class) on relevant outcome variables.

The major limitation of cross-sectional studies has been when differences among younger and older respondents were erroneously attributed to growing old; for example, some researchers have found that the older the respondent, the lower his or her score on intelligence tests. As a result, cognitive abilities have been misinterpreted as declining with age. In fact, such differences may be due to the lower educational levels and higher text anxiety of this cohort of elderly compared to younger adults, not to age.

Similarly, in studying individuals' values about the meaning of money and personal savings, for example, it is important to know whether differences between age groups are due to chronological age per se (e.g., whether the younger respondents would eventually think like the older ones as they reached that age), or to differences arising from the historical periods in which the different age groups have lived (known as environmental factors or *period effects*). It is difficult to distinguish period effects from age differences in a cross-sectional research design. As an example, the current cohort of elderly have all lived through and been affected by the Great Depression. The financial burdens imposed by this period in American history probably have affected their values about frugality in saving. In contrast, people whose childhood years occurred during the post–World War II economic boom in this country have adopted less cautious values about saving and investing their earnings. A cross-sectional study would not capture the reasons for these differences. Because many issues in social gerontology center on distinguishing age from cohort effects, a number of research designs have emerged that attempt to do this. They include longitudinal and sequential designs.

LONGITUDINAL STUDIES: DESIGN AND LIMITATIONS

Longitudinal designs permit inferences about age changes. They eliminate cohort effects by studying the same people over time. Each row in Table 1–3 represents

TABLE 1–3 Alternative Research Designs in Aging

| Cohort Born in: | Time of Measurement | | | |
	1950	*1960*	*1970*	*1980*
1900	A_1	A_2		
1910		B_1	B_2	
1920		C_1	C_2	C_3
1930				D_4

Cross-sectional: Cohorts A, B, and C are measured in 1960.

Longitudinal: Cohort A is measured in 1950 and 1960; *or* Cohort B is measured in 1960 and 1970; *or* Cohort C is measured in 1960, 1970, and 1980.

Cohort-sequential: Cohort A is measured in 1950 and 1960; Cohort B is measured in 1960 and 1970.

Time-sequential: Cohorts B and C are measured in 1970; Cohorts C and D are measured in 1980.

Cross-sequential: Cohorts B and C are both measured in 1960 and 1970.

Source: Adapted from K. W. Schaie (Ed.), *Longitudinal studies of adult psychological development* (New York: Guilford Press, 1983).

a separate longitudinal study in which a given cohort (e.g., A, B, or C) is measured once every ten years. Despite the advantages of longitudinal designs over the cross-sectional approach, it still has limitations. First, the longitudinal method does not allow a distinction between age and time of testing. For example, if a sample of 55-year-old workers had been interviewed regarding retirement policies in 1975, before the mandatory retirement age was changed to age 70, and again in 1995, long after mandatory retirement was eliminated, it would be difficult to determine whether the changes found in their attitudes toward retirement came about as a result of their increased age and proximity to retirement, or as a result of the modifications in retirement laws during this period. Longitudinal designs cannot separate the effects of events extraneous to the study that influence people's responses in a particular measurement period.

Another problem with longitudinal studies is the potential for practice effects. This problem occurs in studies that administer aptitude or knowledge tests, where repeated measurement with the same test improves the test-taker's performance because of familiarity or practice. For example, a psychologist who is interested in age-related changes in intelligence could expect to obtain improvements in people's scores if the same test is administered several times, with a brief interval (e.g., less than one year) between tests. In such cases, it is difficult to relate the changes to maturation unless the tests can be varied or parallel forms of the same tests can be used.

Longitudinal studies also present the problem of *attrition* or dropout. Individuals in experimental studies and respondents in surveys that are administered repeatedly may drop out for many reasons—death, illness, loss of interest, or frustration with poor performance. To the extent that people who drop out are not different from the original sample in terms of demographic characteristics, health status, and intelligence, the researcher can still generalize from the results obtained with the remaining sample. However, more often it is the case that dropouts differ significantly from those who stay until the end. As we shall see in Chapter 7, those who drop out of longitudinal studies tend to be in poorer health, score lower on intelligence tests, and are more socially isolated (Riegel, Riegel, and Meyer, 1967; Baltes, Schaie, and Nardi, 1971).

SEQUENTIAL DESIGNS

Some new research designs have emerged in response to the problems of cross-sectional and longitudinal methods. One is the category of sequential designs (Schaie, 1967, 1973, 1977, 1983). These include the cohort-sequential, time-sequential, and cross-sequential methods, which are illustrated in Table 1–3.

A *cohort-sequential* design is an extension of the longitudinal design, whereby two or more cohorts are followed for a period of time, so that measurements are taken of different age groups at different points in time. Thus, for example, an investigator may wish to compare changing attitudes toward federal policies among the cohort born in 1900 and the cohort born in 1910 and follow each one for 10 years, from 1950 to 1960 for the first cohort, 1960 to 1970 for the second. This approach is useful for many social gerontological studies in which age and cohort must be distinguished. However, it still does not separate the effects of cohort from time of measurement.

The *time-sequential* design is useful for distinguishing between age and time of measurement or historical factors. It can be used to determine if changes obtained are due to aging or to historical factors. The researcher using this design would compare two or more cross-sectional samples at two or more measurement periods. For example, a group of 70-year-olds and a group of 60-year-olds might be compared in 1970; the latter could be compared with a new group of 60-year-olds in 1980. Time-sequential designs do not prevent the confounding of age and cohort effects, but it is acceptable to use this method where one would not expect age differences to be confused with cohort differences.

The third technique proposed by Schaie (1983) is the *cross-sequential* design, which combines cross-sectional and longitudinal designs. Thus, for example, the researcher could compare people who were age 40 and 50 in 1960, and again in 1970 when they were age 50 and 60 respectively. This would permit the assessment of cohort and historical factors, because the same cohorts are being compared at two different times, with one providing information on changes from age 40 to 50, and the other representing changes from age 50 to 60. This approach is an improvement over both the traditional cross-sectional and longitudinal designs, but it still confounds age and time of measurement effects. These three sequential designs are becoming more widely used by gerontological researchers. Table 1–4 summarizes potential confounding effects in each of these methods.

Despite the growth of new research methods, much of social gerontology is

TABLE 1–4 Potential Confounding Effects in Developmental Studies

Design	Confounding Effect		
	Age × Cohort Confounded?	Age × Time of Measurement Confounded?	Cohort × Time of Measurement Confounded?
Cross-sectional	Yes	No	No
Longitudinal	No	Yes	No
Cohort-sequential	No	No	Yes
Time-sequential	Yes	No	No
Cross-sequential	No	Yes	No

Source: Adapted from M. F. Elias, P. K. Elias, and J. W. Elias, *Basic processes in adult developmental psychology* (St. Louis: C.V. Mosby, 1977).

based on cross-sectional studies. For this reason, it is important to read carefully in order to make accurate inferences about age changes as opposed to age differences, and to determine whether the differences found between groups of different ages are due to cohort effects or to true effects of aging.

OTHER RESEARCH ISSUES

Aside from these problems unique to gerontology, the basic research tools are similar to those used in sociology and psychology, and include psychological tests, observations, interviews, questionnaires, and case histories. As in all research studies, the measures used must be valid (accurately reflecting the concepts that they are intended to measure) and reliable (yielding the same results from repeated measurements of the same phenomenon).

Accurate sampling can be difficult with older populations. If the sample is not representative, the results are of questionable validity. However, comprehensive lists of older people are not readily available. Membership lists from organizations, such as the American Association of Retired Persons, tend to overrepresent those who are healthy and financially secure. Studies in institutions, such as nursing homes and adult day centers, tend to overrepresent those with chronic impairments. Reaching ethnic minority elderly through organizational lists can be especially difficult.

The problem of selective survival affects all samples of older people. Over time, the birth cohort loses members, so that those who remain are not necessarily representative of all in the original group. Those who survive, for example, probably were healthiest at birth, and maintained their good health throughout their lives—all variables that tend to be associated with higher socioeconomic status.

Even when an adequate sample is located, older respondents may vary in their memories or attention span; such variations can interfere with conducting interviews or tests. Ethical issues and unique difficulties arise in interviewing the frail elderly; Streib (1983) has urged the use of qualitative methods to gather information about this population that has been neglected in gerontological research. An additional problem is that studies of the old-old may be influenced by *terminal drop,* a decline in performance before death (Botwinick, 1984; Palmore and Cleveland, 1976). Since death becomes increasingly likely with age, terminal drop will manifest as a gradual decline in performance test scores with age in cross-sectional designs. In longitudinal studies, this problem may result in an overestimation of performance abilities in the later years because those who survive are likely to represent the physically and cognitively most capable elderly.

Further refinement of research methodologies is a challenging task for social gerontologists. As progress is made in this area, the quality of data with which to study aging will continually improve.

Summary and Implications

Gerontology has grown as a field since early philosophers and scientists first explored the reasons for changes experienced with advancing age. Roger Bacon in the thirteenth century, Adolph Quetelet in the early nineteenth century, Botkin in the late nineteenth century, and Ivan Pavlov and G. Stanley Hall in the early twentieth century made pioneering contributions to this field. During the early 1900s, in Europe and the United States, the impact of an increasing aging population on social and health resources began to be felt. Social gerontological research has expanded since the 1940s, paralleling the rapid growth of the older population and its needs.

A primary reason for the growing interest in gerontology is the increase in the population over age 65. This growth results from a reduction in infant and child mortality and improved treatment of acute diseases of childhood and adulthood, which in turn increases the proportion of people living to age 65 and beyond. In the United States, average life expectancy from birth has increased from 47 years in 1900 to 74.7 in 1984, with women continuing to outlive men. The growth in the population over age 85 has been most dramatic, reflecting major achievements in disease prevention and health care since the turn of the century. Ethnic minority groups in the United States and developing nations have had a smaller growth in the proportion of people living beyond age 65 than whites and industrialized nations, but population projections anticipate a much higher rate of growth for these groups by the early part of the twenty-first century.

Increased needs for health and social services among the old-old population have significant policy implications for American society and that of other industrial nations. For example, Medicare and Medicaid have already begun to experience the strain of an increasing number of older persons with long-term chronic illnesses.

The growing older population, and associated social concerns, have stimulated great interest in gerontological research. However, existing research methodologies are limited in their ability to distinguish the process of aging per se from cohort, time, and measurement effects. Cross-sectional research designs are most often used in this field, but these can provide information only on age differences, not on age changes. Longitudinal designs are necessary for understanding age changes, but suffer from the possibility of subject attrition and the effects of measuring the same individual numerous times. Newer methods in social gerontology, known as cohort-sequential, time-sequential, and cross-sequential designs, test multiple cohorts, or age groups, over time. They also are limited by possible confounding effects, but represent considerable improvement over traditional research designs.

The field of social gerontology will continue to be an important area for research and practice in the future, as the population over age 65, and even more importantly, over age 85, increases. The demographic shifts now in process will demand greater attention from policymakers, program planners, service pro-viders, and researchers in social gerontology. Because research methods in gerontology have improved, today there is a better understanding of many aspects of aging. Research findings to date provide the empirical background for the theories and topics to be covered in the remaining chapters. Despite the recent explosion of knowledge in gerontology, there are many gaps in what is known about older people and the aging process. Throughout the text, we will call attention to areas in which additional research is needed.

References

Baltes, P. B., Schaie, K. W., and Nardi, A. H. Age and experimental mortality in a seven-year longitudinal study of cognitive behavior. *Developmental Psychology,* 1971, 5, 18–26.

Birren, J. E. A brief history of the psychology of aging. *The Gerontologist,* 1961, 1, 69–77, 127–134.

Birren, J. E., and Clayton, V. History of gerontology. In D. S. Woodruff and J. E. Birren (Eds.), *Aging: Scientific perspectives and social issues.* New York: Van Nostrand, 1975.

Botwinick, J. *Cognitive processes in maturity and old age* (3d ed.). New York: Springer, 1984.

Brody, E. Parent care as a normative family stress. *The Gerontologist,* 1985, 25, 19–29.

Crown, W. Some thoughts on reformulating the dependency ratio. *The Gerontologist,* 1985, 25, 166–171.

Elias, M. F., Elias, P. K., and Elias, J. W. *Basic processes in adult developmental psychology.* St. Louis: C.V. Mosby, 1977.

Greene, R. L., and Siegler, I. C. Ethnic groups: Blacks. In E. Palmore (Ed.), *Handbook on the aged in the United States.* Westport, Conn.: Greenwood Press, 1984, 219–233.

Kingson, E. R., Hirshorn, B. A., and Cornman, J. M. *Ties that bind: The interdependence of generations.* Washington, D.C.: Seven Locks Press, 1986.

Longino, C. F. Residential relocation of older people: Metropolitan and nonmetropolitan. *Research on Aging,* 1980, 2, 321–328.

Maddox, G. Sociology of later life. *Annual Review of Sociology,* 1979, 5, 113–135.

Maddox, G. L., and Campbell, R. T. Scope, concepts and methods in the study of aging. In R. H. Binstock and E. Shanas (Eds.), *Handbook of aging and the social sciences* (2d ed.). New York: Van Nostrand Reinhold, 1985, 3–34.

Myers, G. C. Aging and worldwide population change. In R. H. Binstock and E. Shanas (Eds.), *Handbook of aging and the social sciences* (2d ed.). New York: Van Nostrand Reinhold, 1985, 173–198.

Neugarten, B. L. Policy for the 1980's: Age or need entitlement. In B. Neugarten (Ed.), *Age or need? Public policies for older people.* Beverly Hills: Sage Publications, 1982.

NRTA-AARP (National Retired Teachers Association-American Association of Retired Persons). (1981) National survey of older Americans.

Palmore, E., and Cleveland, W. Aging, terminal decline and terminal drop. *Journal of Gerontology*, 1976, *31*, 76–81.

Riegel, K. F., Riegel, R. M., and Meyer, G. A study of the dropout rates in longitudinal research on aging and the prediction of death. *Journal of Personality and Social Psychology*, 1967, *5*, 342–348.

Rosenwaike, I. A demographic portrait of the oldest old. *Milbank Memorial Fund Quarterly: Health and Society*, 1985, *63*, 187–205.

Ryder, N. B. The cohort as a concept in the study of social change. *American Sociological Review*, 1965, *30*, 843–861.

Schaie, K. W. Age changes and age differences. *The Gerontologist*, 1967, *7*, 128–132.

Schaie, K. W. Methodological problems in descriptive developmental research on adulthood and aging. In J. R. Nesselroade and H. W. Reese (Eds.), *Lifespan developmental psychology: Methodological issues*. New York: Academic Press, 1973.

Schaie, K. W. Quasi-experimental research designs in the psychology of aging. In J. E. Birren and K. W. Schaie (Eds.), *Handbook of the psychology of aging*. New York: Van Nostrand Reinhold, 1977.

Schaie, K. W. (Ed.). *Longitudinal studies of adult psychological development*. New York: Guilford Press, 1983.

Schulz, J. H. *The economics of aging*. Belmont, Calif.: Wadsworth, 1984.

Siegel, J., and Davidson, M. Demographic and socioeconomic status of the aging in the United States. U.S. Bureau of the Census, *Current Population Reports*, 1984, No. 138, P-23.

Streib, G. F. The frail elderly: Research dilemmas and research opportunities. *Gerontologist*, 1983, *23*, 40–44.

Suzman, R., and Riley, M. W. (Eds.). Special issue: The oldest old. *Milbank Memorial Fund Quarterly*, 1985, *63*, 177–451.

Torrey, B. B. Demographic shifts and projections: The implications for pension systems. Chapter 4 in *Appendices of the report of the president's commission on pension policy*. Washington, D.C.: The Commission, 1980.

Torrey, B. B. *Technical details on the projection of federal outlays for the older population*. Washington, D.C.: Office of Management and Budget, 1981.

United Nations Secretariat. *World population trends and prospects by country, 1950–2000*. (ST/ESA/SER.R/33), 1982.

U.S. Bureau of the Census. Current Population Reports. *Estimates of the population of the United States by age, sex and race: 1980 to 1985*. Series P-25, No. 985, 1986a.

U.S. Bureau of the Census. Current Population Reports. *State population and household estimates to 1985, with age and components of change*. Series P-25, No. 998, 1986b.

U.S. Senate Special Committee on Aging. *Developments in aging: 1984*. Washington, D.C.: U.S. Government Printing Office, 1985.

U.S. Senate Special Committee on Aging. *Aging America: Trends and projections* (1985–86 ed.). Washington, D.C.: Department of Health and Human Services, 1986.

U.S. Veterans Administration. *Caring for the older veteran.* Washington, D.C.: U.S. Government Printing Office, 1984.

Woodruff, D. Introduction: Multidisciplinary perspectives of aging. In D. Woodruff and J. Birren (Eds.), *Aging: Scientific perspectives and social issues.* New York: Van Nostrand, 1975.

World Health Organization. *World Health Statistics Quarterly,* special issue on public health implications of aging, 1982, *35,* 120–280.

Chapter 2

Historical and Cross-Cultural Issues in Aging

The experience of aging is not the same today as it was in earlier historical periods. The social and economic roles of older persons, their expectations of the social system, as well as what society expects of them, are in many ways profoundly different today from previous generations. Until relatively recently, only a minority of people lived long enough to be considered old. As the number of older people has grown and as social values have changed, the authority and power of the elderly in society have also shifted.

The experience of aging differs cross-culturally as well as historically. That is, in addition to historical changes, there are significant cultural variations that affect the social position of older persons. Perhaps the greatest differences in the elderly's status are between traditional societies and those of the modern Western world, with its rapidly changing values and norms. Examining the different ways that other societies, both historical and contemporary, have dealt with issues affecting the elderly can shed light on the process of aging in our society. The emergence of "comparative sociocultural gerontology" or an "anthropology of aging" has served to refute some of the myths of the "good old days" presumed to exist in historical times and in contemporary nonindustrial societies. It begins to differentiate what aspects of aging are universal or biological as opposed to factors largely shaped by the sociocultural system (Sokolovsky, 1983). Understanding how aging in contemporary American society differs from that experienced elsewhere, and which factors are socioculturally determined, can also suggest strategies for developing better environments in which to grow old.

This chapter briefly examines the extent to which older people were valued in stable, preliterate, or primitive societies and in some other nonwestern cultures. Changes in the social roles of older persons, society's expectations of them, and their expectations of society are considered. In addition, contrasting perspectives are reviewed regarding the impact of modernization on the relationship between older persons and the larger society. These influences are examined first historically and then cross-culturally. Within the constraints of this one chapter, we can only glance at a few other cultures. For a more complete view, we urge you to turn to the developing anthropological works on aging (Amoss and Harrell, 1981; Fry, 1981; Fry and Keith, 1986; Keith, 1982, 1985; Sokolovsky, 1983). While this chapter explores aging cross-culturally and historically, Chapter 15 focuses on the cultural diversity represented by older ethnic minorities within contemporary American society.

Old Age Historically

OLD AGE IN PREHISTORIC TIMES

Although our knowledge of the elderly in prehistoric and primitive societies is limited, we do know that people of advanced age were rare, with most dying before the age of 35. Nevertheless, there were always a few people perceived to be old, although they were probably chronologically relatively young, since maturity and death came quickly in the lives of people struggling to survive in harsh environments. Those few elders were treated with respect, in a manner that reflected a sense of sacred obligation. During ceremonial occasions, elders were seated in positions of high honor (Simmons, 1945).

Even though positive attitudes toward the young-old were widespread, nonsupportive or death-hastening behavior was shown toward those who survived beyond an "intact" stage of life. This stage of old-old age was often referred to as the "sleeping period." No longer able to contribute to the common welfare and look after themselves, the elderly were then viewed as useless, "overaged" or "already dead," and were sometimes treated brutally. Those who outlived their usefulness were a heavy burden in societies that existed close to the edge of subsistence, particularly those in harsh climates or with little horticulture (Glascock and Feinman, 1981, 1986; Simmons, 1945). In some rural areas of ancient Japan, for example, the elderly were carried into the mountains and left there to die. It was not unusual for aged Eskimos to walk off into the snow when famine and disease placed great burdens on the tribe (Amoss and Harrell, 1981). This practice of *geronticide* or *senecide*—the deliberate destruction of aged community members—was viewed as functional and, for many traditional societies, often carried out with great reverence or ceremony. In a minority of primitive tribes, the frail were killed outright; in most, they were abandoned, neglected, or encouraged to commit suicide, and the burial place was converted into some sort of shrine. Consistent with the coexistence of positive attitudes toward the old along with their nonsupportive treatment, geronticide in many societies often occurred under the older person's direction and by a close relative, usually a son (Glascock and Feinman, 1981).

OLD AGE IN GREEK AND ROMAN CULTURE

In Greek and Roman classical cultures, 80 percent of the population perished before reaching the stage of life that we now consider to be middle-age. Nevertheless, our chronological conception of age, with *old* defined as age 60 and over, began during this period. Age implied power in the ancient cities, which were ruled by councils of elders who derived their authority from their years. Within the family, the eldest male's authority was nearly absolute, and the young were dependent on the old by custom and by law. However, only the elite members of society, not the peasants, benefited from the respect accorded age by the community.

Some idea of the changing status of older people in ancient Greek society can be obtained by analyzing how old and young were depicted in Greek tragedy. In her book, *Time in Greek Tragedy*, de Romilly (1968) points to an evolution of views about age from Aeschylus in the late sixth and early fifth centuries

B.C., to Euripides in the mid- to late fifth century B.C. For Aeschylus, age brought with it wisdom, especially about justice and prudence. Although he refers to the destructive influences of age, particularly loss of physical strength, Aeschylus insists that such physical decline has no impact on the older person's mind or spirit. In contrast, Sophocles' tragedies, which were written during the middle of the fifth century, depict old age as distasteful, a time of decline in physical and mental functioning. For Sophocles, youth is the only period of life of true happiness. Later, in Euripides' plays, older people are both wise and weak. Older characters of Euripides long for eternal youth; old age is described as miserable, bitter, and painful. The shift from Aeschylus' admiration of old age to the exaltation of youth and denigration of old age by Sophocles and Euripides may be a reflection of the growth of democracy in fifth-century Greece (and, consequently, a growing belief in social equality) as well as the heroism of young men in the wars of that era.

OLD AGE IN MEDIEVAL EUROPE   1500's

Little is known about the role of older people during the medieval period, except that life expectancy was even shorter than in the Greek and Roman eras (Angel, 1954). To a large extent, increasing urbanization and related problems of sanitation and disease were responsible for the high death rates before people reached old age. The nobility lived longer than the common people during the Middle Ages, mostly because of better standards of living. Furthermore, the general populace was more likely to die of war or the numerous diseases that plagued this era. The nobility had the freedom to flee such conditions. For the small proportion of poor who *did* manage to survive, old age was a cruel period of life.

To the extent that the prevailing attitudes toward older persons in that historical period can be inferred from a poet or playwright, Shakespeare's description of the seven ages of man in his play *As You Like It* provides such a glimpse. Youth evolves from an impulsive boy to soldier, to the fifth age "full of wise saws and modern instances." The sixth age is depicted as weak, with "his big manly voice, turning again toward childish treble." The seventh and final stage "is second childishness and mere oblivion, sans teeth, sans eyes, sans taste, sans everything." Thus, Shakespeare's view of old age is that of decline and uselessness; this may reflect the attitude of sixteenth-century Europe that the old were a burden to a community struggling with food shortages and high death rates among its infants and young soldiers. Perhaps most striking is Shakespeare's attribution of wisdom and perspective to middle-age, in contrast to the ancient Greek writers' beliefs that old age was the time of greatest wisdom.

OLD AGE IN COLONIAL AMERICA

In seventeenth- and eighteenth-century America, old age was treated with deference and respect, in part because it was so rare. This attitude has been described as one of veneration, an emotion closer to awe than affection and a form of worship deeply embedded in the Judeo-Christian ethic of early America (Fischer, 1978). The Puritans, for example, viewed old age as a sign of God's favor and assumed that youth would inevitably defer to age. Old men occupied the highest public offices, as well as positions of authority within the family, until they died; fathers waited until their sixties before giving their land to their eldest son. Church seats were given to the old. The primary basis of the power enjoyed by the elderly in colonial times was their control of property, especially productive property in farmland. In this agricultural society, such control amounted to the ability to dominate all key institutions—the family, the church, the economy, and the polity (Achenbaum, 1985).

Even though the old were exalted by law and custom in colonial times, they received little affection or love from younger people; in fact, most were kept at an emotional distance. In reserving power and prestige for the elderly, society in many ways created this separation between young and old. Elders frequently complained that they had lived to become strangers in their communities. Old age was not a time of serenity, but rather anxiety about adequately fulfilling social obligations and keeping faith with God (Fischer, 1978).

This pattern persisted until about 1770, when attitudes toward the elderly began to change and the relative status of youth was elevated. There are a number of indications of this change: church-seating arrangements that had favored the old were abolished; the first mandatory retirement laws for legislators were passed; and the eldest son no longer automatically inherited the family property. New fashions were introduced that flattered youth rather than the white wigs and broad-waisted coats that favored older men. Words that negatively portrayed elders, such as *codger* and *fuddy-duddy*, appeared in dictionaries in the nineteenth century. In family portraits, all members of the family were placed on the same horizontal plane rather than positioning the oldest male members to stand over women and children (Fischer, 1978).

A major demographic change occurred in approximately 1810, when the median age began to rise, creating a greater percentage of the population older than the typical "old" age of 40 or 50. This was due primarily to a declining birth rate, not a falling death rate. After 1810, the median age advanced at a constant annual rate, approximately 0.4 percent per year, until about 1950 (Fischer, 1978). Fischer (1978) attributes this to reductions in the impact of diseases. A dramatic change was that parents began to live beyond the period of their children's dependency, for the first time historically experiencing a time when their children had left the home and they were still healthy.

THE EFFECTS OF MODERNIZATION

As the foregoing historical examples suggest, definitions of old age, as well as the authority that older people exercised, largely rested on the material and political resources controlled by the elderly. Examples of these resources are traditional skills and knowledge, security from property rights, civil and political power, food from communal sharing, information control, and general welfare from routine services performed by older people (e.g., child care) (Simmons, 1945; Maxwell and Silverman, 1970). Within the constraints set by the social environment and its ideology, the elderly's social rank was generally determined by the balance between the cost of maintaining them and the societal contributions they were perceived to make (Amoss, 1981). As age became a less important criterion for determining access to and control of valued resources, the elderly's status and authority tended to decline.

A number of explanations have been advanced for the declining status of the old in our society. One major explanation is modernization theory. One of the first comparative analyses that raised this issue was reported by Leo Simmons in *The Role of the Aged in Primitive Society* (1945). He noted that the status of older persons, as reflected in their resources and the honor bestowed upon them, varied inversely with the degree of technology, social and economic diversity, and occupational specialization (or modernization) in a given society. As society becomes more modernized, according to this theory, older people lose political and social power, influence, and leadership. These social changes also may lead to disengagement of aging persons from community life. In addition, younger and older generations become increasingly separated socially, morally, and intellectually. Youth is glorified as the embodiment of progress and achievement, as well as the means to attain such progress.

Modernization theory has been advanced primarily by Cowgill and Holmes (1972; Cowgill, 1974a; 1974b). Modernization is defined by Cowgill (1974a) as:

> The transformation of a total society from a relatively rural way of life based on animate power, limited technology, relatively undifferentiated institutions, parochial and traditional outlook and values, toward a predominantly urban way of life, based on inanimate sources of power, highly differentiated institutions, matched by segmented individual roles, and a cosmopolitan outlook which emphasizes efficiency and progress (p. 127).

The characteristics of modernization that contribute to lower status for the elderly were identified by Cowgill and Holmes as (1) health technology, (2) scientific technology as applied in economic production and distribution, (3) urbanization, and (4) literacy and mass education.

According to Cowgill and Holmes, the application of *health technology* has reduced infant mortality and maternal deaths, and prolonged adult life, thereby increasing the number of older persons in the population. With more older people in the labor market, competition for jobs between generations has intensified, and retirement has developed as a means of forcing older people out of the labor market.

Scientific technology creates new jobs primarily for the young, with the elderly more likely to remain in traditional occupations that become obsolete. The rapid development of industries that rely on high technology in the twentieth century and the gap between generations in using computers illustrate this phenomenon. Unable to perform the socially valued role of contributors to the workforce, many retirees feel marginal and alienated.

In the early stages of modernization, when the society is relatively rural, young people are attracted to urban areas, whereas older parents and grandparents remain on the family farm or in rural communities. The resulting residential segregation of the generations has a dramatic impact on family interactions. The geographical and occupational mobility of the young, in turn, leads to increased social distance between generations and to a reduced status of the aged.

Finally, modernization is characterized by efforts to promote *literacy and education,* which tend to be targeted toward the young. As younger generations acquire more education than their parents, they begin to occupy higher status positions. Intellectual and moral differences between the generations increase, with the elderly experiencing reduced leadership roles and influence (Cowgill, 1974a, 1974b).

This theory has received some empirical support. Using a series of socio-economic measures, Palmore and Whittington (1971) found that the status of the elderly, compared to the younger population, had generally declined in the United States from 1940 to 1969. Watson and Maxwell (1977), in their study of the ethnographic records of 26 different societies in Europe and Asia, reported that as the use of technology increased, the elderly's control of important information and the esteem and deference accorded them declined. In a cross-cultural study of 31 countries at different stages of modernization, Palmore and Manton (1974) found that the elderly's relative employment status was lower in the more modernized societies, due primarily to the increased education of the young and a shift away from agriculture as an economic base. Occupation and education, however, had a reversed J-shaped relationship to modernization; that is, in the early phases of rapid social change (illustrated by nations such as Iran, El Salvador, and the Phillipines), the occupational and educational status of the aged declined, but then later improved (exemplified by New Zealand, Canada, and the United States). This suggests that as societies move beyond an initial state of rapid modernization, status differences between generations decrease and the relative status of the elderly may rise, particularly when reinforced by social policies such as Social Security (Cowgill, 1974a). Similarly, Pampel (1981) documented improvement in the relative financial status of the elderly in our country since

World War II. Both Calhoun (1978) and Pampel maintain that societies in advanced stages of modernization become more aware of the older population's devalued status. Thus, through public education, social policies, and the media, they attempt to create more opportunities and positive images of the elderly. This has already begun in the United States, with advertising and television programs increasingly portraying older persons as vital, active, and involved, with many local governments encouraging employers to hire older workers, and with colleges opening their doors to older students.

ALTERNATIVES TO MODERNIZATION THEORY:

More recent analyses of older people's status in nonindustrial societies have found that conditions for high status did not always apply. For example, differences often existed between the prestige of the old and the way they were actually treated; over 80 percent of the 60 nonindustrial societies in Glascock and Feinman's (1981, 1986) sample had some form of nonsupportive treatment (ranging from insults to killing) for the old, even though older members were also respected. Most societies have some norms of favorable treatment toward the elderly, but considerable variability in practice. For example, filial piety in China and Taiwan was not always manifest, but affected by family resources and number of living children (Ikels, 1980). The coexistence of high status and bad treatment in many traditional societies can be partially explained in terms of differential behavior toward the young-old versus old-old, noted in our earlier discussion of traditional societies that abandoned or murdered their frail elderly (Keith, 1985).

Class and sex differences also come into play. For instance, the norms of filial piety were more often practiced by the well-to-do in traditional rural China. Despite the Confucian reverence for age, older people in lower class families had fewer resources to give them status (Cherry and Magnuson-Martinson, 1981; Ikels, 1980). The importance of women's household responsibilities throughout life may explain their relatively higher status in old age than men's (Cool and McCabe, 1983).

IDEAL OF EQUALITY VERSUS STATUS OF AGE IN AMERICA

Besides modernization, Fischer (1978) has formulated other reasons for explaining changes between generations in American society. He argues that these changes cannot be attributed to modernization, because the decline in older people's status occurred before industrialization and urbanization. He also contends that the increase in numbers of older people does not fully explain the shifts in attitudes toward the old. Instead, he suggests that the emphasis on youthfulness that characterizes our society can be partially attributed to our cultural values of liberty and equality. Both of these values run counter to a hierarchy of authority based on age.

According to Fischer, the elevated status of older persons in earlier historical periods gradually became supplanted in the late eighteenth and early nineteenth centuries by an emerging ideal of age equality. The fundamental change was caused by the social and intellectual forces unleashed by revolutions in America and France. The spirit of equality was dramatically expressed in public fetes borrowed from the French Revolution, where a symbolic harmony of youth and age was celebrated in elaborate rituals of young and old exchanging food (Fischer, 1978).

However, although our society's ideology was egalitarian, economic inequalities actually grew in the nineteenth century. For example, economic status became the basis of seating arrangements in public meetings. Individualistic pursuits of wealth created countervailing forces to a sense of community that had previously been founded on the power of elders (Fischer, 1978). Thus, the age equality that had initially replaced veneration of elders was later supplanted by a celebration of youthfulness and a derogation of age. Inequalities based on age reemerged, but this time to the advantage of youth. Growing contempt toward the elderly in the mid-1800s is vividly illustrated by Thoreau's (1856) conclusion, "Age is no better, hardly so well qualified for an instructor of youth, for it has not profited as much as it has lost." Heroes and legends centered on younger men, such as Daniel Boone. Social trends in the early twentieth century, such as the development of retirement policies, mass education, and residential segregation of generations, furthered perceptions of the elderly as useless, with the cult of youth reaching its peak in the 1960s. One irony was that as the economic and social conditions of many elderly declined in modern America, their ties of family affection, especially between grandparents and grandchildren, often grew stronger (Fischer, 1978).

OTHER PERSPECTIVES ON HISTORICAL CHANGE

Historians and gerontologists have questioned whether a "revolution" in age relations occurred between 1770 and 1830 (Achenbaum, 1985). Achenbaum (1978), for example, has taken a position somewhere between Fischer's view and modernization theory regarding the change in status of the elderly in America. He has identified social trends similar to those documented by Fischer, stating that prior to the middle of the nineteenth century, the elderly were venerated because of their experiences and were actively involved in socially useful roles. A decline in the status of the elderly, Achenbaum asserts, occurred during the post-Civil War era. The growing emphasis on efficiency and impersonality in bureaucracies, along with increased misperceptions about senility, furthered a perception of old age as obsolescence. Both Fischer and Achenbaum suggest that it is not possible to establish a firm relationship between modernization and the elderly's status;

rather, they maintain that Americans have always been ambivalent about old age. Shifting beliefs and values are viewed as more salient in accounting for loss in status than changes in the economic and political structures that occurred with modernization.

These contrasting perspectives of social gerontologists and anthropologists suggest that there is not a simple "before and after" relationship in the meaning and significance of old age between pre-industrial and modern societies (Achenbaum, 1985). People in pre-industrial societies who, by reason of social class, lacked property and power undoubtedly suffered from loss of status, regardless of their age. For such persons, modernization brought less improve-ment in status than for the elderly who were better educated and of higher socioeconomic background. Such inequities continue to be problematic, par-ticularly among ethnic minorities within our society (Fry, 1980; Palmore and Manton, 1974). Achenbaum and Stearns (1978) have emphasized that moderniza-tion is not a linear process, but proceeds at different rates and through varied stages, each of which may have a different impact on older people's status.

In addition, cross-cultural evidence shows that cultural values can mitigate many of the negative effects of modernization on the elderly. This is illustrated in modern, industrialized, and urban Japanese society where, some research suggests, values of filial piety and ancestor worship have helped to maintain the relatively high status of older persons and their integration in family life (Palmore, 1975c). Political ideology may also be an intervening variable, as illustrated by the effect of Communist party policies of age equality on reducing the status of the aged in China prior to modernization (Cherry and Magnuson-Martinson, 1981). In sum, the effects of modernization historically do not appear to be uniform nor unidirectional. As shown in the next section, many contemporary cultures are still struggling to define satisfying roles for their rapidly increasing populations of older people. Changing values and declining resources result in conflicting attitudes toward the elderly in many transitional societies.

A Cross-Cultural View of Old Age in Contemporary Societies

As we have discussed, every society defines people as old on some basis, whether chronological, functional, or generational, and assigns that group a particular set of rights, privileges, and duties that differ from those of its younger members. For example, older persons in our society today qualify for Social Security and Medicare on the basis of their age. In some religious groups, only the oldest members are permitted to perform the most sacred rituals. Societies generally distinguish two classes of elders: (1) those who are no longer fully productive economically, but are physically and mentally able to attend to their daily needs; and (2) those who are totally dependent, who require custodial care, and who are regarded as social burdens and thus may be negatively treated. A third group of elderly exists in many societies: those who continue to participate actively in the economy of the social system, through farming or self-employment, through care of grandchildren, or through household maintenance while younger adults work outside the home.

Older people who can no longer work but who control resources essential to fulfill the needs of younger group members generally offset the societal costs incurred in maintaining them. In some social systems, political, judicial, or ritual power and privileges are vested in older people as a group, and this serves to mediate social costs. For instance, in societies such as those of East Africa, politically powerful positions are automatically assigned to men who reach a certain age (Spencer, 1965). In other societies, the old do not inherently have privileges, but gain power as individuals, often through diplomatic skills and contacts with powerful others. The following examples from other cultures illustrate the balance between the costs and contributions made by the aged.

In the subsistence society of the Chipewyan Indians of Canada, older men are accorded low status, and old age is despised and feared; this is primarily because older men, who are no longer able to hunt, are perceived as unproductive, costing

Native American women often perform valued functions within their culture.

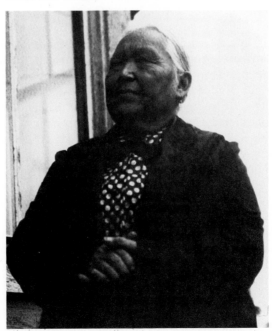

society more than they contribute. Dependent on the contributions of each tribal member, the Chipewyans have sometimes been forced to abandon their old when faced with a choice between the death of older men and that of the entire tribe. Unlike the older men, Chipewyan older women are still able to perform customary domestic and gathering tasks that do not require physical vigor. As a result, aging does not produce as substantial a decline in the status of older women as in that of older men (Sharp, 1981).

Unlike Chipewyan men, older men among the Asmats of coastal New Guinea are able to assert political leadership in kinship and local groups even after their hunting skills have deteriorated. The primary reason for this difference is that the Asmat economy is less precarious, so that older men can still acquire resources to protect their position in old age (Amoss and Harrell, 1981).

IMPORTANCE OF SOCIAL POSITION AND THE CONTROL OF PROPERTY

The control of property is a means of achieving power in most societies. Both in past and present times, the elderly have used their rights over property to guarantee their security by compelling others to support them or to provide them with goods and services. For example, among the Etal Islanders in Micronesia, the old try to keep enough property to ensure continued care by younger members who hope to inherit it (Nason, 1981). In the Gwembe Tonga tribe in Zambia, males were formerly able to secure their position by accumulating land and livestock. As their lineage land became covered by water, however, forced relocation cost many older people their exclusive control of property, and the old became dependent on sons and nephews, who acquired better land at the time of flooding (Colson and Scudder, 1981).

In other societies, the leadership of males derives from their positions within the family. The traditional Chinese extended household is an example. The position of the aging father in the Chinese family depends almost entirely on the political and economic power he wields (Harrell, 1981). As noted earlier, elders in wealthy Chinese households enjoy higher status within the family and are better able to control the lives of their adult children than those in poor households (Ikels, 1980). Both China and India illustrate substantial class differences in the elders' power, as well as the persistence of the extended family structure that confers status on older members, even in the face of modernization. As economic resources decline and class differences disappear in these cultures with increasing modernization, the traditions of filial piety may become undermined. For example, the growing pressures of limited housing and low income in China appear to be having a negative effect on younger generations' attitudes toward old people. In such instances, increased provision of public housing, an old age pension scheme, and policies that support the families' care of elders may serve to reduce tensions between generations (Chow, 1983).

KNOWLEDGE AS A SOURCE OF POWER

Control over knowledge, especially ritual and religious knowledge, is another source of power. The aged Shaman is an example, revered in many societies for knowledge or wisdom. The importance of the elderly in maintaining cultural values is illustrated in India, where traditional Hindu law prescribes a four-stage life cycle for high-caste men: student, householder, ascetic, and mendicant. In the last two stages, older religious men are expected to renounce worldly attachments to seek enlightenment in isolated retreats. This practice ensures that the pursuit of the highest form of knowledge is limited to older men of higher castes (Sokolovsky, 1983). As another example, the !Kung Bushmen value the story-telling ability of people age 45 and over, because the stories are considered to contain the accumulated knowledge of the people. Information and stories are the elderly's resource which can be exchanged for food and security (Biesele and Howell, 1981).

Knowledge as the basis of the elders' power has been challenged in many traditional societies by Western technological and scientific expertise (Goode, 1963; Cowgill, 1974a). For example, the aged farmer who passes on to his children traditional methods of growing crops may be dismayed to find that they ignore this advice and rely on new agricultural methods and products. Examples in which the relevance of traditional knowledge declines with modernization abound in many fields: farming, fishing, construction, housekeeping, even childrearing. They include the Tong elderly of Zambia who lost status due to the flooding of their old habitat and the outmoding of their specialized knowledge (Colson and Scudder, 1981), the elderly in Taiwan who are less knowledgeable in new commercial and industrial contexts (Harrell, 1981), and many native North American groups faced with changing patterns of production and consumption (Amoss, 1981). Among Western Irish peasants, the once dignified movement of the older couple to the sacred "west room" of the house, which signified high esteem, has been replaced by "warehousing" of the elderly in institutions (Scheper-Hughes, 1983).

Among some cultural groups, however, such as the Coast Salish Indians of Washington, a revival of interest and pride in native identity and religion has occurred, thus raising the esteem of elders who possess ritual knowledge (e.g., they are the only ones who know the words and dance steps) (Amoss, 1981; Amoss and Harrell, 1981). Knowledge of the group's culture, particularly traditional arts and handicrafts, and native songs and epics, has enhanced the social status of older persons in these societies; furthermore, the traditions of reverence for old age and wisdom remain strong, overriding the impact of modernization on older people's roles.

The growing desire for ethnic or tribal identity among many Native Americans, which has led to a conscious restoration of old forms, illustrates that modernization does not automatically erode the status of the elders. Similarly, the search for one's heritage or roots has led to increased contacts between younger generations seeking this information from older persons who often are a great repository of family histories.

Cultural and historical factors can also mitigate the presumed negative consequences of modernization for the elderly. For example, in Samoa, despite the influx of U.S. aid, industries, and educational programs designed to promote modernization, the cultural system has been flexible enough to maintain the elderly as a viable part of society. This has largely been due to the persistence of the traditional *matai* family system, which involves the elders in leadership roles within large bilateral kinship groups, and a village council that accords the elders respect and power (Holmes and Rhoads, 1983). The traditional family system has combined with Samoan values of reciprocity in social relationships and an acceptance of dependency in old age to retain high status among Samoan elders (Rhoads, 1984).

EFFECTS OF CULTURE AND MODERNIZATION ARE STILL CHANGING

In other situations, the buffering effects of culture on modernization are less distinct. There are contrasting views, for example, on the issue of modernization and aging in contemporary Japan. As noted earlier, Palmore (1975b) has described the high status and prestige of the elderly in Japan. Buddhism has been viewed as linking the aged to a family system that emphasizes filial devotion, in which the dependence of elders in this "second privileged period" is accepted. More recently, demographic and economic changes appear to have altered traditional conceptions of old age and reduced the positive influences of cultural values. For instance, the modernization of Japanese society has resulted in increased economic demands on the nuclear family; accordingly, the old-old, becoming more dependent on family who have fewer resources to care for them, have sometimes prayed for a quick death in Buddhist temples (Plath, 1983). The unprecedented higher percentage of older people has increased the societal costs of maintaining elders and has created dilemmas for younger family members responsible for their support. The majority of middle-aged persons still believe that care of older parents is the children's responsibility. Nevertheless, the number of nursing homes and long-stay hospitals in Japan has grown rapidly, which suggests that traditional customs of caring for aging parents in adult children's homes are changing. At the same time, the family's capacity to provide care has decreased, due to urbanization, industrialization, the growing numbers of employed women, and the declining number of children since 1950 (Maeda, 1983). As the elderly become more numerous, they may increasingly require goods and services at the perceived expense of younger members of society.

Summary and Implications

These brief examples illustrate how each society responds to its aging members within the constraints set by both the natural environment and the larger human environment of social and technological change. A basic principle governing the status of the aged appears to be the effort to achieve a balance between older people's contributions to the society and the costs of supporting them. As will be discussed in detail in Chapter 10, however, the family can play an important role in supporting the old. Historical and cross-cultural evidence also suggests that maximum social participation of the elderly is the preferred route for public policy.

The extent to which the elderly are engaged in society appears to vary with the nature of their power resources, such as their material possessions, knowledge, and social authority (Dowd, 1980). In most of their exchanges, older people seek to maintain reciprocity and to be active, independent agents in the management of their own lives. That is, they prefer to give money, time, or other resources in exchange for services or materials. This theoretical perspective, which will be described in more detail as social exchange theory in Chapter 3, suggests that modern society should seek ways of increasing the elderly's exchange resources so that they are valued by society. For example, maximizing the social value of the old in our society might include retraining and educational programs and part-time employment. (See Chapter 14.)

Control of resources as a basis for social interactions between members of a society is important throughout the life cycle. However, it becomes even more crucial in old age, because retirement generally results in a decline in one's level of control over material and social resources. As their physical strength diminishes and their social world correspondingly shrinks, many older people face the challenge of altering their environments and using their capacities in ways that will help them to maintain reciprocal exchanges and to protect their competence and independence. These attempts to maintain control over one's environment in the face of changing personal capacities, consistent with the person-environment model presented in Chapter 1, will be discussed in detail in subsequent chapters on biological, psychological, and social changes with aging. The next chapter reviews social theories of aging that offer some explanation of the various ways in which people interact with the larger society as well as their immediate social environments as they age.

References

Achenbaum, W. A. *Old age in the new land: The American experience since 1790.* Baltimore: The Johns Hopkins Press, 1978.

Achenbaum, W. A. Societal perceptions of aging and the aged. In E. Shanas and R. Binstock, *Handbook of aging and the social sciences* (2d ed.). New York: Van Nostrand, 1985, 129–148.

Achenbaum, W. A., and Stearns, P. Old age and modernization. *The Gerontologist*, 1978, *18*, 307–312.

Amoss, P. Coast Salish elders. In P. Amoss and S. Harrell (Eds.), *Other ways of growing old*. Stanford, Calif.: Stanford University Press, 1981, 227–248.

Angel, J. L. Human biology, health, and history in Greece from the first settlement until now. *American Philosophical Society Yearbook*, 1954, 171–172.

Biesele, M., and Howell, N. The old people give you life: Aging among !Kung hunters-gatherers. In P. Amoss and S. Harrell (Eds.), *Other ways of growing old*. Stanford, Calif.: Stanford University Press, 1981, 77–99.

Calhoun, R. *In search of the new old: Redefining old age in America, 1945–1970*. New York: Elsevier, 1978.

Cherry, R., and Magnuson-Martinson, S. Modernization and the status of the aged in China: Decline or equalization? *Sociological Quarterly*, 1981, 22, 253–261.

Chow, N. The Chinese family and support of the elderly in Hong Kong. *The Gerontologist*, 1983, *23*, 584–588.

Colson, E., and Scudder, T. Old age in Gwemba District, Zambia. In P. Amoss and S. Harrell (Eds.), *Other ways of growing old*. Stanford, Calif.: Stanford University Press, 1981, 125–154.

Cool, L., and McCabe, J. The "scheming hag" and the "dear old thing." The anthropology of aging women. In J. Sokolovsky (Ed.), *Growing old in different cultures*. Belmont, Calif.: Wadsworth, 1983, 56–68.

Cowgill, D. Aging and modernization: A revision of the theory. In J. F. Gubrium (Ed.), *Late life communities and environmental policy*. Springfield, Ill.: Charles C. Thomas, 1974a, 123–146.

Cowgill, D. The aging of populations and societies. In F. Eisele (Ed.), *Political consequences of aging. The annals of the American Academy of Political and Social Science*, 1974b, 415, 1–18.

Cowgill, D., and Holmes, L. *Aging and modernization*. New York: Appleton-Century-Crofts, 1972.

de Romilly, J. *Time in Greek tragedy*. Ithaca, N.Y.: Cornell University Press, 1968.

Dowd, J. J. Social exchange: Class and old people. In J. Dowd (Ed.), *Stratification among the aged*. Monterey, Calif.: Brooks Cole, 1980.

Fischer, D. H. *Growing old in America*. Oxford, Eng.: Oxford University Press, 1978.

Fry, C. (Ed.). *Aging in culture and society: Comparative viewpoints and strategies*. New York: J. F. Bergin, 1980.

Fry, C., and Contributors. *Dimensions: Aging, culture and health*. New York: J. F. Bergin, 1981.

Fry, C., and Keith, J. (Eds.). *New methods for old age research: Strategies for studying diversity*. South Hadley, Mass.: Bergin and Garvey, 1986.

Glascock, A., and Feinman, S. Social asset or social burden: Treatment of the aged in nonindustrial societies. In C. Fry (Ed.), *Dimensions: Aging, culture and health.* New York: J. F. Bergin, 1981, 13–31.

Glascock, A., and Feinman, S. Treatment of the aged in non-industrial societies. In C. Fry and J. Keith (Eds.), *New methods for old age research: Strategies for studying diversity.* South Hadley, Mass.: Bergin and Garvey, 1986.

Goode, W. *World revolution and family patterns.* New York: Free Press, 1963.

Harrell, S. Growing old in rural Taiwan. In P. Amoss and S. Harrell (Eds.), *Other ways of growing old.* Stanford, Calif.: Stanford University Press, 1981, 193–210.

Hendricks, J., and Hendricks, C. D. *Aging in mass society: Myths and realities.* Cambridge, Mass.: Winthrop, 1981.

Holmes, L., and Rhoads, E. Aging and change in Samoa. In J. Sokolovsky (Ed.), *Growing old in different societies.* Belmont, Calif.: Wadsworth, 1983, 119–130.

Ikels, C. The coming of age in Chinese society. In C. Fry (Ed.), *Aging in culture and society.* New York: Praeger, 1980, 80–101.

Keith, J. *Old people as people: Social and cultural influences on aging and old age.* Boston: Little, Brown, 1982.

Keith, J. Age in anthropological research. In R. H. Binstock and E. Shanas (Eds.), *Handbook of aging and the social sciences* (2d ed.). New York: Van Nostrand, 1985, 231–263.

Maeda, D. Family care in Japan. *The Gerontologist,* 1983, *23,* 579–583.

Maxwell, R., and Silverman, P. Information and esteem. *Aging and Human Development,* 1970, *1,* 361–392.

Nason, J. D. Respected elder or old person: Aging in a Micronesian community. In P. Amoss and S. Harrell (Eds.), *Other ways of growing old.* Stanford, Calif.: Stanford University Press, 1981, 155–175.

Palmore, E. *The honorable elders.* Durham, N.C.: Duke University Press, 1975a.

Palmore, E. The status and integration of the aged in Japanese society. *Journal of Gerontology,* 1975b, *30,* 199–208.

Palmore, E. What can the U.S.A. learn from Japan about aging? *The Gerontologist,* 1975c, *15,* 64–67.

Palmore, E., and Manton, K. Modernization and the status of the aged: International comparisons. *Journal of Gerontology,* 1974, *29,* 205–210.

Palmore, E., and Whittington, F. Trends in the relative status of the aged. *Social Forces,* 1971, *50,* 84–91.

Pampel, F. *Social change and the aged: Recent trends in the United States.* Lexington, Mass.: Lexington Books, 1981.

Plath, D. Ecstasy years—Old age in Japan. In J. Sokolovsky (Ed.), *Growing old in different societies.* Belmont, Calif.: Wadsworth, 1983, 147–154.

Rhoads, E. Reevaluation of the aging and modernization theory: The Samoan evidence. *The Gerontologist,* 1984, *24,* 243–250.

Scheper-Hughes, N. Deposed kings: The demise of the rural Irish gerontocracy. In J. Sokolovsky (Ed.), *Growing old in different societies.* Belmont, Calif.: Wadsworth, 1983.

Sharp, H. Old age among the Chipewyan. In P. Amoss and S. Harrell (Eds.), *Other ways of growing old.* Stanford, Calif.: Stanford University Press, 1981, 99–110.

Simmons, L. W. *The role of the aged in primitive society.* New Haven, Conn.: Yale University Press, 1945.

Sokolovsky, J. (Ed.). *Growing old in different societies.* Belmont, Calif.: Wadsworth, 1983.

Spencer, D. *The Samburu: A study of gerontology in a nomadic tribe.* Berkeley: University of California Press, 1965.

Thoreau, H. D. *Walden.* New York: New American Library, 1856, Chapter 1, p. 8.

Waring, J. Social replenishment and social change: The problem of disordered cohort flow. *American Behavioral Scientist,* 1975, *19,* 237–256.

Watson, W. H., and Maxwell, R. J. (Eds.). *Human aging and dying: A study in sociocultural gerontology.* New York: St. Martin's Press, 1977.

Chapter 3

Social Theories
of Aging

Why Study Social Theories of Aging?

The notion of developing and verifying a *theory* of aging may seem unnecessary or overly academic. We all grow older. Our bodies change with age, and so do our interests and lifestyles—not just theoretically, but in fact. Yet in a very informal and often unconscious way, we all develop theories from our own experiences. We observe older people in our families and communities and make generalizations about them. In a sense, the stereotypes of older people, sometimes labeled *ageist,* are the result of unconscious theorizing about the meaning of growing old.

The scientific approach to theory development is different in that it is a conscious and methodical attempt to explain why an event or set of events occurs. A scientific theory is based on a logically related set of statements, called *propositions* or *hypotheses,* each of which is subjected to testing through empirical research.

Propositions may be either statements of existing knowledge or predictions based on that knowledge. Each theory is based on not one but a series of such propositions, any one of which may be partially in error. Scientists never entirely prove or disprove a theory. Instead, through empirical research, they gather evidence that may strengthen their confidence in it or move them closer to rejecting the theory by proving that parts of it are untrue. The possibility always exists that with the next empirical test, the theory will not be supported.

Such scientific theories are valuable because they allow us to accumulate knowledge and make sense of the world, to see more coherently and logically what we might otherwise only vaguely perceive, and thus they serve as guides to further research. They may predict what might happen in the future as well as point to unanswered questions or potential changes.

This chapter focuses on social theories—explanations of the changes in social relationships that occur in late adulthood. In effect, these theories attempt to answer questions we all wonder about: What makes for successful aging? What should the elderly do? What should our society be doing with regard to the elderly? Should we force older people to retire or will they be more satisfied if they continue to work? Is it beneficial for the elderly to be active in the community? All of these theories address the basic issue of determining the optimal way for older people to relate to their environments.

As noted in Chapter 1, early research in the field of social gerontology tended to be applied rather than theoretical in nature, primarily because many older people were facing problems requiring immediate solutions. Since the 1950s and 1960s, however, researchers have been addressing broader theoretical questions regarding how people adapt to the changes characteristically associated with aging. Because the resulting proliferation of theoretical perspectives is relatively recent, the theories advanced by sociologists and psychologists tend to be more descriptive than explanatory; most are unable to explain how and why associations occur among the concepts being studied. None of the theories discussed in this chapter has been sufficiently tested to be rejected or to provide accurate predictions about the behavior of individuals. However, each theory suggests some important factors that may be related to aging and thus serves as a guide for further inquiry and possible intervention in the aging process. The theoretical perspectives examined in this chapter with reference to their gerontological applications are: role, activity, disengagement, and continuity theories, the elderly as a subculture, age stratification, interactionist perspectives, social exchange theory, and the political economy framework. All of these have their foundations in basic sociological and psychological models.

Role Theory

One of the earliest attempts by social gerontologists to explain how individuals adjust to aging involved an application of role theory (Cottrell, 1942). People play a variety of social roles in their lifetimes, such as student, mother, wife, daughter, businesswoman, consultant, grandmother, and so on. Such roles identify and describe a person as a social being and are the basis of self-concept. They are organized sequentially into a life course; each social role is associated with a certain age or stage of life. In most societies, particularly Western ones, chronological age is used to determine eligibility for various positions, to evaluate the suitability of different roles, and to shape expectations of people in social situations. Some roles have a reasonable biological basis related to age (e.g., the role of mother), but many could be filled by individuals of a wide age range (e.g., the role of volunteer). Age alters not only the roles expected of people, but also the manner in which they are expected to play them. For example, a family's expectations of a 32-year-old mother are quite different from their expectations of her at age 62. How well individuals adjust to aging is assumed to depend on how well they accept the role changes typical of the later years.

Age norms serve to open up or close off the roles that people of a given chronological age can play. Age norms are assumptions of age-related capacities and limitations—beliefs that a person of a given age can and ought to do certain things. As an illustration, an older widower who starts dating and staying out late at night may be told by a disapproving family member that he should "act his age." Norms may be formally expressed through social policies and laws (e.g., laws against discrimination and mandatory retirement policies). More often, however, they operate informally. For example, even though employers cannot legally refuse to hire a 55-year-old woman because of her age, they can assume that she is too old to train for a new position. Their business norm is to hire younger workers. In such instances, age norms seem unjust and often have detrimental psychological consequences for older persons, causing them to feel worthless, angry, and depressed. In addition, such norms reinforce ageist stereotypes among younger people who are then more likely to assume that older workers are less productive and unreliable. Individuals also hold norms about the appropriateness of their own behavior at any particular age, so that "social clocks become internalized and age norms operate to keep people on the time track" (Hagestad and Neugarten, 1985). Most men in our society, for example, have expectations about the appropriate age at which to graduate from school, start working, marry, have a family, reach the peak of their career, and retire. These expectations have been shifting among younger cohorts, however. For instance, more men in their forties and fifties are entering second or third careers, rather than assuming they must work at their first jobs until they retire.

Every society conveys age norms through socialization, a lifelong process by which individuals learn how to perform new roles, adjust to changing roles, relinquish old ones, and thereby become integrated into society. We tend to think of socialization as occurring primarily in childhood, but we are constantly adjusting to new roles throughout our lives; older adults become socialized to numerous roles that accompany old age.

ROLE DILEMMAS OF LATE ADULTHOOD

Older adults face a number of role dilemmas. With age, people are more likely to lose roles they have filled in the past than to acquire new ones; in addition, the most common role losses are largely irreversible, for example, the loss of the spouse role with widowhood or of the worker role with retirement. Although some older widows remarry and some retirees return to work that they find satisfying, the majority do neither, nor do they develop new roles to replace those they have lost. Since roles are the basis of an individual's self-concept, role loss can lead to an erosion of social identity and self-esteem (Rosow, 1985). Some early research found that the role losses of retirement and widowhood were related to maladjustment, as measured by self-reports about the amount of time devoted to daydreaming about the past, thinking about death, and being absent-minded (Phillips, 1957). Later research has provided less support for this conclusion (Lemon, Bengtson, and Peterson, 1972).

With age, roles also tend to become more ambiguous. Guidelines or expectations about the requirements of roles, such as that of family authority or nurturing parent, become less clear to the elderly themselves as well as to others (Rosow, 1985). Burgess (1960) maintained that the role of the retired person is "roleless." This means that older individuals lack a consensus about societal rules to guide their behavior, which serves to exclude them from socially meaningful activity. Norms that do exist for older adults in our society tend to reflect "middle-aged" standards related to independence and social activity (Bengtson, 1973; Rosow, 1985). This can actually hinder socialization to old age.

Without clear-cut norms to measure conformity to or deviation from a role, there are few rewards for performing a role successfully. This, in turn, can deprive older people of the motivation to master new roles (e.g., role of volunteer) or maintain existing ones (e.g., role of helpful neighbor). Furthermore, the many older people who are unwilling to take on the diminished status and "uselessness" of the retiree role face a lack of desirable role options and models. Others, particularly women and ethnic minorities, may lack the resources to move into new roles or to emulate younger, more physically attractive role models.

The lack of appropriate role models is partially due to the fact that, until this century, most people did not live to old age. Not only did few role models exist, but those in the media and the public realm tended to be youthful in appearance and behavior, maintaining middle-age standards which can actually hinder socialization to old age. With the growing numbers and visibility of older people, middle-aged persons today have more role models to emulate than they did in the past. In addition, more attention has recently been paid to alternative roles that older people can play in our society—trends that may serve to reduce role ambiguity for future cohorts of older people.

Another dilemma is that the transition from the worker role to the retiree role is characterized by role discontinuity, whereby what is learned at one age level may be useless or conflicting at the next age level. For example, learning to be highly productive in the workplace may be antithetical to adjusting to leisure time in retirement. Most workers have few opportunities to prepare for the new, more leisurely lifestyle of retiree, either through retirement planning programs or through interactions with retirees while in occupational roles. Institutions or situations that help people prepare for role changes with age have been limited in our society.

CHANGES ON THE HORIZON?

Although the framework of role theory can help us understand why some older people have difficulties in adjusting to aging, the rapid increase in the number of elderly may change this. In the future, roles appropriate to old age may become clearer, more continuous with past roles, and more satisfying. Future cohorts of older people may be better prepared for the role changes that often accompany the aging process; a growing number of interventions, such as preretirement counseling and widows' support groups, may help to smooth role transitions.

As the number of active, healthy, older people grows, our perception of the role changes that accompany old age may also be altered. Although old age is a time of role loss, it can also encompass role gains, such as volunteer, part-time worker, grandparent, and so on. Other roles, such as neighbor, friend, or parent, generally continue throughout life, although the particular individuals involved and the conception of the roles may shift over time. The role of neighbor, for example, may assume greater importance to the older retiree in good health who now has more time to help others, by watching over neighborhood children, assisting less healthy neighbors, or participating in neighborhood crime watch programs.

There is also growing recognition that the role of "dependent person" is not inevitable with age. Rather, the life course is characterized by varying periods of greater or lesser dependency in social relationships, with most people being emotionally dependent on others regardless of age. Even a physically impaired older person may still continue to support others emotionally (e.g., through a telephone reassurance program), and may be able to devise creative adaptations to ensure competence at home. Current efforts to maintain older people in their own homes as alternatives to institutionalization reflect an awareness of the need to preserve autonomous roles as long as possible.

Role changes experienced by the elderly underlie two of the most widely debated theories of successful aging: activity theory and disengagement theory. Both were based on the Kansas City Study of Adult Life (Havighurst, 1968), but they reached fundamentally different conclusions about successful aging. That this debate continues is illustrated by the standing-room-only crowd that attended the session entitled "Old Theories Never Die" at the 1985 Annual Scientific Meetings of the Gerontological Society of America. To some extent, these theoretical perspectives have also served to legitimize some of the social policies designed to meet the needs of the older population (Minkler and Estes, 1984).

Activity Theory

Activity theory is a dominant theoretical perspective in social gerontology; to a large extent, it is a commonsense theory. It was developed from Robert Havighurst's (1963, 1968) analyses of the Kansas City Study of 300 people—primarily white, middle class, healthy, ranging from 50 to 90 years of age—who were interviewed at regular intervals over a six-year period. It assumes that older people who are active will be more satisfied and better adjusted than less active elderly. Since activity theory presumes that a person's self-concept is validated through participation in roles characteristic of middle age, it is seen as desirable for older people to maintain as many middle-age activities as possible, and to substitute new roles for those that are lost through widowhood or retirement (Lemon, Bengtson, and Peterson, 1972). In order to minimize society's withdrawal from the elderly, which occurs against older people's will or desire, older people must deny the existence of old age by maintaining middle-age lifestyles as long as possible: remain active, keep busy, and stay young! Behavior inappropriate to middle age is considered to be maladaptive.

To a large extent, this perspective is consistent with our society's value system, which emphasizes work and productivity. It has resulted in policies that stress continued social activities as a way to assist the elderly's social integration. Such a perspective is reflected in gerontological practitioners' efforts to develop new roles for older people that involve responsibilities and obligations. The activity perspective is perhaps most strikingly apparent in the numerous recreation events, travel tours, and classes sponsored by retirement communities and senior centers.

CRITIQUE OF ACTIVITY THEORY

Empirical support for activity theory is mixed. Informal social activity with friends has been found to be somewhat related to well-being (Lemon, Bengtson, and Peterson, 1972). The Second Duke Longitudinal Study found that being active in organizations and physical activity were two major predictors of successful aging (Palmore, 1979). Other studies, however, identified a negative association between formal group activity and life satisfaction (Longino and Kart, 1982), which suggests that variables other than level of activity, such as opportunities to interact intimately with others, are needed to explain life satisfaction. Although some studies found that active people have better physical and mental health and take greater satisfaction in life than do the inactive, such people are generally better educated and have more money and options than those less active (Havighurst et al., 1969; Palmore, 1974; Thurmond and Belcher, 1980–81). Therefore, socioeconomic, lifestyle, and generational variables may be more important than maturational ones in the associations found between activity and life satisfaction, health, and well-being.

Activity theory tells us little about what happens to people who cannot maintain the standards of middle-age. By failing to acknowledge a personality dimension, it does not explain the fact that some older persons are passive and happy while others are highly active and unhappy. Another limitation is its assumption that people want to continue their same pattern of activity (Longino and Kart, 1982). Many elderly who were active during middle-age may no longer want to sustain their activity level and, in fact, may value the opportunity to curtail their social involvements. Some older people may simply want to have time to "do nothing," to "sit and rock," and to engage in solitary pursuits. The value placed by older people on being active probably varies with their lifelong experiences, personality, and needs. Havighurst himself (1968) later acknowledged the importance of personality in predicting the association between activity levels and life satisfaction; thus, people who have been active, achieving, and outward-directed in middle-age will probably be satisfied to continue this into old age, whereas those who have been passive, dependent, and home-centered may be content to sustain this contrasting pattern later in life. This perspective has led other sociologists to argue that, rather than remaining active, good adjustment to the aging process involves disengagement.

Disengagement Theory

Disengagement theory, one of the most widely known and controversial theories in social gerontology, was first formulated by Elaine Cumming and William Henry in 1961. Their book, *Growing Old,* challenges the assumption that older people have to be active in order to be well adjusted. Instead, the process whereby older people decrease their activity levels, seek more passive roles, interact less frequently with others, and become increasingly preoccupied with their inner lives is viewed as normal, inevitable, and personally satisfying. Disengagement has its basis in the assumption of an inevitable decline in abilities with age and the universal expectation of death. The process of disengagement may be started either by the older person or by society. Regardless of how the withdrawal process is initiated, it is presumed to be mutual, having positive consequences for both society and the individual.

According to this theory, older people, experiencing losses of roles and energy, want to be released from societal expectations that they be productive and

Some older people derive great satisfaction from more reflective activities.

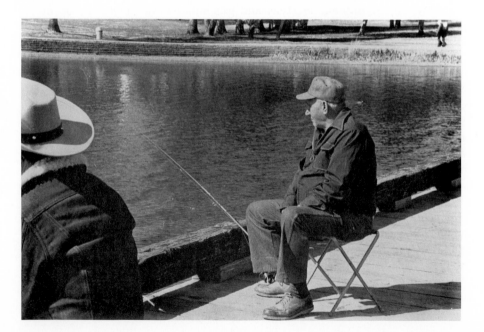

competitive. Disengagement is thus viewed as adaptive behavior, allowing older people to maintain a sense of worth and tranquility while performing more peripheral social roles. For example, Cumming and Henry argued that disengaged older people, freed from the demands of employment roles, are better able to participate in satisfying family relationships than those who remain occupied with work. For men, the process of disengagement tends to be abrupt, as they forfeit their occupational roles. For women, the transition from what is often their central role as parent is more gradual and smooth; however, future cohorts of employed women may experience this transition period differently.

Disengagement is presumed not only to be adaptive for older people, but also to be functional or useful to society. According to Cumming and Henry, all societies need orderly ways to transfer power from older to younger generations. Retirement policies, for example, are assumed to be a way to ensure that younger people with new energy and skills will move into occupational roles. When the elderly have disengaged from the mainstream of society, their deaths are also thought to be less disruptive to society's optimal functioning. Thus, disengagement theory holds that social services, if provided at all, should not seek to revitalize the aged, but rather to encourage their withdrawal.

CRITIQUE OF DISENGAGEMENT THEORY

This theoretical perspective has been widely criticized for assuming that disengagement is inevitable, functional, and universal. Critics point to other cultures where the elderly move into new roles of prestige and power. Likewise, not everyone in our culture disengages, as evidenced by the growing numbers of older people, many in their eighties, who are employed, healthy, and politically and socially active. As with activity theory, disengagement theory fails to account for variability in individual preferences.

The extent to which a person disengages may vary with the individual's position in the social structure. A retired college professor, for example, has more opportunities to remain professionally involved than a retired steel worker. Disengagement also does not appear to be uniform within the individual. A person may disengage socially (e.g., attend fewer social events), but remain fully engaged psychologically (e.g., continue to read about and discuss current events). In addition, what may appear to be disengaged behavior to an outsider may have a very different meaning for the aging person. An older person who sits by a window for hours may not necessarily be disengaged, but may fully enjoy the changing street scenes.

Disengagement theory has also tended to ignore the part that personality plays in the way a person adjusts to aging. People who have always been active, assertive, and socially involved probably will not retreat as they age, but rather will maintain typical ways of adapting to their environments. Similarly, some people always have been withdrawn or passive; hence, disengagement may represent for them a natural transition or continuation of their previous lives rather than the culmination of a process characteristic of all aging individuals (Maddox, 1968). When older people have disengaged, this may not represent personal preference but rather the failure of our society to provide opportunities for continued engagement. For instance, the lack of meaningful part-time jobs is a better explanation of the decline in employment among the elderly than is their personal preference not to work part-time; it makes a difference whether disengagement is forced or freely chosen.

Lastly, it cannot be assumed that older people's withdrawal from useful roles is necessarily good for society. For example, disengagement theory may be seen as legitimizing the earlier mandatory retirement laws and other policies that foster the separation of the elderly from others in society (Minkler and Estes, 1984). Yet policies that have encouraged early retirement have had negative societal consequences. For example, as more people have retired earlier, proportionately fewer workers are available to support those retired persons, thereby straining pension systems. Likewise, the workplace has been deprived of older workers' skills and knowledge. At the same time, a number of social trends are counteracting forces that previously might have led to disengagement, including advances in preventive medicine, growing economic security for older people, and the expansion of leisure roles and options for retirees (Rose, 1965).

In response to such criticisms, Cumming (1963) reformulated the theory to give more consideration to the relationship between personality and disengagement. This reformulation acknowledged that not everyone disengages; rather, adaptive behavior in old age varies widely. Two modes of interacting with the environment were distinguished: impinging and selecting. Impingers were defined as assertive and active in their interactions, whereas selectors tend to be more passive and restrained in their social relations, waiting for others to confirm preexisting assumptions about themselves. Both assertive and passive coping styles were viewed as ways for older people to protect themselves from contradictory or negative social messages, and thus to preserve their self-worth. Cumming (1975) also maintained that misinterpretations of disengagement as isolation, loneliness, and passivity overlook ways that disengaged behavior can be adaptive.

Disengagement is a broad theory encompassing many elements, yet it has been tested only in parts; thus, the controversy over disengagement theory remains unresolved. The theory has generally not been supported by empirical research (Prasad, 1964; Youmans, 1967; Palmore, 1968; Tallmer and Kutner, 1970), although some researchers have found differential disengagement (occurring in some older individuals at different rates and in different aspects of behavior) to be useful (Williams and Wirth, 1965; Streib and Schneider, 1971; Cumming, 1975). Several studies have shown disengagement to be linked to a variety of individual and environmental variables. Differences in environmental opportunities have been found to produce different patterns of engagement and disengagement among the aged (Carp, 1968). It has been suggested that the increased physical and social stress that often accompanies aging, not age per se, may produce disengagement (Tallmer and Kutner, 1970). It also makes intuitive sense that some people will disengage from unsatisfying contacts and maintain satisfying ones; they may also put up with less than satisfying relationships in order to remain engaged (Brown, 1974). More research is needed to investigate variability in disengagement levels, the factors that affect the occurrence of these levels, and the meaning of both engagement and disengagement for individuals (Hochschild, 1975). For example, the societal aspect of the theory, why and how society withdraws from the elderly and with what consequences, has not been empirically studied.

Clearly, neither activity nor disengagement theory fully explains successful or well-adjusted aging. Neither adequately addresses the social structure or cultural and historical contexts in which the aging process occurs. Minkler and Estes (1984) maintain that theories that focus only on what older people do, without considering the social conditions and policies that cause them to act as they do, are inadequate. For example, rather than study individual adjustment in retirement, researchers might explore the possible association between the larger political and economic context and unemployment among older people. These theories have also been criticized as blaming the elderly for their condition and legitimizing incrementalist, individualistic approaches to social policy (Levin and Levin, 1980).

A potential danger of both theories is that society, as well as older individuals, may interpret them as prescriptive; for example, older people may believe that they are supposed to behave in certain ways. Both theories may be described more appropriately as philosophical recommendations about how to live during the later years rather than explanations of the aging process. More variables need to be examined before we can explain why some people are happy in an active old age while others are content to narrow their activities and involvement.

Continuity Theory

The evident shortcomings of the disengagement and activity theories led to the emergence of a third social-psychological theory of adaptation in old age. According to continuity theory, the aging person substitutes new roles for lost ones, and continues to maintain typical ways of adapting to the environment (Neugarten, Havighurst, and Tobin, 1968). Its basic tenets are that people, whether young or old, have different personalities and lifestyles, and that personality plays a major role in adjusting to aging. People who have always been passive or withdrawn are unlikely to become activists upon retirement. Similarly, those who have always been active, assertive, and socially involved are unlikely to sit quietly at home in their old age. Basically, this perspective states that, with age, we become more of what we already were when younger. Central personality characteristics become even more pronounced and core values even more salient with age. An individual ages successfully if she or he maintains a mature, integrated personality while growing old. This, according to continuity theory, is the basis of life satisfaction (Neugarten, Havighurst, and Tobin, 1968). Individuals, therefore, provide their own standards for successful aging rather than try to adjust to a common norm. This subject will be discussed further in Chapter 8.

CRITIQUE OF CONTINUITY THEORY

Although continuity theory has some intuitive appeal and appears to overcome the weaknesses of activity and disengagement theories, it also has limitations. One is that it may not have ecological validity. That is, it places earlier stages of development as the criteria for successful aging, and assumes that individuals seek to maintain a particular pattern of behavior throughout life. It can only be inferred that the lifestyles observed in old age were developed earlier in life and continued into old age. Lifestyles observed in old age may be a response to growing old, rather than reflections of lifelong patterns.

The need for continuity may reduce an individual's self-esteem in the later years when poor health or limited finances may require modifications in one's earlier lifestyle. In fact, maintaining previous patterns can be maladaptive (Fox, 1981–82). There is evidence that the need for continuity may also interfere with an individual's desire to remove himself or herself from disliked roles and behaviors. Research shows that freeing oneself from former roles may have positive effects (Gutmann, 1974; Gutmann, Grunes, and Griffin, 1980; Neugarten, Crotty, and Tobin, 1964). For example, many women adopt more typically "masculine" personality traits as they age; and some aging men act on tendencies in themselves that are generally identified as "feminine." It appears that the elderly most satisfied with their lives are those who have not rigidly conformed to traditional sex roles, but have integrated traits culturally defined as masculine with those culturally defined as feminine (Reichard, Livson and Peterson, 1962; Neugarten, Crotty, and Tobin, 1964; Sinnott, 1977).

The complexity of continuity theory makes it difficult to test empirically, since an individual's reaction to aging is explained through the interrelationships among biological and psychological changes, the continuation of lifelong patterns, and so on. Because it focuses primarily on the individual as the unit of analysis, overlooking the role of external social factors in modifying the aging process, policies based on continuity theory could rationalize a laissez-faire or "live and let live" approach to solving individual problems facing the elderly. The multiple variations in the aging processes of different individuals could be assumed to make concerted policy interventions unfeasible.

The Elderly as a Subculture

In contrast to activity theorists, proponents of a subculture of aging believe that older people maintain their self-concepts and social identities through their membership in a subculture (Rose, 1965). A subculture is formed when particular members within a society interact more with each other than they do with others in the society. Such interaction is presumed to occur when persons within a group develop an affinity for each other through shared backgrounds, problems, and interests, and are simultaneously excluded from interacting with other members of the population.

A number of social and demographic trends are viewed as increasing the opportunities for the elderly to identify with each other and to separate them from the mainstream of American society. These trends include: the increasing numbers of older people; the self-segregation of older people within retirement communities; the "involuntary" segregation of elderly in inner cities and rural areas, due primarily to younger people leaving these areas; and the growing dependence of some older persons on social services and on other people as they withdraw from occupational roles. The formation of an aging subculture is viewed as having two significant consequences for older people: an identification of themselves as old, and thus socially and culturally distant from the rest of our youth-oriented society; and a growing group consciousness that creates the potential for political power and social action.

A variation of the view that elderly persons constitute a subculture is the identification of the aged as a minority group, with problems similar to those of ethnic minority groups (Breen, 1960; Blau, 1981; Busse and Pfeiffer, 1977). From this theoretical perspective, the elderly are viewed as discriminated against because of a shared biological characteristic (age), which is readily visible to others. In common with ethnic minority groups, members of the older population tend to have low social and economic status and unequal opportunities, especially in the employment arena. Society's prevailing negative evaluation of the elderly may lead older people to feelings of self-hatred, but may also serve to unify them politically. According to this perspective, residents of age-segregated retirement communities are especially likely to exhibit characteristics typical of minority groups.

CRITIQUE OF THE SUBCULTURE PERSPECTIVE

Although the concepts of the elderly as a subculture or minority group provide descriptive guides for understanding the role and status of older people in our society, they have limited power to predict behavior and have been widely criticized. Clearly, the concept of a disadvantaged subculture does not apply to all situations nor to all older people. In some settings, older people have high status; the seniority system in Congress, for example, favors age. In addition, many older people are financially well off; most still live in age-integrated neighborhoods; and most interact across generations within their families—forces contrary to the formation of a cohesive subculture. Partially as a result of such contacts with people of other ages, the elderly have not organized in a single, unified way to advance their own interests. Instead, a variety of groups are organized around aging interests, ranging from the age-integrated Gray Panthers to large organizations such as the American Association of Retired Persons (AARP), which attracts members, in part, through its financial benefits. As will be seen in Chapter 13, the question of whether the elderly form a subculture with a collective age identity is closely related to debates about the political influence of age-based organizations and voting blocs.

Streib (1965) has been the most vocal critic of the view of the elderly as a minority group. He maintains that, compared to ethnic minorities, most older people are not systematically deprived of power and privileges, nor do they regard themselves as objects of collective discrimination by a hostile, controlling outgroup. Moreover, membership among the elderly population is not exclusive or permanent, but rather awaits all who live long enough. He suggests that the most realistic view of older people is as a status group similar to other such groups in our society (Streib, 1985). This concept is discussed below in terms of the theory of age stratification.

Age Stratification Theory

Age stratification is less a formal theory than a conceptual framework for viewing societal processes and changes that affect aging. Proponents Matilda White Riley (1971, 1972, 1985) and Ann Foner (1975) maintain that an approach similar to that used in sociological analyses of class stratification is useful to understanding the position of age groups and the meaning of age within a particular social context. Just as societies are stratified in terms of socioeconomic class, every society divides people into categories or strata according to age—"young," "middle-aged," and "old" (Riley, Johnson, and Foner, 1972). That is, people are defined in terms of social roles and responsibilities, not just chronologically.

The sociology of age stratification is concerned with the relationships within and across all age strata, not only the older ones. The basic assumption is that age is a universal criterion by which people's roles, rights, and privileges are distributed as they move from one stratum to the next (Riley, Johnson, and Foner, 1972). Age may be linked directly to social roles (e.g., through legal criteria for voting or retirement) or indirectly, when socially prescribed parameters exist for given roles (e.g., the appropriate ages for dating and marriage).

Each age stratum can be evaluated according to the roles its members typically play and the extent to which these roles are valued by society. Some age strata have more valued qualities than others. Such age grading commonly occurs in the workplace, for example, where younger workers are viewed as more productive and desirable than older employees. The fact that social roles are age graded within an age stratification system produces structured inequalities between age groups, such as between younger and older workers. Age stratification of roles both frees and limits the elderly in modern society. Older retirees, for instance, are freed from many obligatory adult roles. However, norms for age-appropriate behavior also discourage them from choosing such options as returning to school or working part-time.

Because of the variety of physical, social, or psychological factors that affect the aging process, age strata differ in age-related capacities. As we observe daily, people of different ages tend to behave differently and are assigned dissimilar roles; they may be motivated by diverse political and social attitudes, generally have varied organizational attachments, and may be treated differently by other age strata (Riley and Foner, 1968).

Such differences between strata partially result from the processes of allocation and socialization. *Allocation* is the process of assigning and reassigning people of various ages to suitable roles as a way to meet society's needs. For example, age as a criterion for retirement is related to overall employment patterns in the society. *Socialization,* the other intervening process, serves to smooth the transition of individuals from one age status to the next. Age stratification necessitates socialization throughout a lifetime, because, as noted in our discussion of role theory, people move into and out of a succession of roles as they age.

COHORT AND LIFE COURSE EFFECTS

The members of one strata differ from each other in both their stage of life (young, middle-aged, or old), and in the historical periods they have experienced. The two factors, the life course dimension and the historical dimension, explain many differences in how people behave, think, and, in turn, contribute to society. According to the life course dimension, age strata may be defined by chronological age or by stages in the life cycle (e.g., infancy, childhood, adolescence, early adulthood, etc.). Chronological age is important not in an absolute sense, but as an approximate indicator of an individual's personal experiences (biological, psychological, and social) and the varying probabilities of resultant behavior and attitudes. Individuals in the same stage of the life course have much in common: their biological development, the kinds of roles they have experienced (e.g., worker, spouse, or parent), the number of years behind them, and the potential years ahead. Likewise, people at different life stages differ in these respects.

Other differences between age strata are due to the historical dimension, to what is termed *cohort flow*. As we saw in our discussion of research designs (Chapter 1), people who were born at the same time period (cohort) share a common historical and environmental past, present, and future. They have been exposed to similar events, conditions, and changes. Think about some of the major events of this century, such as the two World Wars, the Depression, the Civil Rights Movement, the Vietnam War, human explorations into space, and technological developments that have had a differential impact on different cohorts, often creating wide variations in values, attitudes, and behaviors (the so-called "generation gap"). Riley (1971) referred to the behavior and attitudes that developed from a particular intersection of the life course and historical dimension as "cohort-centric." What this means is that people who are in a similar place on the life course dimension (in the same age stratum) experience historical events similarly and may come to see the world in a like fashion. For example, older people who were at the early stages of their occupational and child-rearing careers during the Depression tend to value economic self-sufficiency and "saving for a rainy day," compared to younger cohorts who experienced periods of economic prosperity during early adulthood. Cohort-centrism solidifies age strata by encouraging the selection of friends from among age-mates, who have similar values and behaviors as a result of common experiences.

The metaphor of people stepping on an escalator at birth has been used to illustrate the process of cohort flow (Riley, Johnson, and Foner, 1972). How many and what types of people step on are never identical, although those who begin at the bottom at the same time move up collectively. The number of people stepping on (i.e., the size of any age stratum) is determined by rates of fertility, age-specific mortality, and migration in and out of a country. The age group does not remain stable as they move along, however. Instead, people acquire distinctive social attributes that enhance or impede the likelihood of their staying on the escalator for the full ride. Some get off, particularly men, by dying. Eventually, fewer people are left in the cohort, until all those who began together are dead.

A DYNAMIC PROCESS

The complex, dynamic nature of the system of age stratification is illustrated by how it influences and is influenced by the changing social-political-economic fabric of society. For example, the trend toward early retirement among the age 55–65 cohort has had an impact on Social Security, on our pension systems, and on the "leisure industry." As more people have chosen early retirement, they have faced living on lower, fixed incomes, at a time when medical, housing, and food costs have rapidly risen. In turn, some elderly have worked through age-based organizations to try to influence retirement policies, which has led to some public perceptions that the older population is financially secure. In sum, socioeconomic factors assure that different cohorts grow old in different ways as they "move up the escalator."

Another illustration of the dynamic nature of age strata involves individual mobility across the strata. In contrast to class mobility, age mobility is universal, inevitable, and irreversible. In other words, although people age in different ways and at different rates, no one can become younger, stop the flow of time, or achieve downward age mobility. All people shift to different age strata with advancing age.

As cohorts "move up the escalator," they may collectively influence age stratification (Waring, 1975). When there is a lack of fit in terms of the roles available to them, cohort members may challenge the existing patterns of age stratification. For example, successive cohorts in this century have experienced increased longevity and formal education levels, which, in turn, have changed the nature of how they age, how they view aging, and the age stratification system itself. Because of their particular relationship to historical events, the people in the old age stratum today are very different from older persons in the past or in the future, and experience the aging process differently. The cohort retiring in the 1980s tends to be oriented more positively toward retirement and leisure than the cohort that retired in the early 1950s. They have also been more likely to challenge restrictions on their roles as workers and community participants through age discrimination suits, legislative action, and political organization than cohorts 10 or 20 years their seniors. These variations, in turn, will affect the experiences and expectations of future cohorts as they age. In other words, as successive cohorts move through the age strata or "up the escalator," they alter conditions to such a degree that later groups never encounter the world in exactly the same way, and therefore age in different ways.

Age stratification also interacts with socioeconomic, ethnic, and sex stratification to determine differences in roles. Just as women and men generally play different roles throughout the life cycle, the nature of their aging experience tends to differ, with women undergoing fewer abrupt transitions in their roles. The timing of life events has been found to vary by social class, with middle- and upper-class individuals tending to marry and have children later than working-class persons (Neugarten, Crotty, and Tobin, 1964). Indeed, there are many ways in which different status or social classes cause people to age differently. For example, older people who have lifelong wealth or who were politically influential have higher status than younger persons without wealth or political power.

CRITIQUE OF AGE STRATIFICATION THEORY

Age stratification theory has been criticized for too narrowly assessing age primarily in terms of chronology or life stage, while giving little consideration to the importance of physical appearance, length of time that a person has been in a given position, and level of physical, mental, and social functioning. As will be shown throughout this text, functional differences in physiological, psychological, and social aging must be taken into account in any theory of aging. These different ways of assessing age make it harder to defend the concept that birth cohorts remain cohesive. Because the diversity of levels of physical appearance and functioning increases with age, cohorts probably become less cohesive as they grow older, not more unified. Another limitation of this theoretical perspective is that family background, sex, ethnic minority status, social class, and the political and economic structure may all be more salient in defining people's roles than age stratification itself (Minkler and Estes, 1984; Atchley and Seltzer, 1976). In fact, some social gerontologists contend that we are moving toward an "age-irrelevant" society, with age-based constraints weakening and socioeconomic status becoming more salient (Hagestad and Neugarten, 1985).

Age strata, cohort succession, historical time, and the life course are all somewhat abstract, global concepts, which thus far have yielded few empirical studies. Because of its focus on structural, demographic, and historical characteristics, age stratification theory is not useful in explaining an individual's behavior as he or she ages. But it can help us understand the ways in which society uses age to fit people into structural niches in the social world, and to observe that this age structure changes with the passage of time. By viewing age groups as members of status groups within a social system, as well as active participants in a changing society, stratification theory is conducive to sociological explanations of age cohorts' behaviors and values, and as such, it deserves further empirical testing.

Interactionist Perspectives

Consistent with the person-environment perspective outlined in the Introduction, recent efforts among social gerontologists have focused on the person-environment transactional process. In particular, symbolic interaction, labeling, and social breakdown theories all emphasize the dynamic interaction between older individuals and their social world. These theories implicitly assume that older people must adjust to ongoing societal requirements. When confronted with change, whether relocation to a nursing home or learning to use a computer, older individuals are expected to try to master the changing situation while extracting from the larger environment what they need to retain a positive self-concept.

The *symbolic interactionist* view of aging argues that the interaction of such factors as the environment, individuals, and their encounters in it can significantly affect the kind of aging process people experience (Gubrium, 1973). Changes in these interactional variables may produce results that are erroneously attributed to inherent maturational changes. For example, the older person who becomes confused following a move to a new apartment may mistakenly be labeled as *senile*. Efforts to ease the stress of moving could minimize resulting confusion. Similarly, apparent disengagement, low self-esteem, and dissatisfaction may result from how other people interpret the elderly's behavior. For instance, the older person who sits and reads may be defined by others as disengaged, yet he or she may actually be very involved in reading about and discussing current events.

Both the self and society are viewed by symbolic interactionists as able to create new alternatives. Therefore, low morale and withdrawal from social involvement are not inevitable with aging, but are one possible outcome of an individual's interactions that can be altered. Policies based on the symbolic interactionist framework optimistically assume that both environmental constraints and individual needs can be changed. An environmental intervention, for example, is the elimination of age discrimination in employment, whereas the individual's decision to pursue leisure rather than paid employment is an attempt to modify personal needs.

Labeling theory, derived from symbolic interaction theory, states that people derive their self-concepts from interacting with others in their social milieu. In other words, we all tend to think of ourselves in terms of how others define us and react to us. Once others have defined us into distinct categories, they react to us on the basis of these categorizations, and as a result, our self-concept and behavior change. For example, this labeling process occurs when someone who is about to retire starts to behave as others have defined retirees: nonproductive, useless, and inactive. Or the older person who forgets to turn off the stove burner is likely to be labeled by concerned relatives as *senile,* yet a younger person's forgetfulness will be explained as being busy and preoccupied. You can probably think of numerous other examples where older persons' behaviors depended largely on the reactions of significant others.

The theories of *social breakdown* and *social reconstruction* are outgrowths of the labeling perspective. The social breakdown syndrome initially referred to the negative feedback generated by a person already susceptible to psychological problems. For example, friends of a person who was once hospitalized for depression may overreact to the slightest indication of another depressive episode, so that what might be a normal grief reaction to a loss becomes labeled as "depression." Once the cycle is initiated, it reinforces others' perception of incompetence, which then ensures even more difficulties (Zusman, 1966). A similar process is assumed to occur among older people who are experiencing role loss and ambiguity; as discussed under role theories, older people faced with changes such as retirement or widowhood reach out for specific cues for how they should act. Should they sell their house? Should they move in with their children? Others, frequently well-intentioned children, react to their reaching out as a sign of their failing capacities. Thus, an adult child who is accustomed to his or her father decisively handling finances may interpret his indecision following his wife's death as a cause for concern rather than as a normal part of grieving. The father may react to such concern by greater indecisiveness, eventually perceiving himself as less competent and turning all decision making over to others. In other words, older persons who accept negative labeling are then inducted into a negative, dependent position. As they learn to behave in ways that older people are "supposed" to act in our society, previous skills of independence atrophy. They perceive themselves as inadequate, and a negative spiral is set into motion (Kuypers and Bengtson, 1973).

The social reconstruction model suggests ways to intervene in this negative cycle (Kuypers and Bengtson, 1973). This model asserts that even small changes in restructuring the environment can provide a more satisfying life among older people. One way to improve the larger society is to provide older people with frames for self-judgment that are more humanitarian than the work ethic that prevails in our society. Another intervention is to provide publicly funded services to address problems of inadequate housing, poor health care, and poverty. Older persons could also be provided with opportunities to develop greater self-confidence and autonomy by involving them in the planning and delivery of such services. These suggestions for altering the environment are consistent with the concept of environmental press, as discussed in the Introduction.

An underlying assumption of the social reconstruction model is that resources that allow older people to exert control over their physical and social environments are not distributed equally across all social classes. Socioeconomic class imposes a structured inequality which limits an individual's mastery over life (Tindale and Marshall, 1980). For example, individuals from lower socioeconomic classes pass from young to middle to old age at a younger chronological age than those from higher socioeconomic backgrounds. Lacking the valued resources that are required for upward mobility, lower income individuals tend to be less healthy, have less access to health care, have children and grandchildren earlier in the life cycle, and so on—all factors that may make them appear older than they are chronologically.

The interactionist perspective has been criticized for focusing on how individuals react to aging rather than on the broader sociostructural factors that shape the experience and management of aging in our society (Minkler and Estes, 1984). This critique is further developed by the political economy theorists, described later in this chapter.

Social Exchange Theory

With roots in behavioral psychology and utilitarian economics, social exchange theory attempts to explain the structured inequality that exists among different age strata. Simone de Beauvoir (1972) asserted that aging is a struggle between classes. Taking this further, Dowd (1980) maintains that definitions of age stratification are incomplete without reference to power, since unequal access to resources as a basis of power determines social status and opportunities. According to social exchange theory, a key factor in defining the elderly's status is the balance between their contributions to society, which are determined by their control of power resources, and the costs of supporting them. Social class predetermines the elderly's possession or absence of valued resources. Through the possession of material goods, abilities, achievements, and other qualities defined by society as desirable, individuals are able to exert power in their social relationships. Because some elderly in our society possess fewer power resources than younger people, their status has declined accordingly. Public attitudes about the costs of supporting the elderly are illustrated by those who misperceive the elderly as the underlying cause of rising health, social service, and long-term care costs. Yet, Dowd would argue that the dominant groups within a society attempt to sustain their own interests by perpetuating institutional arrangements. From this perspective, scapegoating of the elderly for "breaking the federal budget" serves the dominant groups' interests.

Exchange theory was not originally formulated by gerontologists, but as a sociological theory first advanced by Homans (1961) and Blau (1964). It includes four basic premises:

1. Individuals and groups act rationally to maximize rewards and minimize costs to themselves, including those of time, energy, effort, and wealth. These transactions are not only economic, but also encompass intrinsic psychological satisfaction. Individuals attempt to choose interactions from which they "profit" in some way. Profit can be in the form of increased social opportunities, enhanced sense of self-worth, or accomplishment. The principle of reciprocity is implicit in these interactions: people should help those who have assisted them, and should not injure them or retaliation may result.

2. Individuals use their past experiences to predict the outcomes of similar exchanges in the present. An assessment of the benefits and costs involved includes appraising alternatives for reaching the same goal.

3. An individual will maintain an interaction as long as it continues to be more rewarding than costly. If the rewards become devalued relative to their cost (what must be done or forfeited in order to attain them), social interactions will cease.

4. When one individual is dependent on another, the latter accrues power. In other words, power is derived from imbalances in the social exchange, with the individual who values the rewards more highly losing power as the other participant gains power.

Research on family visiting patterns was one of the first applications of social exchange theory to the study of older people (Martin, 1971). Older family members whose only source of power is to remind others of their obligation to visit are put in a dependent and deferent position. Visitors experience little pleasure and satisfaction when faced only with the older person's complaints about their not visiting enough. On the other hand, older family members who have other sources of power, such as a potential inheritance or interesting anecdotes to tell, actually hold the power position, placing the relatives in a dependent position.

The most general and extensive application of exchange theory to explain the status of the elderly has been made by Dowd (1975). He began by criticizing disengagement and activity theories for not addressing the question of why social interaction and activity often decrease with age.

Exchange theory, like activity or disengagement theory, predicts decreasing participation with age in major social interactions. The basis of this prediction, however, is distinct from the other theoretical approaches. First, the explanation of decreasing social integration of the aged is located in the social system via major social institutions as older people are systematically deprived of valued resources needed for favorable social exchanges. Second, the explanation at the level of individual behaviors does not rely on categorizing the elderly as a unique group. Rather, the processes and outcomes identified could be relevant to any individual experiencing comparable changes in resources. Finally, exchange theory suggests possible remedies to ameliorate the existing low resource condition for many older people.

According to Dowd, reciprocal benefits cannot be assumed in social exchanges; rather, both parties to a social transaction must be examined to determine who is benefiting more and why. Loss of power or the ability to control one's environment is offered as the explanation of why older people, left only with the capacity for compliance, disengage. Older people disengage not because it is mutually satisfying, but because society enjoys a distinct advantage in the power relationship. This power advantage is reflected in the economic and social dependency of older people who have outmoded skills. With little to exchange that is of value, they are forced to accept the retirement role in exchange for limited social services, retirement pensions, and Medicare. Unable to participate in labor markets, they are limited in their access to two valued power resources: material possessions and positions of authority.

The other power resources identified by Dowd are personal characteristics, such as beauty, strength, and intelligence; relational characteristics, such as influential friends or caring children; and generalized reinforcers, such as respect, approval, recognition, and support. All these power resources tend to favor the young. For example, aging generally results in a decline of strength and beauty, as defined by the larger society, reducing the elderly's power in intergenerational interactions. Dowd maintains that the only major source of power left untouched by the aging process is the category of generalized reinforcers. However, because generalized reinforcers such as respect and approval are more readily available, they are also less valued than other resources, permitting the elderly only minimal ability to influence exchange rates. Dowd (1980) has emphasized the concepts of dependence and deference as indicators of power: power is acquired through the ability to satisfy one's needs without having to depend on or become indebted to other people. For many older people without resources as a basis of power, deference predominates in their interactions.

Despite their limited resources, most older people seek to maintain some degree of reciprocity and to be active, independent agents in the management of their own lives. Dowd suggests that a principle for the development of policies and services for older people should be a quest for strategies to maximize their resources that are valued by our society. In this model, adaptability is a dual process of influencing one's environment as well as adjusting to it. The elderly are presumed to be able to maximize their power through withholding anticipated rewards and developing their sense of political efficacy and age consciousness. More empirical research is essential to attempt to determine the value of exchange theory as an explanation of the aging process. First, more work is needed in order to quantify the somewhat abstract concepts that form this theoretical perspective.

Political Economy of Aging

The argument that social class is a structural barrier to older people's access to valued resources and that dominant groups within society try to sustain their own interests by perpetuating class inequities is basic to the formulation of the political economy of aging (Minkler and Estes, 1984; Walker, 1981). This perspective is less a theory of individual attributes and processes than a macro analysis of structural properties that determine how people adapt in old age. Estes argues that social, political, and economic conditions affect how social problems, including those of the elderly, are defined and treated. Therefore, the major problems faced by the elderly are socially constructed as a result of our societal conceptions of aging and the aged. These social constructions then take on an objective quality because people act as if they point to concrete realities. The process of aging itself is not the problem; the problems are societal conditions facing older people without adequate income, health care, or housing—needs that a capitalist society has created. Second, national social and economic policies are the key determinants of the elderly's life conditions. These policies, in turn, reflect the dominance of certain values and normative conceptions of social problems and of how benefits and privileges are distributed. "Solutions," such as Social Security, Medicare, and Medicaid, are viewed as a means of social control designed to meet the dominant needs of the economy (Minkler and Estes, 1984). Social policies are also directly influenced by the state of the economy. In a time of shrinking resources, for example, the federal government has reduced its role in addressing problems faced by the elderly. Instead, local responsibility has been emphasized, and problems have been defined as the need for more efficient coordination of fewer resources.

According to Estes, our society's view of the elderly has tended to set them apart to be a dependent group with needs requiring special policies and programs. The fact that most gerontological research has focused on individual biological and psychological changes has resulted in the characterization of old age as a time of inevitable physical decline. This characterization, in turn, justifies the stigmatization and continuing marginality of the elderly. This process, whereby gerontologists stereotype the elderly in terms of the least capable and healthy, has also been referred to as the "New Ageism" (Kalish, 1979). The marginality of the older population is furthered by the development of the "Aging Enterprise," a service industry of agencies, providers, and planners that reaffirms the outgroup status of the elderly in order to maintain their own jobs (Estes, 1979; Kalish, 1979). Policy solutions tend to focus on integrating and socializing the elderly to adapt to their status, rather than efforts to fundamentally alter social and economic conditions. Such policies also serve to maintain social harmony; for example, services such as senior centers are viewed by Estes (1979) as benefiting middle- and upper-income groups and thus preserving social class differences. Similarly, policies such as Social Security, Medicare, and tax credits do not benefit all older people but only the "deserving" elderly—upper-income and downwardly mobile middle-income groups—and thus perpetuate class inequities (Crystal, 1982; Minkler and Estes, 1984; Nelson, 1982).

More recently, the problems of old age have been defined as a crisis that is the result of declining birth rates, increased longevity, and earlier retirement, not the outcome of prior social inaction or economic policy. This definition has resulted in a "scapegoating" of the elderly, blaming them for rising health care and Social Security costs (Kalish, 1979). Estes argues that fundamental policy changes are necessary in order to shift perceptions and structural alignments. For example, policies are needed that would not separate the elderly because of their age. Instead, policies should alter both the elderly's objective conditions, as well as the social processes by which policies are made and implemented. For instance, the status of the elderly can be understood within the context of the labor market and the social relations it produces, and how these change with age. Policy interventions from this perspective would be directed toward institutionalized structures, particularly the labor market. The major contribution of Estes's work has been her critical analysis of the larger sociopolitical conditions that generate the necessity for separate social policies for groups such as the elderly. The major limitation of her radical critique to date is the lack of empirical research.

Summary and Implications

These theoretical perspectives, often drawing on shared concepts such as role loss, all aim to explain the aging process and why some people age more successfully than others. Role theory suggests that the ease with which individuals adjust to aging depends on how they adapt to role changes, such as role ambiguity and discontinuity, that frequently characterize the later years. Activity theory predicts that the elderly who maintain active roles characteristic of middle-age will be more satisfied than less involved older people. In contrast, disengagement theory maintains that withdrawal from such active roles is conducive to satisfaction in old age, as well as beneficial for society. The viewpoint that the elderly form a subculture is focused less on the types of roles performed by older people than on their frequent interaction with one another, which forms the basis for a homogeneous subculture of the aged. Presumably isolated from the mainstream of society, the elderly have been perceived by some theorists as exhibiting characteristics and problems similar to those of ethnic minority groups.

Age stratification theory builds on the basic sociological constructs of role, status, norms, and socialization to provide a framework for understanding the position of older people in society. Age is viewed as one criterion for assigning roles to individuals, with the result that people are divided into age strata. Within the age stratification system, both individual lives and social structures are subject to change. Since age strata have differential access to rewards, structured inequality exists among different age strata.

Interactional perspectives emphasize the interrelationship of individuals with their physical and social environments. Labeling and social breakdown theories describe a cycle in which the older person, who is defined in a negative or limiting way by society, begins to internalize and to act on those definitions, and thus reinforces the initial stereotype. An interactional approach to intervention, such as the social reconstruction model, involves altering the environment to make adaptation easier.

The concept that unequal access to power resources determines social status and life changes is fundamental to social exchange theory. From this perspective, lesser access to power resources underlies the elderly's declining status, rather than their desire to disengage or their inability to remain active in roles characteristic of middle-age.

The political economy theory attributes problems of aging to social constructs and public policies. It argues that current academic and governmental approaches to aging tend to preserve, rather than challenge, underlying social and economic inequities. Solutions must involve fundamental policy changes to alter both social perceptions and objective conditions of the aged.

Thus far, none of these theories adequately explains social aging, but rather describes different aspects of older people's roles in our society. Another limitation is that none of these theories is universal. As we have noted, not all older people disengage or lose power as they age. Nor do any of these theoretical perspectives fully account for the wide variations or multiple dimensions in aging experiences. Yet the growth of these theoretical models has laid the framework for future research directions. As the social, economic, and political conditions affecting older people change, new theoretical perspectives must be developed or older ones revised through the process of empirical research in a variety of sociocultural contexts.

We now turn to reviewing age-related physical and psychological changes that may create both constraints and opportunities for how people age socially.

References

Atchley, R., and Seltzer, M. *The sociology of aging: Selected readings.* Belmont, Calif.: Wadsworth, 1976.

Bengtson, V. *The social psychology of aging.* Indianapolis, Ind.: Bobbs-Merrill, 1973.

Blau, P. *Exchange in power in social life.* New York: John Wiley and Sons, 1964.

Blau, Z. *Aging in a changing society* (2d ed.). New York: Franklin Watts, 1981.

Breen, L. The aging individual. In C. Tibbitts (Ed.), *Handbook of social gerontology.* Chicago: University of Chicago Press, 1960, 157.

Brown, A. S. Satisfying relationships for elderly and their patterns of disengagement. *The Gerontologist,* 1974, *14,* 258–262.

Burgess, E. W. *Aging in western societies.* Chicago: University of Chicago Press, 1960, 20.

Busse, E., and Pfeiffer, E. (Eds.). *Introduction: Behavior and adaptation in late life.* Boston: Little, Brown, 1977.

Carp, F. M. Some components of disengagement. *Journal of Gerontology,* 1968, *23,* 382–386.

Cottrell, L. The adjustment of the individual to his age and sex roles. *American Sociological Review,* 1942, *7,* 617–620.

Crystal, S. *America's old age crisis.* New York: Basic Books, 1982.

Cumming, E. Further thought on the theory of disengagement. *International Social Science Journal,* 1963, *15,* 377–393.

Cumming, E. Engagement with an old theory. *Aging and Human Development,* 1975, *6,* 187–191.

Cumming, E., and Henry, W. E. *Growing old.* New York: Basic Books, 1961.

DeBeauvoir, S. *The coming of age.* New York: Putnam and Sons, 1972.

Dowd, J. J. Aging as exchange: A preface to theory. *Journal of Gerontology,* 1975, *30,* 584–594.

Dowd, J. J. *Stratification among the aged.* Monterey, Calif.: Brooks/Cole, 1980.

Estes, C. *The aging enterprise.* San Francisco: Jossey Bass, 1979.

Foner, A. Age in society: Structures and change. *American Behavioral Scientist,* 1975, *19,* 289–312.

Foner, A., and Kertzer, D. Transitions over the life course: Lessons from age-set societies. *American Journal of Sociology,* 1978, *83,* 1081–1104.

Fox, J. H. Perspectives on the continuity perspective. *International Journal of Aging and Human Development,* 1981–82, *14,* 97–115.

Gubrium, J. F. *The myth of the golden years.* Springfield, Ill.: Charles C. Thomas, 1973.

Gutmann, D. L. Alternatives to disengagement: Aging among the Highland Druze. In R. LaVine (Ed.), *Culture and personality: Contemporary readings.* Chicago: Aldine, 1974.

Gutmann, D. L., Grunes, J., and Griffin, B. The clinical psychology of later life: Developmental paradigm. In N. Datan and N. Lohman (Eds.), *Life span developmental psychology: Transitions of aging.* New York: Academic Press, 1980.

Hagestad, G., and Neugarten, B. Age and the life course. In R. H. Binstock and E. Shanas (Eds.), *Handbook of aging and the social sciences* (2d ed.). New York: Van Nostrand Reinhold, 1985.

Havighurst, R. J. Successful aging. In R. Williams, C. Tibbits, and W. Donahue (Eds.), *Processes of aging* (Vol. 1). New York: Atherton Press, 1963.

Havighurst, R. J. Personality and patterns of aging. *The Gerontologist,* 1968, *8,* 20–23.

Havighurst, R. J., Munnichs, J. M. A., Neugarten, B. L., and Thomae, H. *Adjustment to retirement.* The Netherlands: Van Goreum and Comp., N.V., 1969.

Havighurst, R. J., Neugarten, B. L., and Tobin, S. S. Disengagement and patterns of aging. In B. L. Neugarten (Ed.), *Middle age and aging.* Chicago: University of Chicago Press, 1968, 161.

Hochschild, A. Disengagement theory: A critique and proposal. *American Sociological Review,* 1975, *40,* 553–569.

Homans, G. *Social behavior: Its elementary forms.* New York: Harcourt, Brace and World, 1961.

Kalish, R. The new ageism and the failure models: A polemic. *The Gerontologist,* 1979, *19,* 398–402.

Kuypers, J. A., and Bengtson, V. L. Social breakdown and competence: A model of normal aging. *Human Development,* 1973, *16,* 181–201.

Lemon, B., Bengtson, V., and Peterson, J. Activity types and life satisfaction in a retirement community. *Journal of Gerontology,* 1972, *27,* 511–523.

Levin, J., and Levin, W. C. *Ageism: Prejudice and discrimination against the elderly.* Belmont, Calif.: Wadsworth, 1980.

Longino, C. F., and Kart, C. S. Explicating activity theory: A formal replication. *Journal of Gerontology,* 1982, *37,* 713–722.

Maddox, G. Persistence of life-style among the elderly: A longitudinal study of patterns of social activity in reaction to life satisfaction. In B. L. Neugarten (Ed.), *Middle age and aging.* Chicago: University of Chicago Press, 1968, 181–183.

Martin, J. D. Power, dependence, and the complaints of the elderly: A social exchange perspective. *Aging and Human Development,* 1971, *2,* 108–112.

Minkler, M., and Estes, C. *Readings in the political economy of aging.* Farmingdale, N.Y.: Baywood, 1984.

Nelson, G. Social class and public policy for the elderly. *Social Science Review,* 1982, *56,* 85–107.

Neugarten, B., Crotty, W., and Tobin, S. S. Personality types in an aged population. In B. Neugarten (Ed.), *Personality in middle and late life.* New York: Atherton Press, 1964.

Neugarten, B., Havighurst, R. J., and Tobin, S. S. In B. L. Neugarten (Ed.), *Personality and patterns of aging in middle age and aging.* Chicago: University of Chicago Press, 1968, 173–177.

Neugarten, B., and Moore, J. The changing age-status system. In B. Neugarten (Ed.), *Middle age and aging.* Chicago: University of Chicago Press, 1968.

Palmore, E. The effects of aging on activities and attitudes. *The Gerontologist,* 1968, *8,* 259–263.

Palmore, E. (Ed.). *Normal aging II: Reports from the Duke longitudinal study.* Durham, N.C.: Duke University Press, 1974.

Palmore, E. Predictors of successful aging. *The Gerontologist,* 1979, *19,* 427–431.

Phillips, B. A role theory approach to adjustment in old age. *American Sociological Review,* 1957, *22,* 212–217.

Prasad, S. B. The retirement postulate of the disengagement theory. *The Gerontologist,* 1964, *4,* 20–23.

Reichard, S., Livson, F., and Peterson, P. *Aging and personality.* New York: John Wiley and Sons, 1962.

Riley, M. W. Social gerontology and the age stratification of society. *The Gerontologist,* 1971, *11,* 79–87.

Riley, M. W. Age strata in social systems. In R. H. Binstock and E. Shanas (Eds.), *Handbook of aging and the social sciences* (2d ed.). New York: Van Nostrand Reinhold, 1985, 369–414.

Riley, M. W., and Foner, A. *Aging and society: An inventory of research findings.* New York: Russell Sage Foundation, 1968.

Riley, M. W., Johnson, J., and Foner, A. *Aging and society (Vol. 3): A sociology of age stratification.* New York: Russell Sage Foundation, 1972.

Rose, A. M. The subculture of the aging: A framework in social gerontology. In A. M. Rose and W. A. Peterson (Eds.), *Older people and their social worlds.* Philadelphia: F. A. Davis, 1965.

Rose, A. M. A current theoretical issue in social gerontology. In A. M. Rose and W. A. Peterson (Eds.), *Older people and their social worlds.* Philadelphia: F. A. Davis, 1965.

Rosow, I. Status and role change through the life cycle. In R. H. Binstock and E. Shanas (Eds.), *Handbook of aging and the social sciences* (2d ed.). New York: Van Nostrand Reinhold, 1985, 62–93.

Sinott, J. D. Sex-role inconstancy, biology, and successful aging: A dialectical model. *The Gerontologist,* 1977, *10,* 317–320.

Streib, G. F. Are the aged a minority group? In A. W. Gouldner and S. M. Miller (Eds.), *Applied sociology.* New York: The Free Press, 1965.

Streib, G. F. Social stratification and aging. In R. H. Binstock and E. Shanas, (Eds.), *Handbook of aging and the social sciences* (2d ed.). New York: Van Nostrand Reinhold, 1985, 339–363.

Streib, G. F., and Schneider, C. J. *Retirement in American society.* Ithaca, N.Y.: Cornell University Press, 1971.

Tallmer, M., and Kutner, B. Disengagement and morale. *The Gerontologist,* 1970, *10,* 317–320.

Thurmond, G., and Belcher, J. Dimensions of disengagement among black and white rural elderly. *International Journal of Aging and Human Development.* 1980–81, *12,* 245–265.

Tindale, J. A., and Marshall, V. W. A generational conflict perspective for gerontology. In V. W. Marshall (Ed.), *Aging in Canada: Social perspectives.* Don Mills, Ontario: Fitzhenry and Whiteside, 1980, 43–50.

Walker, A. Toward a political economy of old age. *Aging and Society,* 1981, *1,* 73–94.

Waring, J. M. Social replenishment and social change. The problem of disordered cohort flow. *American Behavioral Science,* 1975, *19,* 237–256.

Williams, R. H., and Wirth, C. G. *Lives through the years.* New York: Atherton Press, 1965.

Youmans, E. G. Disengagement among older rural and urban men. In E. G. Youmans (Ed.), *Older rural Americans.* Lexington: University of Kentucky Press, 1967.

Zusman, J. Some explanations of the changing appearance of psychotic patients: Antecedents of the Social Breakdown Syndrome Concept. *The Milbank Memorial Fund Quarterly.* 1966.

Part II

The Physiological Context of Social Aging

If we are to understand what makes older people different from younger age groups, and why the field of gerontology has evolved as a separate discipline, we must first review the changes in biological and physiological structures that affect the day-to-day functioning of the elderly. Part II provides this necessary background. Normal changes in major organ systems and how they influence the older person's ability to perform daily tasks and to interact with their social and physical environments are described in Chapter 4. This area of research has received considerable attention as scientists have explored the basic processes of aging. Numerous theories have been developed to explain observable changes such as wrinkles, gray hair, stooped shoulders, and slower response time, as well as other biological functions that can only be inferred from tests of physiologic function. These include changes in the heart, lungs, kidneys, and bones. There are many normal changes in these organ systems that do not imply disease, but in fact may slow down the older person. Furthermore, significant differences have been observed among people and among organ systems in the degree of change experienced. The implications of these changes for the maximum life span of humans are discussed.

Age-related changes in the five major senses are the focus of Chapter 5. Because sensory functions are so critical for our daily interactions with our social and physical environments, and because many of the declines observed in sensory systems are a model of changes throughout the body, it is useful to focus on each sensory system and its role in linking individuals with their environments. The implications of biological changes in each system for older individuals' abilities to adapt to and interact with the world around them are also discussed in Chapter 5. Recommendations are made for modifying the environment and for communicating with older people who are experiencing significant declines in vision, hearing, taste, smell, touch, and even in their kinesthetic sense.

Chapter 6 focuses on diseases of the organ systems described in Chapters 4 and 5, and how these diseases can affect older people's social functioning. Acute and chronic diseases are differentiated, and the impact of these diseases on the demand for health and social services is presented. Chapter 6 also provides some striking statistics on older people's use of health services, barriers to their use, and recommendations for enhancing utilization. Most existing medical, dental, and mental health services do not adequately address the special needs of the older population. As a result, older people who could benefit most from the services fail to use them. The dynamic interactions between older people and their environments are acknowledged in a theoretical model that explains differences in the use of health services. According to this model, some segments of the older population are unable or unlikely to use existing services because the services are not appropriate for their physical and economic needs and abilities. As a result, it is important to design health services that fulfill the needs of frail, low-income, and ethnic minority elderly in order to maximize use among these groups, who have traditionally underutilized services.

Throughout Part II, the tremendous variations in how people age physically are emphasized. Because of genetic, lifestyle, and environmental factors, some people will show dramatic declines in all of their organ systems at a relatively early age. Most older people, however, will experience varied rates of decline in different systems. For example, some people may suffer from chronic heart disease, yet at the same time maintain strong bones and muscle strength. In contrast, others may require medications for painful osteoarthritis, but their heart and lungs remain in excellent condition. The following vignettes illustrate these variations:

A Healthy Older Person

Mrs. Hill is an 84-year-old widow. She has been slightly deaf all her life, has some recent loss of vision, and has to watch her blood pressure, primarily by paying attention to her diet. Despite her minor physical limitations, Mrs. Hill is able to get around to visit her many friends, neighbors, and family in the community. She is still able to drive, walk to the local grocery store almost daily, and take bus trips to visit her grandchildren. Active in the local senior center, she was one of the first participants in a health promotion project for older adults at the center. Now she exercises at the center three times a week and tries not to miss the lunches on Mondays and Wednesdays. She rarely visits the doctor except for an annual check-up. She does admit to getting frustrated by her reduced energy and the need to slow down, but, for the most part, she accepts these changes and adjusts her physical activities accordingly. Her son-in-law has made some minor modifications in her home, especially in the height and location of kitchen shelves, so that her daily routine is an easy one for her. Friends and relatives are frequently telling her how she does not look her age; she, in turn, becomes impatient with older people who stay home all the time, watch TV, and complain. She is usually optimistic about her situation, believing that throughout life a person has to accept the bad with the good.

An Older Person with Chronic Illness

Mr. Jones, age 69, had a stroke at age 64 and is paralyzed on his left side, so he is unable to walk. The stroke has also left him with slightly slurred speech and some personality changes. His wife states that he is not the kind, gentle man she used to know. He has to be lifted from bed to chair and recently became incontinent. His wife first tried to care for him at home, but after he became incontinent, she felt she could no longer handle the responsibility and made the difficult decision to institutionalize him. Both Mr. and Mrs. Jones are having difficulty adjusting to the nursing home placement. Since Mr. Jones remains mentally alert and aware of all the changes, he continually expresses his frustration with his physical limitations and with his forced retirement and reduced income. Their children live in another state and have been unable to help their mother with the daily care or the financial burden of the nursing home. In fact, the children are critical of their mother's decision to institutionalize their father because they think she should have kept him at home, no matter what. As their financial resources dwindle, Mr. and Mrs. Jones are facing the need to apply for Medicaid to cover nursing home costs. Mr. Jones starts to cry easily, sobbing that he is losing control of his life and that his life was never meant to be like this. Mrs. Jones feels angry that her caregiving efforts have not been appreciated and that her husband is so difficult.

These two vignettes point to the complexity of physiological aging. Chrono-logical age is often a poor predictor of health and functional status, as illustrated by Mrs. Hill's excellent functional and emotional health, and Mr. Jones's situation of physical dependency, even though he is 15 years younger than Mrs. Hill. Part II describes these variations in physical health and sensory function that are related to normal aging, contrasts these with changes due to disease, and presents factors that influence older people's health care behavior.

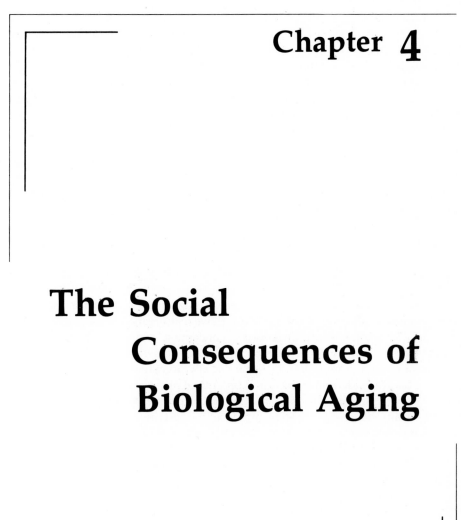

Chapter 4

The Social
Consequences of
Biological Aging

When asked to describe the physical aspects of aging, most people think only of the visible signs—graying hair, balding among some men, wrinkled skin, stooped shoulders, and a slower walk or shuffling gait. Although these are the most visible signs of old age among humans, there are numerous other changes that occur in our internal organs—the heart, lungs, kidneys, stomach, bladder, and central nervous system. These changes are not as easy to detect because they are not visible. In fact, x-rays and computer-assisted images of organ systems are not very useful for showing most changes that take place. It is primarily by measuring the functional capacity of these systems (i.e., the performance capacity of the heart, lungs, kidneys, and other organs) that their relative efficiency across the life span can be determined.

Biological aging, or *senescence*, can be defined as the normal process of changes over time in the body and its components, a process that eventually affects an individual's functioning vis-à-vis the environment but does not necessarily result in disease or death. As noted in the Introduction, this process is gradual and common to all living organisms. It is not, in itself, a disease, but aging and disease are often linked in most people's minds, since declines in organ capacity and internal protective mechanisms do make us more vulnerable to sickness. Because certain diseases such as Alzheimer's, arthritis, and heart conditions have a higher incidence with age, we may erroneously equate age with disease. However, a more appropriate conception of the aging process is a gradual accumulation of irreversible functional losses to which the average person tries to accommodate in some socially acceptable manner. Individual differences are evident in the rate and severity of physical changes, as illustrated by the vignettes of Mrs. Hill and Mr. Jones. Not all people show the same degree of change in any given organ system, nor do all the systems change at the same rate and at the same time. Individual aging depends largely on genetic inheritance, nutrition and diet, physical activity, and environment.

In this chapter, normal age-related changes in major organs of the human body are reviewed. The implications of these changes for older people's ability to interact with their social and physical environments, and the impact of system deterioration and disease on life expectancy, are examined within the context of personal competence vis-à-vis the environment. In the next chapter, the diseases of aging that may impair organ functions more than would be expected from normal aging will be discussed. First, it is useful to examine the major theories of biological aging that have been advanced to explain the changes in all living organisms over time.

Biological Theories of Aging

The process of aging is complex and multidimensional, involving significant loss and decline in some physiological functions, and minimal change in others.

Scientists have long attempted to find the causes for this process. A theme of some theories is that aging is a process that is programmed into the genetic structure of each species. Other theories state that aging represents an accumulation of stimuli from the environment that produce stress on the organism. Any theory of aging must be based on the scientific method, using systematic tests of hypotheses and empirical observations; in addition, biological theories must meet the following three criteria (Rockstein and Sussman, 1979):

1. The aging phenomenon described must be evident in all members of a given species.

2. The process must progress with time.

3. The process must have a deteriorating effect on the organism, leading finally to organ or system failure.

Each of the theories described below meets these criteria, although the evidence to support them is not always clear. Although these theories help our understanding of aging, none of them is totally adequate for explaining what causes aging.

The Wear and Tear Theory suggests that, with time, the organism simply wears out (Wilson, 1974). In this model, aging is a pre-programmed process; that is, each species has a biological clock that determines its maximum life span and the rate at which each organ system will deteriorate. This process is compounded by the effects of external stress on the organism (e.g., nutrient deficiencies). Cells continually wear out, and existing cells cannot repair damaged components within themselves. This is particularly true in tissues that are located in the striated skeletal and heart muscle and throughout the nervous system; these tissues are composed of cells that cannot undergo cell division. As we will see later, these systems are most likely to experience significant decline in their ability to function effectively with age.

The Autoimmune Theory proposes that aging is a function of the body's immune system becoming defective and attacking not just foreign proteins, bacteria, and viruses, but also producing antibodies against itself. This explanation of the immune system is consistent with the process of many diseases that increase with age, such as cancer, diabetes, and rheumatoid arthritis (Walford, 1969). Nevertheless, this theory does not explain why the immune system becomes defective with age; only the *effects* of this change are described.

The Cross-Linkage Theory (Bjorksten, 1974) focuses on the changes in *collagen* with age. Collagen is an important connective tissue found in most organ systems. As a person ages, there are clearly observable changes in collagen, for instance, wrinkling of the skin. These changes lead to a loss of elasticity in blood vessels, muscle tissue, skin, the lens of the eye, and other organs, and to slower wound healing. Another visible effect of changes in collagen is that the nose and ears tend to increase in size. Bjorksten (1974) suggests that these changes are due to the binding of essential molecules in the cells through the accumulation of cross-linking compounds, which in turn slows the process of normal cell functions.

A special case of the cross-linkage theory is the *Free Radical Theory* of aging (Harman, 1956, 1981). Free radicals are highly reactive chemical compounds possessing an unpaired electron. Produced normally by the use of oxygen within the cell, they interact with other cell molecules and may cause DNA mutations, cross-linking of connective tissue, changes in protein behavior, and other damage. Such reactions continue until one free radical pairs with another or meets an antioxidant, which can safely absorb the extra electron. It has been proposed that the ingestion of antioxidants such as vitamin E and carotene can inhibit free radical damage; this can then slow the aging process by delaying the loss of immune function and reducing the incidence of many diseases associated with aging (Cutler and Cutler, 1983; Harman, 1981; Harman, Heindrick and Eddy, 1977). However, research evidence for this theory has been inconclusive.

The Cellular Aging Theory suggests that aging occurs as cells slow their number of replications. Hayflick (1970) reported that cells grown in culture (i.e., in controlled laboratory environments) undergo a finite number of replications, approaching 50 doublings. Cells from older subjects replicate even fewer times, as do cells derived from individuals with *progeria,* a rare condition in which aging is accelerated and death may occur by age 15 to 20. In addition, proponents of this theory point out that each cell has a given level of DNA that is eventually depleted.

Studies of Vitamin E and Aging

Vitamin E is a fat-soluble substance that has long been known to be important for membrane structure and metabolism, and more recently as a natural antioxidant. It has been suggested that antioxidants can slow cellular aging, and thereby extend the life span through the process of depressing appetite, reducing food intake, in this manner delaying growth and matura-tion. Antioxidants have also been hypothesized to suppress tumor growth and slow the decline of immune processes. Animal studies that have tested the addition of vitamin E to mice diets have found some increases in survival. It has been found to reduce the levels of lipofuscin in the heart, liver, and testes of mice. Well-controlled studies with human populations are lacking; therefore, it is too early to conclude that antioxidants such as vitamin E can slow the aging process in humans. However, consumption of very high levels of vitamin E (greater than 1,000 international units per day) has been associated with increased mortality in some groups of people over age 65 (Schneider and Reed, 1985).

This in turn reduces the production of RNA, which is essential for producing enzymes necessary for cellular functioning. Hence, the loss of DNA and subsequent reduction of RNA eventually results in cell death.

Of all the theories of physiological aging, the cellular theory appears to hold the greatest promise for explaining the causes and processes of aging. The role of cell replication and RNA production in aging is widely accepted in the scientific community. It should not be assumed, however, that the step from understanding to reversing the process of aging will be achieved soon. It is often erroneously assumed that scientific discoveries of the *cause* of a particular physiological process or disease can immediately lead to *changing* or reversing that condition. Unfortunately, that step is a difficult one to make, as evidenced by research progress in cancer. Scientists have long observed the structural changes in cancer cells, but the reasons for these changes are far from being understood. Without a clear understanding of why a particular physiological process takes place, it is impossible to move toward reversing that process.

Research on Physiological Changes with Age

It is difficult to distinguish normal, age-related changes in many human functions from changes that are secondary to disease or other factors. Until the 1940s, much of our knowledge about aging came from cross-sectional comparisons of healthy, young persons with institutionalized or community-dwelling elderly who had multiple health problems. These comparisons led to the not surprising conclusion that the organ systems of older persons function less efficiently than those of younger persons.

Since the 1940s, a series of longitudinal studies have been undertaken with healthy younger and middle-aged persons who have been followed for several years to determine changes in various physiological parameters. The first of these studies began in 1946 at the Gerontology Research Center in Baltimore, and is described in Chapter 1. The initial sample of 600 healthy males between the ages of 20 and 96 was expanded in 1978 to include females. Today, many of the people in the original sample are still participating in the study. The second study was undertaken in 1955 at Duke University's Center for the Study of Aging, with a sample composed entirely of older adults. Some of these individuals were followed for more than 20 years (Palmore, 1974, 1985). Many other researchers around the country are now examining physiological functions longitudinally. The information in this chapter is derived from their work.

AGING IN BODY COMPOSITION

Although individuals vary greatly in body weight and composition, there is a general decline in the proportion of body weight contributed by water for both men and women: on the average, from 60 percent to 54 percent in men, and from 52 percent to 46 percent in women (Kenney, 1982). Lean body mass in muscle tissue is lost, whereas the proportion of fat increases (see Figure 4–1). Because of an increase in fibrous material, there is a loss of elasticity and flexibility in muscle tissue. After age 50, the number of muscle fibers steadily decreases, although exercise can still increase muscle tone. These changes in body composition have a significant effect on older people's ability to metabolize many medications.

FIGURE 4–1 Distribution of Major Body Components

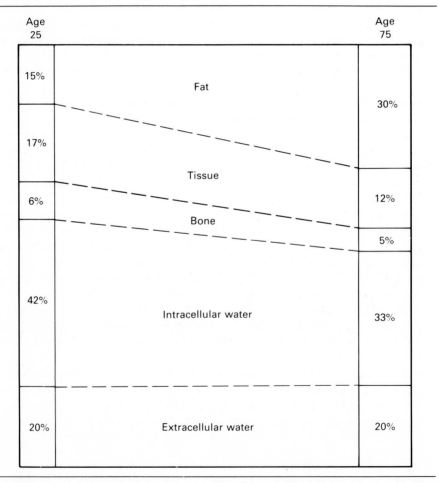

Source: Reprinted with permission from the American Geriatrics Society, Speculations on vascular changes with age, by R. J. Goldman (*Journal of the American Geriatrics Society,* Vol. 18, p. 766, 1970).

With advanced old age, there is a tendency toward weight loss. This is why we rarely see people in their eighties and nineties who are obese. The balance of sodium and potassium also changes, with the ratio of sodium increasing by 20 percent from age 30 to 70. Changes in body composition also have implications for the diet of older people; although older people generally need fewer total calories per day than active younger people, it is important for them to consume a higher proportion of protein, calcium, and vitamin D (Guigoz and Munro, 1985). However, many elderly do not change their diet during the later years unless advised specifically by a physician. Others, especially those living alone, eat poorly balanced meals.

CHANGES IN THE SKIN

As stated at the beginning of this chapter, changes in the appearance and texture of skin and hair are often the most visible signs of aging. These also tend to have deleterious consequences on how older people view themselves and are perceived by others. The human skin is unique among all other mammals in that it is exposed directly to the elements, with no protective fur or feathers that shield other animals from the direct effects of sunlight. In fact, ultraviolet light from the sun, which damages the elastic fibers beneath the skin's surface, is probably most directly responsible for the wrinkled, dried, and tougher texture of older people's skin. This is evident when one compares the appearance of the skin of two 75-year-old people—one a retired farmer who has worked under the sun most of his life, the other a retired office worker who has spent most of his years indoors. The farmer generally will have more wrinkles; darker pigmentation known as *melanin*, which has been produced by the body to protect it from ultraviolet rays; and drier skin with a leathery texture. He is also more likely to have so-called *age spots* or *liver spots*—harmless from a health standpoint but of concern sometimes for their appearance. As one might expect, people who spend most of their lives in sunny climates are more prone to these changes. Recently, there has been growing concern about the negative consequences of extensive exposure to the sun, such as premature wrinkling and the disease state of skin cancers.

Besides these environmental factors, the human body itself is responsible for some of the changes in the skin with age. The outermost layer of skin, the *epidermis,* constantly replenishes itself by shedding dead cells and replacing them with new cells. As the person gets older, the process of cell replacement is slowed, up to 50 percent between ages 30 and 70 (Leyden, McGinley and Grove, 1978). More importantly, the connective tissue that makes up the second layer of skin, the *dermis,* becomes less elastic with age. This results in reduced elasticity and thickness of the outer skin layer, longer time for the skin to spring back into shape, and increased sagging and wrinkling. Women often experience these problems earlier than men, sometimes as early as their twenties and thirties. This is because women tend to have less oil in the sebaceous glands. However, there is considerable variation in the process of skin change, depending on the relative amount of oil in the glands, exposure to the sun, and heredity. Despite its changing appearance, the skin can still perform its protective function throughout old age. Wound healing is also slower in older persons. Thus, people over age 65 require 50 percent more time than those under age 35 to form blisters as a means of closing a wound, and more time to form new epithelial tissue to replace blistered skin (Gilchrest, 1982).

The sebaceous and sweat glands, located in the dermis, generally deteriorate with age. Changes also occur in the deepest, or *subcutaneous*, skin layers which tend to lose fat and water. This can damage the effectiveness of the skin's temperature regulatory mechanism and make older people more sensitive to hot and cold temperatures. As a result, older persons' comfort zone for ambient temperature is generally three to five degrees warmer than that for younger persons. It also takes longer for an older person to adjust after being exposed to extreme temperatures, either hot or cold (Fox, Woodward, Exton-Smith, Green, Donnison and Wicks, 1973; Collins, 1986). This leaves the older individual much more vulnerable to hypothermia (low body temperature, sometimes resulting in brain damage and death) and hyperthermia (heat stroke), as evidenced by reports of increased accidental deaths among the elderly during periods of extremely cold winter weather and during prolonged heat spells (Kolanowski and Gunter, 1981; Applegate et al., 1981). It is recommended that indoor temperatures be set at 68°–70°F in older people's homes, and that humidity be minimized (Collins, 1986).

CHANGES IN THE HAIR

As we age, we also experience changes in the appearance and texture of our hair. Hair is thickest in early adulthood and decreases by as much as 20 percent in diameter by age 70. This is why so many older people appear to have fine, limp-looking hair. This change is compounded by the increased loss of hair with age. Although we lose up to 60 strands of hair daily during youth and early adulthood, the hair is replaced regularly through the action of estrogen and testosterone. As we age, however, more hairs are lost than replaced, especially in men. Some men experience rapid hair loss, leading to a receding hairline or even complete baldness by their mid-forties. Reasons for the observed variation in hair loss are not clear, but genetic factors appear to play a role.

Gray hair is a result of loss of pigment in the hair follicles. As we age, there is less pigment produced at the roots, so that eventually all the hair becomes colorless, or white in appearance. The gray color of some people's hair is an intermediate stage of pigment loss. In fact, some people may never experience a total loss of pigment production, but will live into an advanced old age with relatively dark hair. Others may experience graying in their twenties. In our

---

Symptoms of Hypothermia and Hyperthermia

Hypothermia is defined as body temperatures below 95° Fahrenheit over a long period. It occurs when an individual's shivering response cannot be activated because of systemic changes or because it is ineffective after prolonged exposure to cold. Symptoms of hypothermia can appear in just a few hours, or over several days. These include confusion and forgetfulness, problems with speaking or breathing, shivering, sleepiness, poor coordination, a puffy face, and a stomach that is cold to touch (Avery, 1984). Body heat is lost faster than it can be replaced, resulting in an inability to raise one's body heat, loss of functional capacities, confusion, disorientation, and, in extreme cases, death. Older people who cannot afford to keep their homes heated in the winter are at higher risk for hypothermia.

Hyperthermia, on the other hand, occurs when body temperature rises above normal and cannot be relieved by sweating, which results in heat exhaustion, heat stroke, heart failure, and stroke. Dizziness, nausea, vomiting, dry skin, cramps, fainting, and confusion may be initial symptoms. The problem is aggravated in older persons because of a reduced efficiency in their sweating response (Foster, Ellis, and Dore, 1976). Those who are overweight or have kidney problems, high blood pressure, poor circulation, diabetes, or emphysema are more vulnerable to hypothermia than healthy older people. Older people with low income levels who live in houses with no air conditioning are at great risk for hyperthermia in climates where temperatures exceed 90° Fahrenheit for several days in a row.

---

society, graying of hair tends to have more stigma associated with it for women than for men.

CHANGES IN THE MUSCULO-SKELETAL SYSTEM

Stature or height declines an average of three inches with age, although the total loss varies across individuals and between men and women. We reach our maximum size and strength at about age 25, after which our cells decrease steadily in number and size. This decline occurs in both the trunk and the extremities, and may be attributable to the loss of bone mineral. The spine becomes more curved and discs in the vertebrae become compacted. Such loss of height is intensified for individuals with *osteoporosis,* a disease that makes the bones less dense, more porous, and hence more prone to fractures following even a minor stress. For older people who have no natural teeth remaining, it is not unusual to lose a considerable volume of bone in the jaw or alveolar bone. This results in a poor fit

With osteoporosis, both trabecular and cortical bones become more brittle and lace-like.

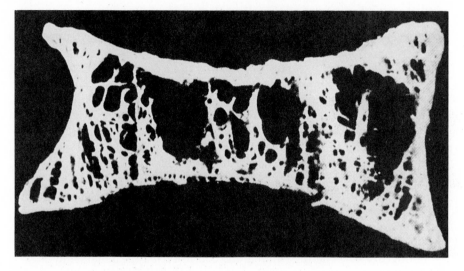

of dentures, and a painful feeling when chewing or biting with dentures. The loss of bone mass characteristic of osteoporosis is *not* a normal process of aging, but a disease that occurs with more frequency among older women, as will be discussed in Chapters 6 and 16.

Another normal change with aging is that shoulder width decreases as a result of bone loss, weakened muscles, and loss of elasticity in the ligaments. Crush fractures of the spine cause the vertebrae to collapse, such that over time, some older people (especially women) appear to be stoop-shouldered or hunched—a condition known as *kyphosis*. Stiffness in the joints is also charac-teristic of old age; this occurs because cartilage between the joints wears thin, and the fluid that lubricates them decreases. Strength and stamina also decline with aging. Maximum strength at age 70 has been found to be 65 to 85 percent of the maximum capacity of a 25-year-old. This drops to 50 percent by age 80, although older persons who maintain an active physical fitness program show much less decline in strength.

These musculo-skeletal changes make it difficult for older people to perform some tasks of daily living. For example, it may be difficult to get out of a chair or bed, or to reach up or deep inside a cabinet located overhead. The older person may attempt to accommodate to the latter situation by climbing on a chair or footstool in the kitchen to reach objects on top shelves. This is a dangerous way to solve the problem, because of the loss of balance that often accompanies the aging process and the increased brittleness of bones that some older people experience. These changes contribute to a higher incidence of falls and hip fractures in older people, which in turn may produce long-term disability and even death. Minor modifications around the home can reduce the risk of falls, for instance, installing handrails and grab bars, and making sure that surfaces are smooth and secure.

AGING IN THE RESPIRATORY SYSTEM

Almost every organ system shows some decline in functional or reserve capacity with age, as illustrated by several physiological indices in Figure 4–2. Complex functions that require the integration of multiple systems experience the most rapid decline. For example, maximum breathing capacity—which requires coordination of the respiratory, nervous, and muscular systems—is greatly decreased. Accordingly, normal changes in the respiratory and cardiovascular system become most evident with age. These changes are responsible for an individual's declining ability to maintain physical activity for long periods and the

FIGURE 4–2 Aging in Organ Systems

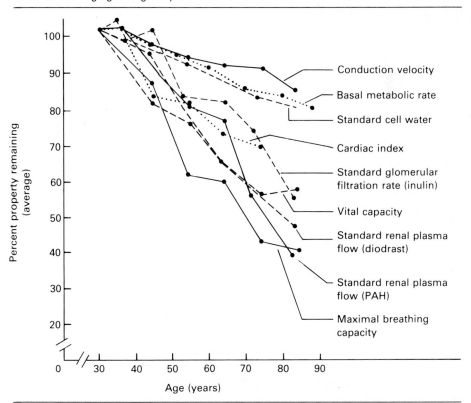

Source: N. W. Shock, The physiology of aging. *Scientific American,* Vol. 206, p. 110. Copyright 1962. Reprinted by permission of the publisher and the author.

increasing tendency to fatigue easily. With aging, the muscles that operate the lungs lose elasticity so that respiratory efficiency is reduced. Vital capacity, or the maximum amount of oxygen that can be brought into the lungs with a deep breath, declines. In fact, it has been estimated that the average decline for men is 50 percent at age 70 from age 25, the peak of a healthy man's lung function, or a decline from six quarts of air to three quarts. Breathing may become more difficult after strenuous exercise or after climbing up several flights of stairs, but it does not necessarily impair the older person's daily functions. It may simply mean that the person has to move more slowly or rest on the stairway landing. However, the rate of decline in vital capacity has been found to be slower in physically active men than in sedentary healthy men. Indeed, longitudinal studies have consistently found the former to have twice the vital capacity of the latter in middle-age (Dehn and Bruce, 1972; Dill, Robinson, and Ross, 1967; Bruce, 1984).

Of all the body systems, the respiratory system suffers the most punishment from environmental pollutants and infections (Rockstein and Sussman, 1979). For this reason, it is difficult to distinguish normal, age-related changes from pathological or environmentally induced diseases. *Cilia*, which are hairlike structures in the airways, are reduced in number and are less effective in removing foreign matter. This diminishes the amount of oxygen available. This, combined with declining muscle strength in the chest that impairs cough efficiency, makes the older person more susceptible to chronic bronchitis, emphysema, and pneumonia. Older people can avoid serious loss of lung function by remaining active, attempting to pace their tasks, and taking part in activities that do not demand too much exertion. Avoiding strenuous activity on days when the air quality is poor can also reduce the load on an older person's lungs.

CARDIOVASCULAR CHANGES AND THE EFFECTS OF EXERCISE

Structural changes in the heart and blood vessels include a reduction in bulk, a replacement of heart muscle with fat, a loss of elastic tissue, and an increase in collagen. Within the muscle fibers, an age pigment composed of fat and protein, known as *lipofuscin,* may take up 5 to 10 percent of the fiber structure (Pearson and Shaw, 1982). These changes produce a loss of elasticity in the arteries, weakened vessel walls, and varicosities, or abnormal swelling, in veins that are under high pressure (e.g., in the legs). In addition to loss of elasticity, the arterial and vessel walls become increasingly lined with lipids (fats), creating the condition of *atherosclerosis,* which makes it more difficult for blood to be pumped through the vessels and arteries. It should be noted that this buildup of fats and lipids occurs to some extent with normal aging, but it is exacerbated in some individuals whose diet includes large quantities of saturated fats. In Chapter 6, such lifestyle risk factors for heart disease will be reviewed.

Blood pressure is expressed as the ratio of systolic to diastolic pressure. The former refers to the level of blood pressure (in mm.) during the contraction phase (systole), whereas the latter refers to the stage when the chambers of the heart are filling with blood. For example, a blood pressure of 120/80 indicates that the pressure created by the heart to expel blood can raise a column of mercury 120 mm. During diastole, in this example, the pressure produced by blood rushing into the heart chambers can raise a column of mercury 80 mm. Both systolic and diastolic blood pressure tend to increase with normal aging, but the elevation of the former is greater (see Figure 4–3). As with changes in the heart, extreme elevation of blood pressure is not normal and is associated with diet, obesity, and lifestyle, all of which have cumulative effects over the years. The negative effects of abnormally high or low blood pressure are examined in Chapter 6.

The maximum heart rate achievable by sustained exercise is directly associated with age; the formula is: 220 minus age in years. For example, a 25-year-old could expect a maximum heart rate of 195 (220−25), whereas a 70-year-old could achieve 150 (220−70) beats per minute. However, there is some

FIGURE 4–3 Effect of Age on Systolic Blood Pressure

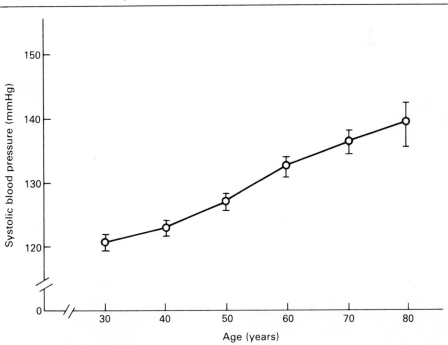

Source: J. D. Tobin, Physiological indices of aging. In D. Danon, N. W. Shock, and M. Marois (Eds.), *Aging: A Challenge in Science and Society.* Vol. 1. New York: Oxford University Press, 1981.

variation across individuals, with the heart rate remaining relatively high in physically active older persons. Resting heart rates also decrease with aging, although physically well-conditioned older people tend to have heart rates more similar to the average younger person.

These changes in the heart and lungs result in less efficient utilization of oxygen. This, in turn, reduces an individual's capacity to maintain physical activity for long periods. Nevertheless, physical training for older persons can significantly reduce blood pressure and increase their aerobic capacity (DeVries, 1970; Shephard, 1978). Recent studies of older men described as "master athletes"— individuals who have continued to participate in competitive, aerobic exercise (running, bicycling, swimming) into the later years—have shown that physical training results in a greater volume of oxygen, more lean body weight, and lower percent of fat than in untrained older persons. However, these levels were found to be poorer than in younger athletes, underscoring the reality that normal changes in the body's physiology and its operation cannot be eliminated completely. Even in healthy persons there is some loss of strength and stamina.

Nevertheless, the positive effects of exercise on slowing these changes are becoming widely recognized. Researchers have found a significant increase in aerobic capacity as measured by maximum volume of oxygen uptake, and a

Organized sports activities such as the San Francisco Bay to Breakfast Walk provide opportunities for aerobic exercise.

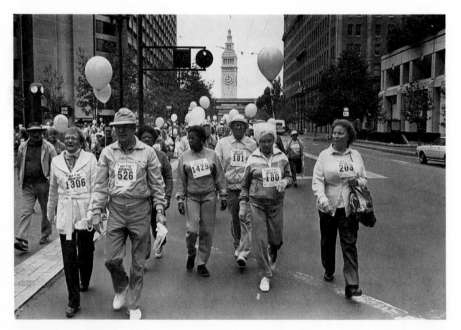

reduction in fat composition among sedentary older persons after six months of low-intensity exercise training (e.g., walking for 20–30 minutes), followed by six months of high-intensity training (e.g., jogging for 20–30 minutes) (Ehsani, 1984; Hagberg, 1984; Seals, Hagberg, Hurley, Ehsani, and Holloszy, 1984). High-intensity exercise resulted in significant weight loss, but low-intensity exercise did not. However, high-intensity training resulted in more orthopedic injuries than did low-intensity training among older participants. This research also suggests that exercise may not be sufficient for reducing cholesterol and triglyceride levels, both of which have been associated with heart disease. Instead, reduced intake of fats and carbohydrates appears to be essential. While there are limitations, these findings justify optimism that physical health can be considerably improved through some lifestyle changes.

These findings regarding the benefits of regular exercise for older people raise the concept of active life expectancy, that is, the portion of remaining life during which one is independent and not living a disabled existence. Thus, for a sedentary 65-year-old, *active* life expectancy has been calculated to be 10 years of the remaining 16.5 years life expectancy for that age (Katz, Branch, Branson, Papsidero, Beck, and Greer, 1983). Aerobic exercise and a healthy lifestyle can significantly increase active life expectancy by postponing and shortening the period of morbidity (e.g., days of sickness) that one can expect in the later years. The significance of certain lifestyle habits for maintaining good health in old age will be discussed in more detail in Chapters 6 and 19.

CHANGES IN THE URINARY SYSTEM

Both kidney and bladder function change with age. The kidneys play an important role in regulating the body's internal chemistry by filtering blood and urine through an extraordinary system of tubes and capillaries, known as glomeruli. As blood passes through these filters, it is cleaned, and the necessary balance of ions and minerals is restored. In the process, urea (e.g., water and waste materials) are collected and passed through the ureter and the bladder, where they are excreted in the form of urine. With age, the kidneys decrease in volume and weight, and the total number of glomeruli correspondingly decreases by 30 percent from age 30 to age 65. As a result, renal function, defined by the rate at which blood is filtered through the kidneys, declines by up to 50 percent with age (Rockstein and Sussman, 1979). These changes have significant implications for an older person's tolerance for certain medications such as penicillin, tetracycline, digoxin, and others that are cleared by glomerular filtration. These drugs remain active longer in an older person's system and may be more potent, indicating a need to reduce drug dosage and frequency of administration.

The kidneys also lose their capacity to absorb glucose, as well as their concentrating and diluting ability, contributing to increased problems with dehydration and hyponetremia (i.e., a loss of salt in the blood). Of any organ system, renal function deteriorates most dramatically with age, irrespective of disease.

Compounding this problem, bladder function also deteriorates with age. The capacity of the bladder may be reduced by as much as 50 percent in some persons older than age 65. At the same time, however, the sensation of needing to empty the bladder is delayed (Rockstein and Sussman, 1979). The latter condition may be more a function of central nervous system dysfunction than changes in the bladder. As a result, urinary incontinence is common in the elderly. The problem may be made worse by a stroke, dementia, or other diseases associated with the nervous system, such as Parkinson's.

Because of these changes in the kidney and the bladder, older people may be more sensitive to the effects of alcohol and caffeine. Both of these substances inhibit the production of a hormone that regulates urine production. Ordinarily, this hormone, known as antidiuretic hormone (ADH), signals to the kidneys when to produce urine in order to keep the body's chemistry balanced. When it is temporarily inhibited by the consumption of alcohol, coffee, or tea, the kidneys no longer receive messages and, as a result, produce urine constantly. This in turn dehydrates the body. It appears that ADH production is slowed with aging, so substances that inhibit its production increase the load on the kidneys and the bladder. Because of these changes, older people may start to avoid social outings, even a trip to the grocery store, out of fear that they may not have access to a bathroom. Possible treatments for urinary incontinence, as well as ways that older people can alter their daily habits to accommodate bladder problems, are discussed more fully in Chapter 6.

SEXUAL CHANGES

Men and women experience changes in their sexual organs as they age, but these do not necessarily lead to sexual incapacity. The normal physiological changes that characterize men's aging alter the nature of the sexual response, but do not interfere with men's sexual performance. These changes include: (1) slower response to sexual stimulation, with a longer time needed to obtain an erection, (2) less full erections, (3) decreased volume and force of ejaculation, (4) occasional lack of orgasm during intercourse, and (5) increased length of time between orgasm and subsequent erections. Impotence is the most common sexual disorder among men over age 45. What is unclear is the extent to which there may be a physical basis for impotence, such as the effects of drugs (especially antihypertensives, antidepressants, and tranquilizers), prostate disorders, alcohol, or diabetes. Fear of failure, which is created by psychosocial factors rather than physiological changes, appears to underlie many cases of impotence. Even chronic disease does not necessarily eliminate sexual capacity. For example, many older persons, after adequate medical consultation, can resume sexual activity following a heart attack.

Changes in prostatic cells with age result in an enlargement of the prostate in more than 90 percent of men over the age of 80; by age 40, 10 percent of men already have enlarged prostates. In fact, one investigator has suggested that the prostate will deteriorate in all men if they live to be very old (Silber, 1981). Surgery may be required in some of these cases (Boss and Seegmiller, 1981).

Older women's sexuality may be influenced more by sociocultural expectations than older men's, primarily because of the limited number of male partners and the common cultural definition of older women as asexual and unattractive. Accordingly, the majority of sexual disorders experienced by older women are psychological in origin, not physical. From a physical point of view, no impediment exists to full sexual activity after menopause. Kinsey, Pomeroy, Martin and Gebhard (1948), in fact, established that women experience only a slight decline in their capacity for sexual pleasure throughout life.

Physiological changes do occur, however, primarily due to the loss of estrogen, which is manifest approximately five years after the menopause. The common changes experienced by women are the thinning of the vaginal walls, increased length of time for vaginal lubrication to occur, and loss of vaginal elasticity. (Urinary tract infections may occur more frequently because of thinning vaginal walls which offer less protection to the bladder and urethra.) While these changes may render intercourse somewhat less pleasurable, they can be minimized by sexual regularity.

A woman's capacity for orgasms may be slowed, but not impaired. Generally, an older woman's sexual response cycle has all the dimensions of the response of her younger counterpart, but the time it takes for her to respond to sexual stimulation gradually increases. The intensity of her sexual response may gradually decrease, with the orgasm becoming shorter and less pronounced (Masters and Johnson, 1970). Overall, the greatest barrier to women's sexual pleasure is the lack of socially approved partners and the societal double standard of aging, which defines the older man as distinguished and attractive, and the older woman as a "has been."

There are a variety of ways that older couples can adapt to these changes in sexual functioning. For both older men and women, long leisurely foreplay can enhance their sexual response. Avoiding alcohol use prior to sexual activity can be helpful, since alcohol increases desire, but decreases sexual ability. For women, consistent sexual activity, including masturbation, maintains vaginal lubricating ability and vaginal muscle tone, reducing discomfort during intercourse. Water-soluble lubricants, such as KY jellies and vaginal creams that can be purchased over the counter in drug stores, are also helpful in enhancing vaginal lubrication. Health professionals need to be alert to medications that adversely affect sexual functioning, such as antihypertensives, tranquilizers, and antidepressants. Simply knowing more about normal age-related sexual changes may help older people to maintain their sexual self-esteem.

CHANGES IN THE GASTROINTESTINAL SYSTEM

The gastrointestinal system includes the esophagus, stomach, intestines, colon, liver, and biliary tract. Although the esophagus does not show age-related changes in appearance, there are some changes in its function in some elderly. These may include a decrease in contraction of the muscles and more time for the cardiac sphincter (a valvelike structure that allows food to pass into the stomach) to open, thus taking more time for food to be transmitted to the stomach. The result of these changes may be a sensation of being full before having consumed a full meal. This in turn may reduce the pleasure a person derives from eating, and result in inadequate nutrient intake. This sensation also explains why older people may appear to eat such small quantities of food at mealtimes.

Secretion of digestive juices in the stomach apparently diminishes after age 50, especially among men. As a result, older people are more likely to experience the condition of atrophic gastritis, or a chronic inflammation of the stomach lining. Gastric ulcers are more likely to occur in middle-age than in old age, but older people are at greater risk for colon and stomach cancer. Because of this risk, older people who complain of gastrointestinal discomfort should be urged to seek medical attention for the problem, instead of relying on home remedies or over-the-counter medications.

As with many other organs in the human body, the small and large intestines decrease in weight after age 40. There are also functional changes in the small intestine, where the number of enzymes is reduced, and simple sugars are absorbed more slowly, resulting in diminished efficiency with age. The smooth muscle content and muscle tone in the wall of the colon also decrease. Anatomical changes in the large intestine are associated with the increased incidence of chronic constipation in older persons.

However, behavioral factors are probably more important than organic factors in the development of constipation. These will be discussed in more detail in Chapter 6. Spasms of the lower intestinal tract are an example of the interaction of physiological with behavioral factors. Although they may occur at any age, such spasms are more common among older persons. These spasms are a form of functional disorder, that is, a condition without any organic basis, often due to psychological factors. Many gastrointestinal conditions that afflict older persons are unrelated to the anatomical changes described above. Nevertheless, they are very real problems to an older person who experiences them.

The liver also grows smaller with age, by about 20 percent, although this does not appear to have much influence on its functions. However, there is a deterioration in ability to process any medications that are dependent on liver function. Jaundice occurs more frequently in the elderly, and may be due to changes in the liver or to the obstruction of bile in the gall bladder. In addition, high alcohol consumption may put excessive strain on the older person's liver.

AGING IN THE NERVOUS SYSTEM

The brain is composed of billions of neurons, or nerve cells, which are lost as we grow older. Neuronal loss begins at age 30, well before the period termed *old*. It is compounded by alcohol consumption, cigarette smoking, and breathing polluted air. The frontal lobe has been found to experience a greater loss of cells than other parts of the brain (Brody, 1973). A moderate degree of neuronal loss does not create a major decline in brain function, however. In fact, contrary to popular belief, we can function with fewer neurons than we have, so their loss is not the reason for mild forgetfulness in old age. Even in the case of Alzheimer's disease and other dementias, severe loss of neurons may be less significant than changes in brain tissue, blood flow, and receptor organs.

Other aging-related changes in the brain include a reduction in its weight by 10 percent, an accumulation of lipofuscin (e.g., an age pigment composed of fat and protein), and slower transmission of information from one neuron to another (Goldman, 1970). The reduction in brain mass occurs in all species, and is probably due to loss of fluids. The gradual buildup of lipofuscin, which has a yellowish color, causes the outer cortex of the brain to take on a yellow-beige color with age. As with the moderate loss of neurons, these changes do not appear to alter brain function in old age. That is, difficulties in solving problems or remembering dates and names cannot be attributed to these slight changes in the size and appearance of the brain.

In contrast, the change in neurotransmitters and in the structure of the synapse (the junction between any two neurons) does affect cognitive and motor function. Electroencephalograms, or readings of the electrical activity of the brain, show a slower response in older brains than in the young. These changes may be at least partially responsible for the increase in reaction time with age. Other hypotheses include neuronal loss and reduced blood flow; however, available data are inconclusive. Reaction time is a complex product of multiple factors, primarily the speed of conduction and motor function, both of which are slowed by the increased time needed to transmit messages at the synapses.

The reduced speed with which the nervous system can process information or send signals for action is a fairly widespread problem, even in middle-age when people begin to notice lagging reflexes and reaction time. As a result, such tasks as responding to a telephone or doorbell, crossing the street, completing a paper and pencil test, or deciding among several alternatives generally take longer for older people than for the young. Most people adjust to these changes by taking more time to do a task and avoiding rush situations; for example, an older person may compensate by leaving the house one hour before an appointment instead of the usual 15 minutes, shopping for groceries during times when stores are not crowded, or shopping in smaller stores. Such adaptations are perhaps most pronounced in the tasks associated with driving. The older driver tends to be more cautious, to slow down well in advance of a traffic signal, to stay in the slower lane, and to avoid freeways during rush hour. Although younger drivers may become impatient with the slowness of older drivers, their accident rates tend to be lower than the young. On the other hand, older people do have more accidents per mile driven (Waller, 1986).

Changes in the central nervous system that accompany aging also affect the senses of hearing, taste, smell, and touch. Despite these changes, intellectual and motor function apparently do not deteriorate significantly with age. The brain has tremendous reserve capacity that takes over as losses begin. It is only when neuronal loss, inadequate function of neurotransmitters, and other structural changes are severe that the older person experiences significant loss of function. The changes in the brain that appear to be associated with Alzheimer's disease will be discussed in Chapter 9.

Summary and Implications

As shown by this review of the major biological systems, the aging process is gradual, beginning in some organ systems as early as the twenties and thirties, and progressing more rapidly after age 70, or even 80, in others. Even with 50 percent deterioration in many organ systems, an individual can still function adequately. The ability for human beings to compensate for age-related changes attests to their significant amount of excess reserve capacity. In most instances, the normal physical changes of aging need not diminish a person's quality of life. Since many of the decrements are gradual and slight, older people can learn to modify their activities to adapt to their environments, for example, by pacing the amount of physical exertion throughout the day. Family members and professionals can be supportive by encouraging modifications in the home, such as minimizing the use of stairs, moving the focus of the older person's daily activities to the main floor of the home, and reinforcing the older person's efforts to cope creatively with common physical changes.

There are significant differences in the rate and severity of decline in various organ systems, with the greatest deterioration in functions that require co-ordination among multiple systems, muscles, and nerves. Similarly, there are wide variations across individuals in the aging process, springing from differences in heredity, diet, exercise, and living conditions. Many of the physiological functions that were once assumed to deteriorate and to be irreversible with normal aging are being reevaluated by researchers in basic and clinical physiology, as well as by health educators. Even people who begin a regular exercise program late in life have experienced significant improvements in their heart and lung capacity. The role of preventive maintenance and health promotion in the aging process will be discussed in Chapter 19.

Finally, we should note the implications of improved health for maximum human life span. Life expectancy for humans (the average expected longevity) has increased in most countries around the world due to significant reductions in infant mortality and some adulthood diseases, such as tuberculosis. However, it is unlikely that the maximum life span will increase beyond the generally accepted period of about 110–120 years (see Table 4–1). This is because, as implied by many of the physiological theories reviewed earlier in this chapter, there appears to be a maximum biologically determined life span for human cells, tissues, and the organs that they comprise. For these reasons, more and more persons will expect to live longer, but the maximum number of years they can expect to live will not be increased in the foreseeable future unless, of course, some extra-ordinary and unanticipated biological discoveries occur (Fries, 1980; Fries and Crapo, 1981).

Perhaps the most important goal of health planners and practitioners should be to approach a rectangular survival curve. That is, as seen in the survival curve in Figure 4–4, developments in medicine, public hygiene, and health have already increased the percentage of people surviving into the later years. The ideal situation is one where all people would survive to the maximum life span, creating a "rectangular curve." We are approaching this ideal curve, but it will not be achieved until the diseases of youth and middle-age—including cancer, heart disease, diabetes, and kidney diseases—can be prevented altogether, or at least managed as chronic conditions.

TABLE 4–1 Maximum Recorded Life Spans for Selected Species

Species	Types	Maximum Life Span (years)
Primates	Rhesus monkey	29
	Gorilla	39
	Human	115
Carnivores	Domestic cat	28
	Domestic dog	20
Rodents	Black rat	5
	Gray squirrel	15
Birds	Golden eagle	46
	Domestic dove	30
Reptiles	Snapping turtle	58+
	Galapagos turtle	100+

Source: Adapted from: T.B.L. Kirkwood, Comparative and evolutionary aspects of longevity. In C. E. Finch and E. L. Schneider (Eds.), *The Handbook of the Biology of Aging,* 2nd edition. New York: Van Nostrand Reinhold, 1985, p. 34. Reprinted by permission of the author and publisher.

FIGURE 4–4 Increasing Rectangularization of the Survival Curve

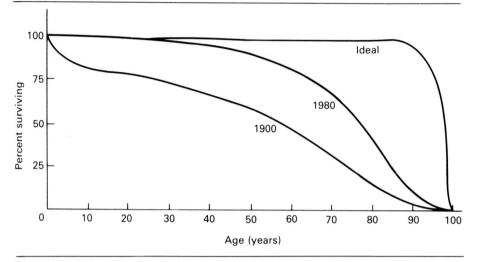

Source: Adapted from L. Hayflick, The cell biology of human aging. *Scientific American,* 1980, p. 60, by permission of the publisher.

References

Applegate, W. B., Runyan, J. W., Brasfield, L., Williams, M. L., Konigsberg, C., and Fouche, C. Analysis of the 1980 heat wave in Memphis. *Journal of the American Geriatrics Society,* 1981, *29,* 337–342.

Avery, W. M. Hypothermia and heat illness. *Aging,* 1984, *8,* 43–47.

Bjorksten, J. Crosslinkage and the aging process. In M. Rockstein, M. L. Sussman, and J. Chesky (Eds.). *Theoretical aspects of aging.* New York: Academic Press, 1974.

Boss, G. R., and Seegmiller, J. E. Age-related physiological changes and their clinical significance. *The Western Journal of Medicine,* 1981, *135,* 434–440.

Brody, H. Aging of the vertebrate brain. In M. Rockstein (Ed.), *Development and aging in the nervous system.* New York: Academic Press, 1973, 121–134.

Bruce, R. A. Exercise, functional capacity and aging—Another viewpoint. *Medical Science Sports Exercise,* 1984, *16,* 8–13.

Collins, K. J. Low indoor temperatures and morbidity in the elderly. *Age and Ageing,* 1986, *15,* 212–220.

Cutler, E. D., and Cutler, R. G. Tissue auto-oxidation, antioxidants, and life span potential. *The Gerontologist,* 1983, *23* (Special Issue), 194.

Dehn, M. M., and Bruce, R. A. Longitudinal variations in maximal oxygen intake with age and activity. *Journal of Applied Physiology,* 1972, *33,* 805–807.

DeVries, H. A. Physiological effects of an exercise training regime upon men aged 52–88. *Journal of Gerontology,* 1970, *25,* 325–336.

Dill, D. B., Robinson, S., and Ross, J. C. A longitudinal study of 16 champion runners. *Journal of Sports Medicine*, 1967, 7, 4–32.

Ehsani, A. A. Effects of exercise training on myocardial function and oxygenation in patients with ischemic heart disease. Paper presented at meetings of the Gerontological Society of America, San Antonio, Texas, 1984.

Foster, K. G., Ellis, F. D., and Dore, L. Sweat responses in the aged. *Age and Ageing*, 1976, 15, 91–95.

Fox, R. H., Woodward, P. M., Exton-Smith, A. N., Green, M. F., Donnison, D. V., and Wicks, M. H. Body temperatures in the elderly. *British Medical Journal*, 1973, 1, 200–206.

Fries, J. F. Aging, natural death, and the compression of morbidity. *New England Journal of Medicine*, 1980, 303, 130–135.

Fries, J. F., and Crapo, L. M. *Vitality and aging.* San Francisco: W. H. Freeman, 1981.

Gilchrest, B. A. Skin. In J. W. Rowe and R. W. Besdine (Eds.), *Health and disease in old age.* Boston: Little, Brown, 1982, 381–392.

Goldman, R. J. Speculations on vascular changes with age. *Journal of the American Geriatrics Society*, 1970, 18, 765–779.

Guigoz, Y., and Munro, H. N. Nutrition and aging. In C. E. Finch and E. L. Schneider (Eds.), *Handbook of the biology of aging* (2d ed.). New York: Van Nostrand Reinhold, 1985, 878–893.

Hagberg, J. M. Physiological and metabolic status of master athletes. Paper presented at meetings of the Gerontological Society of America, San Antonio, Texas, 1984.

Harman, D. A theory based on free radical and radiation chemistry. *Journal of Gerontology*, 1956, 11, 298.

Harman, D. The aging process. *Proceedings of the National Academy of Science*, 1981, 78, 7124–7128.

Harman, D., Heindrick, M. L., and Eddy, D. E. Free radical theory of aging: Effect of free radical-reaction inhibitors on the immune response. *Journal of the American Geriatrics Society*, 1977, 25, 400–407.

Hayflick, L. Aging under glass. *Experimental Gerontology*, 1970, 5, 291–303.

Katz, S., Branch, L. G., Branson, M. H., Papsidero, J. A., Beck, J. C., and Greer, D. S. Active life expectancy. *New England Journal of Medicine*, 1983, 309, 1218–1224.

Kenney, R. A. *Physiology of aging: A synopsis.* Chicago: Year Book Medical Publishers, 1982.

Kinsey, A. C., Pomeroy, W. B., Martin, C. E., and Gebhard, P. H. *Sexual behavior in the human male.* Philadelphia: W. B. Saunders, 1948.

Kirkwood, T. B. L. Comparative and evolutionary aspects of longevity. In C. E. Finch and E. L. Schneider (Eds.), *Handbook of the biology of aging* (2d ed.). New York: Van Nostrand Reinhold, 1985, 27–44.

Kolanowski, A., and Gunter, L. Hypothermia in the elderly. *Geriatric Nursing*, 1981, 2, 362–376.

Leyden, J. J., McGinley, K. J., and Grove, G. L. Age-related differences in the rate of desquamation of skin surface cells. In R. D. Adelman, J. Roberts, and V. J. Christafalo (Eds.), *Pharmacological interventions in the aging process.* New York: Plenum Press, 1978.

Masters, W. H., and Johnson, V. *Human sexual inadequacy.* Boston: Little, Brown, 1970.

Palmore, E. (Ed.). *Normal aging: Reports from the Duke Longitudinal Study, 1955–1969.* Durham, N. C.: Duke University Press, 1970.

Palmore, E. (Ed.). *Normal aging II: Reports from the Duke Longitudinal Study, 1970–1973.* Durham, N. C.: Duke University Press, 1974.

Palmore, E. (Ed.). *Normal aging III: Reports from the Duke Longitudinal Study.* Durham, N. C.: Duke University Press, 1985.

Pearson, D., and Shaw, S. *Life extension.* New York: Warner Books, 1982.

Rockstein, M., and Sussman, M. *Biology of aging.* Belmont, Calif.: Wadsworth, 1979.

Schneider, E. L., and Reed, J. D. Modulations of aging processes. In C. E. Finch and E. L. Schneider (Eds.), *Handbook of the biology of aging* (2d ed.). New York: Van Nostrand Reinhold, 1985, 45–78.

Seals, D. R., Hagberg, J. M., Hurley, B. F., Ehsani, A. A., and Holloszy, J. O. Endurance training in older men and women. *Journal of Applied Physiology,* 1984, *57,* 1024–1029.

Shephard, R. J. *Physical activity and aging.* Chicago: Croon Helm, 1978.

Shock, N. W. The physiology of aging. *Scientific American,* 1962, *206,* 100–110.

Silber, S. J. *The male: From infancy to old age.* New York: Charles Scribner and Sons, 1981.

Walford, R. L. *The immunological theory of aging.* Baltimore: Williams and Wilkins, 1969.

Waller, J. A. The older driver. *Generations,* Fall 1986, 36–38.

Wilson, D. L. The programmed theory of aging. In M. Rockstein, M. L. Sussman, and J. Chesky (Eds.), *Theoretical aspects of aging.* New York: Academic Press, 1974, 11–21.

Chapter **5**

Sensory Changes and Their Social Consequences

There is a popular belief that, as we get older, we cannot see, hear, touch, taste, or smell as well as we did when we were younger, and it appears to be true. The decline in all our sensory receptors with aging is normal; in fact, it begins relatively early. We reach our optimum capacities in our twenties, maintain this peak for a few years, and gradually experience a decline, with a more rapid rate of decline after the ages of 45 to 55. Having said this, we should note that there is tremendous diversity among individuals in the rate and severity of sensory decline, as illustrated earlier by Mrs. Hill and Mr. Jones. Some older persons may have better visual acuity than most 25-year-olds; there are many 75-year-olds who can hear better than most younger persons. Think about the wine taster who, in old age, may still be considered the master of his trade, doing a job that requires excellent taste discrimination.

Although age per se does not determine deterioration in sensory functioning, it is clear that many internal changes do take place. (The older person who has better visual or hearing acuity than a 25-year-old probably had even better sensory capacities in the earlier years.) It is important to focus on *intraindividual* changes with age, not *interindividual* differences, when studying sensory and perceptual functions. Unfortunately, most of the research on sensory changes with age is cross-sectional, that is, based on comparing different persons who are older and younger. For this reason, the reader needs to be aware that there are tremendous individual differences in how much and how severely sensory functions deteriorate with age.

In this chapter, changes are examined that have been found to occur with aging in the structure and function of all the sensory organs. Both normal and disease-related changes in the eye, the ear, the taste and smell receptors, as well as in the skin and the temperature-regulating system, are reviewed. Some implications of these changes for older people's social functioning are suggested, in order to enhance their competence vis-à-vis their environments. Likewise, the importance of recognizing these sensory changes in designing appropriate environments for older persons is considered.

Normal Changes with Age

Changes in different senses occur at varied rates and to different degrees. Thus, the person who experiences an early and severe decline in hearing acuity may not have any deterioration in visual functioning. Some sensory functions, such as hearing, may show an early decline, yet others, such as taste and touch, change little until well into advanced old age. Over time, however, sensory changes affect an older person's interactions with the social and physical environments.

Because these changes are usually gradual, people adapt and compensate by using other, still-intact sensory systems. For example, they may compensate by standing closer to objects and persons in order to hear or see, by using nonverbal cues such as touch and different body orientations, or by utilizing technical devices such as bifocals or hearing aids. To the extent that people can control their environment and make it conform to their changing needs, sensory decline need not be incapacitating. However, if the environment does not allow for modification to suit individual needs, if the decline in any one system is severe, or if several sensory systems deteriorate at the same time, it becomes much more difficult for individuals to use compensatory mechanisms. Such problems are more likely to occur in advanced old age.

Before reviewing the major changes in sensory processes that accompany aging, it will be helpful to clarify some terminology. *Sensation* is the process of taking in information through the sense organs. *Perception* is a higher function in which the information received through the senses is processed in the brain. *Sensory threshold* is the minimum intensity of a stimulus that a person requires in order to detect the stimulus. This differs for each sensory system. *Recognition threshold* is the intensity of a stimulus needed in order for an individual to identify or recognize it. As might be expected, a greater intensity of a stimulus is necessary to recognize than to detect it. *Sensory discrimination* is defined as the minimum difference necessary between two or more stimuli in order that a person be able to distinguish between them. There is considerable evidence that, with normal aging, a decline occurs in all sensory systems (Ordy and Brizzee, 1979). That is, sensory and recognition thresholds increase, and discrimination between multiple stimuli demands greater distinctions between them.

Changes in Vision

Although the proportion of blind persons in old age is not significantly higher than among younger persons, the rates of impairments that affect some aspects of visual functioning increase with age. As a result, older persons are more likely to experience problems with daily tasks that require good visual skills.

ANATOMY AND PHYSIOLOGY OF THE EYE

Before reviewing the changes in visual function that occur with age, it will be useful first to describe how the eye works. As shown in Figure 5–1, the eye is composed of several elements that work in harmony to transmit visual images from the external world to the brain, which in turn translates them into meaningful stimuli for understanding the environment. The process of seeing begins when light enters through the cornea, passes the pupil and the lens, which refracts light rays into angles that then reach the retina. The lens is shaped in such a way as to allow refraction, or scattering of light at specific angles to form an

FIGURE 5–1 The Eye

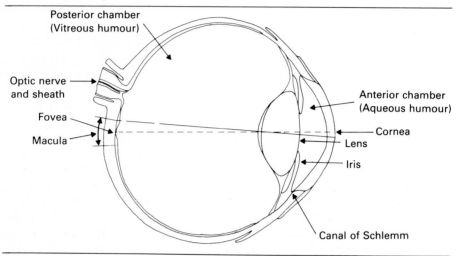

image on the retina; many age-related changes affect the shape of the lens, as will be noted later. Images formed on the retina, which covers more than two-thirds of the eye, are transformed into messages that can be carried by the optic nerve to the brain. The richest concentration of blood vessels in the retina is in the macula. This part of the eye allows us to see fine detail and provides central vision. Located in the retina are the rods and cones, visual receptors that respectively allow the functioning of vision at low light levels and the ability to discern colors. As the person moves from a dimly lit situation to bright light, there is a shift in the retina from rod to cone vision. This change, undetected by the individual, allows a person to see under different conditions of light and dark. Note also that there are chambers in front of and behind the lens, filled with a clear viscous fluid that regulates the amount of pressure on the optic nerve.

Most age-related problems in vision are attributable to changes in parts of the eye. However, there is growing evidence that these problems are aggravated by changes in the central nervous system which block the transmission of stimuli from the sensory organs (Weale, 1975; Ordy and Brizzee, 1979). Changes in the visual pathways of the brain and in the visual cortex may be a possible source of some of the alterations that take place in visual sensation and perception with age.

EFFECTS OF STRUCTURAL CHANGES IN THE CORNEA AND PUPIL

The cornea is usually the first part of the eye to be affected by age-related changes. The surface of the cornea thickens with aging, and the blood vessels become more prominent. The smooth, rounded surface of the cornea becomes flatter and less smooth, and may take on an irregular shape. The older person's eye appears to lose its luster and is less translucent than it was in youth. In some cases, a fatty yellow ring, known as the *arcus senilis*, may form around the cornea. This is not a sign of impending vision loss; in fact, it has no impact on vision. It is sometimes associated with increased lipid deposits in the blood vessels.

At its optimal functioning, the pupil is sensitive to light levels in the environment, widening in response to low light levels, contracting when light levels are high. With aging, the pupil appears to become smaller and more fixed in size. The maximum opening of the pupil is reduced in old age, commonly to about two-thirds the original maximum. That is, the older person's pupil is less able to respond to low light levels by dilating or opening to the extent needed. The eye also responds more slowly to changes in light conditions. This problem is compounded by a slower shift from cones to rods under low-light conditions. As a result, the older person may have considerable difficulty functioning in low-light situations, or in adjusting to significant changes in ambient light. In fact, older people may need three times more light than young persons to function effectively (Pastalan, 1976). These changes may also reduce the older person's ability to discern images in conditions of poor light contrast (e.g., driving at twilight or under foggy or rainy conditions), and to detect details in moving objects (Sekuler and Owsley, 1982; Sekular, Owsley, and Hutman, 1982). For these reasons, older people may choose to avoid such activities, especially driving among fast-moving traffic, on freeways, at night when bright headlights create glare against asphalt surfaces, and in rain. This is a safe approach for coping with age-related difficulties in low-light situations, but older people must be encouraged to maintain their activity level and not become isolated because of declines in visual function. In such instances, families and professionals may have to encourage older people to use other forms of transportation, such as buses and taxis, thereby avoiding the problem of too little environmental stimulation relative to the person's competence.

As another illustration, many older people may feel frustrated when they go to a special restaurant for an evening dinner, only to find that the tables are lit by candles. This makes it difficult to read the menu, to see the way to the table, even to have eye contact with dinner companions. It may also be frustrating for family and friends in such situations if they do not understand that the older person's complaints about the restaurant stem from these changes in vision, not from their lack of appreciation for their efforts. Some older people cope with these problems by avoiding such restaurants altogether or going there only during daylight hours.

PROBLEMS RELATED TO OXYGEN AND FLUID LEVELS

Problems in rod and cone function may be related to a reduced supply of oxygen to the retina (McFarland and Fisher, 1955); oxygen is necessary for the production of rhodopsin, which is a critical element in the functioning of rods. Some researchers have suggested that the slowing of rhodopsin production may be due to a deficiency of vitamin A. However, there is little research evidence to suggest that increased intake of vitamin A in old age can improve visual functioning under low-light conditions.

As stated earlier, there are two fluid-filled chambers in the eye; aqueous humor fills the anterior or front portion of the eye, and vitreous humor is found in the posterior chamber, behind the lens. The aqueous humor drains through the Canal of Schlemm. In the disease state known as *glaucoma,* there may be less efficient drainage, or perhaps excessive production of the aqueous humor. Glaucoma occurs more frequently after middle-age and can be managed with regular medications. More severe cases may require surgery or, more recently, the use of laser treatment. In its later stages, glaucoma may result in tunnel vision, which is a gradual narrowing of an individual's field of vision, such that peripheral vision is lost, and the individual can focus only in the center. Untreated glaucoma is the third leading cause of blindness in the United States (Kornzweig, 1977; Leibowitz et al., 1980), and increases in frequency with aging (see Table 5–1).

Unlike the aqueous humor, which drains and is replenished throughout life in healthy persons, the vitreous humor remains constant. With aging, it may thicken and shrink. Lumps of collagen, the primary content in this fluid, may be formed. Older persons who complain of "floaters" in the eye are responding to these free-floating formations in the front chamber of the eye. These changes, which cannot be prevented or stopped, are often upsetting to individuals. Those who experience them should be assured that floaters do not cause blindness. Frequent examinations by an ophthalmologist are useful in the later years to check for such conditions and to determine if they may be caused by other diseases.

TABLE 5–1 Framingham Eye Study: Prevalence of Major Diseases of the Eye

	Senile Cataract (%)*	Senile Macular Degeneration (%)*	Diabetic Retinopathy (%)*	Open-Angle Glaucoma (%)*
Total	15.5	8.8	3.1	3.3
Age 52–64	4.5	1.6	2.1	1.4
Age 65–74	18.0	11.0	2.9	5.1
Age 75–85	45.9	27.9	7.0	7.2

*Statistically significant increase with age (P < .01)

Source: M. M. Kini, H. M. Leibowitz, T. Colton, R. J. Nickerson, J. Ganley, and T. R. Dawber, Prevalence of senile cataract, diabetic retinopathy, senile macular degeneration and open-angle glaucoma in the Framingham Eye Study. *American Journal of Ophthalmology* 85 (1978): 31. Published with permission from The American Journal of Ophthalmology. Copyright by The Ophthalmic Publishing Company.

EFFECTS OF AGING ON THE LENS

Perhaps the greatest age-related changes in the eye occur in the lens. In fact, it has been suggested that the lens is a model system for studying aging because it contains some of the oldest cells in the body, formed during the earliest stages of the development of the embryo (Vaughan, Schmitz, and Fatt, 1979). Furthermore, the lens is a relatively simple structure biochemically; all of its cells are of the same type, composed of protein.

Collagen is the primary protein in the lens, and makes up 70–80 percent of the total tissue composition of the entire body. As with collagen in other parts of the body, the lens tissue thickens and hardens with age. This makes the lens less elastic, thereby reducing its ability to change form (i.e., from rounded to elongated and flat) as it focuses from near to far. Muscles that help stretch the lens also deteriorate with age, thereby compounding the problem of changing the shape of the lens. This process, known as *accommodation*, begins to deteriorate in middle-age and is manifested in increasing problems with close vision. (We all are familiar with people even in their forties and fifties who need to hold their reading material at arms length!) As a result, many persons in their forties may need to use reading glasses or bifocals. By age 60, accommodative ability is significantly deteriorated (Borish, 1970). Decrements in accommodation may cause difficulties for the older person when shifting from near to far vision; for example, when looking across a room, while walking up or down stairs, when reading and looking up, and when writing notes while looking up at a blackboard or a lecturer.

The hardening of the lens due to changes in collagen tissue does not occur uniformly. Rather, there is differential hardening, with some surfaces allowing more light to enter than others. This results in uneven refraction of light through the lens and onto the retina. When combined with the poor refraction of light through the uneven, flattened surface of the cornea, extreme sensitivity to glare often results. This problem becomes particularly acute in environments with a single source of light aimed at a shiny surface, such as a large window at the end of a long, dark corridor with highly polished floors, occasional street lights on a rain-slicked highway, or a bright, single, overhead incandescent light shining on a linoleum floor. These conditions may contribute to older people's greater caution, and often anxiety, while driving or walking.

From childhood through early adulthood, the lens is a transparent system through which light can easily enter. With normal aging, the lens becomes more opaque, and less light passes through, compounding the problems of poor vision in low light that were described earlier. Some older persons experience a more severe opacification (clouding of the lens) to the point that the lens prevents light from entering. This condition, known as a *cataract*, is the second leading cause of blindness in the United States (Kornzweig, 1978). Its incidence increases significantly with age. Thus, for example, in the Framingham Eye Study (Kini, Leibowitz, Colton, Nickerson, Ganley, and Dawber, 1978), 4.5 percent of the sample aged 52–64 had at least one senile cataract. Among those aged 75–85, 45.9 percent had a cataract in one or both eyes; this represents a tenfold difference between the two age groups (see Table 5–1).

A cataract may occur in any part of the lens, in the center, the peripheral regions, or scattered throughout. A scattered cataract produces extreme opacity in various parts of the lens and causes light to refract at varying densities, resulting in severe problems with glare. If the lens becomes totally opaque, cataract surgery may be required to extract the lens. One of the most frequently performed types of eye surgery, it carries relatively little risk, even for very old persons. A lens implant in place of the extracted lens capsule is a common treatment, but a contact lens or special cataract glasses are alternative treatments. The advantage of the implant is that it does not require the older person to have good finger dexterity to put the lens in the eye and take it out. The implant is particularly useful for the person who still has one natural lens, because it allows an image to form at the same distance in both eyes. When the older person first obtains a substitute lens, it takes some time to adjust to performing daily activities, especially if the artificial lens is not an implant, and the images form on different planes for the two eyes.

In addition to getting harder and more opaque, the lens becomes yellower with age. This is also due to changes in the collagen tissue that makes up the lens. The yellow lens acts as a filter to screen out some wavelengths of light, thus reducing the individual's color sensitivity. This makes it particularly difficult to discriminate among colors that are close together in the color spectrum, especially those in the blue-green-violet range. Older people may have problems selecting clothing in this color range, sometimes resulting in their wearing poorly coordinated outfits. Deterioration in color discrimination may also be due to age-related changes in the visual and neural pathways.

The physical environment can be redesigned to accommodate the older person's competence in this area. For example, older people can benefit from rooms and hallways that use widely contrasting colors on opposite ends of the color spectrum, such as red and yellow, green and orange. Generally, blue and green should not be used to define adjoining spaces, such as stairs and stair landings, floors and ramps, and curbs and curbcuts. This is particularly important when the junction of those spaces represents different levels, so that not seeing these leaves a person at risk of an accident.

OTHER CHANGES IN VISION

Depth and distance perception also deteriorate with aging, because of a loss of convergence of images formed in the two eyes. This is caused by differential rates of hardening and opacification in the two lenses, uneven refraction of light onto the retina, and reduced visual acuity in aging eyes. (The problem of depth perception becomes compounded for people who have had cataract surgery and must use contact lenses or cataract glasses.) As a result, there is a rapid decline after age 75 in the ability to judge distances and depths, particularly in low-light situations and in the absence of orienting cues. Examples of situations with inadequate cues include stairs with no color distinctions at the edges, and pedestrian ramps or curbcuts with varying slopes and no cues to guide the user. The older driver who is undergoing changes in depth perception experiences increased problems when driving behind others, approaching a stop sign, or parking between other cars.

Another change in the visual system that normally occurs with age is narrower peripheral vision (the ability to see on either side without moving the eyes or the head). The field of vision may be as wide as 270° in some young persons, and as narrow as 120° in some older adults. This is because the fovea (or blind spot) increases in size between ages 60 and 90, and retinal metabolism deteriorates, especially in the peripheral region where there are fewer nerve endings. The problem of reduced peripheral vision becomes particularly acute when driving. An older person may not see cars approaching from the left or right at an intersection. Combined with reduced reaction time and age-related musculo-skeletal changes that make turning the neck difficult, older drivers experience greater risks. These changes are often of great concern to family members and friends who worry about whether and how to convince an older person to stop driving.

Some elderly persons experiencing senile macular degeneration may have the opposite problem: loss of the central visual field. The macula is that point in the retina with the best visual acuity, because it has the highest concentration of cones. *Macular degeneration,* the fourth major cause of blindness in the United States, occurs if the macula receives less oxygen than it needs, resulting in destruction of the existing nerve endings in this region. The incidence of macular degeneration, like cataracts, increases with age, but even more dramatically. Of those men and women aged 52–64 in the Framingham study, 1.6 percent had signs of macular degeneration, compared to 27.9 percent of those in the 75–85 age group (Kini et al., 1978).

The early stages of macular degeneration may begin with a loss of detail vision; then central vision gradually becomes worse, so that in severe cases, the older person has poor central vision, but adequate peripheral vision. Total blindness rarely occurs. Older persons with this condition may compensate by using their remaining peripheral vision. They may then appear to be looking at the shoulder of someone they are addressing, but actually be relying on peripheral vision to see the person's face.

Some older people experience reduced secretion of tears, often associated with diseases such as Sjögren's Syndrome. These individuals, most often postmenopausal women, complain of "dry eyes." Unfortunately, this condition has no known cure, but it does not cause blindness and it can be managed with artificial tears to prevent redness and irritation. Artificial tears can be purchased at most drugstores.

The muscles that support the eyes, similar to those in other parts of the body, deteriorate with age. In particular, two key muscles atrophy. These are the elevator muscles, which move the eyeball up and down within its socket, and the ciliary muscle, which aids the lens in changing its shape. Deterioration of the elevator muscles results in a reduced range of upward gaze. This may cause problems with reading overhead signs and seeing objects that are placed above eye level, such as on high kitchen shelves. Weakening of the ciliary muscles contributes to the problem of poor accommodation in the later years.

ASSISTING ADAPTATION THROUGH ENVIRONMENTAL MODIFICATIONS

Because of declining vision, an older person may feel compelled to give up valued social activities, such as playing cards, participating in reading clubs, driving, cooking, and hobbies such as sewing, leathercrafts, and stamp collecting. Abandoning these activities often produces a sense of loss and isolation. Furthermore, the environment outside the home can become too demanding and difficult to negotiate safely. Family and friends can assist by providing psychological support and by improving the physical environment to support rather than hinder an older person who is experiencing these changes.

In terms of maintaining person-environment congruence and psychological well-being, an aging person should be encouraged to maintain social contacts, even if new activities must be substituted for old. Older people can take advantage of large-print newspapers and books, as well as "talking books" that are available in many community libraries. Playing cards with large letters also can be beneficial for the person who wishes to continue participating in bridge club activities. Local agencies serving the visually impaired often provide low-vision aids at minimal cost. These include needle threaders for sewing; templates for rotary telephones, irons, and other appliances; large-print phone books, clocks, and calendars; and magnifying glasses for situations where large-print substitutes are unavailable.

Family and friends also can help by improving the physical environment inside and around an older person's home. These changes may be as simple as replacing existing lightbulbs with higher wattage bulbs and putting large-print labels on prescription bottles, spices, and cooking supplies. Other environmental modifications may be more costly or require the use of a professional architect. Contrasting color strips on stairs, especially on carpeted or slippery linoleum stairs, are beneficial in aiding the older person's depth perception. Color and light coding of ramps and other changes in elevation also can be valuable. Increasing the number of light sources and installing nonslip and nonglossy floor coverings can reduce the problem of glare. An even better architectural solution is to use indirect or task lighting (e.g., reading lamps, countertop lamps).

All these solutions can go a long way to enhance the competence of a person who is experiencing gradual declines in visual functions. Age-related changes in vision need not handicap people if they can be encouraged to adapt their usual activities to their current level of visual functioning. Friends, family, and professionals can also aid the elderly in adapting their environments to fit their needs. An older person who is having difficulty adjusting to losses produced by vision decrements may initially resist such changes. One way to address this resistance is for family members and professionals to involve the older person in decisions about environmental modifications and alternative activities.

Changes in Hearing

In terms of survival, vision and hearing are perhaps our most critical links to the world. Whereas vision is important for negotiating the physical environment, hearing is vital for communication. Because hearing is closely associated with speech, its loss disrupts a person's understanding of others and even the recognition of one's own speech. Consider some ways in which we rely on our hearing ability in everyday life: in conversations with family, friends, and co-workers; in localizing the sound of approaching automobiles as we cross the street or drive; and in interpreting other people's emotions through their tone of voice and use of language.

How does a person function if these abilities gradually deteriorate? Clearly, an older person who is experiencing hearing loss learns to adapt and make changes in behavior and in social interactions, so as to reduce the detrimental social impact of hearing loss. Many younger hearing-impaired persons learn sign language or lip reading. But these are complex skills requiring extensive training and practice. Those who experience gradual hearing loss late in life are much less likely to learn them.

THE ANATOMY AND PHYSIOLOGY OF THE EAR

It is useful to review the physiology of the ear in order to understand where and how auditory function deteriorates with age. The auditory system has three components, as illustrated in Figure 5–2. The outer ear begins at the pinna, that visible portion that is identified as the ear. The auditory canal is also part of the outer ear. Note the shape of the pinna and auditory canal; it is a most efficient design for localizing sounds.

The eardrum, or tympanic membrane, is a thin membrane that separates the outer ear from the middle ear. This membrane is sensitive to air pressure of varying degrees and vibrates in response to a range of loud and soft sounds. In the middle ear are located three bones: the malleus, the incus, and the stapes, more commonly known as the hammer, the anvil, and the stirrup (so named because of their shapes). These very finely positioned and interrelated bones carry sound vibrations from the middle ear to the inner ear—that snail-shaped circular structure called the cochlea. Amplified sounds are converted in the cochlea to nerve impulses which are then sent through the internal auditory canal and the cochlear nerve to the brain, where they are translated into meaningful sounds.

FIGURE 5–2 The Ear

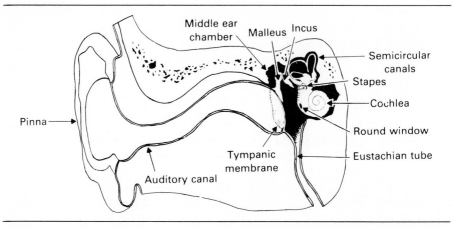

The cochlea is a fluid-filled chamber with thousands of hair cells that vibrate two parallel membranes to move sound waves. Low-pitched sounds stimulate hair cells at the base of the cochlea; high-pitched sounds stimulate hair cells at the apex. The vibration of these hair cells is one of several factors involved in the perception of pitch (or frequency) and loudness (intensity) of a sound.

AGE-RELATED CHANGES

The pinna appears somewhat elongated and rigid in some elderly. These changes in the outer ear, however, have no impact on hearing acuity. The supporting walls of the external auditory canals also deteriorate with age, as is true for many muscular structures in the human body, including, as we have seen, the muscles of the eye. Arthritic conditions may affect the joints between the malleus and stapes, making it more difficult for these bones to perform their vibratory function. Otosclerosis is a condition in which the stapes becomes fixed and cannot vibrate. It is sometimes found in young persons, but more frequently occurs in the later years.

The greatest decline with age occurs in the cochlea, where structural changes result in *presbycusis,* or age-related hearing loss. Changes in auditory thresholds can be detected by age 30 or even younger, but the degeneration of hair cells and membranes in the cochlea is not observed until much later (Ordy, Brizzee, Beavers, and Medart, 1979). It is estimated that 13 percent of the population age 65 and older in the United States suffer from advanced presbycusis. Another 40 to 50 percent have mild to moderate loss of hearing (Corso, 1977; Stevens-Long, 1979; Rockstein and Sussman, 1979).

As with studies regarding changes in the visual system, researchers in the area of auditory perception have suggested that changes in the brain are responsible for the deterioration in auditory functioning. These may include cellular deterioration and vascular changes in the major auditory pathways to the brain (Corso, 1977).

Hearing Loss and Personality Change

Some researchers have suggested that hearing problems lead to social isolation and reduced intellectual functioning (Granick, Kleban, and Weiss, 1976; Hull and Traynor, 1977; Rockstein and Sussman, 1979; Gilhome-Herbst and Humphrey, 1980). However, it is difficult to distinguish the effect of hearing acuity from true intellectual functioning, since most tests of cognitive function demand some hearing ability. A recent study found that elderly with hearing loss did not do as well on verbal tests of cognition as older persons with no hearing loss. The researchers found no differences in nonverbal tests (Thomas, Hunt, Garry, Hood, Goodwin, and Goodwin, 1983). Emotional stability and social integration were also found to be unaffected by hearing loss. In another study, Norris and Cunningham (1981) questioned fifty older persons with high-frequency hearing loss about their social interactions and organizational involvement and found no association between hearing loss and social involvement. These findings support the results of a study by Powers and Powers (1978), who found that hearing loss does not significantly affect older people's social involvement.

There is some clinical evidence that older persons with a diagnosis of paranoia are more likely to have severe hearing problems than are normal elderly. This appears to be particularly true among paranoid persons who have had the hearing loss since middle-age. Some research with hospitalized aged psychiatric patients supports these clinical observations (Cooper and Curry, 1976). In contrast, Moore's (1981) study of elderly psychiatric patients in the United Kingdom revealed no association between deafness and paranoid disorders. It should be noted that this latter study did not obtain information on the duration of the deafness or the psychiatric disorder. A study of community elderly has confirmed the lack of association between hearing disorders and emotional distress (Thomas et al., 1983).

It is important to note that these are *correlational* findings; that is, the finding that some elderly who have psychiatric symptoms are also hearing impaired does not provide sufficient evidence to conclude that hearing impairments that begin in middle-age will cause paranoid reactions in old age. Other reports of the *co-existence* of hearing loss and psychiatric disorders in older populations (Gilhome-Herbst and Humphrey, 1980; Eastwood et al., 1985) must also be interpreted with caution because the data are correlational. In summary, we cannot conclude that there is a causal relationship between hearing loss and cognitive or affective disorders in old age.

Tinnitus is another problem that affects hearing in old age. This is a high-pitched "ringing" that is particularly acute at night or in quiet surroundings. It may occur bilaterally or in one ear only. The incidence increases from 3 percent for younger adults to 9 percent for middle-aged persons and 11 percent among those aged 65 to 74 (Rockstein and Sussman, 1979).

In contrast to visual changes, hearing loss appears to be significantly affected by environmental causes. People who have been exposed to high-volume and high-frequency noise throughout their lives (e.g., urban dwellers, factory workers) experience more hearing decrements in old age than do those from rural, low-noise environments. Women generally show less decline than men (see Figure 5–3). It is interesting to speculate why these sex differences appear. Are they due to variations in noise exposure or to hormonal differences between men and women? The fact that severe hearing loss is found in some women suggests that the former hypothesis may be more likely.

COMPENSATION AND ADAPTATION

Hearing loss can be of several types, involving limited volume and range or distortion of sounds perceived. Older persons who have lost hearing acuity in the range of speech (250–3,000 Hz.) have particular difficulties distinguishing the sibilants or high-frequency consonants such as *z, s, sh, f, p, k, t*, and *g*. Their speech comprehension deteriorates as a result, which may be the first sign of hearing loss. An individual experiencing increased problems with hearing may compensate by raising the volume of the TV and radio, moving closer to the TV, or even by listening to other types of music made by lower pitched instruments such as an organ. When this occurs, it is imperative to determine whether a hearing loss exists, to identify the cause, and to fit the individual with an appropriate hearing aid, if that is possible. A hearing aid increases the volume of sound. This may compensate for loss of higher frequency sounds, but hearing aids cannot completely obliterate the problem of presbycusis. In fact, they often result in such major adaptation problems that many older persons stop wearing them after several months of frustrated attempts to adjust to the device. A major difficulty with hearing aids is that the volume of background noise is raised, in addition to the sound that the user of the device is trying to hear. There is also a greater social stigma associated with wearing a hearing aid than with wearing glasses. These are undoubtedly some of the reasons why relatively few older people who are hearing-impaired use them.

If an older person feels stigmatized by the hearing aid, emotional support from others can be useful in easing the adjustment. If the hearing aid does not appear to fit an older person's needs, a replacement should be sought. Fortunately, developments in hearing aid technology are resulting in custom-made designs that amplify only those frequencies that an individual user has trouble hearing, without magnifying background noises. These newer designs also are less obtrusive and fit well inside the ear.

FIGURE 5–3 Sex Differences in Hearing Thresholds

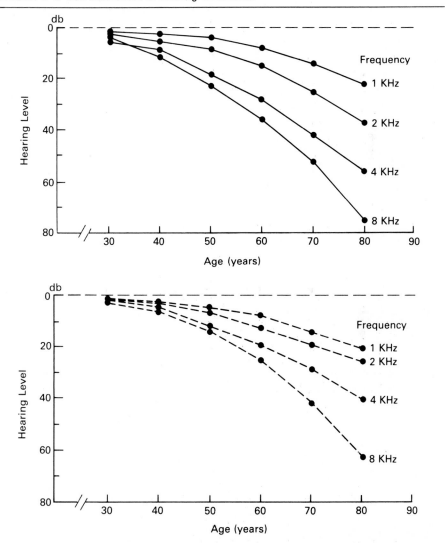

Source: J. M. Ordy, K. R. Brizzee, T. Beavers, and P. Medart. In J. M. Ordy and K. R. Brizzee (Eds.), *Sensory systems and communication in the elderly* (New York: Raven Press, 1979), p. 156. Reprinted with permission of the author and publisher.

   Other means of compensating for hearing loss are to design environments that dampen background noises or to select such settings for communicating with older persons. Soundproof rooms are beneficial, particularly if housing for older people is built on busy streets or near freeways, but this is a costly alternative. Clinics and offices of health professionals should have at least one quiet area where an older patient can communicate with professionals without being distracted by background noises. Older people who are experiencing auditory decline can also benefit from new designs in telephones with volume adjusters and lights that blink when the phone rings.

When conversing with people who are experiencing age-related hearing loss, the following hints can help both younger and older persons enjoy their communication:

1. Face an older person directly.
2. Sit somewhat close.
3. Do not cover the face with hands or objects when speaking.
4. Speak slowly and clearly, but without exaggerating speech.
5. Do not shout.
6. Avoid distracting background noises by selecting an appropriate place away from other people, machines, and traffic sounds.
7. Speak in a lower, but not monotonic, tone of voice.
8. Repeat key points in different ways.

One of the most frustrating experiences for some older people is the simultaneous deterioration of both hearing and vision. Although it is relatively rare for aging to result in significant declines in both these functions, family members, friends, and professionals must be especially sensitive to the communication techniques described earlier. When talking with an older person who is impaired in both hearing and vision, touching his or her hand, arm, or shoulder may aid communication.

Changes in Taste and Smell

Although many older people complain that food does not taste as good as it once did, research findings about taste and smell sensitivity in old age are less conclusive than those regarding vision and hearing. Some studies have suggested higher recognition thresholds among older persons for the taste of sucrose and sodium chloride (Bourliere, Cendron, and Rapaport, 1958; Byrd and Gertman, 1959; Cooper, Bilash, and Zubek, 1959; Richter and Campbell, 1940). However, more recent research has shown only minimal changes with age (Hermel, Schonwetter, and Samueloff, 1970; Kranz, Berndt, and Wagner, 1977; Murphy, 1979; Weiffenbach, Baum, and Burghauser, 1982). It is difficult to conclude with certainty that changes in taste sensitivity are a normal process of aging because individual variability is so much greater in older people than among younger people. External factors such as smoking and medications contribute to these differences. The varied findings across studies may also be due to a lack of control for response criteria or salivary changes which could affect taste acuity (Weiffenbach, Baum, and Burghauser, 1982).

There is more evidence for reduced sensitivity to smell among older persons, and this, in fact, may be the cause of lowered taste discrimination. The olfactory, or smell receptors, are located in the upper part of the nasal cavity. These receptors show some deterioration with age, although this does not necessarily cause a loss of olfactory sensitivity. Individuals who have acute olfactory sensitivity in their youth apparently retain this in their later years; in a unique study of healthy perfumers aged 70 to 78, olfactory acuity was very high (Schiffman, 1979).

Certain problems are associated with reduced sensitivity to taste and smell. For example, declines in the recognition and identification of odors, especially the odor of gas, has been found in people over age 80 (Anand, 1964). This raises an important safety concern with this age group. Some older people compensate for losses in taste sensitivity by increasing their salt intake. This is not only harmful for individuals with hypertension, but it is also ineffective if the lack of taste is really due to reduced sensitivity to the smell of food. Other older people may find that food is so unappetizing that they lose interest in it, and eat only when they are very hungry. This is risky because it may result in poor nutrition. A better approach is to enhance the flavor of foods with herbs and spices, and with

Cooking classes can enhance the enjoyment of food.

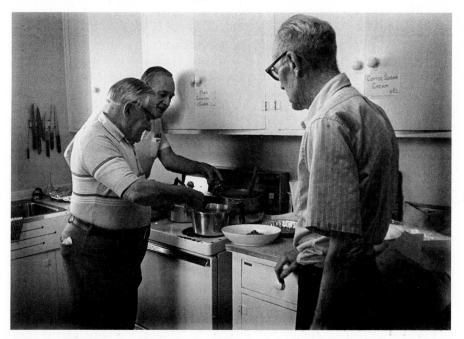

pleasant aromas (e.g., basil, tarragon, cinnamon) that do not disturb the older person's digestive system, and may actually enhance the digestive process. Classes in cooking with herbs and spices can be valuable for older people who are experiencing changes in their taste and olfactory abilities. Along with cooking techniques, the nutritional value of each ingredient, and the benefits and potential harm of each spice and herb should be reviewed in these classes. These activities can also help older people in sharpening their sensitivity to tastes and odors.

Changes in the Sense of Touch

Somesthetic or touch sensitivity also deteriorates with age. This is partially due to changes in the skin (see Chapter 4) and partially to a loss with age in the number of nerve endings. Reduced touch sensitivity is especially prevalent in the fingertips and palms, and in the lower extremities (Whanger and Wang, 1974; Kenshalo, 1979; Verillo, 1980).

An important aspect of touch sensitivity is pain perception. The elderly tend to be less able to discriminate among levels of perceived pain than young respondents. Studies of age differences in threshold levels of pain, however, have produced mixed results (Harkins and Warner, 1980).

It is important to distinguish between pain perception and pain behavior. Tolerance for pain is a subjective experience, which has been found to be related to cultural and personality factors (Zborowski, 1952). In older people, increased complaints of pain may be a function of depression and psychosomatic needs. On the other hand, some people may attempt to minimize their pain by not reporting above-threshold levels of unpleasant stimuli. This is consistent with a frequently observed attitude among many older persons that pain, illness, and discomfort are necessary corollaries of aging. In fact, most elderly probably underreport actual pain experienced. For example, an older person may not report symptoms of a heart attack unless or until it is severe. This has significant implications for health-seeking behaviors among older persons, as will be discussed in Chapter 6.

Changes in Mobility and the Kinesthetic Sense

Although the incidence of mobility problems is greater among the elderly, aging per se is not the cause of motor disabilities. Disease states such as arthritis, stroke, some cardiac disorders, and damage to the kinesthetic sense may affect both the peripheral and central mechanisms responsible for mobility. Other factors limiting mobility include stiffness of joints, reduced ability to raise or turn the neck, and difficulty in gait and posture. Arthritis is a common chronic disease in older people that has a major impact on daily functioning, as will be discussed in

Chapter 6. Simple tasks, such as reaching cupboards and overhead shelves, may become more difficult for an older person with arthritis or *kyphosis* (i.e., curvature of the spine due to osteoporosis). These conditions occur more frequently in older women. Combined with declines in the visual system that limit peripheral vision and upward gaze, an older person experiencing stiffness of neck joints and kyphosis must make adjustments while driving. Environmental modifications, such as a driver's seat that tilts back and raises to fit an older driver's special needs, can be useful.

The kinesthetic system lets an individual know his or her position in space; adjustments in body position become known through kinesthetic cues. Because of age-related changes in the central nervous system, which controls the kinesthetic mechanism, as well as in muscles, older people demonstrate a decreased ability to orient their bodies in space and to detect externally induced changes in body position. Other physiological and disease-related changes, such as damage to the inner ear, may exacerbate this problem. Researchers who have

---

An Older Person with
Multiple Sensory Impairments

Mrs. Wilson is an 82-year-old widow who has lived on her own for the past 20 years since her husband died. She had cataract surgery 12 years ago in her left eye, and began wearing a hearing aid 10 years ago. She has adjusted quite well to these changes in her vision and hearing, and remains active in her monthly bridge club and volunteering at the local library. The only situations she avoids are large gatherings, such as lunch at the senior center where it always seems to be too noisy for her to enjoy conversations with her friends. More recently, Mrs. Wilson has stopped driving at night because of increasing sensitivity to glare and problems with finding her way on the poorly lit rural roads near her home. She enjoys gardening and is proud of her rose garden with its varied fragrances in the summer. Recently she has noticed a slight loss of her well-honed skills in telling apart one variety of rose from another by their fragrances, but she remains better at it than her children and grandchildren! She also plants aromatic herbs in her garden so she can use them to perk up her cooking. The medications she has been taking over the past several years seem to have affected her taste sensitivity, so she enjoys cooking with herbs and spices for herself and her friends. Mrs. Wilson realizes that her vision, hearing, taste, and smell have all declined as she has aged, but she is determined to make the best use of her remaining abilities in these senses. The changes she has made in her environment, such as avoiding night driving and using more herbs in cooking, are examples of Mrs. Wilson's attempts to maintain person-environment congruence.

compared old and young subjects have found that older persons need more external cues to orient themselves in space, and can be incorrect by 5 to 20 degrees in estimating their position.

Not surprisingly, these changes in motor functioning and in the kinesthetic system result in greater caution among older persons, who then tend to take slower, shuffling, and more deliberate steps. Older people are more likely to seek external spatial cues and supports while walking. As a result, they are less likely to go outside in inclement weather for fear of slipping or falling. Some may complain of dizziness and vertigo. These normal, age-related changes combine with the problems of slower reaction time, muscle weakness, and reduced visual acuity to make it far more likely for older people to fall and injure themselves.

Summary and Implications

Changes in sensory function with age do not occur at a consistent rate in all senses and for all people. Some people show rapid declines in vision while maintaining their hearing and other sensory abilities. Others experience an early deterioration in olfactory sensation, but not in other areas. All of us experience some loss in these functions with age, but interindividual differences are quite pronounced.

Normal age-related declines in vision reduce the ability to respond to differing light levels, to function in low-light situations, to see in places with high light contrast with glare, to discern color tones, especially in the green-blue-violet range, and to judge distances and depth. Peripheral vision becomes somewhat narrowed with age, as does upward and downward gaze. Older people have more diseases of the eye, including glaucoma, cataracts, and macular degeneration; if these diseases are not treated, blindness can result. The older person who experiences significant declines in visual function with age should be encouraged to maintain former levels of activity, either by adapting the environment to fit changing needs or by substituting new activities for those that have become more difficult. Some older people prefer to withdraw from previous activities, thereby becoming more isolated and at risk of depression.

Decline in auditory function generally starts earlier than visual problems, and affects more people. Significant impairments in speech comprehension often result. Although hearing aids can frequently help improve hearing in the speech range, many older people feel uncomfortable and even stigmatized when using them. Hence, the solutions to communicating with hearing-impaired older people may lie mostly within the environment, not within older persons themselves. These include changes in communication styles, such as speaking directly at an older person in a clear voice, but not shouting; speaking in a lower tone; repeating key points; and sitting closer to a hearing-impaired person.

Environmental aids such as soundproof or quiet rooms and modified telephones can also be invaluable for older people who are experiencing significant hearing declines.

Although many older people complain that food does not taste as good as it once did, there are only minimal changes with age in taste acuity, despite a significant loss in the number of taste buds. The decline in olfactory receptors with age is more significant than in taste receptors, and may be responsible for the perception of reduced taste acuity. These changes are more pronounced in people who smoke or drink heavily, and in those who use certain medications. There is less change in people who have sharpened their taste and olfactory sensitivity, such as professional winemakers and perfumers. This pattern suggests that older people should be encouraged to participate in activities that enhance their taste and olfactory functions.

Age-related changes in touch sensitivity can affect pain perception and produce reduced sensitivity in the extremities (e.g., fingertips, palms, toes). This could place an older person at greater risk of scalding because of an inability to detect high water and surface temperatures. Slower reaction times and poorer kinesthetic responses with aging often result in slower movement and greater caution in older people, especially in unfamiliar environments or where surfaces are slippery or wet.

As we have seen in previous chapters, normal aging does not lead to disability. However, the changes that occur with normal aging, as noted here and elsewhere, are likely to result in a slowing of functions, increased caution, and a reduction of physical activity. This should not be considered a sign of disease but a recognition of the older person's sensory and physical limitations and capabilities.

Older people should be encouraged to maximize use of all their functions, so that deterioration does not occur more rapidly than necessary. Unfortunately, the fear of not being able to hear, see, or maintain their balance keeps many older people tied to their homes and increases the risk of social isolation. It is important for people of all ages to maintain their activity levels because those who use their neuromuscular functions, sensory capacities, and cognitive skills regularly can prevent premature deterioration of these functions. Hence, the recognition of and use of one's capacities to the fullest should begin early in life and continue into advanced old age.

As we learn more from studies of sensory changes with aging, reports that once appeared definitive are found to be less so, and a complete understanding of some areas is shown to be lacking. This is particularly true in the areas of taste, smell, and pain perception. Research is needed to distinguish normal changes in these areas from those that are related to disease, and those that can be prevented. Longitudinal research would help to answer many of these questions. Finally, research that examines the impact of sensory deterioration on the older person's interactions with the environment is also needed.

References

Anand, M. P. Accidents in the home. In W. F. Anderson and B. Isaacs (Eds.), *Current achievements in geriatrics*. London: Cassell, 1964.

Applegate, W. B., Runyan, J. W., Brasfield, L., Williams, M. L., Konigsberg, C., and Fouche, C. Analysis of the 1980 heat wave in Memphis. *Journal of the American Geriatrics Society*, 1981, *29*, 337–342.

Avery, W. M. Hypothermia and heat illness. *Aging*, 1984, *344*, 43–47.

Borish, J. M. *Clinical refraction* (3rd ed.). Chicago: Professional Press, 1970.

Bourlière, F., Cendron, H., and Rapaport, A. Modification avec l'age des senils gustatifs de perception et de reconnaissance aux saveurs salée et sucrée chez l'homme. *Gerontologie*, 1958, *2*, 104–112.

Bradley, R. M., Stedman, H. M., and Mistretta, C. M. A quantitative study of lingual taste buds and papillae in the aging rhesus monkey tongue. In R. T. Davis and Charles W. Leathers (Eds.), *Behavioral pathology of aging in rhesus monkeys*. New York: A. R. Liss, 1985.

Byrd, E., and Gertman, S. Taste sensitivity in aging persons. *Geriatrics*, 1959, *14*, 381–384.

Cooper A. F., and Curry, A. R. The pathology of deafness in the paranoid and affective psychoses of later life. *Journal of Psychosomatic Research*, 1976, *20*, 97–105.

Cooper, R. M., Bilash, I., and Zubek, J. P. The effect of age on taste sensitivity. *Journal of Gerontology*, 1959, *14*, 56–58.

Corso, J. F. Auditory perception and communication. In J. E. Birren and K. W. Schaie (Eds.), *Handbook of the psychology of aging* (1st ed.). New York: Van Nostrand Reinhold, 1977.

Eastwood, M. R., Corbin, S. L., Reed, M., Nobbs, H., and Kedward, H. B. Acquired hearing loss and psychiatric illness: An estimate of prevalence and co-morbidity in a geriatric setting. *British Journal of Psychiatry*, 1985, *147*, 552–556.

Foster, K. G., Ellis, F. P., Doré C., Exton-Smith, A. N., and Weiner, J. S. Sweat responses in the aged. *Age and Ageing*, 1976, *5*, 91–101.

Gilhome-Herbst, K., and Humphrey, C. Hearing impairment and mental state in the elderly living at home. *British Medical Journal*, 1980, *281*, 903–905.

Granick, S., Kleban, M. H., and Weiss, A. D. Relationships between hearing loss and cognition in normally hearing aged persons. *Journal of Gerontology*, 1976, *31*, 434–440.

Harkins, S. W., and Warner, M. H. Age and pain. In C. Eisdorfer (Ed.), *Annual review of gerontology and geriatrics* (vol. 1). New York: Springer, 1980.

Hermel, J., Schonwetter, S., and Samueloff, S. Taste sensation identification and age in man. *Journal of Oral Medicine*, 1970, *25*, 39–42.

Hull, R., and Traynor, R. Hearing impairments among aging persons in a health care facility. *American Health Care Association Journal*, 1977, *3*, 14–18.

Kenshalo, D. R. Changes in the vestibular and somesthetic systems as a function of age. In J. M. Ordy and K. R. Brizzee (Eds.), *Sensory systems and communication in the elderly*. New York: Raven Press, 1979.

Kini, M. M., Leibowitz, H. M., Colton, T., Nickerson, R. J., Ganley, J., and Dawber, T. R. Prevalence of senile cataract, diabetic retinopathy, senile macular degeneration and open-angle glaucoma in the Framingham Eye Study. *American Journal of Ophthalmology,* 1978, *85,* 28–34.

Kolanowski, A., and Gunter, L. Hypothermia in the elderly. *Geriatric Nursing,* 1981, *2,* 362–365.

Kornzweig, A. L. Visual loss in the elderly. *Hospital Practice,* 1977, *12,* 51–59.

Kranz, D., Berndt, H., and Wagner, H. In J. E. Birren and K. W. Schaie (Eds.), *Handbook of the psychology of aging.* New York: Van Nostrand Reinhold, 1977.

Leibowitz, H. M., Krueger, D. E., Maunder, L. R., Milton, R. C., Kini, M. M., Kahn, H. A., Nickerson, R. J., Pool, J., Colton, T. L., and Ganley, J. P. The Framingham Eye Study Monograph. *Survey of Ophthalmology* Supplement, 1980, *24,* 335–610.

McFarland, R. A., and Fisher, M. B. Alterations in dark adaptation as a function of age. *Journal of Gerontology,* 1955, *10,* 424–428.

Mistretta, C. M. Aging effects on anatomy and neurophysiology of taste and smell. *Gerodontology,* 1984, *3,* 131–136.

Moore, N. C. Is paranoid illness associated with sensory defects in the elderly? *Journal of Psychosomatic Research,* 1981, *25,* 69–74.

Murphy, C. The effect of age on taste sensitivity. In S. Han and D. Coons (Eds.), *Special senses in aging.* Ann Arbor: Institute of Gerontology, University of Michigan, 1979.

Murphy, C. Effects of aging on food perception. *Journal of the American College of Nutrition,* 1982, *1,* 128.

National Center for Health Statistics. Current estimates from the national health interview survey. *Vital and Health Statistics,* 1975, Series 10, No. 115.

Norris, M. L., and Cunningham, D. R. Social impact of hearing loss in the aged. *Journal of Gerontology,* 1981, *36,* 727–729.

Ordy, J. M., Brizzee, K. R., Beavers, T., and Medart, P. Age differences in the functional and structural organization of the auditory system in man. In J. M. Ordy and K. R. Brizzee (Eds.), *Sensory systems and communication in the elderly.* New York: Raven Press, 1979.

Ordy, J. M., and Brizzee, K. R. (Eds.). *Sensory systems and communication in the elderly.* New York: Raven Press, 1979.

Pastalan, L., et al. *Age-related vision and hearing changes: An empathic approach.* Slide-tape program developed at the University of Michigan, Ann Arbor, 1976.

Powers, J. K., and Powers, E. A. Hearing problems of elderly persons: Social consequences and prevalence. *Journal of the American Speech and Hearing Association (ASHA),* 1978, *20,* 79–83.

Richter, C. P., and Campbell, K. H. Sucrose taste thresholds of rats and humans. *American Journal of Physiology,* 1940, *128,* 291–297.

Rockstein, M., and Sussman, M. *Biology of aging.* Belmont, Calif.: Wadsworth, 1979.

Schiffman, S. Changes in taste and smell with age: Psychophysical aspects. In J. M. Ordy and K. R. Brizzee (Eds.), *Sensory systems and communication in the elderly.* New York: Raven Press, 1979.

Sekuler, R., and Owsley, C. The spatial vision of older humans. In *Aging and human visual function*. New York: Alan R. Liss, 1982.

Sekuler, R., Owsley, C., and Hutman, L. Assessing spatial vision of older people. *American Journal of Optometry and Physiological Optics*, 1982, *59*, 961–968.

Stevens-Long, J. *Adult life*. Palo Alto, Calif.: Mayfield, 1979.

Thomas, P. D., Hunt, W. C., Garry, P. J., Hood, R. B., Goodwin, J. M., and Goodwin, J. S. Hearing acuity in a healthy elderly population: Effects on emotional, cognitive and social status. *Journal of Gerontology*, 1983, *38*, 321–325.

Vaughan, W. J., Schmitz, P., and Fatt, J. The human lens: A model system for the study of aging. In J. M. Ordy and K. R. Brizzee (Eds.), *Sensory systems and communication in the elderly*. New York: Raven Press, 1979.

Venstrom, D., and Amoore, J. E. Olfactory threshold in relation to age, sex or smoking. *Journal of Food Science*, 1968, *33*, 264–265.

Verillo, R. T. Age-related changes in the sensitivity to vibration. *Journal of Gerontology*, 1980, *35*, 185–193.

Weale, R. A. Senile changes in visual acuity. *Transactions of the Ophthalmological Societies of the U.K.*, 1975, *95*, 36–38.

Weiffenbach, J. M., Baum, B. J., and Burghauser, R. Taste thresholds: Quality specific variation with human aging. *Journal of Gerontology*, 1982, *37*, 372–377.

Whanger, A. D., and Wang, H. S. Clinical correlates of the vibratory sense in elderly psychiatric patients. *Journal of Gerontology*, 1974, *29*, 39–45.

Zborowski, A. Cultural components in response to pain. *Journal of Social Issues*, 1952, *8*, 16–30.

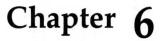

Chapter 6

Health, Chronic Diseases, and Use of Health Services

No aspect of old age is more alarming to many of us than the thought of losing our health. Our fears center not only on the pain and inconvenience of illness, but also on its social-psychological consequences, such as loss of personal autonomy and financial burdens we may face. Poor health, more than any other change commonly associated with aging, can reduce a person's competence in dealing with his or her environment.

This chapter examines social and psychological factors that affect perceptions of health and use of health services, looking first at definitions of good health and how the social context, especially stress, affects it. Chronic and acute health problems are then differentiated, followed by a discussion of the most common chronic diseases experienced by older people and some of their social consequences. The remainder of the chapter is devoted to utilization of health care by the elderly, including descriptions of three models for predicting and analyzing health behavior. Health promotion programs are briefly described as a way to reduce the incidence of chronic diseases, primarily through altering health behaviors.

Defining Health

It is not necessary to argue that good health is valued, but what do we mean by *good health*? Most people would agree that health is something more than the mere absence of disease or infirmity. As defined by the World Health Organization in 1947, health is a state of complete physical, mental, and social well-being. Thus, health implies an interaction and integration of body, mind, and spirit, a perspective that is reflected in the growth of health promotion programs with the elderly.

As used by health care workers and researchers, the term *health status* refers to: (1) the presence or absence of disease, and (2) the degree of disability in an individual's level of functioning (Branch, 1980; Kane and Kane, 1981; World Health Organization, 1974). Thus, activities that older people can do, or think they can do, are useful indicators of both how healthy they are and the services and environmental changes they need in order to cope with their impairments. Older people's ability to function independently at home is of primary concern. The most commonly used measure of this ability, termed the *Activities of Daily Living* (ADL), summarizes an individual's performance in personal care tasks such as bathing, dressing, using the toilet, eating, getting in or out of a bed or chair, caring for a bowel control device, as well as such instrumental activities as managing money, shopping, light housework, meal preparation, making a phone call, and taking medications (Jette and Branch, 1981; National Center for Health Statistics, 1982).

Less than 20 percent of older people are estimated to have a mild degree of disability in their ADL. Only a small proportion—approximately 4 percent—are severely disabled (Manton and Liu, 1984). The more disabled elderly are limited in their amounts and types of major activities and mobility, such as eating, dressing, bathing, or toiletry. Severely disabled persons are often unable to carry on major activities without the assistance of family or professionals. The extent of disabilities and need for help in personal care activities increase with age, as shown in Figure 6–1. Those aged 85 and older are four to six times more likely to be disabled and to require assistance than those aged 65 to 74. About 46 percent of persons over age 85 are disabled, compared to about 13 percent of those aged 65 to 74, and 25 percent aged 75 to 84 (Manton and Liu, 1984). In 1985, approximately 5.2 million persons 65 years or older were estimated to need assistance in order to remain in the community. This figure is expected to reach 7.2 million by the year 2000, 10.1 million by 2020, and 14.4 million by 2050 (U.S. Senate Special Committee on Aging, 1986).

FIGURE 6–1 Percent of the Population with Severe Activity Limitation: 1982

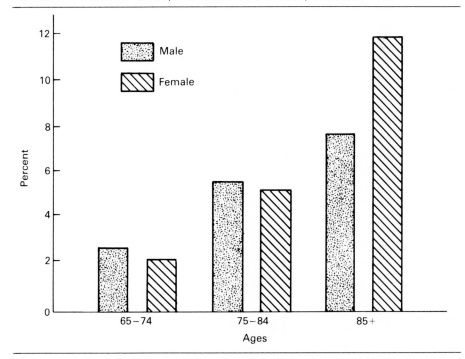

Source: National Center for Health Statistics, *Preliminary Data from the 1982 Long Term Care Survey.* Comparison percent of their age counterparts with incomes less than $7,000, 1982.

The Social Psychological Context of Health

Societal values affect our attitudes toward loss of health. In our own culture, these attitudes tend to be negative. The importance placed by our culture on being independent and highly active may underlie the relative inability of North Americans to accept illness graciously, as compared with the Danes and the British, for example (Shanas et al., 1968). Such values may also explain why healthy elderly often do not want to share housing or recreational activities with those who have mental or physical disabilities.

Yet the fear of declining health may trouble us more than the actual experience of it. Although younger people assume that health issues are older people's greatest preoccupation, only 21 percent of the elderly in a 1981 Harris poll considered this to be the case (Harris et al., 1981). In fact, most older people appear to be fairly positive about their health. A 1982 survey by the National Center for Health Statistics indicated that 65 percent of elderly in the community described their health as excellent, very good, or good compared to their age peers, while only 35 percent reported their health as fair or poor (National Center for Health Statistics, 1982). In an earlier survey, older persons with long-term chronic disabilities rate their overall health as much better than those who were just beginning to experience chronic illness (Shanas, 1962). Even institutionalized older persons tend to rate their health positively (Ferraro, 1980; Fillenbaum, 1979). These positive ratings, despite health problems, have been explained in terms of comparison to peers, a sense of accomplishment from having survived to old age, and a perception of competence to meet environmental demands (Myles, 1978). Most older people appear to adjust their perceptions of their health in response to the aging process (Cockerham, Sharp, and Wilcox, 1983).

Perceptions of good health tend to be associated with other measures of well-being, particularly life satisfaction. Older persons who perceive themselves as reasonably healthy tend to be happier, more satisfied, more involved in social activities, and less tense and lonely. In turn, lower life satisfaction is associated with lower levels of self-perceived health (Cockerham, Sharp, and Wilcox, 1983).

Social and psychological factors undoubtedly influence people's assessments of their physical well-being. An older person's position in the social structure—for example, whether one is male or female, black or white, high or low income—affects perceptions of health. Thus, while 69 percent of white persons age 65 and older rate their health as good or excellent, only 54 percent of Blacks and 65 percent of Hispanics that age do so. More than 40 percent of persons aged 65 and older with incomes over $25,000 rate their health as excellent, compared with 25 percent of their age counterparts with incomes less than $7,000 (National Center for Health Statistics, 1981). In most cases, these self-assessments are fairly accurate, since ethnic minority and lower-income elderly do, in fact, have poorer health, as is discussed later in this chapter. The historical time period through which a person has lived and in which one is living may also have an effect. A reliable evaluation of health takes into account not only a physician's assessment of a patient's physical condition, but the older person's self-perceptions, observable behavior, and life circumstances. Some studies have found that older people's self-perceptions of health are fairly accurate and correlate reasonably well with physicians' ratings and with more objective indices (Ferraro, 1980; Fillenbaum, 1979).

Effects of Stress on Health

As the previous discussions suggest, health status involves the dynamic interplay among physical, social, and psychological forces. Environmental factors affect both perceptions of and actual degree of physical well-being. One of the most significant environmental factors is stress.

Individuals are subject to different degrees of stress from their environments, with diverse consequences for their overall physical and mental health. In this context, *stress* can be defined as the gamut of social psychological stimuli that produce physiological responses of shallow, rapid breathing, muscle tension, increased blood pressure, and accelerated heart rate. The literature on social stress and health emphasizes that stress has broad physiological effects on the body, thereby predisposing people to a wide range of diseases (Cassel, 1976). How people cope with stress, however, affects the likelihood of deleterious consequences, as will be seen in the discussion of adaptation in Chapter 8 (Holmes and Masuda, 1974; Hamburg, 1982). Hypertension, cardiovascular disease, and cancer have been correlated with particular risk factors, such as stressful lifestyles, cigarette smoking, drinking, and being overweight (Abramson and Hopp, 1976; Wiley and Camacho, 1980). Health risk factor analyses move beyond assessments of possible differences in genetics and in health care to variations in health behaviors and lifestyles that can affect the outcome of stressful life events. Although definitive proof from large-scale controlled studies is not available, considerable evidence suggests that the control of multiple risk factors can reduce such potentially fatal conditions as cardiovascular disease (Multiple Risk Factor Intervention Trial Research Group, 1982). Possible health promotion interventions to minimize stress are discussed later in this chapter as well as in Chapter 19.

Studies concerning stressful life events and health are especially relevant to older people. As people age, they are more likely to experience events involving loss, especially loss of health and income. In addition, the cumulative amount of stress they have experienced may increase. This can tax their declining physiological and psychological capacities to the limit, leading to illness, disease, and death. On the other hand, older persons have been found to perceive less stress in every important life domain except health, and to report greater life satisfaction than do their younger counterparts (House and Robbins, 1983). The old-old, in particular, are "survivors" who have coped with multiple stressful social changes, including the Great Depression and two World Wars (Masuda and Holmes, 1978).

The impact of stress on the health of the elderly is as yet unclear. Although the psychological resources gained through older people's life experiences may have important mediating effects, more research is needed to determine whether the findings of reduced stress with age reflect cohort differences or the effects of aging over the life course.

Chronic and Acute Diseases

As noted in Chapter 4, the risk of disease and impairment increases with age; however, the extreme variability in older people's health status, as illustrated by Mrs. Hill and Mr. Jones in the vignette, shows that poor health is not necessarily a concomitant of aging (Fries and Crapo, 1981). The incidence of acute or temporary conditions, such as infections or the common cold, decreases with age. Those acute conditions that occur, however, are more debilitating and require more care, especially for older women. The average number of days of restricted activity due to acute conditions is nearly three times greater for people age 65 and over than it is for those 17 to 44 years old (National Center for Health Statistics, 1984; Jack and Ries, 1981). An older person who gets a cold, for example, faces a greater risk of pneumonia or bronchitis because of changes in organ systems (described in Chapter 4) which reduce the older person's resistance and recuperative capacities. Thus, older people are more likely to suffer restrictions on their social activities as a result of temporary health problems.

They are also much more likely than the young to suffer from chronic conditions. Chronic health conditions are defined as long term (more than three months), often permanent, and leaving a residual disability that may require long-term management or care rather than cure. More than 80 percent of persons age 65 and over have at least one of these, with multiple conditions being common in the elderly (National Center for Health Statistics, 1981). The pattern of illness and disease has changed in the past 80 years. With advances in medical technology and the growth in the percentage of people surviving infectious diseases and accidents and reaching old age, chronic conditions have replaced acute diseases as a major health risk for older people and have increased the need for long-term care services. The societal consequences of this change, especially the effects on health care financing, are discussed at length in Chapter 19.

The most frequently reported chronic conditions causing limitation of activity in persons age 65 and over are arthritis (50 percent), hypertension (39 percent), hearing impairment (30 percent), and heart disease (26 percent). In most cases, the rates for these diseases are much higher for the older population than for persons age 45 to 64. For example, the likelihood of suffering from arthritis is 80 percent higher for those 65 years old and over than for those age 45 to 64 (National Center for Health Statistics, 1982). The differences in *morbidity,* or days of sickness, from the top 10 chronic conditions for older and middle-aged populations per 1,000 persons are shown in Figure 6–2.

Although the nature and severity of any chronic condition varies with the individual, most older persons are capable of carrying out their normal daily

FIGURE 6–2 Morbidity from Top Ten Chronic Conditions—Rates per 1,000 Persons: 1982

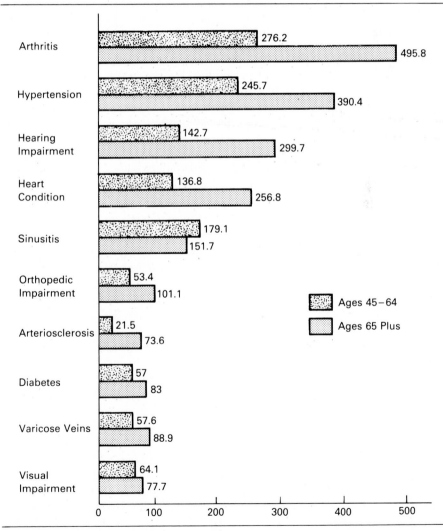

Source: National Center for Health Statistics. 1982 Health Interview Survey.

routines, as noted in our earlier discussion of ADL. For example, chronic heart problems may limit an older person's capacity to jog five miles a day, but he or she may still be able to live at home, visit with friends, and take a daily walk. Only about 2 percent of those age 65 and over are confined to bed by their chronic conditions, and most older people with chronic conditions are not dependent on others for managing their daily routines (Federal Council on the Aging, 1981). On the other hand, the small percentage who do need assistance with care have placed enormous pressures on formal health services as well as on informal caregivers.

INTERACTIVE EFFECTS

Even though the majority of chronic conditions are not severely limiting, they can nevertheless make life difficult and lower older people's resistance to other illnesses. The functional limits imposed by a chronic illness interact with the social limits set by others' perceptions of the illness to influence an older person's daily functioning. Therefore, it is important to look beyond the statistics on the frequency of chronic conditions to the nature of chronic illnesses, the interaction of physical changes with emotional and sociocultural factors, and the physiological differences between younger and older people.

Certain types of chronic diseases (e.g., cancer, anemia, and toxic conditions) may be related to older people's declining immunity, that is, reduced resistance to environmental carcinogens, viruses, and bacteria (Hickey, 1980). The accumulation of long-term, degenerative diseases may mean that a chronic condition, such as bronchitis, can have different and more negative complications than the same disease would have in a younger person. With reduced resistance to physical stress, an older individual may be less able to respond to treatment for any acute disease, such as a cold or flu, than a younger person would. The cumulative effect of chronic illness and an acute condition may become the crisis point where the older person becomes dependent on others for care.

Sociocultural factors also are apparently related to the incidence and severity of chronic conditions; the prevalence of disability is higher among nonwhites, people with low socioeconomic and education status, and those in nonfarm rural areas (Cohen and Brody, 1981). Disabling chronic illnesses tend to occur earlier among Blacks and Native Americans than among whites, resulting in higher rates of hospitalization, longer hospital stays, and a shorter life expectancy (Markides, 1983; Hendricks and Hendricks, 1981). In a survey of Black, Mexican-American, and white residents of Los Angeles County, older ethnic minority respondents were more likely to report poorer health than older whites, even with the effects of socioeconomic status, sex, and income held constant (Dowd and Bengtson, 1978). Poorer self-assessments of health and lower life expectancies have been explained as products of discriminatory policies, where nonwhites have had

Chronic Diseases of Aging

Our society's technological ability to keep people with multiple chronic illnesses alive, who in earlier years would have died of these same conditions, means that many older people survive into advanced old age with some loss of quality of life. As each of these illnesses progresses, the older person adjusts his or her lifestyle and environment accordingly. Consider the case of 82-year-old Mrs. Fox. She is proud that she has run the household of her son and his two children for the past 20 years. Today, as her grandchildren reach adulthood, Mrs. Fox realizes that she can no longer maintain the household and do the shopping and cooking for her family as she once did. Her diabetes, which was first detected 25 years ago, has become more bothersome, depleting her of the energy and stamina that she needs for keeping up her activities. High blood pressure and two heart attacks have placed her in the hospital four times during the past five years. A recent fall in her son's home revealed fractures in her hip and wrist bones that were attributed to osteoporosis. She has recovered from the fall, but now walks slowly with the aid of a cane.

Her doctors suspect that Mrs. Fox's tendency to fall may be due to her heart condition that occasionally leads to blackouts. They have suggested that she may benefit from a pacemaker, and have proposed that she undergo surgery to implant one soon. They have also recommended to Mrs. Fox and her son that she give up her housekeeping functions and move to a retirement apartment. Mrs. Fox has adamantly refused surgery, saying that she is fine now and does not want any artificial extension of her life. She is also determined to maintain her role as the manager of her son's home. In an attempt to accommodate these needs, he has decided to move to a small, one-story home where Mrs. Fox can still run the household, but it will not be so large as to tax her diminishing physical capacities.

lower incomes and inadequate nutrition throughout their lifetimes. An additional factor is that ethnic minorities, because of their cultural values and negative experiences with formal services, are less likely to utilize the health care system. (The effects of ethnic minority status on the incidence of chronic conditions is further discussed in Chapter 15.)

Psychological factors also influence how a person reacts to chronic physical problems. For example, people with a pessimistic outlook toward their health and aging tend to have less physiological reserve capacity, as illustrated by comments such as, "She lost her will to live," or "He stopped fighting and gave up." There are numerous examples of the impact of an optimistic attitude on the outcome of disease, perhaps best exemplified by Norman Cousins's (1979) accounts of the positive effects of humor on curing his potentially fatal disease. Thus, the impact of any chronic condition appears to be mediated by the physiological changes that occur with age, the sociocultural context, and the person's mental and emotional outlook.

Unfortunately, well-intentioned family members and health care professionals may assume that all chronic conditions are disabling or that a certain degree of disability is inevitable with aging. As a result, they may prematurely restrict a person's independence or not use the same treatments that they might administer to younger adults. The following anecdote illustrates how others' perceptions of health typical of old age can be unnecessarily limiting.

> A 101-year-old man went to see a doctor about a pain in his left leg. The doctor said, "It is just a sign of aging," to which the man replied, "But my right leg is the same age, and it feels just fine."

In sum, disabling health changes occur at different rates in different individuals and are not inevitable with age. We turn now to an examination of the most common chronic health problems faced by older people.

TYPES OF CHRONIC CONDITIONS

Heart disease, cancer, and strokes account for over three-quarters of all deaths among people over age 65, as shown in Table 6–1 (National Center for Health Statistics, 1982, 1984). Even though there have been rapid declines since 1968, heart disease remains the major cause of death. It is the number-one risk factor among adults age 65 and over, killing twice as many people as do all forms of cancer combined, and accounting for 20 percent of adult disabilities. Heart disease accounts for 20 percent of hospital admissions, and over 45 percent of deaths that occur among the elderly. Although death rates from cancer, especially lung cancer, continue to rise, it is estimated that eliminating cancer as a cause of death would extend the average life span by only two to three years. Eliminating deaths due to major cardiovascular diseases, however, would add an average of 11.4 years to life at age 65 and would lead to a sharp increase in the proportion of older persons in the total population (U.S. Senate Special Committee on Aging, 1986). The third leading cause of death among the elderly, stroke, has been decreasing since 1968 (National Center for Health Statistics, 1984).

Men have higher rates of heart disease and cancer than women. In fact, sex differences in mortality are due mainly to the greater incidence of coronary heart disease among men (Waldron, 1976). However, women experience more acute and chronic conditions than men, and they have higher rates of arthritis, high blood pressure, strokes, diverticular disease of the colon, hiatus hernia, incontinence, osteoporosis, and senile macular degeneration (Verbrugge, 1983; Women's Health, 1985). These diseases are less likely to result in death than cancer

TABLE 6–1 Mortality Rates for Older Women and Older Men, from All Causes and the Three Leading Causes

	Deaths per 100,000 Population per Year, 1978		
	65–74	*75–84*	*85+*
All causes			
Females	2,138	5,863	13,541
Males	4,185	9,385	17,259
Diseases of heart			
Females	823	2,666	6,674
Males	1,762	4,064	7,991
Malignant neoplasms (cancer)			
Females	589	959	1,139
Males	1,077	1,849	2,137
Cancer of lung			
Females	85	87	70
Males	389	479	317
Cerebrovascular diseases (strokes)			
Females	208	866	2,298
Males	290	984	2,244

Source: Vital and Health Statistics, Series 3, No. 22. Hyattsville, Md.: National Center for Health Statistics, 1982.

and heart disease, but they may lead to nearly as many days spent in bed. In other words, older women are more likely to be bothered by chronic conditions and to be ill and in bed at home, but they are less likely to be seriously sick, to be hospitalized, or to face life-threatening diseases than are older men (Lewis, 1985). These differences imply a reduction in the quality of life for women who live to advanced old age.

Heart Disease and the Cardiovascular System   Heart disease is a condition in which blood to the heart is deficient because of a narrowing or constricting of the cardiac vessels that supply it. This narrowing may be due to *atherosclerosis,** in

---

*The terms *atherosclerosis* and *arteriosclerosis* are often used interchangeably, causing confusion regarding their distinction. Arteriosclerosis, a generic term, sometimes called hardening of the arteries, refers to the loss of elasticity of the arterial walls. This condition occurs in all populations, and can contribute to reduced blood flow to an area. In atherosclerosis, the passageway of the large arteries narrows as a result of the development of plaques on their interior walls; atherosclerosis has been found to be age-related and of higher incidence in industrialized populations. Arteriosclerosis and atherosclerosis can be superimposed, but there is not a causative relationship between the degree of atherosclerosis and the loss of elasticity (arteriosclerosis) (Kart, Metress, and Metress, 1978; Boss and Seegmiller, 1981).

which fatty streaks or plaque formation begins early in life and accumulates to reduce the size of the passageway of the large arteries. A number of factors have been found to increase the risk of atherosclerosis. These include: hypertension or high blood pressure, elevated blood lipids (resulting from a dietary intake of animal products high in cholesterol), cigarette smoking, diabetes mellitus, obesity, inactivity, stress, and family history of heart attack. People in industrialized nations have higher levels of atherosclerosis, but the extent to which this is due to lifestyle factors in developed countries is unknown.

As the reduced blood flow caused by atherosclerosis becomes significant, angina pectoris may result. The symptoms are shortness of breath and pain from beneath the breastbone, in the neck, and down the left arm. For older individuals, these symptoms may be absent or may be confused with signs of other disorders, such as indigestion or gallbladder diseases. Treatment includes rest and nitro-glycerine, which serves to dilate the blood vessels.

If deficient blood supply to the heart persists, heart tissue will die, producing a dead area known as an *infarct.* In other words, coronary artery disease can lead to a myocardial infarction, or heart attack. Acute myocardial infarction results from blockage of an artery supplying blood to a portion of the heart muscle. The extent of heart tissue involved determines the severity of the episode. Heart attacks may be more difficult to diagnose in older people, since the symptoms in the elderly are often a generalized state of weakness, dizziness, confusion, or shortness of breath rather than the chest and back pains or numbness in the arms that characterize heart attacks in younger people. Symptoms in the elderly may also merge with other problems, so that a heart attack may not be reported or treated until it is too late for effective help. Although women are less likely to have heart attacks than men, once women develop a myocardial infarction, they fare less well than men, as evidenced by their higher mortality within the first year (Kannel and Brand, 1983).

The term *congestive heart failure,* or heart failure, indicates a set of symptoms related to the impaired pumping performance of the heart, so that one or more chambers of the heart do not empty adequately during the heart's contractions. Heart failure does not mean that the heart has stopped beating, but that its pumping efficiency has decreased. This results in shortness of breath, reduced blood flow to vital body parts, including the kidneys, and a greater volume of blood accumulating in the body tissues, causing edema (swelling). Treatment involves drugs, dietary modifications (e.g., salt reduction), and rest.

Most cardiovascular problems can be treated with rest, drugs, and appropriate diet, and thus do not prevent older people from carrying out modified daily routines. Preventive steps are most important, however. For example, hyper-tension, or high blood pressure, has been found to be the major risk factor in the development of cardiovascular complications and can be affected by preventive actions (Kannel and Gordon, 1978; Sheehy, 1980; Kannel, 1985). The risk of hypertension is greater for women than men aged 55 and over, with the difference becoming more pronounced with age (Kannel and Brand, 1983). This may partially explain why the incidence of coronary heart disease and strokes increases with age among women, although women on the average still live longer than men.

As noted in Chapter 4, blood pressure often increases with age, from an average of 120/70 to 130–140/80, but increases greater than this represent a definite hazard. Among the elderly, the risk of coronary heart disease, stroke, and death rises progressively with increasing blood pressure (Kannel, 1985). The rates of high blood pressure, or *hypertension,* are higher among Blacks than whites. About 56 percent of the Black population over age 65 is affected, compared to about 45 percent of older whites (USDHEW, 1979).

Significant increases in blood pressure should never be considered normal. In some isolated, primitive populations, a rise in pressure with age does not occur (Page, Damon, and Moellering, 1974). Although genetic factors may come into play, this difference suggests that individuals can make lifestyle changes that may reduce their vulnerability to high blood pressure. The preventive measures most likely to reduce cardiovascular risk are weight control; physical activity; treatment of diabetes; reduced intake of salt, saturated fats, and cholesterol; and avoidance of cigarette smoking and excessive alcohol intake (Abramson and Hopp, 1976; Kannel and Brand, 1983). For most people, hypertension can be controlled by medications and/or changes in the health habits described above (Tucker, 1980; Borhani, 1986; Kirkendall, 1986).

Another cardiovascular problem, which is less frequently addressed than hypertension, is *hypotension* or low blood pressure. Yet hypotension, characterized by dizziness and faintness from exertion after a period of inactivity and frequently related to anemia, is actually more common among the elderly. Problems with hypotension may be more pronounced for an older person after sitting or lying down for a long time (postural hypotension) or suddenly standing, after which a person may appear to lose balance and sway. Hypotension is not in itself dangerous, but can increase the risk of falls. Older people who have a history of low blood pressure or who are taking some types of antihypertensive medications need to move more slowly.

Strokes and Other Cerebrovascular Problems   We have seen how heart tissue can be denied adequate nourishment because of changes in the blood vessels that supply it. Similarly, arteriosclerotic and atherosclerotic changes in blood vessels that serve the brain can reduce its nourishment and result in the disruption of blood flow to brain tissue and malfunction or death of brain cells (Kart, Metress, and Metress, 1978). This impaired brain tissue circulation is called *cerebrovascular disease.* When a portion of the brain is completely denied blood, a cerebrovascular accident (CVA), or stroke, occurs. The severity of the stroke depends on the particular areas as well as the total amount of brain tissue involved. Many elderly who have heart problems also are at risk for cerebrovascular disease.

CVAs represent the third leading cause of death. Of the 200,000 deaths from strokes each year, 80 percent occur among persons aged 65 and over (National Center for Health Statistics, 1982). Atherosclerotic changes, in which fatty deposits gradually obstruct an artery in the brain or neck, are a common underlying condition. The most frequent cause of strokes in older persons is a cerebral thrombosis, a blood clot that either diminishes or closes off the blood flow in an artery of the brain or neck. Another cause of stroke is cerebral hemorrhage, in which a weak spot in a blood vessel of the brain bursts. Cerebral hemorrhage is less common in the elderly, although more likely to cause death when it does occur. The risks of stroke appear to be related to social and personal factors, most prominently hypertension, but also age, previous lifestyle, diet, and activity patterns (Kannel and Gordon, 1978). Regular, sustained exercise and low-fat diets are associated with the reduction of fatty particles that clog the blood stream (Abramson and Hopp, 1976).

The area of the brain that is damaged by a stroke dictates which body functions may be affected. For instance, if the speech center of the brain dies, then the stroke victim may be unable to speak or understand speech (aphasia). Another possible effect is paralysis of one side of the body (hemiplagia), which also may be associated with blindness in half of the victim's visual field (heminanopsia).

The treatment for strokes is similar to that for heart attacks and hypertension: modulated activity and supervised schedules of exercise and drugs. Stroke victims may require physical, occupational, and speech therapy, and their recovery process can be slow, frustrating, and emotionally draining for the victim and his or her family. Rehabilitation must address not only physical conditions, but also the psychosocial needs for support and respite of stroke victims and their families. The recognition of this wider range of rehabilitation has led to the creation of stroke support groups in many communities, organized by stroke victims and their families, or by local hospitals and senior centers.

Cancer   Among those 65 years old and over, 19 percent of deaths are due to cancer, especially cancers of the stomach, lungs, intestines, and pancreas. In fact, these malignancies in old age are the second leading cause of death, and 50 percent of all cancer occurs and is diagnosed after age 65. Cancer of the bowel is the most common malignancy in those age 70 and over, and second to lung cancer in cancer-related deaths. Lung cancer has its highest incidence in men age 65 and over, but appears to be associated more with smoking than with age. Cancer of the colon is more common in women, whereas rectal cancer is more frequent in men. Women also face increasing risks of breast and cervical cancers with age (National Center for Health Statistics, 1982). The greater risk of cancer with age may be due to a number of factors, such as the effects of a slow-acting carcinogen, prolonged "development time" necessary for growth to be observable, extended pre-exposure time, and failing immune capacity that is characteristic of increased age

(Weg, 1983). Certain diet and lifestyle factors may also be related to cancer. Diagnosing cancer in old age is often more difficult than at earlier life stages, because of the existence of other chronic diseases and because symptoms of cancer, such as weight loss, weakness, or fatigue, may be inaccurately attributed to aging, depression, or dementia. In addition, the current older generation's fear of cancer may be so great that they do not seek medical help to address their suspicions and fears.

Arthritis   Although not a leading cause of death, arthritis is widespread among the elderly and is a major cause of limited activity. In fact, all persons over age 60 have been estimated to have some physical evidence of arthritis, with over 80 percent having some "rheumatic complaint" (Boss and Seegmiller, 1981). Because arthritis is so common and the symptoms are so closely identified with the normal aging process, older people may accept arthritis as an inevitable accompaniment of a long life. If so, they may fail to seek treatment or to learn strategies to reduce pain and support their independent functioning. Although many treatments are used to control arthritic symptoms, little is known about ways to postpone or eliminate these disorders (National Institute on Aging, 1981).

Arthritis is not a single entity, but includes over 100 different conditions of inflammations and degenerative changes of bones and joints (Cohen, 1982). *Rheumatoid arthritis* is a chronic inflammation of the membranes lining joints and tendons, and is characterized by pain, swelling, bone dislocation, and limitation of motion. It afflicts two to three times more women than men and can cause severe crippling. Rheumatoid arthritis is not associated with aging per se; many young people also have this condition, with initial symptoms most commonly appearing between 20 and 50 years of age. Symptoms of rheumatoid arthritis include malaise, fatigue, loss of weight, fever, joint pain, redness, swelling, and stiffness affecting many joints. The disease is characterized by acute episodes followed by periods of relative inactivity. The cause of rheumatoid arthritis is unknown; treatment includes a balance of rest, exercise, and use of aspirin, which provides relief from pain, fever, and inflammation. Use of other antiinflammatory agents, antimalarials, and corticosteroids, as well as surgical procedures to repair joints and correct various deformities, has been found to be effective for some people.

Osteoarthritis, which is presumed to be a universal corollary of aging, is a gradual degeneration of the joints that are most subject to stress—those of the hands, knees, hips, and shoulders. Pain and disfigurement in the fingers are manifestations of osteoarthritis, but are generally not disabling. Osteoarthritis of the lower limbs, however, can limit mobility. Heredity, as well as environmental or lifestyle factors—particularly obesity, occupational stresses, and wear and tear on the joints—have been identified as causes of osteoarthritis. Some progress has been made in minimizing inflammation and pain through the use of antiinflammatory drugs, mild exercise, heat and cold, and reduction of strain on weight-bearing joints through weight loss and the use of weight-bearing appliances. Surgical procedures may restore function to the hips and knees, but cannot cure the arthritic condition. In addition, long-range effects are unknown since the surgery is usually performed on people over age 70.

The pervasive and unpredictable nature of the pain of arthritis can dominate a person's life and result in frustration and depression. Even on "good days" when pain subsides, an older arthritic may live with the fear of the inevitable "bad day," and may structure daily activities in order to avoid pain. Each day may seem to consist of a succession of obstacles, from getting out of bed and fastening clothing, to opening mail, dialing the phone, and handling dishes for meals. Concentrating on coping with one obstacle after another in the completion of tasks can be exhausting, even when minimal physical exertion is involved in each task.

The prime danger for people with arthritis is reducing their physical activity in response to pain. Movement stimulates the secretion of synovial fluid, the substance that lubricates the surfaces between joints and increases blood flow to joint areas. Movement also tones the muscles that hold joints in place and that shield joints from excessive stress. When someone tries to avoid pain by sitting still as much as possible, the losses in lubricating fluid and muscular protection make movement still more painful. Eventually, the muscles surrounding immobilized areas lose their flexibility, and affected joints freeze into rigid positions called *contractures*. For these reasons, older people need to be encouraged to maintain physical activity in spite of pain. The adage "use it or lose it" has special meaning to an arthritis victim! The environment may need to be restructured in these cases, so that a person with arthritis is able to walk around and keep up with daily activities, but is not burdened by extreme press or demands. For example, a smaller home on one level, such as that selected by Mrs. Fox in our earlier description of multiple chronic diseases, can reduce the environmental press for arthritic elderly.

Osteoporosis   The human body is constantly forming and losing bone through the metabolism of calcium. As noted in Chapter 4, osteoporosis involves a more dramatic loss in bone mass. The increased brittleness of the bones associated with this condition can result in diminished height, slumped posture, backache, and a reduction in the structural strength of bones, making them susceptible to fracture. Compressed or collapsed vertebrae are the major cause of kyphosis, or "dowager's hump," the stooped look that many of us associate with aging.

The primary risk posed by osteoporosis is a fracture of the neck of the femur, or thigh. Many of the falls and associated hip fractures of old age actually represent an osteoporotic femoral neck that broke from bearing weight, causing the individual to fall. Many older people have undiagnosed osteoporosis, often showing no symptoms until a fall or fracture occurs. Typically, no immediate preceding event can be identified as the cause of the fracture. Approximately 25 percent of women and 15 percent of men who are 80 years and older experience a hip fracture. These are of concern because of their impact on mortality; it is estimated that 15 percent of people with a hip fracture die from it or from surgical complications (Nussbaum, 1981; Lindsay, 1981). Those who survive hip surgery face reduced mobility and loss of independence, as well as a fear of further falls and fractures, all factors that may constrict their social worlds. (However, not all falls and fractures among the elderly result from osteoporosis. Cardiovascular disease underlies approximately one-half of them. Others are due to a decline in postural control, produced by impairments of the senses and the central nervous system, changes previously discussed in Chapter 4 [Kerzner, 1983].)

Osteoporosis apparently starts well before old age (perhaps as young as age 35) and is more than four times more common in women than in men. The causes of osteoporosis are unclear, although it may be associated with loss of calcium and estrogen in menopausal women, a sedentary lifestyle, or a genetic factor that determines bone density. For example, Caucasian women are more likely to develop this condition than Black women (Sharpe, 1979; Exton-Smith, 1985).

The goal in treatment is to prevent further bone loss. Increased intake of dietary calcium, vitamin D, fluoride, moderate weight-bearing exercise such as vigorous walking to help retain calcium, and estrogen have been used as therapies (Wheeler, 1976; Weiss, 1980; National Institute on Aging, 1981). Estrogen replacement therapy, however, has been found in some cases to be associated with endometrial, breast, and uterine cancer (Kerzner, 1983). Furthermore, therapy is far less effective if begun long after the menopause than immediately after the menopause. Small, short-stature women who are postmenopausal, have high caffeine intake, smoke cigarettes, and have a family history of osteoporosis appear to be most at risk of cancer associated with estrogen treatments. An additional problem is when estrogen therapy is discontinued, bone loss is more rapid than prior to treatment. Fluoride treatments have also been given, but may have negative side effects of gastrointestinal and rheumatic complaints (Jones and Jones, 1982; National Institute on Aging, 1981).

Certain dietary and exercise habits may help prevent osteoporosis, especially increasing the amount of calcium after age 30 (Gregory, 1982). Physicians recommend increasing daily calcium intake from 800 mg to 1200 mg among postmenopausal women (i.e., by drinking three or more eight-ounce glasses of milk daily, or by using calcium supplements) (Nussbaum, 1981; National Institute on Aging, 1981).

Exercise and calcium do not appear to prevent fracturing after bone loss has occurred. One reason is that an estimated 40 percent of osteoporotic women have a deficiency of the enzyme that is needed to metabolize calcium (lactose), thus making calcium less easily absorbed (Kerzner, 1983). An additional problem is that once one fracture is present, a patient has a 70 to 80 percent chance of developing another (Lindsay, 1981).

Chronic Obstructive Pulmonary Disease or Respiratory Problems   Chronic
bronchitis, fibrosis, asthma, and *emphysema* are manifestations of chronic obstructive
pulmonary diseases that damage lung tissue. They increase with age, develop
slowly and insidiously, and are progressive and debilitating, often resulting in
frequent hospitalizations, major lifestyle changes, and death (Boss and Seegmiller,
1981). In fact, by age 90, most people are likely to have some signs of emphysema,
with shortness of breath and prolonged and difficult exhalation. Getting through
daily activities can be extremely exhausting under such conditions. Causes of
chronic obstructive pulmonary diseases are both genetic and environmental,
especially prolonged exposure to various dusts, fumes, or cigarette smoke. Four
times as many men as women have these diseases (Shephard, 1982), probably
due to a combination of normal age changes in the lung and the effects of cigarette
smoke and air pollution in the community and at the work site. Treatment is
usually continuous, and includes drugs, respiratory therapy, breathing exercises
to compensate for damage, and the avoidance of respiratory infections, smoking,
pollution, and other irritants.

Allergic reactions to bacterial products, drugs, and pollutants also increase
with age. The greater incidence of drug allergies may be a function of both
decreases in physiological capacities and the increased use of many drugs, such as
sedatives, tranquilizers, antidepressants, and antibiotics.

Diabetes   Compared with other systems of the body, the endocrine glands do
not show consistent and predictable age-related changes, other than the gradual
slowing of functioning. However, insufficient insulin, produced and secreted by
the pancreas, can lead to *diabetes mellitus.* Diabetes mellitus is characterized by
above-normal amounts of sugar (glucose) in the blood and urine, resulting from
an inability to use carbohydrates. Diabetics may go into a coma when their blood
sugar levels get very high. Low blood sugar (hypoglycemia) can also lead to
unconsciousness.

Older diabetics include: (1) those who have had the disease since youth; (2)
those who develop it in late middle-age and incur related cardiovascular
problems; and (3) those who develop it late in life and generally show mild patho-
logic conditions. The incidence of newly diagnosed diabetes is highest in the
60- to 80-year-old category (Levin, 1982). Although diabetes can occur at any
age, diabetic problems related to the body's lessened capability to metabolize
carbohydrates can be particularly severe in the elderly. In fact, adult-onset
diabetes is estimated to affect 79.7 per 1,000 older persons. Many cases in the
elderly are associated with being overweight (Marchasseault, 1983; Williams,
1978).

Symptoms of diabetes include excessive thirst, increased appetite and
urination, fatigue, weakness, loss of weight, and decreased wound healing. These
symptoms may not be present in older people, however. Instead, diabetes among

the elderly is generally detected incidentally through eye examinations, hospitalization, and testing for other disorders. Since blood glucose may be temporarily elevated under the stress of illnesses such as stroke, myocardial infarction, or infection, people should not be labeled as diabetic unless the high glucose level persists under conditions of reduced stress (Marchasseault, 1983; Levin, 1982).

The cumulative effect of high blood glucose levels can lead to complications in advanced stages of diabetes. These include infections, nerve damage, blindness, renal disorders, stroke, harm to the coronary arteries, skin problems, and poor circulation in the extremities, leading to gangrene. The interaction of diabetes with ordinary age-related physical problems can result in serious health difficulties and consequent limitations on daily activities. Atherosclerosis and coronary heart disease, for example, are more common in diabetics than in nondiabetics.

Diabetes cannot be cured, but it can generally be managed at home through a diet of reduced carbohydrates and calories; regular exercise; proper care of feet, skin, teeth, and gums; and monitored insulin intake for those who require it. To minimize forgetfulness and treatment errors, older people, especially those who acquire diabetes late in life, may need instruction regarding the importance of diet, daily examination of their bodies, urine testing, and the correct dosage of insulin or other drugs. With proper management, diabetics can live long and useful lives (Kart, Metress, and Metress, 1978).

Problems with the Kidneys and Urinary Tract   The various diseases and disorders of the urinary system characteristic of old age tend to be either acute infections or chronic problems resulting from the gradual deterioration of the structure and function of the excretory system with age. As we have seen in Chapter 4, the kidneys shrink in size, and their capacity to perform basic filtration tasks decreases, leading to a higher probability of disease or infection. One of the most common age-related problems for women is inability of the bladder to empty completely. This often results in cystitis, an acute inflammatory state accompanied by pain and irritation. Cystitis can generally be treated by antibiotics. Older men face an increased risk of diseases of the prostate gland, with cancer of the prostate being the most frequent malignancy of older men. Cancer of the prostate frequently spreads to the bones, but surgery is rarely recommended for men over age 70.

A more difficult, noninfectious, and chronic urinary problem is incontinence (inability to control urine and feces), which has been estimated to occur in 5 to 19 percent of men and 7 to 38 percent of women over age 65 and living in the community (Diokno, Brock, Brown, and Herzog, 1986; Ouslander, 1981). Since older people and their families consider incontinence a taboo topic, they tend to be unaware of methods to cope with and treat incontinence. Most elderly do not discuss the problem with their doctors, and only a small percentage use any protective devices. This widespread reluctance to acknowledge incontinence as a problem can have serious psychological and social implications, particularly on the decision to institutionalize an older person. Accordingly, about half of the elderly living in nursing homes experience at least one episode of incontinence daily (Boss and Seegmiller, 1981; Weiss, 1983).

Incontinence sometimes results from a specific precipitating factor, such as acute illness, infection, or even a change in residence. It can be treated if the cause is known. Temporary incontinence can be caused by bladder or urinary tract infections which may be treated with antibiotics. Prescribed medications can also cause urgent and frequent urination. If informed of the detrimental effects of medication on an older person, a physician may reduce the drug dosage. With age, the bladder and urethra in women commonly descend, resulting in stress incontinence; leaking then occurs with the increased abdominal pressure brought on by coughing, sneezing, lifting, or physical exercise. Chronic functional incontinence often results from neurological changes and accompanies other problems, such as Parkinson's disease and organic brain syndrome. Other physical causes that should be investigated medically are prostate problems, pernicious anemia, diabetic neuropathy, and various cancers.

Since the types and causes of incontinence vary widely, thorough diagnosis and individualized treatment programs are critical. Even habitual incontinence should not be assumed to be irreversible; it may be treated or partially controlled through drugs, dietary changes, exercises, surgical procedures, or behavioral management techniques, such as reducing fluid intake when bathroom access is limited. Even incurable problems can be managed through protective products (e.g., absorbent pads) and catheters (tubes draining the bladder) to reduce complications, anxiety, and embarrassment. In fact, only about 25 percent of older persons with incontinence are so severely disabled that they are unlikely to regain continence and require a catheter or other external applicances to cope with the conditions (Murphy, Lamb, and Duthie, 1983). Physical exercise designed to promote and maintain sphincter muscle tone can also be a means to prevent or reduce age-related incontinence, particularly among older women. All possible treatments, including behavioral techniques and biofeedback, should be explored, since older people's embarrassment and humiliation over their difficulties may result in their avoiding social gatherings out of fear of having their incontinence detected. Support groups, such as "Health for Incontinent People," have chapters nationwide.

Problems with the Intestinal System   Many older people experience problems in digestion and continuing gastrointestinal distress, due particularly to age-related slowing down of the digestive process. Most intestinal problems are, in fact, related to unbalanced diets or diets with limited fiber content. Diverticulitis is one of the most common difficulties, affecting up to 50 percent of persons aged 80 and over, and especially women (Almy and Howell, 1980). It is a condition in which pouches or sacs (diverticula) in the intestines (especially in the colon) result from weakness of the intestinal wall; these sacs become inflamed and infected, leading to symptoms of nausea, abdominal discomfort, bleeding, and changes in bowel function. Management includes a high-fiber diet and antibiotic therapy. Diverticulitis is increasing in industrialized nations, and may be associated with a highly refined diet lacking in fiber (Kart, Metress, and Metress, 1978).

Many older people worry about constipation, but this is not an inevitable outcome of aging, as noted in Chapter 4. Causes of constipation include overuse of cathartics, lack of exercise, psychological stress, gastrointestinal disease, and an unbalanced diet with respect to bulk. Constipation may be a symptom of an underlying disease or obstruction. If this is not the case, treatment commonly includes physical activity, dietary modification, and increased fluid intake. Because many older people are overly concerned about having regular bowel movements, they may become dependent on laxatives, which can, over time, cause problems, such as irritating the colon and decreasing the absorption of certain vitamins. Some older people may become preoccupied with bodily functions, often boring or frustrating family members with detailed accounts.

Hiatus hernia appears to be increasing in incidence, especially among obese women; this occurs when a small portion of the stomach slides up through the diaphragm. Symptoms include indigestion, difficulty in swallowing, and chest pain that may be confused with a heart attack. Medical management includes weight reduction, elevation of the upper body when sleeping, changes in the size and frequency of meals, and medication. Although hiatus hernia in itself is not especially severe, it may mask the symptoms of more serious intestinal disorders, such as cancer of the stomach.

The incidence of gall bladder disease, especially with gallstones, also increases with age and is indicated by pain, nausea, and vomiting, with attacks increasing in number and severity. Most cases in the elderly are asymptomatic, and physicians debate whether to perform surgery or follow a more conservative course of medical management. Medical treatment usually involves a program of weight reduction, avoidance of fatty foods, and use of antacids.

Oral Diseases   The current oral health status of older people in the United States is largely unknown, but there is evidence that several types of oral diseases increase with age. The most visible condition is edentulousness, or loss of teeth. A recent nationwide study showed that 42 percent of adults over age 65 were edentulous (Brunelle, 1987), a rate much lower than that reported in previous years for the U.S. (U.S. Public Health Service, 1974), or the rates for other industrialized countries such as Scotland and the Netherlands (Manderson and

Ettinger, 1975; Swallow, 1978). As might be expected, the rate increases with age. For example, a survey in the state of Iowa (Beck et al., 1982) showed edentulism rates of 33.8 percent among those aged 65–74, and 44.4 percent of those over age 75.

The common problems of dental caries and gum disease also appear to increase with age, although the evidence is limited and less clear. In the Baltimore Longitudinal Study, the rate of root caries was found to be four times greater among subjects over age 60 than in those under age 40 (Baum, 1981). The rate of secondary coronal caries (cavities that develop in the exposed, upper part of the teeth) relative to the number of remaining natural teeth seems to be higher among the elderly (Chauncey, 1978). To what extent the higher rates in adults reflect changes over time in preventive dental care, such as the widespread use of water fluoridation, is unclear. Many studies show an age-related increase in the incidence of periodontitis (or gum disease), although evidence of substantial increases after age 54 is lacking (Beck, 1984).

In contrast, cancers of the lip, tongue, mouth, gum, pharynx, and salivary glands increase with aging, regardless of ethnic minority status or sex (Cutler and Young, 1975). In North America and Western Europe, cancer of the lip is the most frequent and has the highest survival rates among those listed above (between 65 and 90 percent over a five-year period). Presently, very little is known about lifestyle characteristics associated with the development of this disease (Beck, 1984).

Use of Physician Services by Older People

The increased incidence of many chronic and acute diseases among the elderly would seem to predict a striking growth with age in the use of health care services. In fact, however, as shown in Table 6–2, older persons use physician services only

TABLE 6–2 Interval Since Last Physician Visit

Age	Less Than 1 Year	1 to 2 Years	2 to 5 Years	5 Plus Years
	(Percentage)			
All ages	75.4	11.0	9.9	3.7
25 to 44	71.9	12.0	12.0	4.0
45 to 64	74.4	9.4	10.6	4.0
65 to 74	80.2	6.4	7.7	5.7
75 plus	85.4	4.8	5.9	3.9

Source: National Center for Health Statistics, Health Interview Survey. Unpublished tabulation, 1983.

50 percent more than younger people (6.3 visits among those age 65 and older versus 4.0 among the 17–24-year-old group). There is only a slight increase with age in the probability of seeing a doctor at least once in the previous year; 74.4 percent of those aged 45 to 64 reported doing so, compared to 80.2 percent of those aged 65 to 74, and 85.4 percent of persons 75 years or older (National Center for Health Statistics, 1983; U.S. Senate Special Committee on Aging, 1986). This is true even though a variety of medical and dental services aimed specifically at the elderly have developed in recent years, and increasing numbers of specialists are being trained in geriatric health care. Both younger and older people tend to visit physicians primarily for acute symptoms and to receive similar diagnostic and therapeutic services in the doctor's office (Davis, Brody and Cooper, 1980). Apparently, older persons underutilize physician services for chronic conditions and preventive health care (Haug, 1984).

There are several possible reasons for the failure to seek medical help for chronic conditions. One may be the belief among many older persons that these conditions are natural concomitants of aging, and that a physician can do little to relieve or cure them (Nuttbrock and Kosberg, 1980). In addition, older people may not report symptoms and seek help for health problems because they fear the possibility of a serious illness and are concerned about the expense of physician visits, diagnostic tests, and hospitalization (Rowe, 1985). Another barrier may be the negative attitudes of health professionals, some of whom may believe that older patients are difficult to manage and that the diseases associated with aging cannot be reversed (Kosberg and Harris, 1978; Ford and Sbordone, 1980). Clearly, such perceptions by physicians interact with older patients' attitudes in ways that do not enhance the likelihood that the elderly will receive adequate care for serious chronic diseases.

Use of Other Health Services

In contrast to their relative underutilization of physician services, older people are more likely to be hospitalized and to stay longer once they are in the hospital. The average stay for persons over age 65 in 1981 was 14.1 days, more than twice as long as the 6.5 day average among those aged 17 to 24 (National Center for Health Statistics, 1982). However, the length of stay has been reduced since the introduction of Diagnostic Related Groupings for Medicare patients in 1983 (see Chapter 19). Hospital utilization apparently reflects older people's need for health care more accurately than do elective visits to a physician's office.

The use of prescription medications may also be an indication of the elderly's real needs for health care. Although representing only 11.8 percent of the population, older people purchased 25 percent of all prescription medications in 1982. About 25 percent of the elderly take three or more prescription drugs a day, compared to 9 percent of younger people (American Association of Retired

Persons, 1986). As might be expected, most of these drugs are for the chronic health problems that occur with greater frequency in old age (e.g., hypertension, cardiovascular disease, arthritis). In many instances, however, older people may be taking too many or inappropriate drugs.

An area of elective health care, ignored even more than routine medical care, is the use of professional dental services. Although the rate of preventive dental service utilization in the United States has risen significantly over the past 20 years among younger cohorts, the use of dental services by the elderly has increased only slightly. In the latest national survey, older persons continued to be the lowest utilizers of professional dental care; 41.4 percent had not seen a dentist in more than five years in 1981, in contrast to 5.9 percent among the youngest age group and 21.6 percent of those aged 45–64, as shown in Table 6–3 (National Center for Health Statistics, 1985). This rate is incongruent with the level of oral diseases that require professional attention in older persons. Yet, once older persons enter the dental care system, their average number of visits is similar to that of younger people, as shown in Table 6–4.

TABLE 6–3 Time Interval Since Last Dental Visit: 1981

Age	<6 Mos.	6–24 Mos.	2–4 Yrs.	≥5 Yrs.	Never
17–24	40.6%	34.9%	14.5%	5.9%	4.0%
25–44	41.3	33.1	14.5	9.1	2.0
45–64	37.3	25.7	14.4	21.6	1.5
65 plus	**26.5**	**16.6**	**14.4**	**41.4**	**1.2**

Source: National Center for Health Statistics, 1985. Current Estimates from the National Health Interview Survey: U.S., 1981. DHHS Publication No. 82–1569.

TABLE 6–4 Number of Dental Visits in Past Year: 1983

| Characteristic | Total | Number of Visits in Past Year | | | | | |
		None	*1*	*2*	*3*	*4*	*≥5*
All Persons							
18–24 years	100.0	44.1	25.2	15.7	5.2	2.9	6.1
25–34 years	100.0	41.7	23.6	18.3	5.8	3.3	6.7
35–44 years	100.0	40.1	21.9	19.0	6.5	4.4	7.4
45–54 years	100.0	44.7	19.4	17.1	6.1	4.0	7.8
55–64 years	100.0	48.0	16.8	17.3	6.5	4.1	6.3
65 years and over	100.0	60.9	13.9	12.7	4.6	3.0	4.0

Source: Advancedata. From Vital and Health Statistics of the National Center for Health Statistics, Number 122, August, 1986.

Models of Health Behavior

Some older persons do seek regular medical and dental health services. What distinguishes them from the underutilizers? Numerous studies have shown that it is not the severity of the older person's health problems (Wolinsky, 1978; Krout, 1983; Holtzman and Akiyama, 1985). Sometimes an older person with the most serious problems is the least likely to seek care. Researchers who have explored this question have developed a number of predictive models. The most widely used frameworks are the behavioral model and the health belief model.

THE BEHAVIORAL MODEL

The behavioral model (Aday and Andersen, 1974; Andersen, 1968; Andersen and Newman, 1973) suggests that three sets of variables can account for differences in the use of health services. These are predisposing, enabling, and need variables. The first consists of demographic characteristics, such as age, sex, ethnic minority status, education, and occupation of the head of a household which will be discussed below. Age differences already have been noted above.

Predisposing Variables: Sex, Ethnic Minority Status, and Education   Turning to sex differences, females are more likely than males to use medical and dental services at all ages, as shown in Table 6–5. Sex differences in the use of dental services diminish with age, but this may reflect the greater distribution of edentulousness (loss of teeth) among older women. As noted previously, however, females at all ages are less likely to be hospitalized and, once in the hospital, they stay fewer days than males.

Nursing homes are more than twice as likely to be occupied by older women than by men. Two reasons may be cited for this: a greater proportion of women live to be 75 years and older, and there is a greater availability of family members, especially wives, to care for chronically ill older men at home. As a result of smaller family size during the Depression, many women today have outlived a spouse or adult child who could provide help in times of health crises.

This relative availability of family supports may explain differences in the use of nursing home and hospital services by ethnic minority groups. Thus, for example, Native Americans, Blacks, and Hispanics, who tend to have more extensive family networks than many Caucasian ethnic groups, are less likely to use these professional services. However, the differential use of health services may be due to factors other than ethnicity per se. This situation illustrates one of the problems with the behavioral model of health service utilization. It is likely that ethnic minority status interacts with the older person's income, occupation, and perceptions of the health care system; availability of third-party payments (i.e., private and government funded insurance plans) for health care; and

TABLE 6–5 Number of Medical and Dental Visits per Person per Year, by Age and Sex: United States, 1981

Sex	All Ages	17–24 Years	25–44 Years	45–64 Years	65 Years and Over
		Number of Physician *Visits per Person per Year*			
Both Sexes	4.6	4.0	4.4	5.1	6.3
Male	4.0	2.6	3.2	4.7	6.0
Female	5.2	5.4	5.5	5.4	6.6
		Number of Dental *Visits per Person per Year*			
Both Sexes	1.7	1.6	1.8	1.8	1.5
Male	1.5	1.4	1.5	1.8	1.4
Female	1.8	1.8	2.0	1.8	1.5

Source: Unpublished data from the National Health Interview Survey, National Center for Health Statistics, 1983.

professional attitudes toward treating ethnic minorities. Unfortunately, the behavioral model does not consider interactions among the predisposing, enabling, and need variables.

Education is another predisposing variable that predicts differential use of health services. Like ethnicity, however, it probably interacts with occupation, income, availability of health insurance, attitudes, and knowledge about health care. Nowhere is the difference in utilization associated with educational levels more dramatic than in the use of dental services. Across all age groups, families headed by college graduates are two to three times more likely to seek dental services than those headed by an individual with eight years of education or less (HRA, 1977; Kiyak, 1984).

Enabling Variables   The second category in the behavioral model is that of enabling variables: family income, the ability to pay for services, the availability of third-party payments, and community resources. Not surprisingly, family income plays a critical role in the use of all health services. It appears that Medicare and Medicaid can reduce some of the differential effects of income for older persons, but because some health expenses must still be paid out-of-pocket, the poorest elderly remain the least likely to obtain health services. And it is precisely the poorest among the older population who are the most vulnerable to the diseases that increase with age.

The individual's own perception of the ability to pay may be even more important than actual costs in determining use of health services. Regardless of income level, older people who feel that they cannot afford health care (often because they have an exaggerated concept of the expense) will not seek care. Although this may also be true among the younger population, the latter are more likely to be knowledgeable about ways to obtain low-cost health services. As a result, younger people may be less likely to report avoiding health services because of high costs.

Another factor that may affect utilization of health services is their accessibility. It is generally assumed that the relatively fewer services available in rural and nonmetropolitan areas, combined with the greater transportation difficulties, result in lower utilization rates in these areas. However, older persons' utilization of general health services does not differ significantly by community size (Krout, 1983), although hospital admissions are greater among rural elderly (Roos and Shapiro, 1981; Shapiro and Roos, 1984, 1985).

Information about the availability of services, their costs, and criteria for enrolling in special programs is a critical determinant of access to services (Lind, 1978; Ward, 1978; Snider, 1980), especially the utilization of services supported by public funds for special populations. To the extent that older persons have strong informal networks, or are integrated into the community's formal support systems, they are more likely to know about services and to seek additional information. Such knowledge is the first step in entering the health care system. The challenge for health care providers is to understand the factors that determine how older persons enter the health care system and how they make regular use of health services.

Need Variables   The third set of variables in the behavioral model, and perhaps the most important for motivating older persons to use health services, is the need factor. This includes symptoms of health and illness, perceived need for health care, and functional health problems. Studying these variables systematically is difficult, particularly in large-scale national surveys where a detailed assessment of physical symptoms and perceived need for various services is prohibitively expensive. Yet need variables are often the best predictors of utilization. For example, an older person who is reluctant to admit to any pain associated with a physical health condition will not seek health care.

Because of the widespread acceptance by older people of poor health as a concomitant of aging, the physical symptoms of a disease must be accompanied by a perceived need for treatment. Depression is one example of a condition with numerous physical and psychological symptoms (e.g., sleeplessness, loss of appetite, crying spells) that an older person may define as normal, or as something to adapt to; worse yet, an older person may assume that nothing can be done about the problem.

Health care providers and health educators must encourage consistency between older persons' perceptions and actual symptoms of disease. Perceived need depends on the individual's "health IQ," that is, an understanding of the processes of disease and health, an ability to distinguish normal aging from disease, and a psychological willingness to deal with one's health problems. Many older people may deny that they need health care because they are unwilling to view themselves as ill, helpless, or dependent. It is therefore critical to dissociate the need for health care from dependency in the minds of older people, and to reinforce the belief that they can improve their health. These concepts of self-responsibility should be a part of any health education and health promotion program aimed at the elderly, as discussed later in this chapter.

THE HEALTH BELIEF MODEL

Another model of health services utilization is the *health belief model* (Rosenstock 1966, 1974; Maiman and Becker, 1974; Becker, Maiman, Kirscht, Haefron, and Drachman, 1977). This model hypothesizes that people will not seek health services unless they (1) view themselves as vulnerable or susceptible to a disease which they (2) perceive as having severe consequences. In addition, individuals must (3) see an association between performing particular behaviors and outcomes, and must (4) be convinced that the benefits to seeking health care outweigh the barriers. Many older people, for example, believe that a doctor cannot help them or that their illness is not severe enough to require medical attention (Shanas and Maddox, 1985).

This model would predict, for example, that an older woman will be more likely to practice preventive health behavior related to breast cancer if she sees herself susceptible to breast cancer and if she believes that the disease can be fatal, and that monthly breast self-examinations are effective for preventing it. The older woman who does not think she is at risk, or believes that preventive behaviors make no difference because she will get the disease anyway, will be less likely to practice such behavior. Thus, all four elements of the health belief model must operate simultaneously.

An important distinction between this model and the behavioral model described earlier is that the health belief model focuses on the *individual's* perceptions, not on demographic and social conditions that differentially affect groups of people. Thus, the health belief model tends to be more focused on the individual's internal state, that is perceptions, motives, and self-reported likelihood of taking action.

Researchers have used the health belief model to examine retrospectively numerous health behaviors among subjects of varying ages (Eve, Watson, and Reiss, 1980; Ferraro and Mutran, 1983). It is less useful for predicting health behavior (Kegeles, 1969). Some components of the model, particularly the belief that preventive behaviors are effective, are more closely related to actual health service utilization than are other components (Haefner, 1974).

The health belief model appears potentially valuable for changing health behaviors. Attempts to use it in behavior change programs, however, have met with mixed success, and there are no reports of research on its application to older persons' health behaviors specifically. This area deserves further study, considering the significance of perceived need in both the health belief and behavioral models of health care utilization.

THE CONGRUENCE MODEL

An alternative approach to examining health service utilization among the elderly is the person-environment (P-E) congruence model. As briefly described in the Introduction, this model (Lawton and Nahemow, 1973; Kahana, 1975; Kahana, Liang, and Felton, 1980) has been applied to the integration of older persons with their physical and social environments. Health behavior is proposed to be a function of the "fit" or congruence between an individual's perceived and objective health needs, cognitive and physical capacities to deal with the health care system, informal support systems, and the health care delivery system's characteristics, constraints, and opportunities.

On Lok Senior Health Services in San Francisco is an example of modifying health care services to be responsive to the particular needs of Chinese, Filipino, and Italian elderly who do not speak English, and whose health beliefs are often incongruent with the prevailing medical model in the United States. On Lok has utilized informal neighborhood networks, altered traditional methods of financing through the use of waivers and health maintenance organizations, and made services accessible in order to maintain the frail elderly in the community. Without the usual fee-for-service limitation, On Lok has the flexibility to provide any service, from meals to acute hospitalization, based on the individual participants' needs. The On Lok model has been able to cut health care costs by reducing the need to use expensive institutional care, while simultaneously providing high-quality services (National Pacific/Asian Resource Center for Aging, 1986).

The congruence model has not been widely tested, but it holds promise for planning alternative health care delivery systems that are most likely to fit the needs of older persons. The greatest strength of a person-environment approach to evaluating health service utilization is that it avoids the pitfall of viewing the environment as static; that is, it suggests that the health care system cannot remain as it has always been, or as it was designed to serve younger people's needs, but that it must be modified if older persons are to utilize services effectively. The other two models focus primarily on characteristics of the person, not on the nature of the service delivery system. This alternative model also minimizes the danger of assuming that some older people just cannot be helped because of demographic and historical characteristics that affect their use of health services. Instead, the emphasis of the congruence model is on developing services that fit the needs of all types of elderly. This model predicts that utilization can be made most effective if two conditions change: (1) patients' attitudes, values, and knowledge about health care can be enhanced; and (2) health care settings can be designed to be more sensitive to the older patients' needs. Only by effecting changes in both of these areas can health practitioners and gerontologists expect to improve older persons' use of all health care services: ambulatory, acute, chronic, and dental services.

Health Promotion with the Elderly

Another intervention to impact older people's health behavior and utilization of health services is health promotion. Health promotion includes ". . . any combination of health education and related organizational, political, and economic changes conducive to health" (Green et al., 1980). This emphasis on the variety of interventions acknowledges the complex social, biological, cultural, and economic factors that influence health and health behavior. Accordingly, this definition includes altering individual health practices, such as diet and exercise, as well as trying to create healthier environments and to change cultural attitudes and expectations toward health (*Healthy People,* 1979). Health promotion repre-sents a shift from a biomedical model that emphasizes the physician's responsi-bility to treat disease, to a model where individuals are responsible for and feel more in control of their own health. Health promotion thus makes explicit the importance of people's environments and lifestyles as major determinants of their health status.

The primary rationale for health promotion programs is to reduce the incidence of chronic diseases, thereby enhancing the elderly's quality of life. As suggested in our earlier discussion of disease, as many as 80 percent of the chronic illnesses that afflict the elderly are estimated to be related to social, environmental, and behavioral factors, particularly poor health habits (Dychtwald, 1983; Filner and Williams, 1979). In addition, 90 percent of fatal and near-fatal episodes of strokes and heart attacks are believed to be preventable. For example, heart disease has been linked to daily stress, sedentary living, weight gain, smoking, and high cholesterol diets. Yet all of these risk factors can be reduced, even in later life, through changes in health habits (e.g., controlling blood pressure and weight, stopping cigarette smoking, reducing cholesterol levels, and engaging in regular, moderate exercise) (Farquhar, 1978). A viable health care goal, as noted in Chapter 1, is therefore the "compression of morbidity," delaying the age at which chronic illness and the infirm period of life begins (Fries, 1980; 1983; 1984). This goal translates into helping people to live as much of the normal life span as possible—that is, to die of old age rather than disease and to enjoy the highest possible quality of life in their later years. This goal seems feasible, given the evidence that individuals over age 75 who followed seven health-enhancing behaviors achieved the same health index ratings as those 30 years younger who followed few or none of these behaviors (Belloc and Breslow, 1972). Other evidence is shown by older runners who steadily improve their running times and become more fit and physically stronger, even as they grow older, although they cannot achieve the maximum capacity attainable in their youth.

The most important elements of a strategy to postpone infirmity are thus prevention and changes in social expectations of older people (Fries, 1984). Accordingly, the theme of health promotion programs is that the later years can be a positive time of personal growth; people of any age can modify their health care practices in ways to enhance their independence and life satisfaction. Health and productivity are viewed as interacting conditions: The unproductive individual is at higher risk of illness and economic dependency, the sick person is limited in productivity, and is therefore at higher risk of dependency (Butler and Gleason, 1985).

THE RELATIONSHIP OF HEALTH PRACTICES TO HEALTH OUTCOMES

Considerable research demonstrates the relationship of personal health habits to health status (Belloc and Breslow, 1972; Kane, Kane, and Arnold, 1985), although more longitudinal research is needed (Branch and Jette, 1984). The following factors have been identified to be related to good health status: not smoking, limiting alcohol consumption, controlling one's weight near ideal, sleeping seven to eight hours per night, and moderate levels of exercise. These relationships have been found to be cumulative and independent of age, sex, and economic status (Wiley and Camacho, 1980). Additional epidemiological evidence demonstrates links between specific health habits and decreased longevity and/or increased health risks. These specific lifestyle factors, discussed briefly below, include alcohol consumption, cigarette smoking, diet, and exercise.

The relationship between drinking alcohol and physical health is U-shaped, with the least healthy tending to be those who drink heavily and those who abstain (Wiley and Camacho, 1980), although abstainers may include former heavy drinkers who have damaged their systems. Excessive drinking (five or more drinks at a single setting) has been found to contribute to poorer than average physical health (Belloc and Breslow, 1972) and to hasten death by eight to 12 years (Cohen and Brody, 1981).

The effects of cigarette smoking, especially in interaction with other risk factors, on heart disease, emphysema, and lung cancer have been extensively documented (Wiley and Camacho, 1980). Smokers who use oral contraceptives, are exposed to asbestos, have excessive alcohol consumption, or are at risk for hypertension have a greater chance of experiencing nonfatal myocardial infarctions (Rosenberg et al., 1980) and are at significant risk for cancers of the oral cavity and lung (Rothman, 1975).

Poor diet has been determined to be related to obesity, cancer, and heart disease, especially among those who are 30 percent or more over their ideal weight (Belloc and Breslow, 1972; Wiley and Camacho, 1980). Obesity carries an increased risk of cardiovascular and pulmonary difficulties, aggravates other conditions such as hypertension, arthritis, and diabetes, and adds risk to surgery. Interpretation of the relationship between obesity and morbidity and mortality is difficult, however, since obesity is correlated with other risk factors, such as high blood pressure.

The relationship between diet, blood cholesterol, coronary heart disease, and stroke has also been suggested in numerous studies. As noted earlier, diets high in fat, sugar, and salt and low in fiber have been found to be associated with a high incidence of coronary heart disease, hypertension, diabetes, obesity, and tooth decay, and certain cancers common among older people (Ahrens, 1979). Most of such evidence, however, is from epidemiologic studies that demonstrate an association between diet and disease, but do not necessarily prove causation. For example, some environmental factors that influence the likelihood of disease are also linked to poor nutrition. These include low socioeconomic status, ill-fitting dentures, eating alone, or a sedentary way of life (*Healthy People*, 1979).

There is considerable evidence of the relationship between exercise and health, particularly between cardiovascular heart disease and sedentary lifestyles (Belloc and Breslow; 1972; Wiley and Camacho, 1980; Kannel, 1967; Palmore, 1970). Many physical changes in older people that are mistakenly attributed to aging are actually due to being physically unfit. Physically inactive people age faster and look older than physically fit persons of the same age (Moritani, 1981). It has been suggested that a goal of physical exercise should be that a 60-year-old is 60 years old in body as well as in time! (Sheehan, 1978). Because the body's adaptability to exercise remains unimpaired by aging, exercise can slow the decline of physiological functions, restore and maintain muscular strength and flexibility, and reduce the risk of hypothermia and accidents (de Vries, 1977). It appears to benefit even those with coronary artery disease, diabetes, hypertension, and pulmonary disorders by causing weight loss; reducing blood sugar, blood fat, and high blood pressure; and improving circulation (Shepard, 1978, 1981).

Psychosocial conditions, particularly a loss of control, excessive stress, and the absence of social supports, have also been linked to decreased longevity and/or poor health (Berkman, 1986; Cohen, Teresi, and Holmes, 1985; Beck, 1982; *Healthy People*, 1979; Petrich and Holmes, 1977). There is relatively strong epidemiologic evidence that persons who are married, have close contacts with friends and relatives, and share common religious, ethnic, or cultural interests with others experience lower morbidity and greater longevity than those without such ties (Blazer, 1982; Cohen and Brody, 1981). Social networks apparently act to buffer the negative effects of stress (Cohen, Teresi, and Holmes, 1985; Berk, 1986). Translating the results of research on social supports into health services has been slow, partly because they do not fit the traditional biomedical model of disease and treatment.

HEALTH PROMOTION GUIDELINES

Given the growing evidence about the relation of health practices to health status, most health promotion programs include components on nutrition, exercise, and stress management. Oral health promotion has also been implemented by some geriatric dentists. An underlying theme is taking responsibility for one's own health, rather than relying on medical professionals. Some programs also include educating participants to change the larger social environment, perhaps through collective action. Several components of health promotion programs are briefly described.

1. *Nutrition.* Although information on older people's dietary needs is incomplete and often contradictory, the basic principles are:

1. Consume a wide variety of foods.

2. Increase consumption of unprocessed foods containing complex carbohydrates (starch and fiber), such as whole grains and legumes.

3. Restrict intake of sugar, fat, cholesterol (less than 10 percent of the total calories consumed should be derived from saturated fat) (Grundy, 1982; Ahrens, 1979; U.S. Senate, 1977).

Unfortunately, there are a number of barriers to adequate nutrition. Some of these result from physical and social changes common to aging and include the following:

1. an inability to chew and swallow due to no teeth, missing teeth, or loose-fitting dentures

2. problems with taste or smell

3. poor digestion of certain foods

4. emotional barriers, such as loneliness, that deprive mealtime of its social satisfactions and may diminish appetite

Others result from societal conditions, such as the expense of particular foods or lack of access to them. Any nutritional assessment of an older person must take account of such factors that can affect the amount and type of food consumed.

2. *Exercise.* Prior to beginning an exercise program, older people should have a thorough medical examination, including a treadmill or other exercise tolerance test to determine their baseline for physical fitness. An ideal exercise program begins with a low level of activity and includes an initial warm-up, with stretching, light calisthenics, and leisurely walking, more strenuous exercise for 20 minutes

Most health promotion programs include an
exercise component.

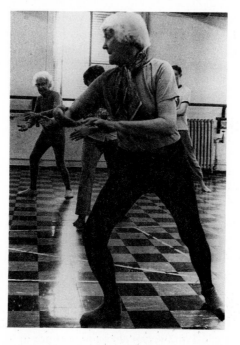

or more, and a relaxing cool-down period of five to 10 minutes of light exercise.
Walking is the safest and best exercise for older people. Most ambulatory older
persons can build up their walking to one or more miles daily, and at a speed of
three or four miles per hour. A healthy older person may be able to undertake a
more vigorous aerobic program, such as swimming, jogging, or bicycling (Harris,
1983).

3. *Stress Management.* Stress-related disorders include emotional disturb-
ances, psychosomatic complaints, headaches, insomnia, hypertension, and certain
types of rheumatic or allergic afflictions as well as cardiovascular and kidney
diseases. As noted earlier, older people may be more susceptible to such negative
effects because of the body's decreased ability to adapt to stress and increased
vulnerability to physiological changes induced by the stress response itself. This
means that the aging process may be accelerated by repeated exposure to stress at
a time of diminished adaptability (DeBerry, 1981–82). Health care professionals
have shown increasing interest in ways to reduce such potential negative effects
through stress management techniques, such as stress alleviation, progressive
muscle relaxation, and clinical biofeedback.

When using techniques to regulate stress, a person focuses on a constant stimulus, such as the repetition of a word or phrase, or fixed gazing at an object. Another self-regulatory approach is progressive muscle relaxation, in which various muscle groups are systematically tensed and then released to achieve a state of deep relaxation. When used with a group of widows, these techniques were found to reduce stress-related psychosomatic symptoms of headaches, insomnia, and nightly awakenings, as well as self-reported tension and anxiety levels (DeBerry, 1981–82). Biofeedback training aims to increase awareness of specific muscle tension, to control that tension through the use of biofeedback equipment in the laboratory, and to transfer that ability from the laboratory to real-life situations. Clinical biofeedback has been used to treat high blood pressure, migraine, and tension headaches. Underlying all these relaxation techniques is an emphasis on quiet attentiveness to a person's bodily sensations. More research is needed, however, on which modalities are most helpful to older people.

ORAL HEALTH PROMOTION

Only a few health promotion programs include preventive dentistry. One reason for this is that dental disease and tooth loss are frequently assumed to be natural concomitants of aging. Once an individual has lost many teeth from poor oral health in the middle years, it is presumed there is little to promote and maintain. Despite this skeptical attitude, held by professionals and older people alike, some oral health promotion efforts have been found to be successful (Kiyak, 1980; Kiyak and Miller, 1982; Price and Kiyak, 1981; Kiyak and Mulligan, 1985).

With increased preventive dentistry in youth and middle-age, tooth loss has become less prevalent in the later years (American Dental Association, 1979). This means that individuals with teeth remaining must perform regular oral health care, including brushing, flossing, and regular visits to a dentist or hygienist. As noted earlier, older people are not only less inclined to use professional dental services, but also less likely to know and value techniques of preventive dentistry (Kiyak and Miller, 1982; Gilmore and Kiyak, 1984). Instead, prevention must be defined differently by age: In younger persons, the initiation of dental disease and tooth loss can be prevented; in the elderly, the goal is to prevent *further* disease, particularly disease caused by poorly fitting dentures and by regimens prescribed for other medical conditions.

HEALTH PROMOTION FOR THE FRAIL ELDERLY

Although preventive efforts have focused on healthy elderly in the community, health promotion principles have been implemented in institutional settings. For example, the concepts of self-responsibility and control have been promoted through giving nursing home residents the care of plants, pets, or bird feeders

(Banziger and Roush, 1983; Beck, 1982; Rodin and Langer, 1977). Range-of-motion exercise for institutionalized older persons has been found under certain conditions to improve muscle tone and enhance feelings of well-being (Allen, 1985). Many chair exercises can be adapted for impaired, even bed-bound, older persons. More work is needed to adapt health promotion materials and techniques to take account of differing incidences of specific conditions, risk factors, or living situations of the frail elderly. Some of the other limitations and barriers to health promotion with the elderly are discussed further in Chapter 19.

Summary and Implications

Although older persons are at risk of more diseases than younger people, most older people rate their own health as satisfactory. Health status refers not only to an individual's physical condition, but also to her or his functional level in various social and psychological domains. It is affected by a person's social surroundings, especially the degree of environmental stress and social support available. Although stress has been found to increase the risk of certain illnesses, such as cardiovascular disease, older people are generally less negatively affected by stress; this may reflect maturity, self-control, or a lifetime of developing coping skills.

Older people are more likely to suffer from chronic or long-term diseases than from temporary, or acute, illnesses. The majority of older persons, however, are not limited in their daily activities by chronic conditions. The impact of such conditions apparently varies with the physiological changes that occur with age, the individual's adaptive resources, and his or her mental and emotional perspective. The type and incidence of chronic conditions also vary by gender.

The three leading causes of death among persons over age 65 are heart disease, cancer, and stroke. Diseases of the heart and blood vessels are the most prevalent. Since hypertension or high blood pressure is a major risk in the development of cardiovascular problems, preventive actions are critical, especially weight control, dietary changes, appropriate exercise, and avoidance of cigarette smoking. Cancers, especially lung, bowel, and colon cancers, are the second most frequent cause of death among older persons; the risk of cancer increases with age. Cerebrovascular disease or stroke is the third leading cause of death among older persons. It may be caused by cerebral thrombosis, or blood clots, and by cerebral hemorrhage. Healthy lifestyle practices are important in stroke prevention.

Arthritis, although not fatal, is a major cause of limited daily activity and is extremely common among older persons. Osteoporosis, or loss of bone mass and the resultant increased brittleness of the bones, is most common among older women. Chronic respiratory problems, particularly emphysema, increase with age, especially among men. Diabetes mellitus is a frequent problem in old age, and is particularly troubling because of the many related illnesses that may result. Problems with the intestinal tract include diverticulitis, constipation, and hiatus hernia. Cystitis and incontinence are frequently occurring problems of the kidneys and urinary system. Although the majority of older persons have some type of incontinence, many kinds can be treated and controlled.

The growth of the older population, combined with the increase in major chronic illnesses, has placed greater demands on the health care system in this country. Nevertheless, older people seek outpatient medical, dental, and mental health services at a lower rate than their incidence of chronic illnesses would predict. Like younger people, the older population is most likely to seek health services for acute problems, not for check-ups on chronic conditions or for preventive care. Beliefs that physicians, dentists, and mental health professionals cannot do much to help their chronic problems may deter many older people from seeking needed care. The problem may be compounded by some health care professionals' attitudes that older people are poor candidates for health services because many of their health conditions cannot be cured. More university and continuing education classes are needed to provide training in geriatrics and gerontology for staff in health care settings and to address their attitudes toward older people.

Three theoretical models identify reasons for utilization and nonutilization of health services by older people. The behavioral model suggests that utilization differs as a function of predisposing variables such as age, sex, race, and occupation; enabling variables such as family income and perceived ability to pay; and need variables (actual and perceived need). This model is useful in describing why some people use health services and others do not, but it does not explain differences within subgroups such as the elderly.

The health belief model predicts that people are more likely to seek health services if they view themselves as susceptible to a disease, believe that it has severe consequences, and are convinced that the benefits of treatment outweigh the barriers. Although this model has been tested mostly in retrospective studies and rarely with older populations, it holds promise for testing different interventions to increase older people's use of health services.

A third approach, the person-environment congruence model, postulates that utilization is a function of the "fit" or integration between individual needs and capacities and the opportunities and constraints of the health care system. Thus, the availability of nearby and physically accessible services with staff who are sensitive to the needs of ethnic minority elderly is critical if utilization rates are to increase dramatically among traditionally underserved populations. As the number of people with more education and experience with the health care system increases, designing specialized health services may be less important. Nevertheless, it is essential that health planners consider the special needs of the aging population in designing appropriate services that fit them.

The elimination or postponement of the chronic diseases that are associated with old age appears to be the major task for both future biomedical researchers as well as health promotion specialists. Treatment methods for all these diseases are changing rapidly with the growth in medical technology and the increasing recognition given to such environmental factors as stress, nutrition, and exercise in disease prevention. If health promotion efforts to modify lifestyles are successful, and if aging research progresses substantially, the chronic illnesses that we have discussed will undoubtedly be postponed and disability or loss of functional status will be delayed.

References

Abramson, J. H., and Hopp, C. The control of cardiovascular risk factors in the elderly. *Preventive Medicine,* 1976, 5, 32–47.

Aday, L. A., and Andersen, R. A framework for the study of access to medical care. *Health Services Research,* 1974, 9, 208–220.

Ahrens, E. H. Symposium report on the task force on the evidence relating six dietary factors to the nation's health. *American Journal of Clinical Nutrition,* 1979, 32, 2621–2748.

Allen, J. The use of isometric exercises in a geriatrics treatment program. *Geriatrics,* 1985, 20, 346–347.

Almy, T. P., and Howell, D. A. Diverticular disease of the colon. *New England Journal of Medicine,* 1980, 202, 324–331.

American Association of Retired Persons. *Survey of 1,000 persons 45 and older.* Washington, D.C., 1986.

American Dental Association. *Prevention and control of dental disease through improved access to comprehensive care.* Chicago: ADA, 1979.

Andersen, R. *A behavioral model of families' use of health services.* Chicago: Center for Health Administration Studies, 1968.

Andersen, R., and Newman, J. Societal and individual determinants of medical care utilization in the United States. *Milbank Memorial Fund Quarterly,* 1973, 51, 95–124.

Avorn, J. Medicine: The life and death of Oliver Shay. In A. Pifer and L. Bronte (Eds.), *Our aging society.* New York: Norton, 1986.

Banziger, G., and Roush, S. Nursing homes for the birds: A control-relevant intervention with bird feeders. *The Gerontologist,* 1983, 23, 527–532.

Baum, B. J. Characteristics of participants in the oral physiology component of the Baltimore Longitudinal Study of Aging. *Community Dentistry and Oral Epidemiology,* 1981, 9, 128–134.

Beck, J. D. The epidemiology of oral diseases in the elderly. *Gerodontology,* 1984, 3, 5–116.

Beck, J. D., Cons, N., Field, H., and Walker, J. *The Iowa survey of oral health: 1980.* Final Report to NIH, University of Iowa College of Dentistry, Iowa City, Iowa, 1982.

Beck, P. Two successful interventions in nursing homes: The therapeutic effects of cognitive activity. *The Gerontologist,* 1982, *22,* 378–383.

Becker, M., Maiman, L., Kirscht, J., Haefner, D., and Drachman, R. Health belief model and prediction of dietary compliance: A field experiment. *Journal of Health and Social Behavior,* 1977, *18,* 348–366.

Belloc, N. B., and Breslow, L. Relationship of physical health status and health practices. *Preventive Medicine,* 1972, *1,* 409–421.

Berkman, L. Social networks, support and health: Taking the next step forward. *American Journal of Epidemiology,* 1986, *123,* 559–562.

Berkman, L., and Breslow, L. *Health and ways of living: The Alameda County study.* New York: Oxford University Press, 1983.

Blazer, D. G. Social support and mortality in an elderly community population. *American Journal of Epidemiology,* 1982, *115,* 684–694.

Borham, N. O. Prevalence and prognostic significance of hypertension in the elderly. *Journal of the American Geriatrics Society,* 1986, *34,* 112–114.

Boss, G., and Seegmiller, J. E. Age-related physiological changes and their clinical significance. *Western Journal of Medicine,* 1981, *135,* 13–19.

Branch, L. Functional abilities of the elderly: An update on the Massachusetts health care panel study. In S. G. Haynes and M. Feinleib (Eds.), *Epidemiology of aging.* NIH Publication No. 80-969, Washington, D.C.: U.S. Government Printing Office, 1980.

Branch, L., and Jette, A. Personal health practices and mortality among the elderly. *American Journal of Public Health,* 1984, *74.*

Brunelle, J. A. Coronal and root surface caries and tooth mortality of U.S. adults. Presented at symposium on NIDR Adult Dental Health Survey, Meetings of the International Association for Dental Research, Chicago, March 1987.

Butler, R., and Gleason, H. *Productive aging: Enhancing vitality in later life.* New York: Springer, 1985.

Cassel, J. The contribution of the social environment to host resistance. *American Journal of Epidemiology,* 1976, *104*(2), 107–123.

Chauncey, H. H. The incidence of coronal caries in normal aging male adults. Paper presented at meetings of the International Association for Dental Research. March 1978.

Cockerham, W. C., Sharp, K., and Wilcox, J. Aging and perceived health status. *Journal of Gerontology,* 1983, *38*(3), 349–355.

Cohen, C., Teresi, J., and Holmes, D. Social networks, stress and physical health: A longitudinal study of an inner-city elderly population. *Journal of Gerontology,* 1985, *40,* 478–486.

Cohen, J. B., and Brody, J. A. The epidemiologic importance of psychosocial factors in longevity. *American Journal of Epidemiology,* 1981, *114,* 451–461.

Cohen, S. Arthritis—But what sort? *Geriatrics,* 1982, *37,* 49–51.

Cousins, N. *Anatomy of an illness.* New York: Bantam Books, 1979.

Cutler, S. J., and Young, J. L. (Eds.). *Third national cancer survey: Incidence data.* National Cancer Institute Monograph E1:1–454, 1975.

Davis, L. J., Brody, E. M., and Cooper, R. H. Problems of urban elderly in utilization of health services. Paper presented at meetings of the Gerontological Society. 1980.

DeBerry, S. An evaluation of progressive muscle relaxation on stress related symptoms in a geriatric population. *International Journal of Aging and Human Development,* 1981–82, *14,* 255–269.

deVries, H. A. Physiology of physical conditioning for the elderly. In R. Harris and L. J. Frankel (Eds.), *Guide to fitness after 50.* New York: Plenum Press, 1977.

Diokno, A. C., Brock, B. M., Brown, M. B., and Herzog, R. Prevalence of urinary incontinence and other urological symptoms in the noninstitutionalized elderly. *Journal of Urology,* 1986, *136,* 1022–1025.

Dowd, J., and Bengtson, V. Aging in minority population: An examination of the double jeopardy hypothesis. *The Journal of Gerontology.* 1978, 33.

Dychtwald, K. Overview: Health promotion and disease prevention for elders. *Generations,* 1983, *7,* 5–7.

Evashwick, C., Rowe, G., Diehr, P., and Branch, L. Factors explaining the use of health care services by the elderly. *Health Services Research,* 1984, *19,* 357–382.

Eve, S. B., Watson, J. B., and Reiss, E. M. Use of health care services among older adults. Paper presented at meetings of the Gerontological Society, 1980.

Exton-Smith, A. N. Mineral metabolism. In C. Finch and E. Schneider (Eds.), *Handbook of the biology of aging* (2d ed.). New York: Van Nostrand, 1985.

Farquhar, J. W. *The American way of life need not be hazardous to your health.* New York: W.W. Norton, 1978.

Federal Council on the Aging. *The need for long-term care: Information and issues.* DHHS Publication Number OHDS81-20704, Washington, D.C., U.S. Department of Health and Human Services, 1981.

Ferraro, K. F. Self ratings of health among the old and old-old. *Journal of Health and Social Behavior,* 1980, *21,* 377–383.

Ferraro, K. F., and Mutran, E. Differences in health care utilization of older men and women. Paper presented at meetings of the Gerontological Society, 1983.

Fillenbaum, G. G. Social contexts and self assessments of health among the elderly. *Journal of Health and Social Behavior,* 1979, *20,* 45–51.

Filner, B., and Williams, T. F. Health promotion for the elderly: Reducing functional dependency. In *Healthy people: The surgeon general's report on health promotion and disease prevention.* Washington, D.C.: U.S. Government Printing Office, 1979.

Ford, C. V., and Sbordone, R. J. Attitudes of psychiatrists toward elderly patients. *American Journal of Psychiatry,* 1980, *137,* 571–575.

Fries, J. Aging, natural death, and the compression of morbidity. *New England Journal of Medicine,* 1980, *303,* 130–135.

Fries, J. F. Aging, natural death, and the compression of morbidity. *Generations,* 1983, Spring, 16–18.

Fries, J. F. The compression of morbidity: Miscellaneous comments about a theme. *The Gerontologist,* 1984, *24,* 354–359.

Fries, J. F., and Crapo, L. M. *Vitality and aging.* San Francisco: W.H. Freeman, 1981.

Gilmore, S. S., and Kiyak, H. A. Predictors of dental behavior among the elderly. *Special Care in Dentistry,* 1984, *5,* 169–173.

Green, L. W., et al. *Health education planning: A diagnostic approach.* Palo Alto, Calif.: Mayfield, 1980.

Gregory, C. A. Possible influence of physical activity on musculoskeletal symptoms of menopausal and postmenopausal women. *Journal of Obstetric and Gynecological Nursing,* 1982, *11,* 103–107.

Grundy, S. M. Rationale of the diet-heart statements of the American Heart Association. *Circulation,* 1982, *65,* 839a–854a.

Haefner, D. P. The health belief model and preventive dental behavior. *Health Education Monographs,* 1974, *2,* 420–432.

Hamburg, D. A. An outlook on stress research and health. In G. R. Elliott and C. Eisdorfer (Eds.), *Stress and human health: An analysis and implications of research.* New York: Springer, 1982.

Harris, L., et al. *Aging in the 80's: America in transition.* Washington, D.C.: National Council on Aging, 1981.

Harris, R. Fitness and exercise: A day in the life of Dr. H. *Generation,* Spring 1983, 23–26.

Haug, M. Doctor and elderly patient relationships and their impact on self-care. Paper presented at meetings of the Gerontological Society. 1984.

Health Resources Administration. *A decade of dental service utilization, 1964–1974.* DHHS Publication #(HRA)80-56, 1977.

Healthy people: The surgeon general's report on health promotion and disease prevention. Washington, D.C.: USGP, DHEW, 1979.

Hendricks, J., and Hendricks, C. D. *Aging in mass society: Myths and realities* (2d ed.). Cambridge, Mass.: Winthrop, 1981.

Hickey, T. *Health and Aging.* Belmont, Calif.: Wadsworth, 1980.

Holmes, T. H., and Masuda, M. Life change and illness susceptibility. In B. S. Dohrenwend and B. P. Dohrenwend (Eds.), *Stressful life events: Their nature and effects.* New York: Wiley, 1974.

Holtzman, J. M., and Akiyama, H. Symptoms and the decision to seek professional care. *Gerodontics,* 1985, *1,* 44–49.

House, J., and Robbins, C. Age, psychosocial stress, and health. In M. W. Riley, B. Hess, and K. Bond, *Aging in society: Selected reviews.* Hillsdale, N.J.: Erlbaum, 1983.

Jack, S., and Ries, P. Current estimates from the National Health Interview Survey: United States, 1979. *Data from the national health interview survey.* 1981, Series 10, No. 136. Rockville, Md.: NCHS.

Jette, A., and Branch, L. The Framingham disability study, II: Physical disability among the aging. *American Journal of Public Health,* 1981, *71,* 1211–1216.

Jones, G. S., and Jones, H. W. *Gynecology.* Baltimore, Md.: Williams and Williams, 1982.

Kahana, E. Matching environments to needs of the aged: A conceptual scheme. In J. Gubrium (Ed.), *Late life: Recent developments in the sociology of aging.* New York: Charles Thomas, 1975.

Kahana, E., Liang, J., and Felton, B. Alternative models of P-E fit: Prediction of morale in 3 homes for the aged. *Journal of Gerontology,* 1980, *35,* 584–595.

Kane, R., Kane, L., and Arnold, S. Prevention and the elderly: Risk factors. *Health Services Research,* 1985, *19,* 945–1006.

Kane, R., and Kane R. *Assessing the elderly: A practical guide for measurement.* Lexington, Mass.: Lexington Books, 1981.

Kannel, W. B. Habitual level of physical activity and risk of coronary heart disease: The Framingham study. *Canadian Medical Association Journal,* 1967, *96,* 811–812.

Kannel, W. B. Hypertension and aging. In C. Finch and E. Schneider (Eds.), *Handbook of the biology of aging* (2d ed.). New York: Van Nostrand, 1985.

Kannel, W. B., and Brand, F. N. Cardiovascular risk factors in the elderly woman. In E. Markson (Ed.), *Older women.* Lexington, Mass.: Lexington Books, 1983, 315–327.

Kannel, W. B., and Gordon, T. Evaluation of cardiovascular risk on the elderly: The Framingham study. *Bulletin of the New York Academy of Medicine,* 1978, *54,* 573–596.

Kart, C. S., Metress, E. S., and Metress, J. *Aging and health: Biologic and social perspectives.* Menlo Park, Calif.: Addison-Wesley, 1978.

Kegeles, S. Field experimental attempt to change beliefs and behavior of women in an urban ghetto. *Journal of Health and Social Behavior,* 1969, *10,* 115–124.

Kerzner, L. Physical changes after menopause. In E. Markson (Ed.), *Older women.* Lexington, Mass.: Lexington Books, 1983.

Kirkendall, W. M. Treatment of hypertension in the elderly. *American Journal of Cardiology,* 1986, *57,* 63C–68C.

Kiyak, H. A. An experimental preventive dentistry program for the elderly. Final report to the National Institute for Dental Research, R23-DE5235, 1980.

Kiyak, H. A. Utilization of dental services by the elderly. *Gerodontology,* 1984, *3,* 17–26.

Kiyak, H. A., and Miller, R. Age differences in oral health behavior and beliefs. *Journal of Public Health Dentistry,* 1982, *42,* 29–41.

Kiyak, H. A., and Mulligan, K. Behavioral research related to oral hygiene practices. In H. Löe and D. Kleinman (Eds.), *Dental plaque control measures and oral hygiene practices.* Oxford, Eng.: IRL Press, 1985.

Kosberg, J., and Harris, A. Attitudes toward elderly clients. *Health and Social Work,* 1978, *3,* 68–90.

Krout, J. A. Knowledge and use of services by the elderly: A critical review of the literature. *International Journal of Aging and Human Development,* 1983, *17,* 153–167.

Lawton, M. P., and Nahemow, L. Ecology and the aging process. In C. Eisdorfer and M. P. Lawton (Eds.), *The psychology of adult development and aging.* Washington, D.C.: American Psychological Association, 1973.

Levin, M. Diabetes: The geriatric difference. *Geriatrics,* 1982, *37,* 41–45.

Lewis, M. Older women and health. *Women and Health,* 1985, *10,* 1–16.

Lind, S. D. Social service utilization: Application of a behavioral model of demand to an elderly population. Unpublished doctoral thesis, Brandeis University, 1978.

Lindsay, R. Osteoporosis. In *Health issues of older women.* State University of New York at Stony Brook, 1981.

Maiman, L. A., and Becker, M. H. The health belief model: Origins and correlates in psychological theory. *Health Education Monographs,* 1974, *2,* 336–353.

Manderson, R. D., and Ettinger, R. L. Dental status of the institutionalized elderly population of Edinburgh. *Community Dentistry and Oral Epidemiology,* 1975, *3,* 29–32.

Manton, K. G., and Liu, K. *The future growth of the long-term care population: Projection based on the 1977 national nursing home survey and the 1982 long term care survey.* Washington, D.C., 1984.

Marchesseault, L. C. Diabetes mellitus and the elderly. *Nursing Clinics of North America,* 1983, *19,* 791–798.

Markides, K. Minority aging. In M. W. Riley, B. Hess, and K. Bond (Eds.), *Aging in society.* Hillsdale, N.J.: Erlbaum, 1983.

Masuda, M., and Holmes, T. H. Life events: Perceptions and frequencies. *Psychosomatic Medicine,* 1978, *40,* 236–361.

Moritani, T. Training adaptations in the muscles of older men. In E. L. Smith and R. C. Serfass (Eds.), *Exercise and aging: The scientific basis.* Hillside, N.J.: Enslow, 1981.

Multiple Risk Factor Intervention Trial Research Group. Multiple risk factor intervention trial. *The Journal of the American Medical Association,* 1982, *248,* 1465.

Murphy, J., Lamb, S., and Duthie, E. Urinary incontinence in the elderly. *Wisconsin Medical Journal,* 1983, *82,* 19–21.

Myles, J. F. Institutionalization and sick role identification among the elderly. *American Sociological Review,* 1978, *43,* 508–521.

National Center for Health Statistics. *Current estimates from the national health interview survey: U.S. 1981.* National Health Survey, Series 10, #141. DHHS Publication #82-1569, 1982.

National Center for Health Statistics. Comparison with their aged counterparts with incomes less than $7000. *Preliminary Data* from the 1982 long-term care survey, 1985.

National Center for Health Statistics. Summary of the national health interview survey. Unpublished tabulation, 1983.

National Center for Health Statistics. Changes in mortality among the elderly, United States, 1940–78 supplement to 1980. *Vital and health statistics,* Series 3. DHHS Publication No. (PHS) 82-1406a, 1984.

National Institute on Aging. *Osteoporosis and aging.* Washington, D.C.: U.S. Department of Health and Human Services, 1981.

National Pacific/Asian Resource Center on Aging. On Lok senior health services. *Update,* 1986, *7,* 1–3.

Nussbaum, S. R. Management of osteoporosis. In A. H. Gorall, L. A. May, and A. G. Mulley (Eds.), *Primary care medicine.* Philadelphia: Lippincott, 1981.

Nuttbrock, L., and Kosberg, J. I. Images of the physician and help-seeking behavior of the elderly: A multivariate assessment. *Journal of Gerontology,* 1980, *35,* 241–248.

Ouslander, J. G. Urinary incontinence in the elderly. *The Western Journal of Medicine,* 1981, *135,* 482–483.

Page, L. B., Damon, A., and Moellering, R. C. Antecedents of cardiovascular disease in six Solomon Island societies. *Circulation,* 1974, *49,* 1132.

Palmore, E. Health practices and illness among the aged. *The Gerontologist,* 1970, Winter, Part I, 313–316.

Petrich, J., and Holmes, T. H. Life change and onset of illness. *Medical Clinics of North America,* 1977, *61,* 825–837.

Price, S., and Kiyak, H. A. A behavioral approach to improving oral health among the elderly. *Special Care in Dentistry,* 1981, *1,* 267–274.

Rodin, J., and Langer, E. J. Long-term effects of a control-relevant intervention with the institutionalized aged. *Journal of Personality and Social Psychology,* 1977, *35,* 897–902.

Roos, N. P., and Shapiro, E. The Manitoba longitudinal study on aging: Preliminary findings on health care utilization by the elderly. *Medical Care,* 1981, *19,* 644–657.

Roos, N. P., Shapiro, E., and Roos, L. L. Aging and the demand for health services: Which aged and whose demand? *The Gerontologist,* 1984, *24,* 31–36.

Rosenberg, L., Hennekins, C. H., Rosner, B., Belanger, C., Rothman, K., and Speizer, F. Oral contraceptive use in relation to nonfatal myocardial infarction. *American Journal of Epidemiology,* 1980, *111,* 59–66.

Rosenstock, J. M. Why people use health services. *Milbank Memorial Fund Quarterly,* 1966, *44,* 94–127.

Rosenstock, J. M. The health belief model and preventive health behavior. *Health Education Monographs,* 1974, *2,* 354–386.

Rothman, K. J. Alcohol. In J. Fraumeni (Ed.), *Persons at high risk of cancer: An approach to cancer etiology and control.* New York: Academic Press, 1975.

Rowe, J. W. Health care of the elderly. *New England Journal of Medicine,* 1985, *312,* 827–835.

Shanas, E. *The health of older people: A social survey.* Cambridge, Mass.: Harvard University Press, 1962.

Shanas, E., and Maddox, G. Health, health resources and the utilization of care. In E. Shanas and R. Binstock (Eds.), *Handbook of aging and the social sciences* (2d ed.) New York: Van Nostrand, 1985.

Shanas, E., Townsend, P., Wedderburn, D., Friis, H., Milhoj, P., and Stehouwen, J. *Old people in three industrial societies.* New York: Atherton, 1968.

Shapiro, E., and Roos, L. Using health care: Rural/urban differences among the Manitoba elderly. *The Gerontologist,* 1984, *24,* 270–274.

Shapiro, E., and Roos, N. P. Elderly nonusers of health care services. *Medical Care,* 1985, *23,* 247–257.

Sharpe, W. D. Age changes in human bone: An overview. *Bulletin of the New York Academy of Medicine,* 1979, *55,* 757–773.

Sheehan, G. *On running and being: The total experience.* Warner Books, 1978.

Sheehy, T. Hypertension in the elderly. *Medical Times,* 1980, *108*(6), 31–37.

Shepard, R. J. *Physical activity and aging.* Chicago: Croom Helm/Year Book Publishers, 1978.

Shepard, R. J. Cardiovascular limitations in the aged. In E. C. Smith and R. C. Serfass (Eds.), *Exercise in aging: The scientific basis.* Hillside, N.J.: Enslow, 1981.

Shephard, R. J. *Physiology and biochemistry of exercise.* New York: Praeger, 1982.

Snider, E. Awareness and use of health services by the elderly: A Canadian study. *Medical Care,* 1980, *18,* 1177–1182.

Swallow, J. N. A survey of edentulous individuals in a district in Amsterdam. *Community Dentistry and Oral Epidemiology,* 1978, *6,* 210–216.

Tucker, R. M. Is hypertension different in the elderly? *Geriatrics,* 1980, *35*(5), 28–32.

USDHEW, National Center for Health Statistics. Current estimates from the national health interview survey: United States, 1977. *Vital and health statistics, No. 126.* Washington, D.C.: Public Health Service, 1978.

USDHEW, National Center for Health Statistics. Current estimates from the national health interview survey: United States, 1977. *Vital and health statistics, No. 130.* Washington, D.C.: Public Health Service, 1979.

U.S. Public Health Service, National Center for Health Statistics. *Edentulous persons, United States, 1971.* Washington, D.C.: DHEW, 1974.

U.S. Senate. *Dietary goals for the U.S.* (2d ed.). Washington, D.C.: USGPO, 1977.

U.S. Senate Special Committee on Aging. *America in transition: An aging society,* 1984–85 edition. Washington, D.C.: U.S. Government Printing Office, 1985.

U.S. Senate Special Committee on Aging. *Aging America: Trends and projections.* Washington, D.C.: U.S. Government Printing Office, 1986.

Verbrugge, L. Women and men: Mortality and health of older people. In M. W. Riley, B. Hess, and K. Bone, *Aging and society.* Hillsdale, N.J.: Erlbaum, 1983.

Waldron, I. Why do women live longer than men? Parts I and II, *Social Science and Medicine,* 1976, *10,* 340–362.

Ward, R. A. Services for older people: An integrated framework for research. *Journal of Health and Social Behavior,* 1978, *18,* 61–70.

Weg, R. Changing physiology of aging: Normal and pathological. In D. S. Woodruff and J. E. Birren (Eds.), *Aging: Scientific perspectives and social issues.* New York: Van Nostrand, 1983.

Weiss, B. D. Unstable bladder in elderly patients. *American Family Physician,* 1983, *4,* 243–247.

Weiss, N. S. Decreased risk of fractures of the hip and lower forearm with postmenopausal use of estrogen. *New England Journal of Medicine,* 1980, *303,* 1195–1198.

Wheeler, M. Osteoporosis. *Medical Clinics of North America,* 1976, *60*(6), 1213–1223.

Wiley, J., and Camacho, T. Life-style and future health: Evidence from the Alameda county study. *Preventive Medicine,* 1980, *9,* 1–21.

Williams, T. F. Diabetes mellitus in older people. In W. Reichel (Ed.), *Clinical aspects of aging.* Baltimore, Md.: Williams and Witkin, 1978.

Wolinsky, F. D. Assessing the effects of predisposing, enabling, and illness-morbidity characteristics on health services utilization. *Journal of Health and Social Behavior,* 1978, *19,* 384–396.

Women's Health. Report of the Public Health Service Task Force on Women's Health Issues. *Public Health Reports,* 1985, *100*(1), 73–92.

World Health Organization. *Planning and organization of geriatric services.* Technical Report, Series 548. Geneva, 1974.

Part III

The Psychological Context of Social Aging

The dynamic interactions between people and their environments as they age, the population trends that have made gerontology such an important concern in the late twentieth century, and the historical background of social gerontology were discussed in Part I. Part II focused on the normal and pathological physiological and sensory changes that take place with aging. The types of chronic and acute health problems that afflict older people were presented. The older population's demands on the health care system and their reasons for using or not using health services were reviewed. Part II concluded with a discussion of the growing field of health promotion, and how improved health behaviors can affect older people's social interactions.

In this section, the focus is on psychological changes with aging—both normal and abnormal—that influence older people's social behavior and dynamic relationships with their physical and social environments. As we have already seen, many changes take place in the aging organism that make it more difficult to perform daily tasks and to respond as quickly and easily to external demands as in youth. Many older people have chronic health problems, such as arthritis, diabetes, or heart disease, that compound the normal changes that cause people to slow down. In a similar manner, some changes in cognitive functioning and personality are a function of normal aging. Other psychological changes may be due to the secondary effects of diseases.

Many researchers have examined changes in intelligence, learning, and memory with aging. The literature in this area, reviewed in Chapter 7, suggests that normal aging does not result in signficant declines. Although older subjects in the studies described do not perform as well as younger subjects, their scores are not so poor as to indicate significant impairments in social functioning. Laboratory tests also may be less than ideal as indicators of cognitive function. Suggestions for improving memory in the later years are discussed in Chapter 7.

Chapter 8 describes personality in old age, psychological models of successful and unsuccessful adjustment to aging, the importance of maintaining self-esteem in the later years, and threats to self-esteem that result from changes in social roles. This chapter also focuses on coping and adaptation in old age. Given the normal age-related changes in physiological, sensory, and cognitive functions, in personality styles, and in older individuals' social networks, some gerontologists have argued that older people experience more stress in a given time period than the young. Furthermore, there has been considerable debate about whether aging results in the use of different types of coping strategies. Older people appear to perceive life events differently from the young, and to attribute less stress to events that they have already experienced. However, there is insufficient longitudinal research in this area to conclude with any certainty that aging is associated with more stressful life events than youth. Coping strategies also appear to remain consistent throughout adulthood and old age.

Some forms of psychopathology, such as manic and antisocial behavior, are more common in youth than in old age. However, some older people are at high risk for major depressive episodes, paranoia, and some forms of dementia. In the case of the dementias, such as Alzheimer's disease, cognitive abilities decline quite dramatically, sometimes within a few years, other times over many years. Older individuals with a diagnosis of dementia experience significant impairments in their ability to interact with other people, and to control their physical and social environments. The impact on family relationships and on the psychological well-being of family caregivers may be so severe as to cause excess stress, often leading to institutionalization of the older person. To the extent that such people do not seek preventive mental health services or obtain these services when they experience depression or paranoia, their social interactions will deteriorate; some may become reclusive and, in the case of severely depressed older persons, at greater risk of suicide. Despite the growing number of studies that support the benefits of therapeutic interventions for older people who are living in the community or in institutions, this segment of the population underutilizes mental health services. Most of the mental health care provided to older people takes place in hospitals, not in community mental health centers nor in private practice.

Perhaps the most important knowledge to be gained in Part III is that aging does not affect all people's psychological functions in the same way. Cognitive declines generally are not so dramatic as to impair older people's social functions. However, some people report mild forgetfulness, a condition known as "benign senescent forgetfulness"; a small segment of the older population experiences Alzheimer's disease or other types of dementia. Personality and patterns of coping also do not change so dramatically as to impair social functioning, although some sex-typed behaviors become less pronounced with age. Coping and adaptation skills do not become impaired with normal aging; styles of coping vary widely among older people. Indeed, aging results in increasing differences in psychological functioning among people, not greater similarity. The following vignettes illustrate the contrasts in psychological aging:

An Older Person with Intact Cognitive Abilities

Mr. Wallace, age 75, is a retired professor in a midwestern community. He retired 10 years ago, after teaching history in a large state university for 40 years. He remains active by doing volunteer work in the local historical society, teaching part-time at the university, and traveling to Europe with his wife for three months every summer, occasionally leading groups of other retirees in tours of medieval European towns. Mr. Wallace's major project that he wishes to complete before he dies is a historical novel about Charlemagne. This is a topic about which he has lectured and read extensively, and one he enjoys investigating in more detail during his trips to Europe. This project occupies much of his remaining time. Mrs. Wallace often remarks that he is busier these days than he was before his retirement. During the first few months after retirement, Professor Wallace experienced a mild bout of depression; it was relieved as he became involved in group therapy with other retirees. Mr. Wallace enjoys intellectual challenges today as much as he did when he was employed, in fact, more so, because he is pursuing these activities without the pressures of a day-to-day job. He vows to keep up his level of activity until he "runs out of energy."

An Older Person with Good Coping Skills

Mrs. Johnson, age 83, has suffered numerous tragedies throughout her life. Born to a poor farming family in Mississippi, she moved North with her mother and eight older sisters and brothers as a child, after her father died and the family farm was lost. The family supported itself through hard work in the factories. Mrs. Johnson married young; she and her husband struggled through the years to own their home and raise their three children. Her husband died 20 years ago, leaving her with a small pension. She worked at a manual labor job until she was 70 years old, when her arthritis made it painful for her to do the heavy work needed on the job. During the past three years, Mrs. Johnson has experienced a series of losses: her son and daughter-in-law died in an auto accident; her last surviving sister died; and her oldest granddaughter, the one on whom she could most depend, moved West to attend medical school. Mrs. Johnson admits these losses are painful, but that it is "God's will" that she experience them. Her strong faith in God helps her accept these changes in her life, and her deteriorating health, as part of a "Master Plan." When she becomes too distraught, she turns to the Bible, and looks forward to visits from her grandchildren and great-grandchildren to keep her busy.

An Older Person with Severe Cognitive Impairment

Mr. Adams is aged 68. Several years ago he started showing signs of confusion and disorientation. He was diagnosed as having Alzheimer's disease at age 64, one year before his retirement. He and his wife had purchased a large motor home in anticipation of traveling during retirement; now all their plans have completely changed. While there have been some brief periods during the past four years where he has seemed to be better, Mr. Adams now is extremely agitated and disoriented, wanders during the night, and is very negative and occasionally abusive to people near him. He often does not know who his wife and children are. The slightest change in routine will upset him. In his lucid moments, Mr. Adams cries and wonders what has happened to his life; at some points, he can also carry on short conversations. His wife is determined to keep him at home, even though he often verbally abuses her and does not recognize or appreciate all that she does for him. She is able to take him to an adult day health center during the day, where the staff try to keep him active and stimulated. He and his wife also attend meetings of ASSIST, the support group for Alzheimer's patients and their families. ASSIST has been a primary support to his wife, where she can often ventilate about how hard things are and then be supported for her efforts. Mr. Adams expresses great fear at the thought of a nursing home, but his wife worries about how long she can manage him at home and their children think that he should be in a nursing home.

The next three chapters describe how the aging process influences cognitive abilities, personality styles, and responses to major life events, and emphasize the wide variations in these processes with aging. Mental health and illness also occur in older people, but sometimes take on different features than in youth. The vastly different psychological states of Mr. Wallace, Mrs. Johnson, and Mr. Adams reflect the variations in these major aspects of aging, which will be reviewed next.

Chapter 7

Cognitive Changes
with Aging

One of the most important and most studied aspects of aging is cognitive functioning; that is, intelligence, learning, and memory. These are critical to an individual's performance in every aspect of life, including work and leisure activities, relationships with family and friends, and roles in the community. Older people who have problems in cognitive functioning will eventually experience stress in these other areas as well, along with an increasing incongruence between their competence levels and the demands of their environments. Researchers have attempted to determine whether normal aging is associated with a decline in the three areas of cognitive functioning and, if so, to what extent such a decline is due to age-related physiological changes. Much of the research on these issues has evolved from studies of cognitive development across the life span. Other studies have been undertaken in response to concerns expressed by many older persons or their families that they cannot learn as easily as they used to, or that they have more trouble remembering names, dates, and places than previously.

This chapter reviews the research on cognition and normal aging, the problems of determining why observed changes occur, some of the social consequences of age-related cognitive changes, and some techniques that older persons can use to improve their learning and memory. We examine the three key elements of intellectual processes: intelligence, learning, and memory, and touch upon the issue of creativity.

Intelligence and Aging

The first of the three components of cognition, intelligence, is difficult both to define and to measure. Of all of the elements of cognition, it is least verifiable. We can only infer its existence and can only indirectly measure individual levels. Intelligence has been defined as the "theoretical limit of an individual's performance" (Jones, 1959, p. 700). The limit is determined by biological and genetic factors; however, the ability to achieve the limit is influenced by environmental opportunities, such as a challenging educational experience, as well as by environmental constraints, such as the absence of books or other intellectual stimulation. Huyck and Hoyer (1982) have defined intelligence as a range of abilities, including the ability to deal with symbols and abstractions, to acquire and comprehend new information, to adapt to new situations, and to appreciate and/or create new ideas. Intelligence quotient (or IQ) refers to an individual's relative abilities in some of these areas compared to others of the same chronological age. Unfortunately, most tests of intelligence (IQ tests) do not measure all the components of intelligence. For example, how can a person's creativity be determined and evaluated with sufficient validity? How can criteria of successful adaptation be established that can be measured in paper and pencil form?

Most theorists agree that intelligence is composed of many different components. Perhaps the most complex model is Guilford's (1966, 1967) three-dimensional structure of intellect (see Figure 7–1). The three dimensions represent the content of knowledge (e.g., figures, symbols, words), the operations that an individual must perform with this knowledge (e.g., memorize, evaluate, come up with single or multiple solutions), and the products that are derived from these operations (e.g., relations, systems, implications). A multidimensional structure of intelligence, although not identical to Guilford's model, is assumed by most measures of intelligence, which assess different abilities and types of knowledge.

In contrast, the general factor theory of intelligence, which was first proposed by Spearman in 1927, suggests that there is a general ability that is required for all intellectual tasks, as well as a set of specific abilities that are necessary for some tasks, but not for others. Such a general aspect of intelligence may exist, but it is difficult to measure it independent of the specific abilities that are associated with it.

The work of Thurstone and Thurstone (1941, 1958) gives credence to both

FIGURE 7–1 A Three-Dimensional Model of Intellect

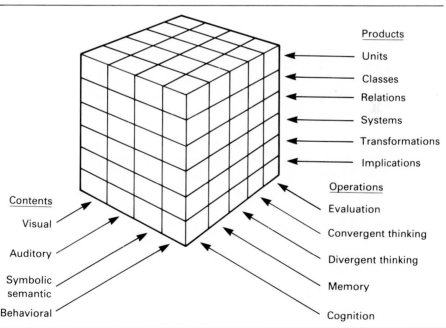

Products
Units
Classes
Relations
Systems
Transformations
Implications

Operations
Evaluation
Convergent thinking
Divergent thinking
Memory
Cognition

Contents
Visual
Auditory
Symbolic semantic
Behavioral

Source: J. P. Guilford, *The nature of human intelligence* (New York: McGraw-Hill, 1967) and J. P. Guilford, *Way beyond the IQ* (Buffalo, N.Y.: Creative Education Foundation, 1977). Reprinted by permission of the author, McGraw-Hill, and the Creative Education Foundation.

positions. They proposed a primary mental abilities model that includes a general intelligence factor, and is composed of five primary and independent abilities: number, word fluency, verbal meaning, reasoning, and space. Although this model was initially developed with young adults, recent work by Schaie and colleagues provides support for this multi-ability model in older adults (Schaie, 1979; Schaie and Labouvie-Vief, 1974; Schaie and Hertzog, 1983). A useful distinction has been made between *fluid intelligence* and *crystallized intelligence* (Cattell, 1963; Horn, 1970; Horn and Donaldson, 1980). Fluid intelligence consists of skills that are biologically determined, independent of experience or learning, and may be similar to what is popularly called "native intelligence." It involves processing information that is not embedded in a context of existing information for the individual. Crystallized intelligence refers to the knowledge and abilities that the individual acquires through education and lifelong experiences. These two types of intelligence have been found to show different patterns with aging, as we will see in the next section.

There has been considerable controversy regarding intelligence in the later years (Botwinick, 1984). Many researchers have found significant differences between young and old persons on intelligence tests, with older persons performing at a much lower level. Others have concluded that aging is not really associated with a decline in intelligence, but that the particular IQ tests and the time pressures on test-takers are more detrimental to older persons than to the young. Still others have pointed to methodological problems in conducting research in this area. Unfortunately, these mixed research findings have served to perpetuate the stereotype that older people are less intelligent than the young.

Many older persons are concerned that their intelligence has declined from when they were young. This concern may loom so large for them that merely taking part in a study intended to "test their intelligence" may provoke sufficient anxiety to affect their performance on the test. Such anxieties may also influence the older person's daily functioning. Research with children has shown that false information given to them about their IQ scores or test performance, whether the information shows that they scored very well or very poorly, leads to future behavior that is consistent with the false test scores. This situation represents a confirmation of expectations or a "self-fulfilling prophecy." In the same way, people who are told by friends, family, test-givers, or society in general that they should not expect to perform as well on intellectual tasks because aging causes a decline in intelligence may, in fact, come to perform more poorly.

The most widely used measure of adult intelligence is the Wechsler Adult Intelligence Scale (WAIS). It consists of 11 subtests, six of which are described as Verbal Scales (which measure, to some extent, crystallized intelligence), and five as Performance Scales (providing some measure of fluid intelligence). Verbal scores are obtained by measuring an individual's ability to define the meaning of words, to explain why such things as social and legal laws are established, to interpret proverbs, and to explain similarities between words and concepts. In this way, accumulated knowledge and abstract reasoning can be tested. Performance tests focus on an individual's ability to manipulate unfamiliar objects and words, often in unusual ways. These include tests of spatial relations and abstract reasoning, and may require an individual to put puzzles together to match a picture, match pictures with symbols or numbers, or arrange pictures in a particular pattern. Both psychomotor and perceptual skills are needed in performing these tasks. In addition, the performance tests on the WAIS are generally timed; the verbal tests are not.

A consistent pattern of scores on these two components of the WAIS has emerged in numerous studies; it has been labelled the *Classic Aging Pattern*. People beyond the age of 65 in some studies, and even earlier in other studies, perform poorly on Performance Scales, but their scores on Verbal Scales remain stable. The tendency to do worse on the performance tasks with aging may reflect age-related changes in noncognitive functions, such as sensory and perceptual abilities, and in psychomotor skills. As we have seen in Chapters 3 and 5, aging results in a slowing down of the neural pathways and of the visual and auditory functions. This slower reaction time, and the delay in receiving and transmitting messages through the sense organs, explain poorer performance on subtests requiring such capabilities. Some researchers have therefore argued for the elimination of time constraints in performance tasks. Studies that have not measured speed of performance have still found significant age differences in these subtests (Botwinick, 1984). Furthermore, when motor speed (i.e., the time to physically perform a task) was measured separately from cognitive components of the task (e.g., visual search, memory, coding), older persons did worse than young test-takers in both components (Storandt, 1976). These results suggest that there is a decline in performance-related aspects of intellectual function, independent of psychomotor or sensory factors. Speed of cognitive processing may also decline with age and, in turn, slow an individual's responses on tests of performance.

Turning to verbal skills, the Classic Aging Pattern suggests that the ability to recall stored verbal information and to use abstract reasoning tends to remain constant throughout life. Declines, where they exist, tend not to show up until advanced old age, or, in the case of cognitive impairment such as the dementias, to begin early in the course of the disease.

Some researchers have argued that this age-related decline in tests of intelligence may reflect a deterioration in complex, formal-logical, and integrative thinking (Denney, 1981, Craik, 1977). That is, older people may be using more concrete, less abstract thought processes than in youth. In contrast, there is some evidence that, when given logically inconsistent statements, older subjects have been found to analyze these inconsistencies on the basis of their own knowledge, whereas younger adults tend to ignore the logic and attempt to reach conclusions (Labouvie-Vief and Blanchard-Fields, 1982). Older subjects have also been found to reject simplified solutions and to prefer a complex analysis of the problem. This finding from laboratory-based research is supported by surveys of attitudes and beliefs among respondents of varying ages. Younger respondents are more willing to provide a direct response, whereas many older persons attempt to analyze the questions and give more contingency responses; that is, analyzing the question and stating that the answer could be x in one situation, y in another, rather than an all-encompassing response. For example, on a measure of environmental preference, the respondent may be asked, "How much privacy do you generally prefer?" A younger respondent is more likely to focus on the "general" situation, whereas the older respondent will be more likely to consider both situations in which privacy is preferred and where it is not. It thus appears important to review older persons' responses to tests of problem solving and abstract reasoning from other perspectives beyond the traditional approaches that are grounded in cognitive theories developed with younger populations.

PROBLEMS IN MEASUREMENT OF COGNITIVE FUNCTION

A major shortcoming of many studies of intelligence in aging is their use of cross-sectional research designs, rather than longitudinal approaches. As we saw in Chapter 1, the former method is used to compare at a single point in time two or more groups defined by age or other characteristics. The latter approach is used to examine the same group (or groups) several times over a period of weeks, months, or years. Age differences that are obtained in cross-sectional studies may be a reflection of cohort or generational differences rather than actual age changes. In particular, changes in educational systems and the development of television, computers, and high-speed travel have had a profound impact on the experiences of today's youth when compared with those of people who grew up in the early twentieth century. These historical factors may then have a greater effect on intelligence scores than age per se.

Critics of cross-sectional methods have pointed to the advantages of following the same individual in longitudinal studies. However, the length of time and cost to complete longitudinal studies may make them impossible in many situations. Another problem is subject attrition, or dropout from such studies. Researchers who have conducted longitudinal research on intelligence have found a pattern of selective attrition, whereby the people who drop out tend to be those who have performed less well, who perceive their performance to be poor, or whose health status and ambulatory abilities are worse than average (Riegel and Riegel, 1972; Siegler, 1975; Botwinick, 1977). The people who stay in the study (i.e., "the survivors") performed better in the initial tests than did dropouts. This is consistent with our earlier observation that older persons often become unduly anxious about poor performance on tests of intellectual function. Hence, the results become biased in favor of the superior performers, indicating stability or improvement over time, and do not represent the wider population of older adults, whose performance might have shown a decline in intelligence.

LONGITUDINAL STUDIES OF INTELLIGENCE

Several major longitudinal studies have examined changes in intellectual function from youth to old age (Schaie, 1983). The Iowa State Study of intellectual development began as a cross-sectional assessment of 363 male college freshmen in 1919. The first longitudinal follow-up took place in 1950 with 127 of the men who could be located. In 1961, 96 men were retested (Owens, 1953, 1966; Cunningham and Owens, 1983). Using the Army Alpha Test of intelligence, the researchers found general stability in intellectual functioning through middle-age, with a peak in the ages of late forties and fifties. Declines were observed after age 60 in many men, but the degree of change varied widely among the men and across variables. The Iowa State Study is significant as the first major longitudinal assessment of adult intelligence. However, the loss of 75 percent of the original sample by the third follow-up and the selection of college-educated men limit the generalizability of these findings.

The New York State Study of Aging Twins began in 1946 with the goal of examining heredity and aging. Of the original sample of 268 twins (or 134 pairs) over age 60 initially tested between 1947 and 1949 (Kallmann and Sander, 1949), 61 were available for the final follow-up in 1973. This study tested twins five times over this 26-year period on two measures of intelligence and a test of hand-eye coordination. Average performance declined significantly on timed tests, but, as with the Iowa State Study, individual differences were pronounced. Among the individuals who were healthy enough to complete the final follow-up, performance on nonspeeded intelligence tests remained stable until they reached their ninth decade. The greatest declines were observed in the test of hand-eye coordination and in a measure of fluid intelligence. The Aging Twins Study provides valuable information about intellectual function from age 60 to 90. It offers unique insights into the differential effects of heredity and environment on the intellectual function of monozygotic and dizygotic twins, and about the intellectual strength of the old-old (Jarvik and Bank, 1983).

The Seattle Longitudinal Study began in 1956, and collected data on Thurstone's primary mental abilities over 21 years (Schaie, 1983; Schaie and Hertzog, 1983). At each follow-up assessment, individuals who were still available from the original sample were retested, along with a new, randomly selected sample from the same population. This study has provided the basis for the development of sequential research models, described in Chapter 1. Peak performance varied across tests and between men and women, ranging from age 32 on the test of Numbers for men and age 39 for women on the test of Reasoning, to age 53 for Educational Aptitude. A review of age changes for the 128 people who were observed over the entire 21 years of this study reveals significant age decrements after age 60 on tests of word-fluency, space, and numbers. Tests of spatial abilities and inductive reasoning, both indicators of fluid intelligence, showed greater decline with age. However, other primary mental abilities, such as verbal meaning and reasoning, showed *no* declines until the mid-seventies. These results are consistent with cross-sectional results using the WAIS, as we have seen earlier. They suggest that the Classic Aging Pattern holds up in both cross-sectional and longitudinal studies, and that some performance aspects of intelligence may begin to deteriorate after age 60, although major changes are generally rare until the mid-seventies.

The Duke Longitudinal Studies, described in Chapters 1 and 4, assessed intelligence and memory, in addition to many health variables. This series of three longitudinal samples, each measured several times, provides useful information about the relationship between intellectual function and health status, especially cardiovascular disease (Palmore, 1974, 1985; Siegler, 1983). The findings regarding age changes generally are consistent with the other longitudinal studies described in this section; declines in cognitive function were not observed until individuals reached their seventies. Scores on performance tests were found to decline earlier than scores on verbal measures.

FACTORS THAT MAY INFLUENCE INTELLIGENCE IN ADULTHOOD

Researchers who have compared intelligence test scores of older and younger persons have found wide variations in scores of both groups. As described earlier, older test-takers generally have obtained poorer scores, but age per se is only one factor in explaining intellectual functioning.

As mentioned, there is also a biological factor in intelligence, such that some people are innately more intelligent than others. However, it is difficult to determine the relative influence of biological factors, because it is impossible to measure the specific mechanisms of the brain that account for intelligence. There are structural changes in the brain and in neural pathways with aging, as we have seen in Chapter 4. But these changes are generally diffuse and not focused in a particular region of the brain, so that it is impossible to determine what specific changes in the brain and its pathways may account for the age-related deterioration that is observed.

Several other factors may be measured that appear to explain some of the observed differences in intelligence tests between older and younger persons. These include initial level of intelligence, education, occupation, physical health, sensory functions, and test anxiety. In an analysis of WAIS data from people aged 25 to 64, education was found to account for more variance in the general intelligence component of the WAIS than age (Birren and Morrison, 1961). However, age did explain a significant portion of the variance in subtests such as Vocabulary and Digit Symbol, which, as we have already seen, show age-related changes. It is important to statistically control for educational differences when analyzing the relationship between age and intelligence; one study found that the number of significant correlations between age and intelligence test scores was reduced by 30 percent when education was taken into account (Granick and

Friedman, 1967). In a subsequent study, WAIS results of four age groups: 25–29, 35–39, 45–49, and 55–64 were compared (Green, 1969). Consistent with other studies, the Classic Aging Pattern emerged (i.e., verbal scores did not differ across age groups, whereas performance scores consistently declined). However, when age groups were matched on the basis of educational level, there was a significant increase in verbal scores with age, and no differences in performance scores, except on the Digit Symbol, where even in groups with comparable educational achievement, older persons performed more poorly.

Similarly, occupational level, which is generally correlated with educational level, has an impact on a person's intelligence test scores. Older people who still use their cognitive abilities in jobs that require thinking and problem solving (such as Mr. Wallace in the introductory vignette) show less decline on cognitive tests than those who do not keep working. In addition, people whose occupations demand more verbal skills (e.g., lawyers, teachers) may continue to perform very well on these aspects of the intelligence tests; whereas those who use more abstract and fluid skills in their occupations (e.g., architects, engineers) may do well on the performance tests of the WAIS, even into their seventies and eighties. Unfortunately, Green (1969) did not include subjects older than age 64 in his study, but education and occupation probably continue to affect people's WAIS performance into advanced old age.

The effects of declining physical health and sensory losses on intelligence become more severe in the later years, and these factors may displace any positive influence due to education and occupation for people who are 75 years and older. Several studies have identified poorer performance on intelligence tests by elderly in poor health. Even when comparing two groups of healthy men, one in extraordinarily good health and the other with minor medical problems, differences on the performance subtests of the WAIS have been found (Botwinick and Birren, 1963). Older people with cardiovascular problems also tend to do more poorly on tests of intelligence than those without such disorders, particularly in tests that demand psychomotor speed (Hertzog, Schaie, and Gribben, 1978). Changes in WAIS scores were analyzed over a 10-year period among older people whose blood pressure was judged to be normal, borderline, or high. Those who were aged 60 to 69 at the start of the study and had high blood pressure throughout the 10 years declined the most in performance subtests of the WAIS. Those with borderline blood pressure showed the least decline. This may be because mild elevations of blood pressure in older persons are useful for maintaining sufficient blood circulation to the brain (Wilkie and Eisdorfer, 1971).

Another physical health factor that appears to be related to intelligence test scores is an apparent and rapid decline in cognitive function within five years of death. This phenomenon is known as the *terminal drop hypothesis* (Kleemeier, 1961, 1962). Older subjects whose test scores are in the lower range have been found to die sooner than good performers (Jarvik and Falek, 1963). This hypothesis suggests that time since birth (i.e., age) is not as significant in intellectual decline as is proximity to death. Although this phenomenon has been observed in many studies, it has not been researched with large samples of older persons in a longitudinal manner. For this reason, it would be premature to conclude that death could be predicted from intelligence test scores.

As we noted in Chapter 5, hearing loss is common in older persons, especially moderate levels of loss that affect their ability to comprehend speech. The effect of hearing loss on verbal communication may explain findings of poorer scores on verbal subtests of the WAIS among older persons with moderate to high hearing loss. However, there is less association between test scores on performance scales and hearing loss (Botwinick, 1984).

Finally, anxiety may negatively affect older people's intelligence test scores. As shown in the following section, older people in laboratory tests of learning and memory are more likely than the young to express high test anxiety and cautiousness in responding. These same reactions may occur in taking intelligence tests, especially if older people think that the test really measures how "intelligent" they are. Anxieties about cognitive decline and concerns about becoming cognitively impaired may make older people even more cautious, and hence, result in poorer performance on intelligence tests.

The Process of Learning and Memory

Learning and memory are two cognitive processes that must be considered together. That is, learning is assumed to have occurred when an individual is able to retrieve information from his or her memory store. Conversely, if an individual cannot retrieve information from memory, it is assumed that learning has not adequately taken place. Thus, learning is the process by which new information (verbal or nonverbal) or skills are encoded, or put into one's memory. Memory is the process of retrieving or recalling the information stored in the brain when needed. Memory also refers to a part of the brain that retains what has been learned throughout a person's lifetime. For example, a person may have learned many years ago how to ride a bicycle. If this skill has been encoded well through practice, the person can retrieve it many years later from his or her memory store, even if he or she has not ridden a bicycle in many years. Although the exact location in the brain where memories are stored cannot be identified, researchers have attempted to distinguish three separate types of memory: sensory memory, primary or short-term memory, and secondary or long-term memory.

Sensory memory, as its name implies, is the first step in receiving information through the sense organs and passing it on to primary or secondary memory. It is stored for only a few tenths of a second, although there is some evidence that it lasts longer in older persons because of slower reaction times of the senses (Abel, 1972). Sensory memory has been further subdivided into iconic (or visual) and echoic (or auditory) memory. Examples of iconic memory are words or letters that we see, faces of people with whom we have contact, and landscapes that we experience through our eyes. Of course, words can be received through echoic memory as well, such as when we hear others say a specific word, or when we repeat words aloud to ourselves. A landscape can also enter our sensory memory through our ears (e.g., the sound of the ocean), our skin (e.g., the feel of a cold spray from the ocean), and our nose (e.g., the smell of salt-water). To the extent that we focus on or rehearse any information that we receive from our sense organs, it is more likely to be passed into our primary and secondary memories.

Despite significant changes in the visual system with aging (as described in Chapter 5), studies of iconic memory have found only small age differences in the ability to identify stimuli presented briefly. Older people have been found to take longer to identify a single letter or icon (Walsh, Till, and Williams, 1978). In another study, when old and young individuals were tested with seven-letter strings, the former were slower by a factor of 1.3 (Cerella, Poon, and Fozard, 1982), a rate similar to that found with single letters (Walsh et al., 1978). Such modest declines in iconic memory would not be expected to influence observed decrements in secondary or long-term memory. Thus, iconic memory may have little effect on secondary memory.

Although research on iconic memory is limited, there has been even less with echoic memory and less still that has compared older persons with younger. We have all experienced the long-term storage of memories gained through touch, taste, or smell. For example, the odor of freshly baked bread evokes memories in many older people of their early childhood. However, these sensory memories are more difficult to test. As a result, very little is known about any changes experienced with these other modes of sensory memory.

Primary memory is a temporary stage of holding and organizing information, and does not necessarily refer to a storage area in the brain. Despite its temporary nature, primary memory is critical for our ability to process new information. We have all experienced situations where we heard or read a bit of information such as a phone number or someone's name, used that name or number immediately, then forgotten it. In fact, most adults can recall seven, plus or minus two, pieces of information (e.g., digits, letters, words) for 60 seconds or less. It is not surprising, therefore, that local phone numbers in most countries are seven digits or less! In order to retain this information in our permanent memory store (secondary memory), it must be rehearsed actively. In contrast, if we are distracted while trying to retain the information for the 60 seconds that it can last in short-term memory, we immediately forget it, even if it consists of only two or three bits of information. This happens because the rehearsal of such material is interrupted by the reception of newer information in our sensory memory.

As Poon (1985) notes in a recent review of memory function with age, most studies of primary memory have found minimal age differences. For example, people aged 20 to 30 have been found to recall 6 or 7 letters presented auditorily, compared with 5.5 letters by subjects in their seventies (Botwinick and Storandt, 1974). Differences that exist may be due more to increased reaction time with age than to a reduced capacity of primary memory.

True learning implies that the material we have acquired through our sensory and primary memories has been stored in secondary memory. Thus, for example, looking up a telephone number and immediately dialing it does not guarantee that the number will be learned. In fact, only with considerable rehearsal can information from primary memory be passed into secondary memory. This is the part of the memory store in which everything we have learned throughout our lives is kept; unlike primary memory, it has an unlimited capacity.

Age differences in secondary memory appear to be more pronounced than in sensory or primary memory and are often frustrating to older people and their families. Such concern is generally out of proportion to the actual level of decline. These concerns often stem from the fear of dementia, a relatively rare set of conditions that dramatically impair cognitive functions, as we will see in Chapter 9. Older people consistently recall less information than younger people in paired associate tests with retention intervals as brief as one hour or as long as eight months. However, older individuals can benefit significantly from methods to help organize their learning, such as imagery and the use of mnemonics. Examples of such techniques to improve learning and memory are covered later in this chapter.

The Information Processing Model

Figure 7–2 presents the information processing model of memory. This is a conceptual model; that is, it provides a framework for understanding how the processes of learning and memory take place. It is not necessarily what goes on in the neural pathways between the sense organs and the secondary memory store. Having described each of the components in this model, let us review the steps involved in processing some information that we want to retain. One example is the experience of learning new names at a social gathering. Sensory memory aids in hearing the name spoken, preferably several times by other people, and seeing the face that is associated with that name. Primary memory is used to store that information temporarily, so that a person can speak to others and address them by name (an excellent method of rehearsing this information), or manipulate the information in other ways in order to pass it on to secondary memory. This may include repeating the name several times to oneself, trying to isolate some aspect of the person's physical features and relating it to the name, and associating the name with other people one has known in the past who have similar names. In the last type of mental manipulation, information from secondary memory (i.e., names of other people) is linked with the new information. This is a useful

FIGURE 7–2 Schematic Representation of the Information Processing Model

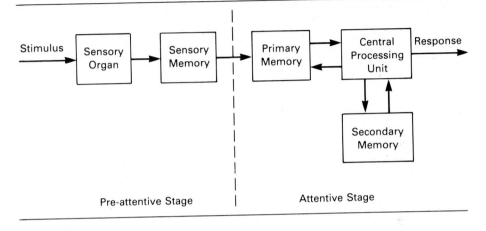

method because the material in secondary memory is permanent, and associating the new information with well-learned information aids in its storage and subsequent recall.

During any stage of this cognitive processing, the newly obtained information can be lost. This may occur if the sensory memory is flooded with similar information; in this case, if a person is being introduced to multiple new names and faces at a party, it is almost impossible to distinguish the names or to associate each name with a face. Information may also be lost during the primary memory stage. In our example, if a person is trying to use the newly heard name and is distracted by other names and faces, or receives unrelated but relevant information (e.g., a telephone call) while rehearsing the new name, the name has not been sufficiently processed to pass into secondary memory.

The learning process may also be disrupted because of inability to retrieve information efficiently from secondary memory. For example, a person may associate the newly heard name with someone known in the past; if he or she has difficulty retrieving the stored name from secondary memory, however, this may be so frustrating as to redirect the individual's attention from the new name to the old name. How often have you ignored everything around you to concentrate on remembering a name that is "on the tip of the tongue" (i.e., in secondary memory), but not easily retrievable? As we will see in the next section, aging appears to reduce the efficiency of processing information in sensory and primary memories, and retrieval from secondary memory. It does *not* influence the storage capacity of primary or secondary memories. That is, contrary to popular opinion, these memory stores are not physical spaces that become overloaded with information as we age.

FACTORS THAT AFFECT LEARNING IN OLD AGE

One problem with assessing learning ability is that it is not possible to measure the process that occurs in the brain while an individual is acquiring new information. Instead, we must rely on an individual's performance on tests that presumably measure what was learned. This may be particularly disadvantageous to older persons, whose performance on a test of learning may be poor because of inadequate or inappropriate conditions for expressing what was learned (Botwinick, 1984). For example, an older person may in fact have learned many new concepts in reading a passage from a novel, but not necessarily the specific concepts that are called for on a test of learning. Certain physical conditions, such as lighting levels, size of print, tone and loudness of the test-giver's voice in an oral exam, and the time constraints placed on the test-taker, may affect performance and thus lead to underestimates of what the older person has actually learned. Consistent with the P-E model, to the extent that the learning environment can be improved with glare-free and direct lighting, lettering of good quality, size, and contrast, a comfortable test-taking situation with minimal background noise, and a relaxed and articulate test-giver, the older learner will learn and recall more on subsequent tests of learning.

Large-print books have enhanced older people's opportunities to learn.

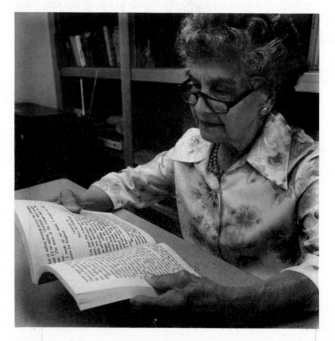

Time constraints are particularly detrimental to older people. Although the ability to encode new information quickly is a sign of learning ability, it is difficult to measure this ability. Instead, response time is generally measured. As we have already seen, psychomotor and sensory slowing with age has a significant impact on the older person's speed in responding. One of the first researchers to test the effect of these conditions on learning was Canestrari (1963). Using a common test of learning, the paired associates task (i.e., linking two unrelated words, letters, digits, or symbols, such as *cat* and *82,* and asking subjects to respond with the second when the first is mentioned), Canestrari presented the paired associates at varying rates, or allowed individuals to pace the task by controlling the visual apparatus themselves. In comparing people aged 60–69 with those aged 17–35, he found striking differences between old and young individuals' performance when the task was paced fast, fewer differences in moderate pacing, and the least differences in self-paced conditions. Young persons did well in all conditions, but older persons in this study benefited the most from self-pacing. Similar results have been reported by Monge and Hultsch (1971), Arenberg (1973), and Smith (1976).

The study by Canestrari, as well as research by Taub (1967) and Botwinick (1978), has shown that older persons make more *errors of omission* than *errors of commission.* That is, older persons are more likely not to give an answer than to guess and risk being wrong. This phenomenon was first recognized in middle-aged and older adults in tests of psychomotor functioning (Welford, 1951). The older the respondent, the more likely he or she was to work for accuracy at the expense of speed. This occurs even when the older learner is encouraged to guess and told that it is acceptable to give wrong answers (i.e., commission errors). Errors of omission may be reduced somewhat by giving rewards for both right and wrong answers (Leech and Witte, 1971).

This tendency toward errors of omission is consistent with studies of cautiousness in older persons, which have yielded some evidence of increased caution and less risk-taking with age. Older people in one study who were given as much time as they wanted to learn a task took the full time and displayed cautiousness in responding. However, when put under a time constraint, they were able to respond almost as accurately within the shorter time (Botwinick, Brinley, and Robbin, 1958). In another study, when hypothetical problems were presented to old and young persons, older men and women were more cautious than the young in financial situations. Older men were more cautious than young men in cases of risking professional failure or one's life. Similarly, older women were found to be more cautious than young women in marriage situations (Wallach and Kogan, 1961). Some studies have used a vocabulary test in which individuals could earn points for defining words, with more points for difficult words. In situations of uncertainty, older persons chose easier words, but did not differ from the young in situations of certainty (Okun and DiVesta, 1976). In a subsequent study, individuals were provided with a rational basis on which they could choose easy or difficult words. In this case, older persons were no more cautious than younger subjects (Okun and Elias, 1977).

These results suggest that in conditions of uncertainty and high risk, older persons are more cautious than the young. Low-risk situations elicit less caution from elderly people and greater willingness to give responses in a learning task. Results of these studies suggest also that the aging process creates an increased need to review multiple aspects of a problem, probably because of past experiences with similar dilemmas.

Verbal ability and educational level are important factors in learning verbal information (Hultsch and Dixon, 1984). Studies that entail learning prose passages have shown age deficits among those with average vocabulary abilities and minimal or no college education. In contrast, older persons with high verbal ability and a college education perform as well as younger subjects in such experiments. This may be due to greater practice and facility with such tasks on the part of more educated persons and those with good vocabulary skills. In fact, education and vocabulary skills are generally correlated, and emerge as better predictors of performance in studies of prose learning than does chronological age (Meyer and Rice, 1983; Rice and Meyer, 1985, 1986).

The conditions under which learning takes place affect older persons more than the young, just as test conditions are more critical. Older persons respond differently to varied testing situations; in one study, those who were tested under challenging conditions ("this is a test of your intelligence") did worse than those in supportive ("the researcher needs your help") conditions, with neutral instructions resulting in scores between these two (Ross, 1968). Positive feedback appears to be a valuable tool for eliciting responses from older adults in both learning and test situations.

It is helpful to pace the information so that it is presented at a rate suitable to the older learner and to give him or her opportunities to practice the new information. Another condition that supports learning is the presentation of familiar and relevant material compared to material perceived by the older learner to be unimportant. Recall of recently acquired information has been found to be worse in older persons than in younger when the new information is unfamiliar or confusing (Hoyer and Plude, 1980; Barrett and Wright, 1981). Similarly, greater age differences have been identified when the material to be learned was low in meaning and personal significance (Fozard, 1980). Laboratory studies of cognitive functioning often seem artificial and meaningless to older people who are unaccustomed to such research methods, and even more so to those with little academic experience. Many people will complain that such tests are trivial, nonsense, or that these tasks have no connection to the "real world." Indeed, it may appear odd to anyone to be learning meaningless words and symbols on a tachistoscope (a screen that is timed to present visual stimuli at a specific pace) or other laboratory device. But for those older people who are unfamiliar with test-taking situations, it may appear particularly foolish and not worth the effort required. This may also serve a useful ego-defensive function for people who feel uncomfortable or threatened by a test-taking situation. It is generally easier for people to blame the environment or the test situation for their poor performance than to accept it as a sign of a decline in their intelligence or their ability to learn.

In an attempt to make learning tasks more meaningful, words in a paired associate task were devised that had more meaning than the typical words used in such situations (e.g., *banker* instead of *insane*). When provided with meaningful associations such as names (e.g., linking the name *Sloan* with the word *banker* helped in recalling the word *banker*), older adults in the study did better than they had with meaningless words and associations. Nevertheless, older people continued to perform more poorly than the young (Hulicka, 1967). A more recent study showed that the use of words familiar to older persons actually resulted in better performance by them than by the young (Barrett and Wright, 1981). For example, when words such as *fedora* (a term with which older persons are more likely to be familiar than the young) were used, the former could recall more words. In contrast, words with which the elderly were less familiar (e.g., *ripoff*) resulted in worse recall.

Most studies of learning focus on verbal information. It is generally assumed that nonverbal information is learned in the same way. In the few studies that have compared the ability of older and younger adults to recognize facial photos, recall has consistently been worse among the former. For example, Ferris and colleagues (1980) showed two age groups (17–39 and 60–88) black and white slides of individual faces. When shown the same slides later, together with other pictures, the elderly recognized fewer faces than the younger people. In an attempt to compare verbal and nonverbal learning, Winograd, Smith, and Simon (1982) showed old and young people black and white drawings of objects and their verbal labels. The ability to recall pictures was better than words for both groups. However, age differences again emerged, such that older adults recalled fewer drawings and verbal labels.

Spatial memory, that is, the ability to recall where objects are in relationship to each other in space (e.g., when finding one's way around a community or using a map), also appears to decline with aging. It is unclear, however, if older people do worse than the young because they have difficulty encoding and processing the information, or if the problem is in retrieval. The possibility of encoding problems as the cause was tested in one study where 48 women aged 60 to 70 were compared with 48 women aged 20 to 30 in their ability to view a three-dimensional model of a town, then to reconstruct the town from memory (Bruce and Herman, 1986). Older women needed two trials to do as well as the young with one trial. They also did better when the buildings and roads were clearly labelled and made distinct with different roof forms and colors than when there were no labels. This study provides support for an age-related decline in encoding ability for spatial information.

Age-Related Changes in Memory

As we have seen, learning involves encoding information and storing it into secondary or long-term memory, so that it can be retrieved and used later. Studies of this process have focused on two types of retrieval: recall and recognition. *Recall* is the process of searching through the vast store of information in secondary memory, perhaps with a cue or a specific, orienting question (e.g., "List the capitals of each state." "Describe how to repair a bicycle." "Give the dates when the U.S. Constitution was signed, when the U.N. Charter was signed," etc.). *Recognition* requires less search. The information in secondary memory must be matched with the stimulus information in the environment (e.g., "Which of these three cities is the capital of New York?"). Recall is demanded in essay exams; recognition is demanded in multiple-choice tests.

Not surprisingly, most researchers have found age-related deficiencies in recall, but few, if any, differences in recognition (Inman and Parkinson, 1983). However, in studies that have tested for recognition ability with multiple response categories, older people do worse when many words or numbers have to be recognized from a large list (Botwinick and Storandt, 1974), or when the word to be identified is included in a list of four rather than just two words (Kausler and Kleim, 1978). Recall tasks have been further divided into free recall and cued recall situations. In the former, no aids or hints are provided for retrieving information from secondary memory. In the latter case, the individual is given some information to aid in the search (e.g., category labels, first letter of a word). Older people tend to do much worse than the young in tests of free recall, but are aided significantly by cueing. In particular, use of category labels (semantic cues) at the learning stage has been found to be more helpful to older persons than the use of structural cues; for example, giving the respondent the first letter of a word to be recalled (Smith, 1977). However, cued recall tests are not as helpful as recognition tests for older learners.

An area of considerable controversy in aging and memory function is the question of whether older people have better recall of events that occurred in the distant past than recent situations. Many events are firmly embedded in secondary memory because they are unique, or so important that subsequent experiences do not interfere with the ability to recall them. The birth of a child, one's wedding ceremony, or the death of a parent, spouse, or sibling are events that most people can recall in detail 40 to 50 years later. This may be because the situation had great private significance or, in the case of world events, such as the bombing of Hiroshima or John F. Kennedy's assassination, had a profound impact on world history. Some distant events may be better recalled because they had greater personal relevance for the individual's social development than recent experiences, or because they have been rehearsed or thought about more. Another possibility is that cues that helped the other person recall events in the past are less effective with recalling recent occasions because of "cue-overload"

(Schonfield and Stones, 1979). That is, the same cues that were once helpful in remembering certain information are also used to recall many recent events. But the cues are so strongly associated with one's older life experiences that the newer information becomes more difficult to retrieve. For example, older people may have difficulty memorizing new phone numbers because the cues that helped them recall phone numbers in the past may be so closely associated with previous ones that they confuse recent phone numbers with the old numbers.

One problem in determining whether recall of distant situations is really better than recall of recent events is the difficulty in validating an older person's memories. In many cases, there are no sources that can be checked to determine the accuracy of an older person's recollections. We can all identify with this process of asking an old friend or family member, "Do you remember the time when . . . ?" If others have no recollection of the event, it may make us wonder if the situation really took place. It may also mean that the event was so obscure that it made no impact on other people. Hence, such memories are difficult to measure accurately.

Some researchers who have tested older persons' recall of historical facts, such as world events that occurred during their youth and middle years, have found that distant events could not be remembered as well as recent ones (Warrington and Silberstein, 1970; Warrington and Saunders, 1971; Squire, 1974). However, other researchers have found the opposite (Botwinick and Storandt, 1974, 1980; Perlmutter, 1978). Indeed, Poon and colleagues (1979) observed that older persons demonstrated better recognition performance than did young subjects when presented with historical events that took place between 1920 and the 1970s. In a study of personally relevant remote events, high-school graduates aged 17 to 74 were shown yearbook pictures and asked to match the photos with names. The researchers controlled statistically for class size and attendance at reunions. Recognition memory was as high as 90 percent in middle-aged subjects; free recall of names was generally worse for all age groups, but even those who had graduated 48 years earlier could remember 20 percent of the names (Bahrick, Bahrick, and Wittlinger, 1975).

Several theories have been offered to explain why older people may have problems with retrieving information from secondary memory. One explanation is that not using the information results in its loss (the disuse theory). This theory suggests that information can fade away or decay unless it is exercised, as in the old adage, "Use it, don't lose it." However, this explanation fails to account for the many facts that are deeply embedded in a person's memory store and that can be retrieved even after years of disuse.

A more widely accepted explanation is that new information interferes with the material that has been stored over a period of many years. As we have noted earlier, interference is a problem in the learning or encoding stage. When the older person is distracted while trying to learn new information, this information does not become stored in memory. Poor retrieval may be due to a combination of such distraction during the learning stage and interference by similar or new information with the material being searched in the retrieval stage. Although researchers in this area have not conclusively agreed on any of these explanations, the interference theory appears to hold more promise than others for explaining observed problems with retrieval.

Researchers have begun to examine older people's feelings about their memory failures and how they cope with these. For example, participants in a recent longitudinal study kept diaries of their experiences with memory. Older adults described more incidents in which they forgot names, objects, locations, and appointments, especially in nonroutine tasks. They also reported feeling more frustrated with a memory failure than did younger people (Cavanaugh, Grady, and Perlmutter, 1983). This may impair the older person's confidence in a learning or test situation, thereby negatively affecting performance in these cases. Indeed, older persons have been found to express less confidence in their responses than the young in tests of recognition and recall (Bahrick, Bahrick, and Wittlinger, 1975).

Improving Memory in the Later Years

There has been considerable experimentation with techniques for improving memory. Although useful at any age, cognitive aids may be particularly helpful for an older person who is experiencing increased problems with day-to-day cognitive functions, such as recalling names, words, phone numbers, and daily chores. Older persons are more likely to use external aids such as notes and lists than they are to use cognitive aids such as imagery and word association. That is, they are more likely to reduce environmental press than to enhance their competence in learning as a means of improving P-E congruence. Many techniques for remembering are acquired as part of a person's formal educational experiences; as a result, an older person who has had minimal educational opportunities will have had less exposure to such techniques. The National Council on the Aging has published an excellent guide for training older people to improve their memory (Garfunkel and Landau, 1981).

Most memory improvement techniques are based on the concept of mediators; that is, the use of visual and verbal links between information to be encoded and information that is already in secondary memory. Mediators may be visual (e.g., the method of locations) or verbal (i.e., the use of mnemonics). The method of locations (or loci) is useful for learning a list of new words, names, or concepts. Each word is associated with a specific location in a familiar environment. For example, the individual is instructed to "walk through" his or her own home mentally. As the person walks through the rooms in succession, each item on the list is associated with a particular space along the way. Older persons using this technique have been found to recall more words on a list than when they used no mediators (Robertson-Tchabo, Hausman, and Arenberg, 1976). One advantage of the method of loci is that learners can visualize the new information within a familiar setting, and can decide for themselves what new concept should be linked with what specific part of the environment. Older learners have been found to recall more information when given the time to develop their own mediators than if the experimenter provides the links for them (Treat and Reese, 1976).

Another way of organizing material to be learned and to assure its storage in secondary memory is to use mnemonics, or verbal riddles, rhymes, and codes associated with the new information. Many teachers use such rhymes to teach their students multiplication, spelling (e.g., "*i* before *e* except after *c*"), and the calendar ("30 days hath September, April, June, and November/ all the rest have 31, except February alone, and that has 28 days clear/ except every leap year"). One of the first mnemonics a music student learns is in conjunction with memorizing the scales (*Every Good Boy Does Fine*). Sailors learn that *r*ed lights in the harbor signify *r*ight and *r*eturn. There are many other mnemonics that we acquire through experience as well as our own efforts to devise ways for ourselves to learn a new concept. Both cognitively intact and impaired elderly have shown improved memory function with the use of mnemonics (Poon, Fozard, Cermak, Arenberg, and Thompson, 1980; Lewinsohn, Danaher, and Kikel, 1977).

Other mediators include using the new word or concept in a sentence, associating the digits in a phone number with symbols or putting them into a mathematical formula (e.g., "the first digit is 4, the second and third are multiplied to produce the first"), placing the information into categories, and using multiple sensory memories. In this last technique, one may write the word (iconic memory), repeat it aloud to oneself (echoic memory), or "feel" the letters or digits by outlining it with one's hand.

Unfortunately, many older persons do not practice the use of newly learned memory techniques. It may be that they are not motivated to use the techniques, which often seem awkward, or they may forget and need to be reminded. Perhaps the fact that these are unfamiliar approaches to the current generation of older people is the major problem. As future cohorts become more practiced in these memory techniques through their educational experiences, the use of such strategies in old age should increase.

Perhaps the most important aspect of memory enhancement is the ability to relax and to avoid feeling anxious or stressed during the learning stage. As noted earlier, many older people become overly concerned about occasional memory lapses, viewing them as a sign of deterioration and possible onset of senile dementia. Thus, a young person may be annoyed when a familiar name is forgotten, but will probably not interpret the memory lapse as loss of cognitive function, as an older person is likely to do. Unfortunately, society reinforces this belief. How often are we told that we are "getting old" when we forget a trivial matter? How often do adult children become concerned that their elderly parent sometimes forgets to turn off the stove, when in fact they may frequently do this themselves?

In addition to mediators, simple devices or *external aids* are often used by older people to keep track of the time or dates, or to remember to turn the stove on or off. For example, placing several large-print calendars around the house, or better yet, using digital clocks that also display the day of the week and the date can be helpful. Older people can develop the habit of associating medication regimens with specific activities of daily living, such as using marked pill boxes and taking the first pill in the morning before their daily shower, or just before or after breakfast, taking the second pill with lunch or before their noontime walk, and so on. These behaviors need to be associated with activities that occur everyday at a particular time, so that the pill-taking becomes linked with that routine. Charts listing an individual's daily or weekly routine can be posted throughout the house. Alarm clocks and kitchen timers also can be placed wherever an older person will be while the oven or stove is in operation. This will help in remembering that the appliance is on without having to stay in the kitchen. Family members with electronic skills could also connect the oven and stove with a red signal light in the older person's bedroom or front entryway. This light would go on everytime the oven or stove was turned on, so that the person would be reminded of this when going to bed or leaving the house. A fire alarm or smoke detector is essential for every older person's home, preferably one for every floor or wing of the house. Finally, for older people who have serious memory problems and a tendency to get lost while walking outdoors, a bracelet or necklace with the person's name, address, and phone number, and relevant medical information listed on it can be a lifesaver.

Wisdom and Creativity

Wisdom and creativity are more difficult to define and measure. Most people have an image of what it means to be wise or creative, but it is impossible to quantify an individual's level of wisdom or creativity. It has been suggested that *wisdom* requires the cognitive development and mastery over a person's emotions that come with age (Clayton and Birren, 1980; Butler and Gleason, 1985). It is a combination of experience, introspection, reflection, intuition, and empathy; these are qualities that are honed over many years and that can be integrated in people's interactions with their world. Thus, younger people may have any one of these skills, but their integration requires more maturity. Wisdom also implies that the individual does not act on impulse and can review all aspects of a given situation objectively. In many cultures, older persons are respected for their years of experience, and the role of "wise elder" is a desired status. Not all elderly have achieved wisdom, however. Indeed, Butler and Gleason (1985) suggest that wisdom requires the ability to transcend the limitations of basic needs such as health, income, and housing, and that the individual must have continued opportunities for growth and creativity. Such older people could play a useful role as "wise elder" in many businesses and government agencies, where their years of experience and ability to move beyond the constraints presumed by others could help such organizations succeed.

Creativity refers to the ability to apply unique and feasible solutions to new situations, to come up with original ideas or material products. A person may be creative in science, the arts, or technology. Although we can point to creative people in each of these areas (e.g., Albert Einstein in science, Wolfgang Amadeus Mozart and Georgia O'Keefe in the arts, Alexander Graham Bell in technology), it is difficult to determine the specific characteristics that make such persons creative. As with intelligence in general, creativity is inferred from the individual's output, but cannot really be quantified or predicted. One measure of creativity is a test of divergent thinking, which is part of Guilford's (1967) structural model of intelligence. This is measured by asking a person to devise multiple solutions to an unfamiliar mental task. Unfortunately, there is no way to know if such a test actually predicts creativity. To date, very few researchers have administered this test to people who are generally considered to be creative. Much of the research on creativity has been performed as analyses of the products of artists and writers, not on their creative process directly. Indeed, no studies have been conducted to compare the cognitive functioning of artists, scientists, technologists, and others who are widely regarded as creative with that of persons not similarly endowed.

Summary and Implications

This chapter presented an overview of the major studies on cognitive functioning in the later years. Researchers have examined age-related changes in intelligence, learning, and memory, and what factors in the individual and the environment affect the degree of change in these three areas of cognitive functioning.

Of all the cognitive functions in aging, intelligence has received the greatest attention and controversy. It is also the area of most concern for many older persons. One problem with this area of research is the difficulty of defining and measuring what is generally agreed to be intelligence. In examining the components of intelligence measured by the Wechsler Adult Intelligence Scale (WAIS), fluid intelligence (as measured by performance scales) has been shown to decline more with aging than verbal, or crystallized, intelligence. This may be due partly to the fact that the former tests are generally timed, the latter are not. However, age differences emerge even when tests are not timed, and when variations in motor and sensory function are taken into account. This decline in fluid intelligence and maintenance of verbal intelligence is known as the Classic Aging Pattern. To the extent that older persons practice their fluid intelligence by using their problem-solving skills, they will experience less decline in this area. In contrast, aging does not appear to impair the ability for word and symbol meanings. This does not imply that the ability to recall words is unimpaired, but when asked for definitions of words, older people can remember their meanings quite readily.

One problem with studying intelligence in aging is that of distinguishing age changes from age differences. To determine changes with age, people must be examined longitudinally. The problems of selective attrition and terminal drop make it difficult to interpret the findings of longitudinal studies of intelligence. These factors may result in an underestimate of the decline in intelligence with aging. The problem of cross-sectional studies of intelligence is primarily that of cohort differences. Even if subjects are matched on educational level, older persons have not had the exposure to computers and early childhood learning opportunities that have become available to recent cohorts. Other factors, such as occupation, sensory decline, poor physical health, and severe hypertension, have been found to have a significant impact on intelligence test scores.

Learning and memory are cognitive functions that are usually examined jointly because tests of memory are actually tests of what a person has learned. According to the information-processing model, learning begins when information reaches sensory memory, then is directed via one or more sensory stores to primary memory. It is in primary memory that information must be organized and processed if it is to be retained and passed into secondary memory. Information is permanently stored in this latter region. Studies of recall and recognition provide evidence that aging does not affect the capacity of either primary or secondary memory. Instead, it appears that the aging process makes us less efficient in "reaching into" our secondary memory and retrieving material that has been stored years ago. Recognition tasks, in which a person is provided with a cue to associate with an item in secondary memory, are easier than pure recall for most people, but especially for older individuals.

The learning process can be enhanced for older people by reducing time constraints, making the learning task more relevant for them, improving the physical conditions by using bright but glare-free lights and large letters, and providing visual and verbal mediators for learning new information. These include mnemonics and the method of loci. Helping the older learner to relax and not feel threatened by the learning task also assures better learning.

This review of the research in cognitive functioning with aging provides considerable evidence of relatively small declines in intelligence, learning, and memory with aging. The declines that do occur begin later in life than generally assumed, and are less dramatic than popularly believed. To the extent that an older person remains healthy and intellectually active, decline in cognitive function is slight, and does not seriously impair an individual's ability to enjoy life in the later years.

Although there is some agreement that wisdom is enhanced by age, there is no conclusive evidence regarding the changes in creativity with age. Indeed, these concepts are more difficult to measure in young and old persons. These and other issues in cognition must be studied more fully with measures that have good construct validity before gerontologists can describe with certainty cognitive changes that are attributable to normal aging.

References

Abel, M. The visual trace in relation to aging. Unpublished doctoral dissertation. Washington University, St. Louis, Missouri, 1972.

Arenberg, D. Cognition and aging: Verbal learning, memory, and problem solving. In C. Eisdorfer and M. P. Lawton (Eds.), *Psychology of adult development and aging.* Washington, D.C.: American Psychological Association, 1973.

Bahrick, H. P., Bahrick, P. P., and Wittlinger, R. P. Fifty years of memory for names and faces: A cross-sectional approach. *Journal of Experimental Psychology,* 1975, *104*, 54–75.

Barrett, T. R., and Wright, M. Age-related facilitation in recall following semantic processing. *Journal of Gerontology,* 1981, *2*, 194–199.

Birren, J. E., and Morrison, D. F. Analysis of the WAIS subtests in relation to age and education. *Journal of Gerontology,* 1961, *16*, 363–369.

Botwinick, J. Intellectual abilities. In J. E. Birren and K. W. Schaie (Eds.), *Handbook of the psychology of aging* (1st ed.). New York: Van Nostrand Reinhold, 1977, 580–605.

Botwinick, J. *Aging and behavior.* New York: Springer, 1978.

Botwinick, J. *Aging and behavior: A comprehensive integration of research findings* (3d ed.). New York: Springer, 1984.

Botwinick, J., and Birren, J. E. Cognitive processes: Mental abilities and psychomotor responses in healthy aged men. In J. E. Birren et al. (Eds.), *Human aging: A biological and behavioral study.* Washington, D.C.: U.S. Government Printing Office, 1963.

Botwinick, J., Brinley, J. F., and Robbin, J. S. The interaction effects of perceptual difficulty and stimulus exposure time on age differences in speed and accuracy of response. *Gerontologia,* 1958, *2*, 1–10.

Botwinick, J., and Storandt, M. *Memory related functions and age.* Springfield, Ill.: Charles C. Thomas, 1974.

Botwinick, J., and Storandt, M. Recall and recognition of old information in relation to age and sex. *Journal of Gerontology,* 1980, *35*, 70–76.

Bruce, P. R., and Herman, J. F. Adult age differences in spatial memory. *Journal of Gerontology,* 1986, *41*, 774–777.

Butler, R. N., and Gleason, H. *Productive aging: Enhancing vitality in later life.* New York: Springer, 1985.

Canestrari, R. E. Paced and self-paced learning in young and elderly adults. *Journal of Gerontology*, 1963, *18*, 165–168.

Cattell, R. B. Theory of fluid and crystallized intelligence: A critical experiment. *Journal of Educational Psychology*, 1963, *54*, 1–22.

Cavanaugh, J. C., Grady, J. G., and Perlmutter, M. P. Forgetting and use of memory aids in 20 and 70-year-olds' everyday life. *International Journal of Aging and Human Development*, 1983, *17*, 113–122.

Cerella, J., Poon, L. W., and Fozard, J. L. Age and iconic read-out. *Journal of Gerontology*, 1982, *37*, 197–202.

Clayton, V., and Birren, J. E. Age and wisdom across the life span: Theoretical perspectives. In P. B. Baltes and O. G. Brim, Jr. (Eds.), *Life-span development and behavior* (Volume 3). New York: Academic Press, 1980.

Craik, F. I. M. Age differences in human memory. In J. E. Birren and K. W. Schaie (Eds.), *Handbook of the psychology of aging* (1st ed.). New York: Van Nostrand Reinhold, 1977.

Cunningham, W. R., and Owens, W. A. The Iowa state study of the adult development of intellectual abilities. In K. W. Schaie (Ed.), *Longitudinal studies of adult psychological development*. New York: Guilford Press, 1983.

Denney, N. W. Adult cognitive development. In D. S. Beasley and G. A. Davis (Eds.), *Aging: Communication processes and disorders*. New York: Grune and Stratton, 1981.

Ferris, S. H., Crook, T., Clark, E., McCarthy, M., and Rae, D. Facial recognition memory deficits in normal aging and senile dementia. *Journal of Gerontology*, 1980, *35*, 707–714.

Fozard, J. L. The time for remembering. In L. W. Poon (Ed.), *Aging in the 1980's: Psychological issues*. Washington, D.C.: American Psychological Association, 1980.

Garfunkel, F., and Landau, G. *A memory retention course for the aged*. Washington, D.C.: The National Council on the Aging, 1981.

Granick, S., and Friedman, A. S. The effect of education on the decline of test performance with age. *Journal of Gerontology*, 1967, *22*, 191–195.

Green, R. F. Age-intelligence relationship between ages sixteen and sixty-four. *Developmental Psychology*, 1969, *1*, 618–627.

Guilford, J. P. Intelligence: 1965 model. *American Psychologist*, 1966, *21*, 20–26.

Guilford, J. P. *The nature of human intelligence*. New York: McGraw-Hill, 1967.

Hertzog, C. K., Schaie, K. W., and Gribbin, K. Cardiovascular disease and changes in intellectual function from middle to old age. *Journal of Gerontology*, 1978, *33*, 872–883.

Horn, J. L. Organization of data on life-span development of human abilities. In L. R. Goulet and P. B. Baltes (Eds.), *Life-span developmental psychology: Research and theory*. New York: Academic Press, 1970.

Horn, J. L., and Donaldson, G. Cognitive development in adulthood. In O. G. Brim and J. Kagan (Eds.), *Constancy and change in human development*. Cambridge, Mass.: Harvard University Press, 1980.

Hoyer, W. J., and Plude, D. J. Attentional and perceptual processes in the study of cognitive aging. In L. W. Poon (Ed.), *Aging in the 1980's: Psychological issues*. Washington, D.C.: American Psychological Association, 1980.

Hulicka, I. M. Age differences in retention as a function of interference. *Journal of Gerontology*, 1967, 22, 180–184.

Hultsch, D. F., and Dixon, R. A. Memory for text materials in adulthood. In P. B. Baltes and O. G. Brim, Jr. (Eds.), *Lifespan development and behavior* (Vol. 6). New York: Academic Press, 1984.

Huyck, M. H., and Hoyer, W. J. *Adult development and aging.* Belmont, Calif.: Wadsworth, 1982.

Inman, V. W., and Parkinson, S. R. Differences in Brown-Peterson recall as a function of age and retention interval. *Journal of Gerontology*, 1983, 38, 58–64.

Jarvik, L. F., and Bank, L. Aging twins: Longitudinal psychometric data. In K. W. Schaie (Ed.), *Longitudinal studies of adult psychological development.* New York: Guilford Press, 1983.

Jarvik, L. F., and Falek, A. Intellectual stability and survival in the aged. *Journal of Gerontology*, 1963, 18, 173–176.

Jones, H. E. Intelligence and problem-solving. In J. E. Birren (Ed.), *Handbook of aging and the individual: Psychological and biological aspects.* Chicago: University of Chicago Press, 1959.

Kallmann, F. J., and Sander, G. Twin studies on senescence. *American Journal of Psychiatry.* 1949, 106, 29–36.

Kausler, D. H., and Kleim, D. M. Age differences in processing relevant versus irrelevant stimuli in multiple item recognition learning. *Journal of Gerontology*, 1978, 33, 87–93.

Kleemeier, R. W. Intellectual change in the senium, or death and the IQ. Presidential Address, American Psychological Association, New York, August 1961.

Kleemeier, R. W. Intellectual change in the senium. *Proceedings of the Social Statistics Section of the American Statistical Association*, 1962, 1, 290–295.

Labouvie-Vief, G., and Blanchard-Fields, F. Cognitive aging and psychological growth. *Ageing and Society*, 1982, 2, 183–209.

Leech, S., and Witte, K. L. Paired-associate learning in elderly adults as related to pacing and incentive conditions. *Developmental Psychology*, 1971, 5, 180–185.

Lewinsohn, P. M., Danaher, B. G., and Kikel, S. Visual imagery as a mnemonic aid for brain-injured persons. *Journal of Consulting and Clinical Psychology*, 1977, 45, 717–723.

Meyer, B. J. F., and Rice, G. E. Learning and memory from text across the adult life span. In J. Fine and R. O. Freedle (Eds.), *Developmental studies in discourse.* Norwood, N.J.: Ablex, 1983.

Monge, R. H., and Hultsch, D. Paired-associate learning as a function of adult age and the length of the anticipation and inspection intervals. *Journal of Gerontology*, 1971, 26, 157–162.

Okun, M. A., and DiVesta, F. J. Cautiousness in adulthood as a function of age and instructions. *Journal of Gerontology*, 1976, 31, 571–576.

Okun, M. A., and Elias, C. S. Cautiousness in adulthood as a function of age and payoff structure. *Journal of Gerontology*, 1977, 32, 451–455.

Owens, W. A. Age and mental abilities: A longitudinal study. *Genetic Psychology Monographs*, 1953, *48*, 3–54.

Owens, W. A. Age and mental ability: A second adult follow-up. *Journal of Educational Psychology*, 1966, *57*, 311–325.

Palmore, E. (Ed.). *Normal aging II: Reports from the Duke longitudinal study*. Durham, N.C.: Duke University Press, 1974.

Palmore, E. (Ed.). *Normal aging III: Reports from the Duke longitudinal study*. Durham, N.C.: Duke University Press, 1985.

Perlmutter, M. What is memory aging the aging of? *Developmental Psychology*, 1978, *14*, 330–345.

Poon, L. W. Differences in human memory with aging: Nature, causes, and clinical implications. In J. E. Birren and K. W. Schaie (Eds.), *Handbook of the psychology of aging* (2d ed.). New York: Van Nostrand Reinhold, 1985, 427–462.

Poon, L. W. Differences in human memory with aging: Nature, causes, and clinical implications. In J. E. Birren and K. W. Schaie (Eds.), *Handbook of the psychology of aging* (2d ed.). New York: Van Nostrand Reinhold, 1985.

Poon, L. W., Fozard, J. L., Cermak, L. S., Arenberg, D., and Thompson, L. W. (Eds.). *New directions in memory and aging: Proceedings of the George A. Talland Memorial Conference*. Hillsdale, N.J.: Erlbaum, 1980.

Reese, H. W. Models of memory development. *Human Development*, 1976, *19*, 291–303.

Rice, G. E., and Meyer, B. J. F. Reading behavior and prose recall performance of young and older adults with high and average verbal ability. *Educational Gerontology*, 1985, *11*, 57–72.

Rice, G. E., and Meyer, B. J. F. Prose recall: Effects of aging, verbal ability, and reading behavior. *Journal of Gerontology*, 1986, *41*, 469–480.

Riegel, K. F., and Riegel, R. M. Development, drop, and death. *Developmental Psychology*, 1972, *6*, 306–319.

Robertson-Tchabo, E. A., Hausman, C. P., and Arenberg, D. A classical mnemonic for old learners: A trip that works. *Educational Gerontology*, 1976, *1*, 215–226.

Ross, E. Effects of challenging and supportive instructions on verbal learning in older persons. *Journal of Educational Psychology*, 1968, *59*, 261–266.

Schaie, K. W. Age changes and age differences. *Gerontologist*, 1967, *7*, 128–132.

Schaie, K. W. Quasi-experimental research designs in the psychology of aging. In J. E. Birren and K. W. Schaie (Eds.), *Handbook of the psychology of aging*. New York: Van Nostrand Reinhold, 1977.

Schaie, K. W. The primary mental abilities in adulthood: An exploration in the development of psychometric intelligence. In P. B. Baltes and O. G. Brim, Jr. (Eds.), *Life-span development and behavior* (Volume 2). New York: Academic Press, 1979.

Schaie, K. W. The Seattle longitudinal study: A 21-year exploration of psychometric intelligence in adulthood. In K. W. Schaie (Ed.), *Longitudinal studies of adult psychological development*. New York: Guilford Press, 1983.

Schaie, K. W., and Hertzog, C. Fourteen-year short-sequential analysis of adult intellectual development. *Developmental Psychology*, 1983, *19*, 531–543.

Schaie, K. W., and Labouvie-Vief, G. V. Generational versus ontogenetic components of change on adult cognitive behavior: A fourteen-year cross-sequential study. *Developmental Psychology,* 1974, *10,* 305–320.

Schonfield, D., and Stones, M. J. Remembering and aging. In J. F. Kihlstrom and F. J. Evans (Eds.), *Functional disorders of memory.* Hillsdale, N.J.: Erlbaum, 1979.

Siegler, I. C. The terminal drop hypothesis: Fact or artifact. *Experimental Aging and Research,* 1975, *1,* 169–185.

Siegler, I. C. Psychological aspects of the Duke longitudinal studies. In K. W. Schaie (Ed.), *Longitudinal studies of adult psychological development.* New York: Guilford Press, 1983.

Smith, A. D. Aging and the total presentation time hypothesis. *Developmental Psychology,* 1976, *12,* 87–88.

Smith, A. D. Adult age differences in cued recall. *Developmental Psychology,* 1977, *13,* 326–331.

Spearman, C. *The abilities of man: Their nature and measurement.* New York: Macmillan, 1927.

Squire, L. R. Remote memory as affected by aging. *Neuropsychologia,* 1974, *12,* 429–435.

Storandt, M. Speed and coding effects in relation to age and ability level. *Developmental Psychology.* 1976, *12,* 177–178.

Taub, H. A. Paired associates learning as a function of age, rate, and instructions. *Journal of Genetic Psychology,* 1967, *111,* 41–46.

Thurstone, L. L., and Thurstone, T. G. *Factorial studies of intelligence.* Chicago: University of Chicago Press, 1941.

Thurstone, L. L., and Thurstone, T. G. *SRA primary mental abilities* (3d ed.). Chicago: Science Research Associates, 1958.

Treat, N. J., and Reese, H. W. Age, pacing, and imagery in paired-associate learning. *Developmental Psychology,* 1976, *12,* 119–124.

Wallach, M. A., and Kogan, N. Aspects of judgement and decision making: Interrelationships and changes with age. *Behavioral Sciences,* 1961, *6,* 23–36.

Walsh, D. A., Till, R. E., and Williams, M. V. Age differences in peripheral perceptual processing: A monoptic backward masking investigation. *Journal of Experimental Psychology: Human Perception and Performance,* 1978, *4,* 232–243.

Warrington, E. K., and Saunders, H. I. The fate of old memories. *Quarterly Journal of Experimental Psychology,* 1971, *23,* 432–442.

Warrington, E. K., and Silberstein, M. A questionnaire technique for investigating very long-term memory. *Quarterly Journal of Experimental Psychology,* 1970, *22,* 508–512.

Welford, A. T. *Skill and age: An experimental approach.* London: Oxford University Press, 1951.

Wilkie, F., and Eisdorfer, C. Intelligence and blood pressure of the aged. *Science,* 1971, *172,* 959–962.

Winograd, E., Smith, A. D., and Simon, E. W. Aging and the picture superiority effect in recall. *Journal of Gerontology,* 1982, *37,* 70–75.

Chapter 8

Personality and
Social Adaptation
in Old Age

We have all had the experience of watching different people respond to the same event in different ways. For example, you probably know some students who are extremely anxious about test-taking while others are calm, and some students who express their opinions strongly and confidently while others rarely speak in class at all. All of these characteristics are part of an individual's personality.

Personality may be defined as a set of innate and learned traits that influence the manner in which each person responds and interacts with the environment. An individual may be described in terms of several personality traits, such as passive or aggressive, introverted or extroverted, independent or dependent. Personality may be evaluated with regard to particular standards of behavior; for example, an individual may be described as adapted or maladapted, adjusted or maladjusted. Personality characteristics affect people's interactions with their environments. This chapter examines changes in personality that influence these interactions.

The purpose of this chapter is to review the research on personality and on how it changes with aging. Theories of personality that have considered age-related changes are examined. The manner in which personality characteristics may change or remain stable are discussed. The following questions are considered: Are personality characteristics both innate and capable of developing throughout life? To what extent does an individual's interactions with the environment change his or her personality or reveal the individual's "true self" that may have been concealed because of social pressures to conform to particular norms? The ways in which self-concept and self-esteem are affected by these normal changes in personality with aging are also reviewed.

Personality styles influence how we cope with and adapt to the changes we experience as we age. The process of aging involves numerous stressful life experiences. How an older person responds to these experiences in an attempt to alleviate such stress has an influence on that individual's long-term well-being. In this chapter we also examine the life events that occur more frequently in old age, and how older people have been found to cope with them.

Innate and Environmental Factors

For many generations, psychologists have considered the issue of nature versus nurture; that is, whether we are born with specific personality traits or whether the environment in which we are raised plus our experiences determine our personality. Studies of twins reared apart and newborn babies suggest that some traits are in fact innate. In spite of differences in the environment in which each twin is raised, they often display behavioral tendencies that are more similar to each other than to siblings raised in the same environment. Furthermore, anyone who has seen a nursery full of infants has seen individual differences in dependency, passivity, and other traits that cannot be attributed solely to environmental influences. Still, personality is shaped by experiences throughout a person's life; in this sense, personality development is mediated by the environment.

The person-environment congruence model presented in this book's Introduction suggests that we are in dynamic interaction with the environment, that our behavior is influenced and modified by the environment, and that we shape the environment around us. This relationship was first proposed by Lewin (1935): $B=f$ (P,E); that is, behavior is a function of the person and his or her environment. An individual's behavior in one situation is often quite different from another, depending on the social norms and expectations of each situation, and on that person's needs and motives. Unfortunately, few researchers have examined this reciprocal relationship in adult development.

Personality Development in Adulthood

ERIKSON'S PSYCHOSOCIAL MODEL

Most theories of personality have emphasized the developmental stages of personality and imply that the social environment influences development. However, there has been disagreement about whether this development continues through adulthood. Sigmund Freud's focus on psychosexual stages of development through adolescence has had a major influence on developmental psychology. In most of his writings, Freud suggests that personality achieves stability by adolescence. Some personality theorists have agreed that personality traits remain stable after these years (see Worchel and Byrne, 1964). In contrast, Erik Erikson, who was trained in psychoanalytic theory, moved away from this approach and focused on psychosocial development throughout the life cycle. According to his model, the individual undergoes eight stages of development of the ego, with the final stage occurring in mature adulthood. At each stage the individual experiences a major crisis or conflict; the conflicts of each stage of development are the foundations of successive stages. Depending on the outcome of the crisis associated with a particular stage, the individual proceeds to the next stage of development in alternative ways.

As shown in Table 8–1, the individual in the last stage of life is confronted with the crisis of ego integrity versus despair. According to Erikson, the individual at this stage of development accepts the inevitability of mortality, achieves wisdom and perspective, or despairs because he or she has not come to grips with death and lacks ego integrity. A major task associated with this last stage is to integrate the experiences of earlier stages and to realize that one's life has had meaning, whether or not it was "successful" in a socially defined sense. Older people who achieve ego integrity feel a sense of connectedness with younger generations, and need to share their experiences and wisdom with them. This

TABLE 8–1 Erikson's Psychosocial Stages

	Stage	Goal
I	Basic trust vs. mistrust	To establish basic trust in the world through trust in the parent.
II	Autonomy vs. shame and doubt	To establish a sense of autonomy and self as distinct from the parent; to establish self-control vs. doubt in oneself.
III	Initiative vs. guilt	To establish sense of initiative within parental limits without feeling guilty about initiating.
IV	Industry vs. inferiority	To establish a sense of industry within the school setting; to learn necessary skills without inferiority or fear of failure.
V	Ego identity vs. role diffusion	To establish identity, self-concept, and role within the larger community, without confusion about the self.
VI	Intimacy vs. isolation	To establish intimacy and affiliation with others, without fearing loss of identity in the process that may result in isolation.
VII	Generativity vs. stagnation	To establish a sense of care and concern for well-being of future generations; to look toward the future and not stagnate in the past.
VIII	Ego integrity vs. despair	To establish a sense of meaning in one's life, versus despair or bitterness that life was wasted.

may take the form of face-to-face interactions with younger people, counseling, sponsoring an individual or group of younger people, or writing memoirs or letters.

Life satisfaction, or the feeling that life is worth living, may be achieved through these tasks of adopting a wider historical perspective upon one's life, accepting one's mortality, sharing experiences with the young, and leaving a legacy to future generations.* Erikson's theory provides a framework for studying personality in late life because it suggests that personality is dynamic throughout the life cycle. Indeed, this theory fits the person-environment model presented in the Introduction; we interact with a variety of other people in different settings, and our personality is affected accordingly.

JUNG'S PSYCHOANALYTIC PERSPECTIVE

Carl Jung's model of personality also assumes changes throughout life, as expressed in the following statement from one of his early writings:

---

*Researchers have found that health, marital, and financial status, as well as the availability of a confidant, are also significant predictors of life satisfaction.

We cannot live the afternoon of life according to the program of life's morning, for what was great in morning will be little at evening, and what in the morning was true will at evening have become a lie (1933, p. 108).

Jung's model emphasizes stages in the development of consciousness and the ego, from the narrow focus of the child to the other-worldliness of the older person. But the development of personality need not always imply maturation and increased wisdom. As Jung (1933) suggests, "the wine of youth does not always clear with advancing years; oftentimes it grows turbid" (p. 105).

Like Erikson, Jung examined the individual's confrontation with death in the last stage of life. He suggested that life for the aging person must naturally contract, that the individual in this stage must find meaning in inner exploration and in an afterlife. In contrast to the young, older persons have "a duty and a necessity to devote serious attention to (themselves). After having lavished its light upon the world, the sun withdraws its rays in order to illuminate itself" (Jung, 1933, p. 109). Jung also focused on changes in archetypes with age. That is, according to Jung, all humans have both a feminine and a masculine side. An archetype is the feminine side of a man's personality (the anima) and the masculine side of a woman's personality (the animus). Both biological and social conditioning have produced these archetypes (Jung, 1959). As they age, people begin to adopt psychological traits more commonly associated with the opposite sex. For example, older men may show more signs of passivity while women may become more assertive as they age, a change that is referred to throughout this text in discussions of gender differences.

EXPERIMENTAL TESTING OF THESE PERSPECTIVES

In testing the validity of these theories, subsequent research has contributed to our understanding of personality development in late adulthood. Many of these studies are cross-sectional; that is, they derive information on age differences, not age changes. There are notable exceptions to this approach, including the Baltimore Longitudinal Studies (described in Chapters 1 and 3) and the Kansas City Studies (described in Chapter 3 and below), which have examined changes in physiological, cognitive, and personality functions in the same individuals over a period of several years. Research by Costa and McCrae (1977, 1980) in the Baltimore studies is related to Erikson's work in that it has emphasized changes in personal adjustment with age. Costa, McCrae, and Norris (1981) tested Erikson's formulation of the last stage of psychosocial development and noted that personal adjustment should be defined in old age as "subjective well-being," or individuals' reports that they are satisfied with their life's accomplishments and have high morale. They found that some personality traits, such as extroversion, are correlated with subjective well-being in old age.

Researchers who have systematically examined personality in middle and old age have found support for Jung's observations regarding decreased sex-typed behavior in old age. David Gutmann (1974a, b; 1980), who has studied personality across the life span in diverse cultures from a psychoanalytic perspective, has found a shift from active mastery to passive mastery as men age. In contrast, women appear to move from passive to active mastery. That is, in most cultures examined by Gutmann, young adult males tend to be more achievement-oriented and concerned with controlling their environments, whereas young adult women tend to be more affiliative and expressive. Gutmann found greater expressiveness, nurturance, and need for affiliation among older males than in younger men, whereas older women tended to be more instrumental and to express more achievement-oriented responses than young women. Gutmann's research also suggests that people may vary with age in their use of magical mastery styles (maladaptive ego responses to stressful situations). He found a smaller proportion of middle-aged persons with this ego style than with active or passive mastery styles. However, magical mastery styles were more frequently observed in men and women beyond age 60. A later analysis of ego styles in other cultures by Gutmann (1977) suggests that this shift toward magical mastery may be more likely to take place among men than women (Gutmann, 1977).

THE KANSAS CITY STUDIES

Longitudinal research by Neugarten, Havighurst, and Tobin (1968) among community-dwelling elderly in Kansas City is consistent with Gutmann's findings and has contributed to our understanding of many other age-related changes in personality and coping. Neugarten found that older men became more accepting of their affiliative, nurturant, and sensual side, while women learned to display the egocentric and aggressive impulses that they had always possessed but had not displayed during their younger years. Neugarten, similar to Jung, has suggested that these characteristics always exist in both sexes, but social pressure and societal values encourage the expression of more sex-typed traits in youth.

The Kansas City studies represented the first major attempt to examine personality longitudinally and provided the empirical basis for activity theory described in Chapter 3. In this important study of adaptation to aging, Neugarten and her associates interviewed 700 residents of Kansas City who were aged 40 to 70, living independently in the community, and relatively healthy in the 1950s; this was then followed with a six-year longitudinal study of 300 persons aged 50 to 90. They found changes in such personality characteristics as nurturance, introversion, and aggressiveness in the later years. Contrary to popular stereotypes, aging was also associated with greater differences (individuation) among individuals; as the people aged, they developed more unique styles of interaction. Neugarten and colleagues (1968) suggested that people do not resemble each other more in old age, but in fact become more differentiated because they grow less concerned about societal expectations.

Other age-related changes observed in the Kansas City studies included shifts toward greater cautiousness and interiority; that is, a preoccupation with one's inner life, and less extroversion. The movement toward interiority does not mean, however, that older persons become more religious, as noted in our discussion of cross-sectional research in Chapter 1. There is very little research evidence that we become *more* religious as we age. It may be that the current cohort of people over age 70 have always been more religious than younger cohorts (see Chapter 13).

The Kansas City researchers also observed decreased impulsiveness, and a movement toward using more sophisticated ego defense mechanisms with age. For example, older persons tended to use less denial and more sublimation. Attitudes toward the world were also likely to change with age, but these were found to relate closely to personal experiences. For instance, people do not necessarily become more conservative as they age. Based on generational (cohort) differences and personal experiences, some persons become more liberal in their social perspective during the later years. Others have been more conservative than younger cohorts throughout their lives. These age-related changes in impulsiveness, types of defense mechanisms used, and attitudes have been supported in studies of personality by researchers examining a diverse variety of cultural and ethnic groups (Thomae, 1980; Shanan, 1978).

Neugarten (1968) categorized the personalities that were observed in the Kansas City studies into four major types:

1. *The Integrated Type:* These are self-actualized elderly who are most satisfied with their lives, and who have complex inner lives and competent egos. They are flexible, realistic, and possess high self-esteem. These persons have come to grips with their mortality and accept death as inevitable. Some integrated elderly may have voluntarily "disengaged" from society and are now concerned about their inner lives. Others, similar to Mr. Wallace in the introductory vignette, are "focused" retirees, or "reorganizers," who shift their energy and interest in retirement to other activities. The first of these may be illustrated by a teacher who retires at age 60, is not involved in many professional or social activities, but is happy with a quiet retirement. The focused retiree may be illustrated by another teacher who retires at age 65, but continues to volunteer for several community organizations and legislative efforts of the local Retired Teachers' Association. Both are happy with their lives because they have chosen to spend their retirement years in a particular style consistent with their needs. Measures of life satisfaction in this group in the Kansas City studies revealed high satisfaction regardless of activity levels.

2. *The Armored-Defensive Type:* These are individuals who are still ambitious and aggressive. Some appear to be fighting an internal battle against aging and death. Such persons often are not introspective and lack insight into their actions. Usually this is not a very successful adaptation to old age but rather expressed in a "holding-on" pattern (i.e., forcing himself or

herself to remain active for fear of becoming dependent). Another expression of this style is the constricted personality, or individuals who are preoccupied with the losses of aging, thereby shutting out new experiences. They often feel angry and resentful toward others. Older persons who refuse to stop working despite poor health and/or problems with psychomotor and intellectual functioning illustrate these aspects of the armored-defensive type.

3. *The Passive-Dependent Type:* Older persons in this category may achieve moderate to high life satisfaction if their dependency needs are met. Included are individuals who relegate all their important tasks to others, let others take care of them, and participate in very few social activities. Neugarten has labeled such persons the "succorance seeking type." This category also includes older persons who are apathetic, withdrawn, and isolated (the "rocking chair" type). Unlike the constricted-defensive individuals described above, this personality type is generally not bitter or resentful toward the rest of the world. Mrs. Johnson in the introductory vignette has some of these characteristics.

4. *The Disorganized (or Unintegrated) Type:* Older persons who fit into this personality category often have a gross deterioration in their cognitive and emotional functions as a result of adult-onset dementia or a personality disorder that has existed since youth (as illustrated by Mr. Adams in the introductory vignette). These individuals generally have poor coping abilities, are only marginally adjusted to their environment, and express little satisfaction with their lives. Contrary to many stereotypes about aging, this group represents a minority of all older persons.

The personality types described above do not encompass all older persons. Many possess characteristics of more than one category; others do not fit into any of the types. Yet these categories are effective in describing widely varying ways in which people age and the effects of poor adaptation. Other researchers have described similar personality types, even in widely divergent cultures (Thomae, 1980; Gaber, 1983; Shanan and Jacobowitz, 1982).

In another classic study of personality in adulthood, interviews were conducted with 87 men aged 55 to 84, who were either retired or anticipating retirement in the near future (Reichard, Livson, and Peterson, 1962). Three of the five personality types identified in this study are comparable to the categories found in the Kansas City studies. These were described as the "mature" (similar to the "integrated" type in the latter study), the "armored" (parallel to the "armored-defensive" type described above), and the "rocking chair" type (representing some groups of passive dependent elderly observed in the Kansas City studies). These three personality types were found to adjust well to retirement. In contrast, elderly men whom they described as "angry" and "self-hating" types were unable to adjust.

DIALECTICAL MODELS OF ADULT PERSONALITY

A more recent model of adult personality development has been proposed by Levinson (1977) and his colleagues (Levinson et al., 1978). This model is based on secondary analyses of American men described in published biographies and in interviews with working-class men. It was only recently tested to determine its applicability to women. In contrast to Erikson, who focused on stages of ego development, Levinson and colleagues have examined developmental stages in terms of life structures, or the underlying characteristics of a person's life at a particular period of time. These life structures include sociocultural features (e.g., social class, ethnic group membership, occupation), one's personal self (e.g., conflicts, fantasies, anxieties), and participation in society (e.g., interaction between the self and society). The choices that individuals make in this participation or interaction with the outside world determine what structure their lives will take. Thus, for example, a man who has anxieties about his role in society and and his identity as a male will select a different occupation and marital situation than one who has no such ego conflicts. Changes in life structure (defined as "eras" by Levinson) represent developmental stages; they generally occur as the individual perceives changes in the self, or as external events such as childbirth and retirement create new demands on one's relationships with others. Levinson and his colleagues have suggested that each era may last as long as 20 years. (See Table 8–2.)

Levinson's model represents an example of a dialectical approach to personality development; it proposes that change occurs because of interactions between a dynamic person (one who is biologically *and* psychologically changing) and a dynamic environment. To the extent that an individual is sensitive to the changing self, he or she can respond to changing environmental or societal conditions by altering something within the self or by modifying some expectations from the environment. This process thereby reestablishes equilibrium with the environment. In previous chapters, we have seen how some normal, age-related changes in physiological functions can slow down older people and affect their activities of daily living. Older persons who deny these biological and physiological changes are more likely to experience problems in modifying their lifestyles and moving into a different developmental phase.

The first researcher to emphasize the importance of the dialectic perspective for adult development was Klaus Riegel (1976). Riegel viewed personality development as a necessary consequence of the conflicts that arise between changing personal needs and abilities and the demands of the social environment. Indeed, growth is defined by Riegel as the resolution of such conflicts and movement to the next stage of greater fit. This approach is quite similar to the person-environment model first presented in the Introduction to this book. As noted earlier, proponents of this model (Lawton and Nahemow, 1973; Kahana, 1973; 1975) argue for the continuing need to maintain congruence between changing personal competence and the demands of the physical and social

TABLE 8–2 Levinson's "Seasons" of Life

Era I	Preadulthood (Age 0–22)
	(An era when the family provides protection, socialization, and support of personal growth)
	*Early Adult Transition (Age 17–22)
Era II	Early Adulthood (Age 17–45)
	(An era of peak biological functioning, development of adult identity)
	Entering the adult world, entry life structure for early adulthood.
	Age 30 transition
	Settling down, culminating life structure for early adulthood.
	*Mid-life transition (Age 40–45)
Era III	Middle Adulthood (Age 40–65)
	(Goals become more other-oriented, compassionate roles, mentor roles assumed; peak effectiveness as a leader)
	Entering life structure for middle adulthood
	*Age 50 transition
	Culmination of middle adulthood
	*Late Adulthood Transition (Age 60+)
Era IV	Late Adulthood Transition (Age 60–65)
	(An era when declining capacities are recognized, anxieties about aging, loss of power and status begins)

Source: D. Levinson, C. M. Darrow, E. B. Klein, M. H. Levinson, and B. McKee, *The seasons of a man's life* (New York: Alfred A. Knopf, 1978). Reprinted with permission of the author and publisher.

environment. The dialectical approach to personality development has received little research attention (except from an environmental design perspective, as we will see in Chapter 12), compared to other theories described earlier.

KOHLBERG'S MODEL OF MORAL DEVELOPMENT

In contrast to models of personality development that focus on growth of the ego across the life span, the work of Lawrence Kohlberg (1969a, 1969b, 1973) and his colleagues (Snarey, Reimer, and Kohlberg, 1985) emphasizes the development of the conscience, or superego, through the acquisition of moral values. By presenting hypothetical moral dilemmas to people and asking them to describe how they would resolve the problem and why, Kohlberg observed six stages of moral development. The first stage is defined by obedience to authority, regardless of the circumstances (e.g., a starving person who has no money and steals food would be perceived as guilty of disobedience by the respondent in this stage of moral development). In the second stage, respondents perceive a need for exchange and reciprocity; they believe that all actions by others—good or bad—demand some reaction. The third stage, described by Kohlberg (1969b) as the "good boy orientation," is defined by a need to meet others' expectations (e.g., completing a job because that is what the teacher or employer expects). Those in the fourth stage focus on the need to maintain social order and to respect authority, and those in the fifth stage expand beyond this to the need to involve all members of society in the maintenance of social order. An individual in this stage recognizes that there must be an arbitrary starting point for rules and expectations of people's behavior, and that one must avoid violating others' contractual or legal rights.

According to Kohlberg, few people reach the sixth stage, which is characterized by a belief in universal logic and ethical principles (e.g., the use of civil disobedience in order to reverse unjust social practices such as discrimination). People at this stage of moral development are directed by their conscience, and by the trust and respect of others. Nobel Peace Prize winners Martin Luther King and Archbishop Desmond Tutu are individuals who may have achieved this ultimate stage of moral development.

Unlike other theories of personality development, Kohlberg's approach is less chronologically oriented. That is, some middle-aged and older people may remain in stage two or three (such as an older person who feels he must seek revenge anytime he is mistreated), whereas a few young persons achieve stage four or five of moral development (such as youths who risk their freedom by protesting against nuclear warfare and unjust wars). Furthermore, Kohlberg's theory does not consider the possibility that some people may be in different stages of moral development simultaneously; for example, an individual may believe that stealing should be punished no matter what (stage one), yet at the same time claim that all people in a democratic society should play a role in devising a social order (stage five). Many moral values held by people may also be contradictory, suggesting that a smooth progression through stages should not be expected in moral development, unlike the development of cognitive abilities and the ego.

Self-Concept and Self-Esteem

A major adjustment required in old age is the ability to redefine one's self-concept or one's image of the self as social roles shift and as new roles are assumed. For example, how does a retired teacher identify himself or herself upon giving up the work that has been that individual's central focus for the past 40 to 50 years? How does a woman whose self-concept is closely associated with her role as a wife express her identity after her husband dies?

As noted in Chapter 3, many older persons continue to identify with the role that they have lost (think of those who continue to introduce themselves as "teacher" or "doctor" long after retiring from those careers). Others experience role confusion, particularly in the early stages, when cues from other people are inconsistent with an individual's self-concept. Still others may undergo a period of depression and major readjustment to the changes associated with role loss.

These persons generally have not established independent self-concepts. To the extent that a person's self-concept is defined independently of particular social roles, one adapts more readily to the role losses that may accompany old age.

In a study of self-concept across the life span, 4,540 persons aged 9 to 89 were measured on four dimensions: achievement-leadership, congeniality-sociability, adjustment, and masculinity-femininity (Monge, 1975). Both age and sex differences emerged on all four components of self-concept. Women in the oldest group (65–89) tended to report more achievement-leadership than women of any other age, except those aged 20 to 34. No significant differences emerged among men of various age groups. Both older men and women had the highest scores on the congeniality-sociability dimension. Adjustment scores remained high in the oldest group. Consistent with Jung's model of adult personality development and the findings of the Kansas City studies, there was a significant decline in self-reported masculinity among men beyond age 50, with a corresponding increase in self-definitions of masculinity among women in midlife.

For an older person whose self-concept is based on social roles and others' expectations, role losses have a particularly significant impact on that individual's self-esteem—that is, evaluation or feeling about his or her identity relative to some ideal or standard. *Self-esteem* is based on an emotional assessment of the self, whereas *self-concept* is the cognitive definition of one's identity. The affective quality of self-esteem makes it more dynamic and more easily influenced by such external forces as retirement, widowhood, health status, and reinforcements (both positive and negative) from others (e.g., respect, deference, ostracism). As a result, alterations in social roles and the loss of status that accompanies some of these changes often have a negative impact on an older person's self-esteem. Think, for example, of an older person whose "ideal self" is as an independent individual. If this person is forced to rely on others for care because of a major debilitating illness such as a stroke or dementia, such an individual is unwittingly robbed of this ideal, and self-esteem may suffer.

An individual who experiences multiple role losses must not only adapt to the lifestyle changes associated with aging (e.g., financial insecurity, shrinking social networks), but must also integrate the new roles with his or her "ideal self" or learn to modify this definition of "ideal." Older persons who are experiencing major physical and cognitive disabilities simultaneously with role losses, or worse yet, whose role losses are precipitated by an illness (e.g., early retirement due to stroke or institutionalization because of Alzheimer's disease) must cope with multiple problems at a time in their lives when they have the fewest resources to resolve them successfully. Depression is not an uncommon reaction in these cases (see Chapter 9). Other older persons may not experience such major emotional upheavals; nevertheless, their self-esteem may be affected. Some studies have shown a generalized decrease in self-esteem from age 50 to 80, although others have found considerable variability in patterns of self-esteem (Kogan and Wallach, 1961; Lowenthal and Chiriboga, 1972).

The following personality factors have been suggested as important to maintaining self-esteem in the later years (Morgan, 1979):

1. Reinterpretation of the meaning of self, such that an individual's self-concept and self-worth are independent of any roles he or she has played ("I am a unique individual" rather than "I am a doctor/teacher/wife"). To the extent that an older person can focus more on internal realities such as personality characteristics, skills, and abilities, and less on external sources of reinforcement, the ego is strengthened and free of environmental influences.

2. Acceptance of the aging process, its limitations and possibilities. That is, individuals who realize that they have less energy and respond more slowly than in the past, but that they can still participate in life will adapt more readily to the social and health losses of old age. It is critical to achieve this level of awareness without giving up on life, as some older persons do. Unfortunately, socialization into old age is not as easy as socialization into other stages, because most people have few appropriate role models that they can emulate (Rosow, 1974). As a result, environmental feedback in the form of television advertising and negative remarks of family and friends may reinforce an individual's internal slowing process and suggest that the older person must withdraw. It therefore appears important for the media and society to provide role models of older people who have adapted successfully to their aging, and how they have done so. (All too often, however, the images of "successful" aging are persons who have unusual athletic, intellectual, or artistic powers, or who have achieved extreme longevity in isolated societies. The typical older person often cannot identify with such people; hence, these "exceptional" people are not used by most individuals as role models of how *they* can adapt to old age.)

3. Reevaluation of one's goals and expectations throughout life. Too often people establish life goals at an early age, and can be constantly disappointed as circumstances change. The ability to respond to internal and external pressures by modifying life goals appropriately reflects flexibility and harmony with one's environment. An older person who has these skills is most likely to adapt successfully to the changes associated with aging.

4. The ability to look back objectively on one's past and to review one's failures and successes. *Life review*, as its name implies, entails an objective review and evaluation of one's life. The individual takes a historical perspective of past experiences and how these have influenced subsequent personality development, behavior, and interpersonal relationships. An older person who has, or who can develop, this ability can call upon coping strategies that have been most effective in the past and adapt them to changed circumstances. We will see in Chapter 9 how life review or reminiscence

therapy has been used successfully as a form of psychotherapy with depressed elderly.

Stress, Coping, and Adaptation

The process of aging entails numerous life changes, as noted in this and previous chapters. These changes, both positive and negative, place demands on the aging person's abilities to cope with and adapt to new life situations. Together with health and cognitive functioning, personality characteristics influence coping responses. Self-concept and self-esteem are two important elements that play a role in coping styles, and may help explain why some older people adjust readily to major life changes, while others have difficulty with such transitions. Indeed, self-esteem, health, and cognitive skills all contribute to an individual's sense of competence. Major life events and situations represent environmental stressors that place demands on an individual's competence. These and other factors that influence adaptation in old age are discussed in this section.

SOME USEFUL DEFINITIONS

Before examining coping and adaptation in old age, it is important to clarify and define some key concepts. The concept of *life events* or *life experiences* forms the basis for this section. These terms refer to internal or external stimuli that cause some change in an individual's daily life. They may be positive or negative, gains or losses, discrete or continuous. Examples of internally created events include changes in eating or sleeping habits, and the effects of a chronic disease such as arthritis or diabetes. Externally initiated events might include starting a new job, losing one's job, or retirement.

Improvement in one's own health or in a family member's health are examples of positive life events, whereas deteriorating health and death are negative events. Life experiences that represent gains include the birth of a grandchild or promotions that lead to increased responsibility and a higher salary. Life events that are losses include the death of a family member or friend, the loss of a spouse through divorce or death, or the loss of the driver role because of declining vision. Some life experiences may have both positive *and* negative aspects. For example, older workers may view their pending retirement with great joy and make numerous plans for the post-retirement years; however, there are some negative consequences as well, including reduced income, unstructured time, and loss of the worker role. Other events with both positive and negative aspects are the purchase of a new home, a vacation, and even a long-awaited family reunion.

One of the problems in assessing the impact of life events is variability in duration. Some events are discrete, such as a vacation or an accident. Others last for long periods, with no distinctive starting and end points. These include changes in eating and sleeping patterns and in health status. Still other events may be discrete but may have long-term antecedents or consequences. Many events experienced by older persons typically have this feature, including retirement, death of spouse, and "the empty nest." Since stress produced by such events is generally ongoing, an individual experiencing them must cope with their diverse aspects over a period of time.

Another distinction to be made is that between *on-time* and *off-time* events (Neugarten, 1979). This concept distinguishes life experiences that a person can anticipate because of one's stage in the life cycle (on-time) from those that are unexpected at a given stage (off-time). Other researchers have used the terms *normative* and *non-normative* events, suggesting that an individual anticipates some life experiences because they are the norm for most people of a given age (Pearlin, 1975; Pearlin and Lieberman, 1979). Thus, for example, a man married to a 75-year-old woman is more likely to expect the death of his wife than is the husband of a 35-year-old woman. A 50-year-old woman is more likely than a 35-year-old to anticipate the onset of menopause and its accompanying physiological and psychological changes. As we will see later in this chapter, researchers have found differences in how people respond to on-time and off-time events.

The concept of *stress* is also important for this chapter. Since Selye's (1946) introduction of this term, many researchers have explored the antecedents, components, and consequences of stress. One problem in understanding this concept has been the diverse definitions given for it. Selye's original definition of stress (which he also calls the "general adaptation syndrome") is the "nonspecific response of the body to any demand made upon it," the goal of which is to prepare the organism for "fight or flight" (Selye, 1946). Fight or flight reactions are the simplest means by which organisms respond to stressful situations. Later in this chapter, we review more complex coping responses used by humans who are experiencing stress. In his early research with rats, Selye found that animals subjected to constant negative external stimuli (e.g., crowding, frustration in finding food) were more likely to develop enlarged adrenal glands and to show physical signs of aging earlier than animals who were not subjected to unpleasant stimuli. In fact, Selye (1970) defined aging as the sum of stresses experienced across one's lifetime.

One recurring problem with the definition of stress is that it has been used to describe both a response (as in Selye's description of perceived tension, enlarged adrenal glands, heightened blood pressure) and a stimulus (labeling a particular event as a stress). In this chapter, the term *stressor* is used to identify stimuli that cause stress or a state of imbalance in the organism, and result in physiological or psychological adaptive responses. Such stimuli may also be described as *stressful.*

It is important to note that not everyone perceives the same events to be stressful. Lazarus and DeLongis (1983) have introduced the concept of *cognitive appraisal;* the way in which a person perceives the significance of an encounter for his or her well-being. Cognitive appraisal serves to minimize or magnify the importance or stressfulness of an event by attaching some meaning to it. If a situation is construed as benign or irrelevant by an individual, it does not elicit coping responses. On the other hand, if a person appraises a situation as challenging, harmful, or threatening, it becomes a stressor, and calls upon the individual's adaptation responses.

It is useful to distinguish between positive and negative stressors such as life events. The concept of cognitive appraisal suggests that a person who perceives a particular situation as a challenge (i.e., a positive stressor) copes differently with it than one who views it as a threat (i.e., a negative stressor). For example, a student who views a final exam as a challenge will prepare for it differently than one who feels threatened by it. The first student will anticipate it as a positive and exciting situation, whereas the second may avoid thinking about, preparing for, or even taking the exam. On the other hand, a student who perceives the exam as irrelevant may do poorly because the situation has not generated enough of a stress response to induce him or her to prepare for or cope with it.

Older people experience similar reactions. An older woman who moves voluntarily to a retirement home may view it as an exciting and much-needed change in her lifestyle, or she may resent the change as too demanding and disruptive. In the former case, she will adapt more readily and will experience less negative stress than in the latter. On the other hand, if this person views the move as totally benign and does not expect it to place any demands on her, she will probably be unpleasantly surprised by the level of stress that she eventually encounters, no matter how minimal.

A certain level of stress is needed in order to stimulate us to perform. Moderate levels of stress are indeed necessary, but too much or too little stress appears to be harmful to emotional and physical well-being. Let us now examine what happens to our stress responses as we age.

AGING AND LIFE EVENTS

There has been much discussion among researchers about the nature of life events in the later years, the older person's ability to cope with them, and whether old age is associated with more or fewer life events than youth. Admittedly, many significant life events tend to occur more often in old age, such as widowhood, retirement, and relocation to a nursing home. Numerous other events generally take place in people's lives during youth and middle-age. As noted earlier, many of these represent role gains or replacement, such as the role of student, voter, homeowner, marital partner, and worker. Both the nature of such roles and the novelty associated with assuming a social role for the first time result in major changes in an individual's daily functioning and demand adaptation to the new situation. Table 8–3, adapted from the work of Pastalan (1977), illustrates the ages when many social roles are generally gained or lost. Note that many social roles

TABLE 8–3 Continuum of Role Gains and Losses

Age	Event*
0 ———	
	Student +
10 ———	
	Consumer +
	Driver +
	Adult +
20 ———	Voter +
	Worker +
	Marital Partner +
30 ———	Parent +
	Home Owner +
40 ———	
	Auditory Decline −
50 ———	Empty Nest −
	Visual Decline −
60 ———	Grandparent +
	Widowhood −
	Tactile Decline −
	Taste Decline −
	Retirement −
70 ———	
	Olfactory Decline −
	Motor Function −
80 ———	Give Up Driving −
	Health −
	Institutionalization −
90 ———	

*+ indicates role gain; − indicates loss.
Source: Adapted from L. A. Pastalan, Designing housing environments for the elderly. *Journal of Architectural Education* 31 (1977).

are rarely lost (e.g., the voter role, the parent role), and some roles, especially those associated with aging, are extensions of others (e.g., becoming a grandparent or parent-in-law). On the other hand, some of the role losses that may occur with aging, such as retirement, are associated with a decline in social status. Few studies have compared the relative stressfulness of role losses, role gains or replacements, and role extensions in old age, although there is extensive research on life stress among younger populations.

Thomas Holmes and his colleagues undertook the first studies of the physiological and psychological impact of increased sources and amounts of stress on humans (Holmes and Rahe, 1967; Rahe, 1972; Holmes and Masuda, 1974). They introduced the concept of life change units, a numerical score indicating the typical level of change or stress that a particular event produces in an individual's day-to-day life. Based on interviews with hundreds of people, Holmes and Rahe derived the Social Readjustment Rating Scale (SRRS). This instrument consists of 43 events, each with an associated change score. The greatest change score is 100, for death of spouse. This is the event that was used as an "anchor point" in the development of the SRRS. That is, respondents were asked to assign life change scores to all other life events, comparing each one with death of spouse, which had been preassigned a score of 100. A copy of the SRRS is presented in Table 8–4. The studies by Holmes and colleagues on young and middle-aged adults revealed that people who experienced multiple events with life change units totalling more than 200 points within a two-year period were more susceptible to physical illnesses.

POTENTIAL PROBLEMS IN MEASUREMENT

It is unclear whether these same life events produce the same level of stress in older persons as they do in younger people. As shown in Table 8–5, many of them are less likely to be experienced in old age (e.g., jail term, marriage, assuming a new mortgage, beginning or ending school). Furthermore, the life change units assigned to some events by the young respondents in Holmes and Rahe's sample may not reflect the degree of stress actually produced by events that they have not yet experienced (e.g., death of spouse).

Eisdorfer and Wilkie (1977) discussed the need to develop appropriate methods for assessing life events in older persons. In response, Amster and Krauss (1974), Muhlenkamp, Gress, and Flood (1975), and Kiyak and Kahana (1975) developed and tested life event scales that are more relevant to the elderly. Whereas the first two studies eliminated many items from the SRRS that were not applicable to older persons, the study by Kiyak and Kahana kept many of the original SRRS items but also added some items that were appropriate for older persons. Comparisons were made between weights assigned to these events by older persons and by college students (median age = 70 and 20, respectively).

Table 8–5 presents comparisons across some items that were common to all four scales. The wide variation in life change scores across these four scales illustrates the problem of relying on absolute scores to determine the stressfulness of an event. However, the relative stress of some items remains constant across the studies; for example, death of spouse received the highest readjustment score in all four. Young and old respondents appear to perceive the stressfulness of an event differently, as illustrated by the significant differences between these groups in the Kiyak and Kahana study. As an illustration, financial problems and death of a close friend were perceived to be more stressful by younger respondents. These findings highlight the need for caution in administering to older persons life events measures that were originally developed with younger samples.

TABLE 8–4 The Social Readjustment Rating Scale

Events	Value
	50
1. Marriage	23
2. Troubles with the boss	63
3. Detention in jail or other institution	100
4. Death of spouse	16
5. Major change in sleeping habits (a lot more or a lot less sleep, or change in part of day when asleep)	
6. Death of a close family member	63
7. Major change in eating habits (a lot more or a lot less food intake, or very different meal hours or surroundings)	15
8. Foreclosure on a mortgage or loan	30
9. Revision of personal habits (dress, manners, associations)	24
10. Death of a close friend	37
11. Minor violations of the law (e.g., traffic tickets, jay walking, disturbing the peace, etc.)	11
12. Outstanding personal achievement	28
13. Pregnancy	40
14. Major change in the health or behavior of a family member	44
15. Sexual difficulties	39
16. In-law troubles	29
17. Major change in number of family get-togethers (e.g., a lot more or a lot less than usual)	15
18. Major change in financial state (e.g., a lot worse off or a lot better off than usual)	38
19. Gaining a new family member (e.g., through birth, adoption, oldster moving in, etc.)	39
20. Change in residence	20
21. Son or daughter leaving home (e.g., marriage, attending college, etc.)	29
22. Marital separation from mate	65
23. Major change in church activities (e.g., a lot more or a lot less than usual)	19
24. Marital reconciliation with mate	45
25. Being fired from work	47
26. Divorce	73
27. Changing to a different line of work	36
28. Major change in the number of arguments with spouse (e.g., either a lot more or a lot less than usual regarding childrearing, personal habits, etc.)	35
29. Major change in responsibilities at work (e.g., promotion, demotion, lateral transfer)	29
30. Wife beginning or ceasing work outside the home	26
31. Major change in working hours or conditions	20
32. Major change in usual type and/or amount of recreation	19
33. Taking on a mortgage greater than $10,000 (e.g., purchasing a home, business, etc.)	31

(Continued)

TABLE 8–4 Continued

Events	Value
34. Taking on a mortgage or loan less than $10,000 (e.g., purchasing a car, TV, freezer, etc.)	17
35. Major personal injury or illness	53
36. Major business readjustment (e.g., merger, reorganization, bankruptcy, etc.)	39
37. Major change in social activities (e.g., clubs, dancing movies, visiting, etc.)	18
38. Major change in living conditions (e.g., building a new home, remodeling, deterioration of home or neighborhood)	25
39. Retirement from work	45
40. Vacation	13
41. Christmas	
42. Changing to a new school	20
43. Beginning or ceasing formal schooling	26

Source: Reprinted with permission from *Journal of Psychosomatic Research,* volume 11, by T. H. Holmes and R. Rahe, "The Social Readjustment Rating Scale," copyright 1967, Pergamon Journals, Ltd.

TABLE 8–5 Comparison of Life Change Units

Event	SRRS	Kiyak and Kahana		Amster and Krauss	Muhlenkamp, Gress, and Flood
		Young	*Old*		
Death of spouse	100	88 *	79	125	73
Marriage	50	78 *	64	50	50
Marital reconciliation	45	65 *	47	39	35
Death of a close friend	37	67 *	47	50	52
Change in residence	20	59	51	43	39
Financial problems	38	68 *	59	56	43
Improved financial status	38	59	48	56	43

*Differences significant at p<.05.

 Another problem with such measures is the implicit assumption that positive and negative life events produce equal levels of stress. When events such as "change in financial status" were split into "problems with finances" vs. "improvements in finances" in the Kiyak and Kahana study, both young and old respondents assigned higher stress scores (life change units) to negative events.

 Most researchers have not explored the impact of previous experience on the life change score assigned by each respondent. In the study by Kiyak and Kahana, scores assigned to three events that had been experienced by older respondents (menopause, retirement, death of spouse) but not by college students were compared. In all three cases, older persons assigned lower readjustment scores than did young students. Other researchers have provided similar evidence. For example, voluntary retirement was not perceived to be highly stressful by older men who had already experienced it (Haynes, McMichael and Tyroler, 1978). Nor is menopause generally recalled as a traumatic event by older women (Neugarten, Havighurst, and Tobin, 1968). Likewise, the event of the "empty nest" has not received high readjustment scores by older parents (Lowenthal and Chiriboga, 1972). These findings support the work of researchers who have argued that the anticipation of an event is more stressful than the actual experience (Neugarten, 1968; Lundberg, Theorell, and Lind, 1975). Previous experiences may also ease an individual's response to subsequent life events. As a result, an older person who has already experienced the death of many friends and relatives may be less stressed by the death of another close friend than an individual, young or old, who has never experienced such an event. This is not to say that an older person will not need to cope with new events as they occur, but the duration and intensity of the stress may be less, thereby alleviating the person's adaptation to a new situation. Thus, research evidence suggests that past experience with similar events enables the older person to cope with a new event.

HISTORICAL, LIFE CYCLE, AND DAILY LIVING FACTORS

As noted earlier, the degree to which a person can anticipate an event may influence the stress produced by it and the ability to cope with it. Life events that are on-time or are expected (e.g., death of spouse following a long illness) are less stressful than unexpected events (Neugarten, 1970, 1979). On the other hand, the loss of a spouse following a long illness has been found to result in more medical problems of the widowed spouse than sudden death or chronic illness of shorter duration (Gerber et al., 1975). This may be due to the cumulative effects of other stressors (e.g., the demands of caregiving) associated with the terminal illness that the surviving spouse could not resolve during the caregiving and anticipatory grieving stages. Thus, the evidence is mixed regarding older people's ability to cope with on-time events. It may be that anticipatory coping does not take the place of coping with an event *after* it occurs. In addition, an individual must cope with other stressors that were not part of the anticipated event.

It is still unclear whether older persons experience more stress in a given period than the young. Some studies provide evidence that older persons are indeed confronted with more stressful live events (Lowenthal and Chiriboga, 1972; Chiriboga and Cutler, 1980; Lieberman, 1975; Hultsch and Plemons, 1979). Others have found the same distribution of such events in young, middle-aged, and older persons, although none of these studies has compared people across a wide age range (Lowenthal, Thurnher and Chiriboga, 1975; Palmore et al., 1979; Lazarus and Delongis, 1983). Still others have argued that older people experience *fewer* stressful life events in a given time period than do the young (Eisdorfer and Wilkie, 1977). These findings point to the need for more longitudinal studies that follow the life experiences of a large sample from middle-age to old age.

It has been argued that the cohort of people aged 65 and older today have experienced more traumatic life events than younger age groups because they lived through the Depression, World War II, and the Korean and Vietnamese Wars. In the Duke Longitudinal Study, such sociohistorical events were probed. Respondents who had lived in the era of such events did not report any trauma associated specifically with them, but many personal and family experiences were influenced by these major occurrences (Siegler and George, 1983). Thus, sociohistorical events form the background for many personal life events, and may even influence an individual's own life (e.g., a war injury, loss of a job during the Depression). These events, however, do not necessarily have long-term effects on a person's adaptation and psychological well-being, unless an individual has experienced them directly (e.g., post-traumatic stress disorder has been identified in some veterans of the Vietnam War).

Although researchers have focused on the stress produced by major life events, Lazarus and Cohen (1977) have suggested that most people experience stress as a result of "chronic daily hassles." Their "hassles scale" measures such day-to-day problems as feelings of loneliness, lack of energy, regrets over past decisions, and concerns about one's current situation. Other emotions that may produce stress for an individual include feelings of powerlessness, normlessness, and social isolation (Seeman, 1976). These are generally not specific events with a beginning or end point, but are chronic and may occur simultaneously with other "hassles." An individual must cope with these emotions, just as with discrete life events. To the extent that an older person feels powerless, lonely, and regretful, feelings of stress will increase, with a corresponding need to adapt to the situation in some way. Lazarus and Cohen have not reported differences in the frequency with which older persons experience such chronic feelings in comparison to younger persons.

One aspect of life events that has not been explored with the elderly, but which may influence psychological well-being, is the impact of anticipated events that do not materialize. That is, how do older persons respond after anticipating a major event, then discovering that it will not take place? One can list many such events, both positive and negative, that may result in stress if they do not occur. For example, anticipating relocation to a nursing home from the hospital, an older person may direct family members to sell his or her home and its furnishings. What happens if a suitable nursing home is not found, and family members put pressure on the person to move in with them? What is the impact of learning just a few days before a major holiday that the family gathering planned by an older person has been cancelled? Variables such as an individual's level of anticipation and availability of optional outcomes undoubtedly play a role in reactions to these situations. Research on how people of different ages cope with such "non-events" is needed.

WHAT DETERMINES STRESS RESPONSES IN OLD AGE?

The manner in which we respond to life events, role changes, and chronic daily hassles depends on many personal and environmental factors. The cognitive appraisal of a situation by an individual as being stressful or not has already been noted to be important. In addition, an event's relative desirability or undesirability, whether or not it is anticipated, and a person's previous experiences with similar events may determine how he or she responds to the situation. The availability of a strong social network that can provide emotional support also has an effect. A person who must face all challenges alone may use different coping strategies than one who has family and friends to turn to in times of crisis.

Both situational and personal factors affect the process of coping with stressful events, sometimes in different ways (Dohrenwend and Dohrenwend, 1980). The former consist of external mediators, such as social and material resources (e.g., friendships and family support, financial adequacy). The latter include the individual's aspirations, values, vulnerabilities, and needs that mediate between a particular stressful situation and its outcomes. For example, an older woman whose husband recently died after a long illness will be more likely to rely on others if she has a strong need for dependency (e.g., Neugarten's passive-dependent type), and if she has family and friends who have previously supported her in crises. If, on the other hand, she is highly independent and/or has no strong social network on which she has relied for past help, she will be more likely to use instrumental, self-initiated coping strategies (e.g., find out more about the problem, learn new skills to solve it), and less likely to ask others to assist her during her grieving. According to these researchers, the outcomes of coping responses may be personal growth, decline, or no change. The type of coping response rarely determines what outcomes will emerge; more often, the outcome varies with the interaction between the nature of the problem and the quality and quantity of internal and external mediators.

Personality styles also may influence how people respond to stress. Earlier in this chapter, Gutmann's (1974a, 1974b, 1977) research on active and passive mastery styles was described. A person with a passive style does not feel powerful enough to directly influence his or her fate, whereas one with an active style tends to rely more on personal abilities and less on others. Differences in responses to stress by older people with these different styles would be expected; however, research has not provided sufficient evidence for such hypothesized variations.

Another personality characteristic that may influence how successfully people respond to stress is *locus of control*. This is the belief by an individual that events in his or her life result from personal actions (internal locus), or are determined by fate or powerful others (external locus). Internal locus of control has been found to be related to successful coping in both young and old (Thomae, 1980). Studies on the stress of relocation have provided additional support for this relationship. Older persons with internal locus of control were found to adjust better to institutional living than those with external locus (Lieberman, 1975; Kivett, 1976; Baker, 1976). These studies have examined the outcomes of reactions to stress; successful adjustment has been defined as survival, satisfaction with living arrangements, and the maintenance of personal identity. In contrast, research on mastery styles has emphasized differences in how persons with active and passive mastery styles respond to stress, without predetermining criteria for success or failure.

COPING

As noted earlier in this chapter, a critical personality feature in the later years is an individual's ability to adapt to major changes in life circumstances, in health and social status, and in social and physical environments. In fact, successful aging requires considerable flexibility in adaptation. This in turn requires awareness of the aging process, acceptance of the limitations that aging places on a person's activities, and an ability to reevaluate life goals and search for alternative means of satisfying needs. An important aspect of adaptation is the ability to use appropriate coping mechanisms when faced with a stressful event.

Does coping change with age? Before answering, we must first define and consider the functions of *coping*. Coping is the manner in which a person responds to stress. It includes cognitive, emotional, and behavioral responses made in the face of internally and externally created events. It differs from defense mechanisms in that people are generally conscious of how they have coped in a particular situation and, if asked, can describe specific coping responses to a given stressor. Indeed, Birren (1969) has emphasized the concept of coping strategy to denote "planful behavior" in response to a stressful situation. *Defense mechanisms*, in contrast, are unconscious reactions that a person adopts to defend or protect the self from impulses and memories that threaten one's identity. Defense mechanisms also have an underlying evaluative quality; some defenses are more primitive or less mature than others (see Table 8–6). Thus, for example, a young child is more likely to use the defense mechanisms of denial and projection, or the need to view threatening impulses as present in others, not in the self. As the individuals mature, so do the defense mechanisms that they use. Vaillant's (1977) longitudinal study of male university graduates provides support for this conclusion. As the graduates reached middle-age, they used fewer primitive mechanisms, such as projection, and more mature mechanisms, such as sublimation (e.g., finding more socially acceptable ways of expressing hostility than through physically threatening behavior).

Unlike defense mechanisms, coping styles cannot easily be categorized as primitive or mature. Some forms of coping, however, are aimed not at resolving the problem, but at providing psychological escape, as illustrated by the categories of coping defined by some researchers (see Table 8–7). For example, an

TABLE 8–6 Major Ego Defense Mechanisms

Defense Mechanism	Example
1. Denial (a premature defense mechanism)	Denying what one really feels to avoid punishment by the super-ego and rejection by others.
2. Projection	Feeling that others are untrustworthy when one feels unsure about one's own trustworthiness.
3. Repression	Forgetting an event that could disturb the feeling of well-being if brought into consciousness.
4. Reaction formation	Extreme display of love and affection toward someone who is actually hated.
5. Regression and fixation	Returning to a comfortable stage of life and/or way of behaving under conditions of anxiety and stress.
6. Displacement	Taking out one's anger and hostility on family because one is afraid of expressing anger toward one's supervisor at work who has humiliated the individual.

older man who is confronted with the news that he has lung cancer may cope by eating or sleeping more, or by taking a vacation to "get away from it all." This response may alleviate the stressful feeling, but it does not aid in the treatment of the cancer. Pfeiffer (1977) has suggested that older persons are more rigid in their thinking than are younger persons, and are therefore prone to use more passive and ineffective coping mechanisms, such as withdrawal, denial, and anxiety. Pfeiffer's description may apply only to a small segment of older persons who are experiencing emotional and cognitive deterioration, however. Other researchers have not found such differences in studies of normal elderly and have not made a distinction between mature and immature coping (McCrae and Costa, 1985).

FUNCTIONS OF COPING

Coping reactions generally serve two functions: to solve a problem that has produced stress for the individual (e.g., a life event, a role loss or gain, a chronic "hassle"), and to reduce the emotional and physiological discomfort that accompanies the stressful situation. These have been defined as problem-focused and emotion-focused coping (Folkman and Lazarus, 1980; Lazarus and Folkman, 1984). In some cases, an individual may focus only on solving the problem *or* dealing with the emotional distress that it creates. In the earlier example, the older

TABLE 8–7 Classification of Coping Responses

General Strategies of Coping

(Lazarus, 1974, 1975a, 1975b; Lazarus and Folkman, 1984; Lazarus and Launier, 1978)

1. Information search in an attempt to understand the situation
2. Direct action to change the situation
3. Inhibition of action
4. Psychological responses to the emotional arousal created by the situation

Coping Responses to Terminal Illness

(Moos, 1977)

1. Searching for information
2. Setting goals
3. Denying or minimizing the problem
4. Seeking emotional support
5. Rehearsing alternative outcomes

Dimensions of Coping

(Kahana and Kahana, 1982)

1. Instrumental (taking action, alone or with the assistance of others)
2. Intrapsychic (cognitive approaches, acceptance of the situation)
3. Affective (releasing tension, expressing emotions)
4. Escape (avoiding or denying the problem, displacement activities such as increased exercise, eating, and smoking)
5. Resigned helplessness (feeling impotent, unable to cope)

---

man who responds to the diagnosis of lung cancer by taking a vacation to get away may address the emotional distress but not the problem per se. Such reactions tend to be incomplete, and do not resolve the problem that is producing stress. In other situations, people may need to deal first with the anxiety produced by a stressful situation, then with the problem itself. For example, upon learning that a close friend has a terminal illness, a person must first cope with shock and helplessness. Only then can rational decisions be made about what to do to help the dying friend through the last months or weeks of life. In most situations, however, emotion-focused and problem-focused coping take place simultaneously. An individual must deal with his or her emotions throughout the course of trying to solve the problem. It has been suggested that coping must fulfill both emotion-regulating and problem-solving functions in order to alleviate stress (Folkman and Lazarus, 1980).

CONSISTENCY VERSUS VARIABILITY IN COPING

Although some researchers have suggested that certain personalities are associated with specific coping styles, there is little evidence for consistency of coping responses in different situations. Indeed, it is difficult to imagine that many situations are similar enough in the types of stress they produce that an individual could use the same responses in all cases. Furthermore, most problems produce multiple demands on a person and evoke diverse emotional reactions. For example, upon learning of a close friend's impending death, a person must cope with the grief, anger, hopelessness, and guilt that such news evokes. An individual may also have to cope with comforting and easing the friend's pain, aiding in financial and funeral plans, and notifying others. How an older person copes with this situation may be somewhat similar to the way he or she copes with an event such as taking a trip to visit children and grandchildren, but the events are so dissimilar that the individual must select appropriate coping strategies for each specific situation.

People may have different repertoires of coping strategies, so that one person is more likely to use a particular set of strategies while another avoids those strategies and uses others. That is, people generally do not cope in just one way, such as only by crying, talking to others or consulting with a professional. We generally express multiple coping responses, sometimes simultaneously, other times in sequence. As stated earlier, we must cope with the emotional stress produced by the problem, *and* with the problem itself.

Many studies have found that certain situations evoke particular coping responses. Consistencies have been identified in how people deal with spinal cord injury (Bulman and Wortman, 1977) and cancer (Weisman and Worden, 1976–77). A widely recognized example of such consistency is the process of coping with one's impending death. As first postulated by Kübler-Ross (1969), an individual experiences five stages in this process that represent different coping responses: (1) denial and isolation, (2) anger and resentment, (3) bargaining and an attempt to postpone, (4) depression, and (5) acceptance. Each of these stages is a way of dealing with the emotions evoked by the knowledge that one will soon die. The issue of coping with the death itself is not addressed by Kübler-Ross's model, although many people do so by using instrumental strategies, such as seeking new medical treatments, getting a second opinion, and planning their funeral. These are responses oriented to dealing with the problem itself, not with the emotions that the problem evokes. These stages, described further in Chapter 14, are mentioned in this context because of the consistency with which diverse people who are confronted with many different situations use these five similar responses to cope with the emotional aspects of death.

Other researchers have noted considerable flexibility in older people's selection of coping responses, based on what is "appropriate" or potentially effective in a given situation. As noted earlier, Pfeiffer (1977) has suggested that aging is associated with a restricted range of coping responses. For example, studies of self-reported coping in response to multiple stressful events support the concept of situational variability (Kahana and Kahana, 1982; Thomae, 1978).

AGING AND COPING STYLES

The question of whether coping styles change with age has not been extensively researched. Some studies of coping among young and middle-aged persons have reported few significant differences (Billings and Moos, 1981; Folkman and Lazarus, 1980), although these groups have generally not been compared with older persons. Older (ages 65 to 91) and middle-aged (ages 50 to 64) respondents in McCrae's (1982) study used more mature coping styles (e.g., problem solving, seeking the advice of family, friends, and professionals) than did younger (ages 24 to 49) respondents. Studies by Kahana and Kahana of older people who move to institutions and by Kiyak and colleagues (1985) of older people who must cope with Alzheimer's disease suggest that older people use a diverse range of coping styles. Similarly, women aged 55 to 65 in stressful situations were likely to use a variety of coping responses, including turning to work or religion, or ignoring the problem (Griffith, 1983). In most cases, these styles are appropriate for the problem at hand and result in successful adaptation. Only in the case of significant cognitive deterioration is there a restriction in the range of an individual's coping responses and a tendency to resort to more primitive reactions, such as denying or ignoring the problem. This small segment of the elderly population may fit Pfeiffer's (1977) description of restricted coping abilities. Nevertheless, the majority of older people appear capable of using a wide repertoire of coping responses and can call upon the most effective ones for a given situation. In sum, the available research suggests that most people maintain their coping styles into old age, and use appropriate responses for the problem at hand.

Even less is known about how gender affects coping. In an eight-year follow-up of older adults in the Duke Longitudinal Study, gender differences were found in the types of life events experienced but not in the coping styles used (Siegler and George, 1983). Older men reported more work and health-related events; women identified more events affecting family members and health problems of significant others. The majority of men and women stated that instrumental strategies (i.e., acting to solve the problem) resulted in better outcomes for most events that occurred to them personally, while palliative coping (i.e., dealing with the emotions created by events) was more helpful for responding to events that affected their families, work, and financial situations.

ADAPTATION TO AGING

To conclude this section, it is important to discuss the implications of older persons' coping responses for their long-term adaptation. *Adaptation* refers to the adjustments that people make in response to changes in themselves and/or their environments, in order to fit themselves to the new conditions. Given older people's numerous experiences with life events, role loss, and environmental changes throughout life, it would appear that adaptation in old age should occur with relative ease. Indeed, in one sense, an individual who has reached age 75 or 80 has proved to be the most adaptable of his or her generation, since the ultimate proof of adaptation is survival. As we have seen thus far, older people continue to face challenges to their well-being in the form of personal and family illnesses, age-related declines in sensory and physiological functions, and changes in their social and physical environments. To the extent that older people are capable of using coping skills that were effective in youth and middle-age, they will continue to adapt to change successfully, thereby maintaining life satisfaction and morale.

Summary and Implications

Personality development in adulthood and old age has received increasing attention over the past twenty years. Earlier theories of personality suggested that development takes place only during childhood and adolescence, and stabilizes by early adulthood. Beginning with Erik Erikson, however, several theorists have suggested that personality continues to change and evolve into old age. According to Erikson's theory of psychosocial development, the individual experiences stages of development, with crises or conflicts at each stage, and the outcome of each has an impact on ego development in the next stage. The eighth and last stage of personality development occurs in old age and poses the conflict of ego integrity versus despair in dealing with one's impending death. Research by Costa, McCrae, and Norris (1981) provides some support for this final stage of ego development.

The work of Carl Jung also emphasizes the growth of personality across the life span but does not specify stages of development. Jung's model, like Erikson's, focuses on the individual's confrontation with death in this last stage. In addition, Jung described a decrease in sex-typed behavior with aging. This has been supported in cross-cultural studies by Gutmann (1974a, 1974b, 1980) and in the longitudinal Kansas City studies by Neugarten and colleagues (1968). These investigators found that men become more accepting of their nurturant and affiliative characteristics as they age, whereas women learn to accept their egocentric and aggressive impulses.

The Kansas City studies have provided other important insights into normal personality development from middle to old age. With aging, people in the sample were found to become more unlike each other. However, some changes in personality were shared by a majority of those studied: increased preoccupation with their inner lives, less extroversion, and a movement toward less impulsiveness and more sophisticated ego defenses. Based on the large number of people interviewed both cross-sectionally and longitudinally in the Kansas City studies, Neugarten described four major personality types in old age: integrated, armored-defensive, passive-dependent, and unintegrated. The majority of people fell into the first two categories and expressed high life satisfaction. Contrary to popular stereotypes, very few older persons could be described as unintegrated.

Other models of adult personality development have been proposed but have received less research attention. Levinson's life structures model is an extension of Riegel's dialectical theory of personality. These approaches emphasize the interaction between an individual and his or her environment as the impetus for development from one level to the next. In Kohlberg's model of moral development (based on theories of cognitive development), the basis for movement from one stage to the next is not specified.

The development of self-concept and self-esteem in old age has been researched even less. It is recognized that older persons' self-concepts must be redefined as they move from traditional roles of worker, spouse, and parent to less well-differentiated roles such as retiree or widow. But the process by which such changes take place and, more importantly, how they influence life satisfaction and self-esteem in old age is unclear.

Somewhat more research has been devoted to age-related changes in the nature of life events and the stress associated with them. Neugarten and others have compared the impact of on-time (or normative) versus off-time (or non-normative) events in terms of older people's ability to cope; anticipating an event such as retirement or menopause may make it less stressful than a situation that is completely unanticipated. However, little is known about how older people cope with an event that is anticipated but fails to occur.

Cognitive appraisal is also an important consideration in understanding people's reactions to life events. To the extent that people perceive a situation as a positive challenge, they experience more positive stress and adapt more readily. If the situation is viewed as a threat, or as a negative stressor, the response may be avoidance or ineffective coping. If a particular life event is viewed as benign or unimportant, coping responses will not be activated. This is fine if the event does not place any demands on an individual, but if it proves to be more stressful than anticipated, an older person will be unprepared to cope with these demands.

The evidence is mixed regarding the question of whether older people experience more major life events in a given period than younger people. The majority of studies have found a similar distribution of stressful events in the lives of young, middle-aged, and aged persons, but more longitudinal studies are needed in this area in order to conclude this with more certainty. The effects of sociohistorical events, such as wars and the Depression, on the current aged cohort's adaptive responses have been found to be relatively minor.

Coping responses are influenced by an individual's access to a support network, cognitive skills, and personality traits such as active versus passive "mastery style" and "locus of control." Although ego defense mechanisms have been observed to become more mature in middle-age and old age, it is difficult to describe coping styles in a similar manner. Age differences in the use of coping styles have not been consistent across studies. Successful aging may be defined as the ability to cope effectively with both major life events and chronic hassles, and to adapt to new situations. An individual who has survived to the age of 75 or older has proved to be adaptable to new situations. Hence, older people who continue to use coping strategies that have proved successful in the past will be likely to maintain their life satisfaction and well-being throughout the later years.

References

Amster, L. E., and Krauss, H. The relationship between life crises and mental deterioration in old age. *International Journal of Aging and Human Development*, 1974, 5, 51–55.

Baker, E. K. Relationship of retirement and satisfaction with life events to locus of control. *Dissertation Abstracts International*, 1976, 37(9B), 4748.

Billings, A. G., and Moos, R. H. The role of coping responses and social resources in attenuating the stress of life events. *Journal of Behavioral Medicine*, 1981, 4, 139.

Birren, J. E. Age and decision strategies. In A. T. Welford and J. E. Birren (Eds.), *Decision making and age*. New York: S. Karger, 1969, 23–36.

Bulman, R. J., and Wortman, C. B. Attributions of blame and coping in the "Real World": Severe accident victims react to their lot. *Journal of Personality and Social Psychology*, 1977, 35, 351–363.

Butler, R. N. *Why survive? Being old in America*. New York: Harper and Row, 1975.

Butler, R. N., and Lewis, M. I. *Aging and mental health* (3d ed.). St. Louis: Mosby, 1983.

Chiriboga, D. A., and Cutler, L. Stress and adaptation: Life-span perspectives. In L. W. Poon (Ed.), *Aging in the 1980's: Psychological issues*. Washington, D.C.: American Psychological Association, 1980, 247–362.

Costa, P. T., and McCrae, R. R. Age differences in personality structure revisited: Studies in validity, stability, and change. *International Journal of Aging and Human Development*, 1977, 8, 261–275.

Costa, P. T., and McCrae, R. R. Still stable after all these years: Personality as a key to some issues in aging. In P. B. Baltes and O. G. Brim (Eds.), *Life-span development and behavior* (Vol. 3). New York: Academic Press, 1980.

Costa, P. T., McCrae, R. R., and Norris, A. H. Personal adjustment to aging: Longitudinal prediction from neuroticism and extraversion. *Journal of Gerontology*, 1981, 36, 78–85.

Cumming, E., and Henry, W. E. *Growing old*. New York: Basic Books, 1961.

Dohrenwend, B. S., and Dohrenwend, B. P. What is a stressful life event? In H. Selye (Ed.), *Seyle's guide to stress research, Volume 1*. New York: Van Nostrand Reinhold, 1980.

Eisdorfer, C., and Wilkie, F. Stress, disease, aging, and behavior. In J. E. Birren and K. W. Schaie (Eds.), *Handbook of the psychology of aging*. New York: Van Nostrand Reinhold, 1977, 251–275.

Folkman, S., and Lazarus, R. S. An analysis of coping in a middle-aged community sample. *Journal of Health and Social Behavior,* 1980, *21,* 219–239.

Gaber, L. B. Activity/disengagement revisited: Personality types in the aged. *British Journal of Psychiatry,* 1983, *143,* 490–497.

Gerber, I., Rusalem, R., Hannon, N., Battin, D., and Arkin, A. Anticipatory grief and aged widows and widowers. *Journal of Gerontology,* 1975, *30,* 225–229.

Griffith, J. W. Women's stress responses and coping: Patterns according to age groups. *Issues in Health Care of Women,* 1983, *4,* 327–340.

Gutmann, D. L. Alternatives to disengagement: Aging among the highland Druze. In R. A. LeVine (Ed.), *Culture and personality: Contemporary readings.* Chicago: Aldine, 1974a.

Gutmann, D. L. The country of old men: Cross-cultural studies in the psychology of later life. In R. A. LeVine (Ed.), *Culture and personality: Contemporary readings.* Chicago: Aldine, 1974b.

Gutmann, D. L. The cross-cultural perspective: Notes toward a comparative psychology of aging. In J. E. Birren and K. W. Schaie (Eds.), *Handbook of the psychology of aging.* New York: Van Nostrand Reinhold, 1977.

Gutmann, D. L. Psychoanalysis and aging: A developmental view. In S. I. Greenspan and G. H. Pollock (Eds.), *The course of life: Psychoanalytic contributions toward understanding personality development. Vol. 3: Adulthood and the aging process.* Washington, D.C.: U.S. Government Printing Office, 1980.

Havighurst, R. J., Neugarten, B. L., and Tobin, S. S. Disengagement and patterns of aging. In J. E. Birren (Ed.), *Relations of development and aging.* Springfield, Ill.: Charles C. Thomas, 1964.

Havighurst, R. J., Neugarten, B. L., and Tobin, S. S. Disengagement and patterns of aging. In B. L. Neugarten (Ed.), *Middle age and aging.* Chicago: University of Chicago Press, 1968.

Haynes, S. G., McMichael, A. J., and Tyroler, H. A. Survival after early and normal retirement. *Journal of Gerontology,* 1978, *33,* 269–278.

Holmes, T. H., and Masuda, M. Life change and illness susceptibility. In B. S. Dohrenwend and B. P. Dohrenwend (Eds.), *Stressful life events: Their nature and effects.* New York: Wiley, 1974.

Holmes, T. H., and Rahe, R. The social readjustment rating scale. *Journal of Psychosomatic Research,* 1967, *11,* 213–218.

Hultsch, D. F., and Plemons, J. K. Life events and life-span development. In P. B. Baltes and O. G. Brim, Jr. (Eds.), *Life-span development and behavior (Volume 2).* New York: Academic Press, 1979.

Jung, C. G. *Modern man in search of a soul.* San Diego: Harcourt Brace and World, 1933.

Jung, C. G. Concerning the archetypes, with special reference to the anima concept. In *C. G. Jung, Collected Works,* Vol. 9, Part I. Princeton, N.J.: Princeton University Press, 1959.

Kahana, E. F. *Matching environments to needs of the aged.* Final Progress Report submitted to NICHD, Fall, 1973.

Kahana, E. F. A congruence model of person-environment interaction. In M. P. Lawton (Ed.), *Theory development in environments and aging.* New York: Wiley, 1975.

Kahana, E. F., and Kahana, B. Environmental continuity, discontinuity, futurity, and adaptation of the aged. In G. Rowles and R. Ohta (Eds.), *Aging and milieu: Environmental perspectives on growing old.* New York: Academic Press, 1982.

Kahana, R. J. Strategies of dynamic psychotherapy with the wide range of older individuals. *Journal of Geriatric Psychiatry,* 1979, *12,* 71–99.

Kivett, V. A. Physical, psychological and social predictors of locus of control among middle aged adults. *Dissertation Abstracts International,* 1976, *37*(5B), 2481.

Kiyak, H. A., and Kahana, E. F. Life events scaling by college students and the elderly. Paper presented at meetings of the American Psychological Association, New York, 1975.

Kiyak, H. A., Montgomery, R., Borson, S., and Teri, L. Coping patterns among patients with Alzheimer's disease and non-demented elderly. Paper presented at meetings of the Gerontological Society, 1985.

Kogan, N., and Wallach, M. A. Age changes in values and attitudes. *Journal of Gerontology,* 1961, *16,* 272–280.

Kohlberg, L. *Stages in the development of moral thought and action.* New York: Holt, Rinehart and Winston, 1969a.

Kohlberg, L. Stage and sequence: The cognitive-developmental approach to socialization. In D. A. Goslin (Ed.), *Handbook of socialization theory and research.* Chicago: Rand McNally, 1969b.

Kohlberg, L. Continuities in childhood and adult moral development revisited. In P. B. Baltes and K. W. Schaie (Eds.), *Life-span developmental psychology* (2d ed.). New York: Academic Press, 1973.

Kübler-Ross, E. *On death and dying.* New York: Macmillan, 1969.

Lawton, M. P., and Nahemow, L. Ecology and the aging process. In C. Eisdorfer and M. P. Lawton (Eds.), *Psychology of adult development and aging.* Washington, D.C.: American Psychological Association, 1973.

Lazarus, R. S. Cognitive and coping processes in emotion. Paper given in a Symposium: Cognitive Views of Motivation, at meetings of the American Association for the Advancement of Science, 1974.

Lazarus, R. S. The self-regulation of emotions. In L. Levi (Ed.), *Emotions—Their parameters and measurement.* New York: Raven Press, 1975a, 47–67.

Lazarus, R. S. Psychological stress and coping in adaptation and illness. In S. M. Weiss (Ed.), *Proceedings of the national heart and lung institute working conference on health behavior.* DHEW Pub. # (NIH) 76-868, 1975b, 199–214.

Lazarus, R. S., and Cohen, J. B. *The hassles scale, stress and coping project.* Berkeley: University of California, 1977.

Lazarus, R. S., and DeLongis, A. Psychological stress and coping in aging. *American Psychologist,* 1983, *38,* 245–254.

Lazarus, R. S., and Folkman, S. *Stress, appraisal and coping.* New York: Springer, 1984.

Lazarus, R. S., and Launier, R. Stress-related transactions between person and environment. In L. A. Pervin and M. Lewis (Eds.), *Perspectives in interactional psychology*. New York: Plenum, 1978, 287–327.

Levinson, D. Middle adulthood in modern society: A sociopsychological view. In G. DiRenzo (Ed.), *We the people: Social change and social character*. Westport, Conn.: Greenwood Press, 1977.

Levinson, D., Darrow, C. M., Klein, E. B., Levinson, M. H., and McKee, B. *The seasons of a man's life*. New York: Knopf, 1978.

Lewin, K. *A dynamic theory of personality*. New York: McGraw-Hill, 1935.

Lieberman, M. A. Adaptive processes in late life. In N. Datan and L. H. Ginsberg (Eds.), *Life-span developmental psychology: Normative life crises*. New York: Academic Press, 1975.

Lowenthal, M. F., and Chiriboga, D. Transition to the empty nest: Crisis, challenge, or relief? *Archives of General Psychiatry*, 1972, 26, 8–14.

Lowenthal, M. F., Thurnher, M., and Chiriboga, D. *Four stages of life*. San Francisco: Jossey-Bass, 1975.

Lundberg, U., Theorell, T., and Lind, E. Life changes and myocardial infarction: Individual differences in life change scaling. *Journal of Psychosomatic Research*, 1975, 19, 27–32.

McCrae, R. R. Age differences in the use of coping mechanisms. *Journal of Gerontology*, 1982, 37, 454.

McCrae, R. R., and Costa, P. T., Jr. Personality, stress, and coping processes in aging men and women. In R. Andres, E. L. Bierman, and W. R. Hazzard (Eds.), *Principles of geriatric medicine*. New York: McGraw-Hill, 1985.

Monge, R. H. Structure of the self-concept from adolescence through old age. *Experimental Aging Research*, 1975, 1, 281–291.

Moos, R. *Coping with physical illness*. New York: Plenum, 1977.

Morgan, J. C. *Becoming old*. New York: Springer, 1979.

Muhlenkamp, A., Gress, L. D., and Flood, M. A. Perception of life change events by the elderly. *Nursing Research*, 1975, 24, 109–113.

National Center for Health Statistics. Advance report of final mortality statistics, 1980. *Monthly Vital Statistics Report*, 32 (4, supplement), 1983.

Neugarten, B. L. Adult personality: Toward a psychology of the life cycle. In B. Neugarten (Ed.), *Middle age and aging*. Chicago: University of Chicago Press, 1968.

Neugarten, B. L. Adaptation and the life cycle. *Journal of Geriatric Psychiatry*, 1970, 4, 71–100.

Neugarten, B. L. Personality change in late life: A developmental perspective. In C. Eisdorfer and M. P. Lawton (Eds.), *The psychology of adult development and aging*. Washington, D.C.: American Psychological Association, 1973.

Neugarten, B. L. Time, age and the life cycle. *American Journal of Psychiatry*, 1979, 136, 887–894.

Neugarten, B. L., Havighurst, R. J., and Tobin, S. S. Personality and patterns of aging. In B. L. Neugarten (Ed.), *Middle age and aging*. Chicago: University of Chicago Press, 1968.

Neugarten, B. L., Wood, V., Kraines, R. J., and Loomis, B. Women's attitudes towards the menopause. In B. L. Neugarten (Ed.), *Middle age and aging.* Chicago: University of Chicago Press, 1968.

Palmore, E., Cleveland, W. P., Nowlin, J. B., Ramm, D., and Siegler, I. C. Stress and adaptation in late life. *Journal of Gerontology,* 1979, 34, 841–851.

Pastalan, L. A. Designing housing environments for the elderly. *Journal of Architectural Education,* 1977, 31, 11–14.

Pearlin, L. Sex roles and depression. In N. Datan and L. Ginsberg (Eds.), *Life-span developmental psychology: Normative life crises.* New York: Academic Press, 1975.

Pearlin, L., and Lieberman, M. Social sources of emotional distress. In R. Simmons (Ed.), *Research in community and mental health.* Greenwich, Conn.: JAI Press, 1979.

Pfeiffer, E. Psychopathology and social pathology. In J. E. Birren and K. W. Schaie (Eds.), *Handbook of the psychology of aging.* New York: Van Nostrand Reinhold, 1977.

Rahe, R. H. Subjects' recent life changes and their near future illness reports: A review. *Annual Clinical Research,* 1972, 4, 393.

Reichard, S., Livson, F., and Peterson, P. G. *Aging and personality.* New York: Wiley and Sons, 1962.

Reigel, K. The dialectics of human development. *American Psychologist,* 1976, 31, 689–700.

Rosow, I. *Socialization to old age.* Berkeley: University of California Press, 1974.

Seeman, M. Empirical alienation studies: An overview. In R. F. Geyer and D. R. Schweitzer (Eds.), *Theories of alienation.* Leiden: Martinus Nijhoff, Social Services Division, 1976.

Selye, H. The general adaptation syndrome and the diseases of adaptation. *Journal of Clinical Endocrinology,* 1946, 6, 117–230.

Selye, H. Stress and aging. *Journal of the American Geriatrics Society,* 1970, 18, 660–681.

Shanan, J. The Jerusalem study of midadulthood and aging. *Israel Journal of Gerontology,* 1978, 2, 37–49.

Shanan, J., and Jacobowitz, J. Personality and aging. In C. Eisdorfer (Ed.), *Annual Review of Gerontology and Geriatrics,* 1982, 3, 148–180.

Siegler, J. C., and George, L. K. The normal psychology of the aging male: Sex differences in coping and perception of life events. *Journal of Geriatric Psychiatry,* 1983, 16, 197–209.

Snarey, J. R., Reimer, J., and Kohlberg, L. Development of social-moral reasoning among Kibbutz adolescents: A longitudinal cross-cultural study. *Developmental Psychology,* 1985, 21, 3–17.

Thomae, H. Reactions to life stress. Paper presented at 11th International Congress of Gerontology, Tokyo, 1978.

Thomae, H. Personality and adjustment to aging. In J. E. Birren and B. Sloane (Eds.), *Handbook on mental health and aging.* Englewood Cliffs, N.J.: Prentice-Hall, 1980.

Vaillant, G. *Adaptation to life.* Boston: Little, Brown, 1977.

Weisman, A., and Worden, J. W. The existential plight in cancer: Significance of the first 100 days. *International Journal of Psychiatry in Medicine,* 1976–77, 7, 1–15.

Worchel, P., and Byrne, D. (Eds.). *Personality change.* New York: Wiley and Sons, 1964.

Chapter **9**

Mental Disorders and the Use of Mental Health Services

As shown in previous chapters, old age is usually accompanied by some deterioration in sensory and cognitive functions, but personality remains relatively stable in normal aging. Nevertheless, personality disorders and psychiatric symptoms may emerge among some older persons who showed no signs of psychopathology earlier in their lives. Although such conditions are not a normal process of aging, in some individuals the stresses of old age may compound any existing predisposition to psychopathology. These stresses may be internal, resulting from the physiological and psychological processes described earlier, or external, which are a function of role losses and the deaths of spouse, friends, and especially one's children. These conditions significantly impact older people's competence, so that they become more vulnerable to environmental press.

The primary affective or emotional disorder of old age is depression, accounting for a significant number of suicides, especially among older men. Alzheimer's disease and other dementias are cognitive disorders that are far more likely to affect the elderly than the young. Alcoholism and drug abuse are less common in older persons, although their effect on the physical health and cognitive functioning of older people is more detrimental than on younger persons. Paranoid disorders and schizophrenia are even less likely to begin in old age; the majority of individuals who have either of these conditions were first diagnosed in youth or middle-age. Each of these conditions is reviewed in this chapter.

Epidemiology of Mental Disorders

The prevalence of psychiatric disorders among older persons who are living in the community ranges from 5 to 45 percent, depending on the population studied and the categories of disorders examined. Even higher rates can be expected in institutionalized elderly, with estimates of 10 to 40 percent of people with mild to moderate impairments, and another 5 to 10 percent with significant impairments (Blazer, 1980). One study found that 22 percent of older persons admitted to a V.A. hospital in one year for acute medical or surgical reasons were also suffering from some form of a mental disorder. The rate was even higher (30 percent) among those admitted to cardiac care units (Schuckit, 1977).

It has been noted that 20 percent of all first admissions to psychiatric hospitals are persons over age 65 (Brody and Kleban, 1983). Older psychiatric patients are more likely to have chronic conditions and to require longer periods of inpatient treatment than is true for younger patients, as evidenced by the fact that 25 percent of all beds in these hospitals are occupied by older persons. Note the discrepancy between this proportion and the proportion of all elderly in the U.S. population—12 percent in 1986. It has been estimated that 100,000 older chronic psychiatric patients live in state mental hospitals, 500,000 in nursing homes, and the remainder (over 1 million) in the community, where they often receive inadequate treatment for their psychiatric condition (Talbott, 1983). As discussed later in this chapter, older persons are less likely to use community mental health services. Older patients comprise less than 6 percent of the load of psychiatric outpatient clinics (Kucharski, White, and Schratz, 1979; Redick and Taube, 1980; Butler and Lewis, 1982).

Older Black psychiatric patients are twice as likely as whites to enter mental hospitals, but far less likely to use nursing home services (Kart and Beckham, 1976). Older Mexican-Americans and Native Americans are less likely to use psychiatric facilities. These lower rates of institutionalization may not reflect differences among ethnic minority groups in incidence of psychiatric disorders; indeed, prevalence data are extremely difficult to obtain for these conditions in older ethnic minorities (Markides, 1986). Few epidemiological studies of late-life psychopathology have examined ethnic minority differences. In one such study, no differences in the rates of psychiatric disorders were found among elderly of different ethnic minority backgrounds (Romaniuk, McAuley, and Arling, 1983).

One problem with describing the prevalence of mental disorders of the elderly is the lack of criteria distinguishing conditions that emerge in old age from those that continue throughout adulthood. In fact, the major classification system for psychiatric disorders, the *Diagnostic and Statistical Manual,* 3rd edition (DSMIII, 1987) of the American Psychiatric Association, makes such a distinction only for dementias that begin in late life. No other mental disorders are distinguished for old age, although other diagnostic categories are described specifically for adulthood as separate from childhood or adolescence. The problem of inadequate criteria for late-life psychopathology is compounded by the lack of age-appropriate psychological tests for diagnosing these conditions. An increasing number of researchers, however, are developing such measures, especially for diagnosing depression and dementia in the elderly.

Depression

The three most prevalent forms of late-life psychopathology are depression, dementia, and paranoia. Of these, depression is the most frequently diagnosed. Epidemiologic surveys have found that 15 to 22 percent of community elderly report depressed moods; 10 to 15 percent have depressions that require clinical interventions (Gurland, Dean, Cross, and Golden, 1980; Blazer and Williams, 1980; Gurland and Cross, 1982). A more recent epidemiologic survey of five communities (Blazer, George, and Landerman, 1986) reported a much lower prevalence of depressive disorders—2.8 percent of a sample of 1,351 community-dwelling persons age 60 and older. This may be due to differences in criteria for depression in these studies. Women tend to report more symptoms of depression in middle-age and early old age, but it may be that more men have clinically diagnosable depression at age 80 and beyond (Gurland et al., 1980).

It is important to distinguish *major depression* from bipolar disorders (that is, ranging from a depressed to a manic state), sadness, grief reactions, and other affective disorders (APA, 1980). Most of the depressions of old age are unipolar; manic-depressive disorders are rare (Post, 1978). Still other cases in late life are *secondary* or *reactive depressions,* which arise in response to a significant life event with which the individual cannot cope. For example, physical illness and the loss of loved ones through death and relocation may trigger depressive reactions in the elderly (Pfeiffer and Busse, 1973).

As described in Chapters 3 and 8, most role *gains* (e.g., worker, driver, voter, spouse, parent) occur in the earlier years, whereas many role *losses* come one after another in the later years, although many older people do experience some role gains. As we have seen, loss of roles may be compounded by decrements in sensory abilities, physical strength, and health. Although depression usually does not result from any one of these alone, the combination of several losses in close sequence may trigger a reactive depressive episode.

The vegetative signs, suicidal thoughts, weight loss, and mood variations from morning to night that are observed in major depression are not found in reactive depression. Environmental and social interventions, as well as psycho- therapy, are more effective than antidepressant medications for secondary depression, as will be seen later in this chapter.

Death rates appear to be greater among elderly with a diagnosis of depression; in one three-year follow-up study, 60 percent of depressed patients had died, compared with only 32 percent among those with no psychiatric diagnosis (Schuckit, Miller, and Berman, 1980). Some specialists have suggested that older persons with depression are more apathetic, less interested in their environments, and more likely to entertain thoughts of suicide than younger depressives (Zung, 1967; Blazer, George, and Landerman, 1986; Mignogna, 1986).

Some of the most obvious signs of depression are reports or evidence of sadness, and feelings of emptiness or detachment. Also common are expressions of anxiety or panic for no apparent cause, loss of interest in the environment, and neglect of self-care, as well as changes in eating and sleeping patterns. The depressed person may complain of vague aches and pains, either generally or in a specific part of the body. Occasional symptoms are not problematic, however. Only when multiple symptoms appear together and persist *for at least two weeks* should an individual and his or her family suspect a depressive episode, especially if an older person speaks frequently of death or suicide. The symptoms of a major depression are listed in Table 9–1.

One problem with detecting depression in the elderly is that they may be more successful than their younger counterparts at masking or hiding symptoms

TABLE 9–1 Summary of DSMIII Criteria for Major Depressive Episode

At least five of the following symptoms present during a two-week period, change from previous functioning, with preexisting illness:

1. Depressed mood
2. Markedly diminished interest or pleasure in activities, apathy
3. Significant weight loss or weight gain, or appetite change
4. Sleep disturbance (awakening early or insomnia)
5. Agitation or retardation of activity
6. Reduced energy level or fatigue
7. Self-blame, guilt, worthlessness
8. Poor concentration, indecisiveness
9. Recurrent thoughts of death, suicide

Source: Adapted with permission from the *Diagnostic and Statistical Manual of Mental Disorders, Third Edition, Revised.* Copyright 1987 American Psychiatric Association, p. 222.

of depression. In fact, many cases of depression in older persons are not diagnosed because the patient either does not express changes in mood or denies them in the clinical interview (Gerner, 1979; Schmidt, 1983). *Masked depression* is one in which few mood changes are reported. Instead, the patient complains of atypical pain and bodily discomfort, is apathetic, and withdraws from others (Gurland and Cross, 1982; Mignogna, 1986).

Health care professionals and family members need to distinguish depression from medical conditions and changes due to normal aging. For example, an older woman with arthritis who complains of increasing pain may actually be seeking a reason for vague physical discomfort that is related to a depressive episode. Similarly, it is important not to dismiss an older person's complaints of increasing sleep disturbance with the assumption that older people merely need less sleep (Shamoian, 1985). People with masked depression are more likely to complain of problems with memory or problem solving. Their denial or masking of symptoms may lead the physician to assume that the individual is experiencing dementia, a condition that is generally irreversible. It is for this reason that depression in older persons is often labeled *pseudo-dementia* (Wells, 1979).

Because of such likelihood of denial, a physician's first goal with an older patient who has vague somatic and memory complaints should be to conduct a thorough physical exam and lab tests, in order to determine if an individual is depressed or has a physical disorder or symptoms of dementia. If the cognitive dysfunction is due to depression, this will improve when the depression is treated. On the other hand, some medical conditions, including Parkinson's, rheumatoid arthritis, thyroid dysfunction, and diseases of the adrenal glands, may produce depressive symptoms. Certain medications may also produce feelings of depression; these include antihypertensives, digoxin, L-dopa, corticosteroids, estrogens, and some antipsychotic drugs. In fact, any medication that has a depressant effect on the central nervous system can produce depressive symptoms in older patients, specifically lethargy and loss of interest in the environment (Schmidt, 1983). For these reasons, it is important for older persons to be examined thoroughly for underlying physical illness and reactions to medications. Physicians must frequently conduct medication reviews to determine if their older patients begin to show side affects to a drug, even after using it for several months or years.

THERAPEUTIC INTERVENTION

It is important to treat both major and secondary depression in the elderly as soon as they are diagnosed, because the older depressed patient is at higher risk of self-destructive behavior and suicide. Several researchers have tested the efficacy of alternative therapies for depression in the elderly. There is some disagreement, however, about the value of such therapies. For example, Epstein (1976) suggests that, although short-term improvements may be achieved through treatment, the long-range prognosis is not very good. Others are more optimistic about the outcomes of treatment if the onset of depression occurs before age 70 (Gerner, 1979; Gallagher and Thompson, 1983; Cadoret, Widner, and North, 1980; Sholomskas, Chevron, Prusoff, and Berry, 1983).

The most common therapeutic intervention with depressed elderly is pharmacological. This has been found to be particularly useful for those experiencing a major depression. Therapy with antidepressants is generally long term. In a series of studies reported by Post (1978), approximately 75 percent of depressed older patients needed continued or intermittent antidepressant medications. Although antidepressants work well for some older persons, many others cannot use these drugs because of other medications they are taking, or because the side effects are more detrimental than the depression itself. These include postural hypotension (i.e., a sudden drop in blood pressure when rising from a prone position), cardiac arrhythmias, urinary retention, disorientation, and dry mouth (Salzman, 1984). Because of these potentially dangerous reactions, it is important to start antidepressant therapy at a much lower dose in the elderly than in younger patients, perhaps doses as low as 50 percent of those used with younger adults for some types of antidepressants (Mignogna, 1986). For these reasons, more and more physicians are, quite appropriately, reluctant to prescribe antidepressants to older persons. Many prefer to try short-term psychotherapy and behavioral therapies first.

Electroshock or electroconvulsive therapy (ECT) is sometimes used in cases of severe depression. ECT is regarded as a quick method for major depression in patients who have not responded to medications, who have a higher risk of suicide, and/or who refuse to eat (Kral, 1976; Merrill, 1978). Older patients with severe agitation, vegetative symptoms, or feelings of hopelessness, helplessness, worthlessness, and delusions often respond well to ECT (Mignogna, 1986). Clinical reports cite the effectiveness of ECT for patients as old as 94 years

(Bernstein, 1972; O'Shea et al., 1987). On the other hand, some psychiatrists have avoided using ECT with older patients because of its potentially harmful effects on memory. It also poses risks for patients with a recent myocardial infarction, stroke, or severe hypertension. Risks to memory function apply in particular when bilateral ECT (i.e., shock to both sides of the brain) is administered. As shown in recent studies (Hirschfeld and Klerman, 1979; Fraser and Glass, 1980; Weeks, Freeman, and Kendall, 1980), unilateral nondominant hemisphere ECT is often preferred because it is capable of alleviating depression without impairing cognitive functioning. Nevertheless, the long-term effectiveness of ECT for elderly depressed persons is not clear.

There have been fewer studies examining the usefulness of psychotherapy with older people. Some researchers have concluded that this method may be successful in combination with pharmacotherapy (i.e., use of antidepressant drugs), but not when it is used alone (Lipman and Covi, 1976; Weissman and Myers, 1978). In particular, secondary depression responds well to supportive psychotherapy that allows the patient to review and come to terms with the stresses of late life. Supportive psychotherapy is useful with older patients because it allows them to reestablish control and emotional stability. Elderly depressed persons appear to benefit from short-term, client-centered, directive therapy more than from therapy that is nondirective or uses free association to uncover long-standing personality conflicts (Gallagher and Thompson, 1983; Sholomskas et al., 1983). These methods can help depressed older patients understand the source of their anxieties, fears, guilt, and apathy that are so detrimental to their interpersonal functioning. The success of a particular treatment strategy may be related to the duration and severity of the depression. Alternative approaches to psychotherapy with older people are discussed later in this chapter.

SUICIDE AMONG OLDER PEOPLE

It has been estimated that 25 percent of all reported suicides occur in persons aged 65 and older (Butler, 1975; Blazer, 1982). In 1980, the national rate was 11.9 suicides per 100,000 population. The rate for persons over age 65 was 17.7 (NCHS, 1983). It is noteworthy that the highest suicide rates in the United States are found among older white males. The prevalence of suicide in this population rises linearly after age 65; almost three times as many suicides occur in white males aged 85 and over as in all other subgroups of elderly combined (Belsky, 1984). According to data compiled by the National Center for Health Statistics (1983), white males over age 85 completed 50 suicides per 100,000 in 1980. In contrast, white females completed 7; nonwhite females 2; and nonwhite males 15 suicides per 100,000 in the same year. Since there are probably a significant number of suicides that appear to be accidents or natural deaths (e.g., starvation, gas poisoning), these statistics may underrepresent the actual incidence of the problem.

One explanation for the higher rates of suicide among elderly white males is that they generally experience the greatest incongruence between their ideal self-image (that of worker, decision-maker, holder of relatively high status in society) and the realities of advancing age (Miller, 1979; Butler and Lewis, 1982). With age, the role of worker is generally lost, chronic illness may diminish one's sense of control, and an individual may feel a loss of status. Social isolation may have an additive effect on the incidence of suicide, which is an important factor in the lives of older white widowed males, who are most likely to lack supportive social networks (Stenback, 1980; Holinger and Offer, 1982). A Japanese study found social isolation to be an important predictor of suicide in older men (Araki and Murata, 1986). Nonwhite elderly males in the United States may be less likely to commit suicide because of more extensive family support systems, described in Chapter 10.

Suicide statistics from 1900 through 1980 show a dramatic decline in suicide rates among the elderly since 1940, although their rates remain highest. In contrast, youths aged 15 to 24 have shown a twofold increase in suicide rates between 1960 and 1980 (McIntosh, 1985). The relative decline in suicide among older persons may be related to an increased use of mental health services or antidepressant medications. It may also reflect the improving economic status of the older population.

There are fewer nonfatal suicide attempts in older men compared to the young. That is, the rate of completed suicides is far greater among older men, 4:1 versus 200:1 in the young (Stenback, 1980; McIntire and Angle, 1981). This difference may be due to the use of more lethal methods of suicide such as shotguns, and a lower likelihood of survival from serious injury.

Because attempts at suicide are more likely to be successful in older men, it is important for family members and professional service providers to be sensitive to clues of an impending suicide. Risk factors include a serious physical illness with severe pain, the sudden death of a loved one, a major loss of independence, or financial inadequacy. Statements that indicate frustration with life and a desire to end it, a sudden decision to give away one's most important possessions, and a general loss of interest in one's social and physical environment must be attended to closely by those who are familiar with the older person. Since older people are less likely to make threats or to announce their intentions than are young people who intend to commit suicide, it is even more important to watch for subtle cues. Clearly, not all older people displaying such symptoms will attempt suicide, but the recognition of changes in an older family member's or client's behavior and moods can alleviate a potential disaster.*

---

*As will be described in Chapter 14, some people believe that suicide for terminally ill older people allows them to maintain control over their death. Groups who adhere to this viewpoint, particularly the Hemlock Society, would be opposed to interventions to stop an older person from choosing suicide.

Dementia

As stated in Chapter 7, normal aging does not result in significant declines in intelligence, memory, and learning ability. Mild impairments do not necessarily signal a major loss but often represent a mild form of memory dysfunction known as benign senescent forgetfulness. Only in the case of the diseases known collectively as the dementias does cognitive function show marked deterioration. Dementia, also referred to as organic brain syndrome or senile dementia, actually includes a variety of conditions that are caused by or associated with damage of brain tissue, resulting in impaired cognitive function and, in more advanced stages, impaired behavior and personality. Such changes in the brain result in progressive deterioration of an individual's ability to learn and recall items from the past. Until recently, it was assumed that all these syndromes were associated with cerebral arteriosclerosis ("hardening of the arteries"). Although it is now known that a number of these conditions occur independently of arteriosclerosis, research on the causes of the deterioration in brain tissue is at an early stage. Some features are unique to each type of dementia, but all dementias have in common a change in an individual's ability to recall events in recent memory, and problems with comprehension, attention span, judgment, and orientation to time, place, and person. The individual with dementia may experience increased concreteness of thought (i.e., be unable to understand abstract thought or symbolic language; for example, he or she cannot interpret a proverb), particularly in the later stages of the disease.

Although not part of normal aging, the likelihood of experiencing dementia does increase with advancing age. Approximately three million persons over age 65 experience some degree of cognitive loss (Busse and Pfeiffer, 1975; Ringler, 1981), and up to 50 percent of institutionalized elderly are estimated to have mild to moderate levels of dementia. As more people live to be over age 70, the number of persons with dementia is expected to increase by 44 percent in whites and 72 percent in Blacks between 1980 and 2005 (Kramer, 1983). This difference by ethnic minority status is attributed to the more rapid growth of Blacks living beyond age 70. However, just as aging and disease are not synonymous, dementia is not inevitable with age.

The major types of dementias are shown in Table 9–2. Note the distinction between *reversible* and *irreversible* dementias. The first refers to cognitive decline, which may be caused by drug toxicity, hormonal or nutritional disorders, and other diseases that may be reversible. Sources of potentially reversible dementias include tumors in and trauma to the brain, toxins, metabolic disorders such as hypo or hyperthyroidism, diabetes, hypo or hypercalcemia, infections, vascular lesions, and hydrocephalus. Severe depression may produce confusion and memory problems in some older people. Some medications may also cause dementia-like symptoms. This problem is aggravated if the individual is taking multiple medications or is on a dosage that is higher than can be metabolized by

TABLE 9–2 Major Dementias of Late Life

Reversible	Irreversible
Drugs	Alzheimer's
Alcohol	Multi-infarct
Nutritional deficiencies	Huntington's Chorea
Normal pressure hydrocephalus	
Brain tumors	Pick's disease
Hypothyroidism/Hyperthyroidism	
Neurosyphilis	Creutzfeldt-Jacob
Depression (pseudo-dementia)	Kuru
	Wernicke-Korsakoff

the older kidney or liver. An individual who appears to be suffering from such reactions should be referred promptly for medical screening.

Irreversible dementias are those that have no discernible environmental cause and cannot yet be cured. Although there is considerable research on the causes and treatments for these conditions, they must be labeled irreversible at the present time. Some of these are more common than others; some have identifiable causes while others do not. Pick's Disease is one of the rarest; in this type, the frontal lobes of the brain atrophy. Of all the dementias, it is most likely to occur in younger persons, and to result in significant personality changes. Creutzfeldt-Jacob and Kuru diseases have been traced to a slow-acting virus. In the former type of dementia, decline in cognitive abilities occurs quite rapidly. The latter type is quite rare, and has been found among some cannibalistic tribes of New Guinea. Huntington's Chorea is a genetically transmitted condition that usually appears in people in their thirties and forties. It results in more neuromuscular changes than do the other dementias.

Multi-infarct dementia has been estimated to represent 15 to 20 percent of all nonreversible dementias (Terry and Wisniewski, 1977). This is the form of dementia that in the past was identified as "senility." In this type, several areas of the brain show infarcts or small strokes that result in damage to one or more blood vessels feeding those areas of the brain. Older people with this condition often have a history of hypertension, strokes, and blackouts. Although multi-infarct dementia may be diagnosed without such a history, such cases are relatively rare, and may indicate another type of dementia, most likely Alzheimer's disease.

The most common irreversible dementia in late life, accounting for 50 to 70 percent of all dementias, is senile dementia of the Alzheimer's type (SDAT, or Alzheimer's disease). Incidence figures are difficult to obtain, but it has been estimated that 5 to 15 percent of all persons over age 65, and over 25 percent in nursing homes have symptoms of SDAT. The prevalence of Alzheimer's disease appears to increase with age; less than 2 percent of the general population under age 60 are affected, whereas rates of 20 percent have been estimated for the population over age 80 (Eisdorfer and Cohen, 1978; Gurland and Cross, 1982). Although a distinction was made in the past between pre-senile (i.e., before age 65) and senile dementia, there is now common agreement that these are the same disease.

Several hypotheses have been proposed to explain the causes of Alzheimer's disease. Some researchers have suggested that it may result from a slow virus, or a virus-like agent called a prion, as in Kuru and Creutzfeldt-Jacob disease (Wurtman, 1985). Others have identified its link with Downs' Syndrome (i.e., a greater frequency in families where Downs' Syndrome has occurred, and a high prevalence in people with Downs' Syndrome by age 40). Multiple occurrences have been found in some families (e.g., two siblings or a parent and child both develop SDAT), which suggests that chromosomal or other genetic factors may play a role in its etiology (Burger and Vogel, 1973; Heston, Mastri, Anderson, and White, 1981). There is increasing evidence for a hereditary type of Alzheimer's disease. Still others have argued that the disease is caused by the accumulation of heavy metals (such as aluminum) in the brain (Crapper, Karlik, and de Boni, 1978; Perl and Brody, 1980). To date, none of these hypotheses has received conclusive support. More recently, emphasis has been placed on the finding of a biochemical imbalance in the brains of SDAT patients, specifically a reduced level of the enzyme choline acetyltransferase (Corkin, 1981; Whitehouse et al., 1981).

As illustrated by Mr. Wallace in the introductory vignette, Alzheimer's disease is characterized by deficits in attention, learning, memory, and language skills. An individual with this condition may also have problems in judgment, abstraction, and orientation. In the earlier stages of the disease, an individual may have difficulties with attention span and with orientation to the environment, increased anxiety and restlessness, and unpredictable changes in mood. Family members may complain that the older person has become more aggressive or, in some cases, more passive than in the past. Depression may set in as the individual realizes that he or she is experiencing these problems. In the more advanced stages of the disease, there may be marked aphasia (i.e., problems recalling appropriate words and labels), perseveration (i.e., repeating the same phrase and thoughts again and again), apathy, and problems with comprehension, such that Alzheimer's victims may not recognize their spouse, children, and long-time friends. However, it is not unusual for some patients in the moderate to advanced stages of SDAT to describe quite articulately and vividly events that took place many years ago. The advanced patient often needs assistance with bodily functions, such as eating and toileting. At autopsy, there is a generalized deterioration of cortical tissue, which appears to be tangled and covered with plaque.

There have been some attempts to determine if SDAT proceeds through a series of stages, such that symptoms become more prevalent and severe. This is a difficult task because the course of SDAT varies so widely. Some patients may experience a rapid decline in memory while their orientation to time, place, and people may remain relatively intact. Others may experience mood and personality changes early, whereas still other patients maintain their pre-morbid personality for many years after the symptoms first appear.

A broad distinction is often made among early, middle, and advanced stages of SDAT. These categories are based on the patient's level of decline in memory, orientation, and activities of daily living. Some psychologists have provided guidelines with the use of assessment tools such as the Mini-Mental Status Exam (Folstein, Folstein, and McHugh, 1975) and the Dementia Rating Scale (Coblentz, Mattis, Zingesser, Kasoff, Wisniewski and Katzman, 1973; Mattis, 1976), which give clues to the patient's level of deterioration on the basis of their test scores. Perhaps the most extensive research to determine the stages of SDAT has been conducted by Reisberg, Ferris, De Leon, and Crook (1982). Based on their observations of functional and cognitive declines in SDAT patients, they have developed a Global Deterioration Scale that delineates seven stages of the disease. These are briefly described in Table 9–3.

Because of recent attention by the media and by researchers on Alzheimer's disease, there is some tendency to overestimate its occurrence, and to assume that it is the cause of all dementias. In many ways, it has taken on the role that multi-infarct dementia had several years ago; that is, the label has been given without a thorough diagnosis. Unfortunately, the most confirmatory diagnosis of Alzheimer's disease may be made only at autopsy, when the areas and nature of damaged brain tissue can be identified. However, several psychological measures of cognitive functioning and a thorough physical exam can provide clues to its existence in the earlier stages, or may indicate that the observed changes in

TABLE 9–3 Global Deterioration Scale

Stage 1:	No cognitive or functional decrements
Stage 2:	Complaints of very mild forgetfulness and some work difficulties
Stage 3:	Mild cognitive impairment on cognitive battery; concentration problems; some difficulty at work and in traveling alone
Stage 4:	Late confusional stage; increased problems in planning, handling finances; increased denial of symptoms; withdrawal
Stage 5:	Poor recall of recent events; may need to be reminded about proper clothing and bathing
Stage 6:	More advanced memory and orientation problems; needs assistance with activities of daily living; more personality changes
Stage 7:	Late dementia with loss of verbal abilities; incontinent; loss of ability to walk; may become comatose

Source: B. Reisberg, S. H. Ferris, M. J. De Leon, and T. Crook, The Global Deterioration Scale for assessment of primary degenerative dementia, *American Journal of Psychiatry, 139,* pp. 1136–1139, 1982. Copyright 1982, the American Psychiatric Association. Reprinted by permission.

behavior and/or personality are due to a reversible condition. Early diagnosis can be made with some certainty with an extensive series of tests. These measures include a medical and nutritional history; laboratory tests of blood, urine, and stool; tests for thyroid function; a thorough physical and psychological examination; and, in some cases, extensive radiological studies, including a CAT (computerized axial tomography) scan or MRI (magnetic resonance imaging) (Eisdorfer, Cohen, and Veith, 1980; Small, Liston, and Jarvik, 1981). In fact, it is primarily through a process of elimination of other conditions that some dementias such as SDAT may be diagnosed. In such diagnoses, it is particularly important to detect depression, drug toxicity, and nutritional deficiencies because, as stated earlier, these conditions may be treated.

THERAPY FOR DEMENTIA PATIENTS

Unfortunately, no completely successful treatment for dementia currently exists. The cognitive functions that are lost with most irreversible forms of dementia cannot be restored through psychotherapy. However, many older persons can benefit from memory retraining and environmental modifications. That is, individual competence can be enhanced somewhat, and the environment simplified considerably in an effort to maintain P-E congruence. The individual's social and home environments can be changed in order to encourage independent functioning (Hiatt, 1980). Written schedules of activities, simplified routes from room to room, and written directions for cooking, bathing, and taking medications can aid a person in finding his or her way around and prevent the frustration that results from getting lost or not recognizing once familiar people and places. It is also important to maintain a regular schedule, to keep the patient active, and to prevent withdrawal from daily interactions. Ultimately, the goal of managing these dementias is to slow the rate of deterioration and to prevent institutionalization for as long as possible. For the SDAT patient who does enter a nursing home, there are a growing number of facilities with special units for elderly with Alzheimer's disease (Peppard, 1986; Rabins, 1986). These units provide a higher staff-to-resident ratio, a safe environment where patients can explore without getting lost, and special services aimed at maintaining the patients' remaining cognitive capacities. A recent study of 32 patients admitted to a special dementia unit found improved mental and physical functioning up to four months later (Benson et al., 1987). However, specialized dementia units are faced with the problem of establishing criteria for selecting residents, recruitment and retention of staff trained in dementia, and the cost of maintaining the necessary staff-to-patient ratio (Rabins, 1986).

One of the most important considerations with Alzheimer's disease and other dementias is to provide social and emotional support to the patient as well as the family. In recent years, there has been a significant growth in family support groups, which now exist in almost every major city and even in smaller

Groups for family members of Alzheimer's patients are an invaluable source of information and support.

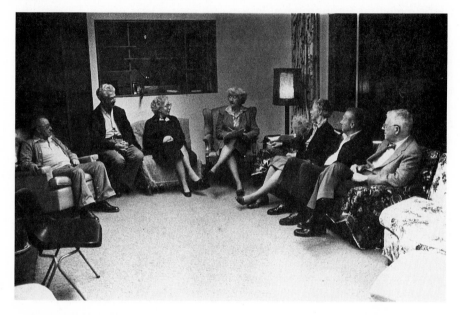

communities. A national organization, Alzheimer's Disease and Related Disorders (ADRDA), serves as a major coordinating body for many of these local groups, and also spearheads attempts to increase research funds to understand and treat this most common form of dementia. The local support groups provide a network of help for families who are faced with the often devastating impact of this disease. Such groups aid their members in coping with the inevitable losses faced by the victims of SDAT, problems such as forgetting where they are when they go for a walk in the neighborhood, not recognizing their own children, not being able to dress themselves, and, in more advanced cases, needing assistance with eating, bathing, and toileting. These groups also provide caregivers with emotional support and respite. The growth of Adult Day Centers has been one response to the need to keep persons with dementia in the community, to help them remain active and retain learned skills, and to provide respite for their family caregivers. As noted in Chapter 19, however, the need for such respite and support is greater than the availability of services.

   Currently, many researchers are testing medications that may improve the cognitive functioning of victims of dementia. These include drugs that restore the activity of neurotransmitters in the brain, and some that even replace neuro-chemicals that are lost. As yet, no medication effectively restores cognitive function in the severely impaired older person for any significant period of time.

As noted earlier, careful screening by a team of physicians, psychologists, and social workers is necessary to determine if the dementia is secondary to a nutritional deficiency, drug toxicity, or physical diseases. If so, treatment should focus on the management of that condition.

Alcoholism

It is difficult to obtain accurate statistics on the prevalence of alcoholism in older people because of the stigma associated with this condition among this cohort. Estimates vary, from 10 to 15 percent of all people over age 55 living in the community (Zimberg, 1974), to less than 10 percent (Siassi, Crocetti, and Spiro, 1973). Surveys of elderly outpatients in general medical hospitals estimate that 15 to 30 percent show symptoms of alcoholism (Moore, 1971; Schuckit and Miller, 1976). A review of national surveys conducted between 1971 and 1982 of drinking patterns among women concluded that women over age 65 report the lowest incidence of alcohol consumption in general, and the lowest incidence of heavy drinking, with 26 to 40 percent stating that they consume any alcohol, and less than 5 percent indicating high consumption (Wilsnack, Wilsnack, and Klassen, 1984). In contrast, widowers and men who have never married are at greater risk for alcoholism (Siassi et al., 1973).

Alcoholics are less likely to be found among the ranks of persons over age 60 because of higher death rates at a young age among alcoholics (Atkinson and Schuckit, 1981). Nevertheless, surveys of alcoholism rates among older persons have revealed approximately equal proportions of those who began to drink heavily before age 40 and those who began in old age. In one study, more than two-thirds of elderly alcoholics had had this problem for many years; others had increased their drinking in response to age-related stressful events (Rosin and Glatt, 1971). This is consistent with the findings of Zimberg (1974).

It is important to distinguish lifelong abusers of alcohol from those who began drinking later in life, often as a reaction to losses and isolation experienced by some older people. Some older persons who are diagnosed as alcoholics have had this problem since middle-age, but increasing age may exacerbate the condition for two reasons. First, the central nervous system, liver, and kidneys become less tolerant of alcohol with age because of the physiological changes described in Chapter 4 (e.g., loss of muscle tissue, reduction in body mass, reduced efficiency of liver and kidney functions). For this reason, a smaller dose of alcohol can be more deleterious in the later years. Second, an individual who has been drinking heavily for many years has already produced irreversible damage to the central nervous system, liver, and kidneys, creating more problems than those due to normal aging alone. It is difficult to determine the incidence of alcoholism among older persons who have no previous history of alcoholism. Physiological evidence is lacking, and drinking is often hidden from friends, relatives, and physicians. The elderly person may justify overconsumption of alcohol on the grounds that it relieves sadness and isolation. Even in cases where family members are aware of the situation, they may minimize it by rationalizing that it is one of the older person's few remaining pleasures.

Physicians may overlook the possibility that alcohol is creating a health problem for the older person, because the adverse effects of alcohol resemble some physical diseases or psychiatric and cognitive disorders that are associated with old age. Older alcoholics may complain of confusion, disorientation, irritability, insomnia or restless sleep patterns, heart palpitations, or a dry cough (Smith-DiJulio, Heinemann, and Ogden, 1977). Beliefs held by health care providers that alcoholism does not occur in older people may also prevent its detection.

In a survey of men in the medical and surgical wards of Veterans Administration Hospitals (Schuckit and Miller, 1976), social disruption such as aggressive behavior toward staff and other patients was found more frequently among long-term alcoholics, but physical health problems were more severe among men who commenced heavy drinking late in life. This same survey revealed greater mental deterioration and more attempts at suicide among older alcoholics compared with age-matched men who had no history of alcohol abuse. However, older women alcoholics have been found to make fewer suicide attempts and to undergo fewer hospitalizations for psychiatric care than elderly male alcoholics (Schuckit and Morrissey, 1976). It is noteworthy that older alcoholics are less likely than young alcoholics to demonstrate a serious personality disorder (Rosin and Glatt, 1971) but are more likely to have symptoms of dementia (Gaitz and Baer, 1971; Ryan and Butters, 1980). Indeed, middle-aged alcoholics have been found to show significant impairments in learning and memory that are more common in advanced old age, suggesting a premature aging phenomenon due to long-term alcohol abuse (Ryan and Butters, 1980). Creutzfeldt-Jacob disease is a form of dementia that is sometimes found in long-term alcoholics. Alcoholism and depression may occur together in the same individual. Heavy drinkers in all age groups have been found to report more depressive symptoms (Wilsnack et al., 1984).

Therapy for geriatric alcoholics has not been differentiated from that for younger alcoholics. However, it is probably more important to focus on the older alcoholic's medical condition because of physical declines that make them more vulnerable to the secondary effects of alcohol. As with younger alcoholics, psychotherapy and occupational and recreational therapy are important for treating older people experiencing alcoholism.

Drug Abuse

Older persons use a disproportionately large number of prescription and over-the-counter drugs, representing approximately 25 percent of all medication costs. In particular, older people are more likely than the young to be using tranquilizers, sedatives, and hypnotics, all of which have potentially dangerous side effects. The use of such medications is even greater in long-term care settings. In a survey of elderly persons residing in the community, 83 percent of the respondents were using two more medications; the average was 3.8 per person (Chien, Townsend, and Townsend, 1978). Older persons have been found to abuse aspirin compounds (Morrant, 1975), laxatives (Cummings, Sladen, James, Sarner, and Misciewiz, 1974), and sleeping pills (Subby, 1975), often because of misinformation about the adverse effects of too high a dosage or too many pills. It is not unusual to hear older patients state that they took twice or three times as much aspirin as they were prescribed because they did not feel their pain was being alleviated with the lower dose. Yet, because of changes in body composition, renal and liver functions with age, combined with the use of multiple medications, older persons are more likely to experience adverse drug reactions. Fortunately there is growing awareness of the effects of "polypharmacy" among health care providers and among older people themselves. There is very little evidence that older persons abuse drugs to the extent that younger populations do, or use illicit drugs such as heroin, cocaine, and marijuana.

Paranoid Disorders and Schizophrenia

Paranoia, defined as an irrational suspiciousness of other people, actually takes several forms. In older persons, paranoia may be due to social isolation, a sense of powerlessness, progressive sensory decline, and problems with the normal "checks and balances" of daily life (Eisdorfer, Cohen, and Veith, 1980). Hearing loss may also be a risk factor in paranoia, although research evidence for this is mixed (see Chapter 5). Still other changes in the aging individual, such as problems with memory, may result in paranoid reactions.

Although the foregoing conditions may produce a genuine paranoid state, some of the suspicious attitudes of older persons may represent accurate readings of their experiences. For example, an older person's children may in fact be trying to institutionalize him or her in order to take over an estate; a nurse's aide may really be stealing from an older patient; neighborhood children may truly be making fun of the older person. It is therefore important to distinguish actual threats to the individual from unfounded suspicions. To the extent that the individual has some control over his or her environment, again consistent with the P-E model, the older person's perception of a threatening situation will be reduced. The diagnosis of paranoid disorders in older people is similar to that in younger patients; the symptoms should have a duration of at least one week, with no signs of schizophrenia, no prominent hallucinations, and no association to an organic mental disorder (APA, 1987).

Schizophrenia is much less prevalent than depression or dementia in old age. It has been estimated that only 1 percent of the population over age 60 living in the community are schizophrenic (Bollerup, 1975). Most elderly persons with this condition were first diagnosed in adolescence or in middle-age and continue to display behavior symptomatic of schizophrenia, although the severity of symptoms appears to decrease with age (Kay, 1972; Lawton, 1972). Late onset schizophrenia with paranoid features has been labeled *paraphrenia* by some psychiatrists, especially in Europe and in Great Britain (Butler and Lewis, 1982).

Many of the current cohort of elderly chronic schizophrenics residing in the community were deinstitutionalized during the early 1960s as part of the national Community Mental Health Services Act of 1963. After spending much of their youth and middle-age in state hospitals, these patients were released with the anticipation that they could function independently in the community with medications to control their hallucinations and psychotic behavior. Although this approach has proven effective for many former schizophrenic inpatients, some have not adjusted successfully to deinstitutionalization, as witnessed by the number of older schizophrenics seen on the streets in most major cities.

THERAPEUTIC INTERVENTIONS

As with depression, psychotherapy can be useful for paranoid older persons. In particular, cognitive behavior-change strategies, in which an individual focuses on changing specific problem areas or misconceptions, may be useful in treating the paranoid older person, because these persons often attribute causality to external factors (e.g., the belief that someone took their pocketbook, that they themselves did not misplace it). Psychotherapy with paranoid elderly may be effective in redirecting beliefs about causality to the individual himself or herself. Pharmacotherapy with antipsychotic medications has been shown to be effective for older schizophrenic patients.

Anxiety

Anxiety disorders are another type of functional disorder or emotional problem with no obvious organic cause. As is true of schizophrenia and paranoid disorders, anxiety disorders are much rarer in older populations than in the young. This may be because the older person develops more tolerance and better ability to manage stressful events. More likely, however, those who have anxiety disorders in middle-age may be less likely to survive to old age (Belsky, 1984).

Psychotherapy with Older Persons

Despite early doubts by Freud (1924) and others about the value of psychotherapy for older patients, many researchers and therapists have proposed and developed psychotherapeutic intervention strategies specifically for this population, or have modified existing approaches. One problem in working with the elderly may be overcoming the misconceptions held by some older about psychotherapy. For this reason, short-term, goal-oriented therapies may be more effective with older patients (Brink, 1979; Zarit, 1980), because they can begin to experience benefits immediately. On the other hand, older patients who are reluctant and unwilling to open up to a therapist may benefit more from long-term treatment in which rapport and trust between the therapist and the client can be established gradually (Mintz, Steuer, and Jarvik, 1981). Several different types of therapy have been explored with this population.

Life review is one therapeutic approach that has been successfully used with older persons. Such therapy encourages introspection through active reminiscence of past achievements and failures, and may reestablish ego integrity in depressed older persons (Lewis and Butler, 1974). This method may also be used effectively by social service providers who are not extensively trained in psychotherapy.

Group therapy has been advocated for older patients experiencing mental disorders, especially depression (Ingersoll and Silverman, 1978; Hartford, 1980). Groups offer the opportunity for peer support, social interaction, and role modeling. Life review may be used effectively as part of group therapy. The opportunity to share life experiences and to learn that others have had similar stresses in their lives appears to enhance insight, self-esteem, and a feeling of catharsis. This was found in a study of a therapy group with older persons who wrote their autobiographies and read these aloud to each other (Birren, 1982).

Groups have also been established for improving memory and enhancing cognitive skills. Groups are an ideal setting for teaching memory skills with the use of games and puzzles, as well as reminiscence exercises. Both reminiscence and learning exercises have been found to improve scores on a test of intelligence; social contact groups showed no change on these tests (Hughston and Merriam, 1982).

More empirical studies have been conducted recently to compare the efficacy of alternative therapeutic interventions. For example, short-term behavioral (i.e., changing maladaptive behavior with operant techniques) and supportive group therapy (i.e., helping the patient to develop ego strength and feelings of control) were found to be equally effective in alleviating secondary depression. The positive impact of treatment continued at the five-week follow-up study (Gallagher, 1981). The effects of a nine-month course of cognitive-behavioral therapy were compared with a psychodynamic approach with depressed persons aged 55 to 78 (Steuer et al., 1984). The former approach consists of active, directive, structured, and time-limited therapeutic modes (Beck, Rush, and Emery, 1979). Its goal is to change behavior *and* self-defeating thought processes. Psychodynamic group therapy uses psychoanalytic concepts such as insight, transference, and the unconscious to relieve symptoms of depression and to prevent its recurrence by understanding why the individual behaves in self-defeating ways. In general, the researchers found that both approaches reduced depression, but that cognitive-behavioral strategies resulted in greater improvements on one of the depression measures. In comparisons of cognitive therapy with behavioral and supportive psychotherapy among depressed older persons, all three approaches were effective in reducing symptoms of depression. However, cognitive and behavioral approaches resulted in continued improvement (i.e., up to one year later), while supportive therapy had less long-term impact (Gallagher and Thompson, 1981). This may be because cognitive and behavioral therapy, alone or in combination, teaches skills that the patient may practice outside the clinical setting.

The therapeutic interventions just described are more frequently used in community settings than with elderly in nursing homes. The latter setting lends itself to more intense, long-term therapies. These include behavior change programs, milieu therapy, reality orientation, and remotivation therapy. Behavior-change techniques using operant reinforcement and token economies have been successfully used in long-term care settings with psychiatrically impaired young and old patients. These methods have been found to increase self-feeding (Baltes and Zerbe, 1976) and self-care (Mishara, 1978; Kiyak, 1980) in older persons, and have been effective in reducing dependency (Sperbeck and Whitbourne, 1981). Milieu therapy is consistent with Lawton and Nahemow's competence model described earlier in this book. This approach focuses on improving the therapeutic environment of the nursing home or enhancing an individual's sense of control over some important aspects of life. One application of principles of milieu therapy has been to encourage older residents to make decisions for themselves in specific domains, such as caring for a pet bird. These elderly were found to remain more active, sociable, and alert than elderly residents who were given no control over their environment (Langer and Rodin, 1976; Langer et al., 1979). In another study aimed at enhancing the perception of control and encouraging cognitive activity among nursing home residents, contingency reinforcement was used to encourage residents to seek out information about their environment and historical events. Memory improvement was found among those in the contingent conditions (Beck, 1982).

Reality orientation was developed by Folsom (1968) to aid confused and disoriented patients in hospital settings. This approach is widely used in nursing homes. Signs and "reality orientation boards" are used to denote the current date, place, and special events. Staff members are encouraged to constantly remind residents of these facts and to use the residents' names during their daily interactions. Unfortunately, studies of reality orientation have provided mixed results. It has not been found to be a valuable therapeutic mode for severely demented older persons.

Remotivation therapy has been used successfully with less confused elderly. Groups of older persons with some cognitive impairment, but more importantly, who are withdrawn from social activities, meet together under the guidance of a trained group leader. The purpose is to discuss events and experiences by bringing all group members into the discussion, emphasizing the event's relevance for each member, and encouraging them to share what they have gained from the session. This approach has been found to be effective in psychiatric hospitals and nursing homes as well as in adult day centers.

There are few systematic comparative studies on the long-term effects of these therapeutic approaches in nursing homes; likewise, the feasibility of instituting such programs within the constraints of nursing homes' policies and procedures has not been examined. Without a commitment to using these therapeutic modes on a long-term basis following successful experimental interventions, nursing home staff cannot expect lasting therapeutic benefits from any of these methods.

Use of Mental Health Services

As noted in Chapter 6, older persons use physician services slightly more than the young, and are hospitalized at a much higher rate. In contrast, mental health services are significantly underutilized by the elderly, especially ethnic minorities. Community-based care is used at a far lower rate than inpatient hospital treatment by older people.

It has been estimated that only 4 to 5 percent of patients using community mental health centers are age 65 or older (Redick and Taube, 1980; Butler and Lewis, 1982), far below their representation in the U.S. population and less than the estimated prevalence of mental disorders among the elderly. Two surveys by the American Psychological Association of community mental health centers, one in 1983 and one in 1985 (Rickards, 1985), provide further evidence for older people's low utilization rates. The surveys revealed that only 6 percent of the client population of these centers was over age 65; an even smaller percentage were ethnic minority elderly. The problem is compounded by poor coordination of activities between mental health centers and senior centers or other programs directed specifically at older persons. Furthermore, a significant portion (44 percent) of community mental health centers reported having no clinical staff trained in geriatrics, and no programs specifically for the older population; an even greater proportion (73 percent) stated that they had no special programs or staff skilled in working with ethnic minority elderly.

A 1976 national survey found that 13 percent of respondents over age 65 had sought professional help for mental disorders (Kulka and Tamir, 1978). This represents a higher rate than the 6 percent reported by Gurin, Veroff, and Feld (1960), and the 3 percent reported more recently by Evashwick, Rowe, Diehr, and Branch (1984). A later epidemiological survey in Baltimore revealed that 4.2 percent of the population aged 65 to 74 had sought treatment for mental disorders during the preceding six months, and only 1.4 percent of those over age 75 had done so. This compared with 8.7 percent of the population under age 65 (German,

Shapiro, and Skinner, 1985). These statistics are particularly striking when compared to the proportion of elderly respondents in that survey who had sought medical treatment during the same six-month period; over 66 percent of the group aged 65 and older had received medical care at least once, compared to slightly more than 50 percent of the population under age 65.

Older persons may be more likely to be hospitalized for mental disorders than to seek community mental health services. Patients over age 65 have been found to account for 3 percent of the outpatient population of hospitals, and 7 percent of the inpatients (Kahn, 1975). A disproportionate number of older persons represent the population of patients in state mental hospitals that house the chronically mentally ill. Despite the deinstitutionalization movement of the 1960s, the great majority of all psychiatric services to the elderly are in such settings.

BARRIERS TO OLDER PERSONS' USE OF SERVICES

In a survey of 88 senior center participants, older persons perceived a general physician to be more effective in treating psychiatric symptoms than mental health professionals (Waxman, Carner, and Klein, 1984). Of this sample, 79 percent would choose general physicians for treatment of depression, and 90 percent for organic brain syndrome. Less than 10 percent thought that a mental health professional would be able to treat the latter condition effectively. This finding is consistent with Lawton's (1979) suggestion and the findings of German and associates (1985) that older adults are generally unwilling to interpret their problems as psychological, preferring instead to attribute them to physical or social conditions or to normal aging. In addition, the current cohort of older persons may be less oriented to the use of mental health services because of societal stigmas, limited knowledge about mental disorders, and a lack of confidence in mental health workers (Kleinman and Clemente, 1976).

Attitudes of physicians and mental health professionals, especially the belief that the elderly cannot benefit from therapy simply because of their age, also have been cited as barriers to older people's obtaining psychiatric services. Butler and Lewis (1982) have labeled such attitudes "professional ageism." These attitudes may partially explain the results of a study in which vignettes of old versus young patients with obvious psychiatric symptoms were presented to 60 general physicians. Whether a general physician referred patients for professional psychiatric treatment depended on the patient's age and the perceived severity of the symptoms (Kucharski, White, and Schratz, 1979). A similar approach has been used with psychologists (Dye, 1978) and with psychiatrists (Ford and Sbordonne, 1980). In both studies, these mental health professionals were not optimistic about the effectiveness of psychotherapy with older patients. This belief, in turn, may affect the decision to use psychotherapy alone or as an adjunct to pharmocotherapy with older patients. However, as more mental health professionals receive specialized training in geriatrics, these stereotypes are expected to be reduced in the future.

Perhaps the greatest barrier to obtaining mental health services is accessibility. In addition to the physical access issues of transportation and architectural barriers, there are significant problems of fragmented services and older people's lack of knowledge about seeking mental health services on their own, or obtaining appropriate referrals from physicians or social service providers. Reimbursement for psychological services is also a problem. For example, Medicare limits outpatient mental health expenditures more than inpatient treatment. Furthermore, co-payment by the subscriber for mental health services is greater than for physical health services. It should be noted that this discrepancy occurs in many health insurance programs used by younger persons as well. Because of attitudes held by older patients toward mental disorders and by therapists toward older clients, however, these reimbursement issues are greater barriers to older persons' use of mental health services than they are for the young. Future cohorts of elderly may be more likely to seek such services in community mental health centers, because of increasing awareness of mental disorders and treatment modalities.

Summary and Implications

The prevalence of mental disorders in old age is difficult to determine, although estimates range from 5 to 45 percent of all elderly. Research in acute and long-term care institutional settings provides higher estimates than epidemiological studies conducted in the community. This is because many older persons with mental disorders are treated in institutional settings rather than seeking care through community mental health services.

The most common mental disorder in late life is depression, although estimates of its prevalence also vary widely, from 2.8 to 22 percent, depending on the criteria used to diagnose depression. Manic-depressive disorders are rare in old age; unipolar depression is more common. Reactive depression that is secondary to major life changes is found frequently in older persons; this condition responds well to environmental and social interventions, whereas antidepressant therapy is more effective for major depression, and electroconvulsive therapy for severe depression in older people who do not respond to other forms of therapy. Diagnosing depression in older people is often difficult. Many deny it, while others attribute it to medical conditions. On the other hand, it is important to screen for medical conditions and medications that may produce depressive symptoms as a side effect.

Depression is a risk factor for suicide in older people, particularly for white men over age 85. Life changes that result in a loss of social status and increased isolation may explain why this group is more likely to commit suicide. The increased risk of suicide in the elderly highlights the need for family members and service providers to be sensitized to clues of an impending suicide.

Dementia includes numerous reversible and irreversible conditions that result in impaired cognitive function, especially recall of recent events, comprehension, learning, attention, and orientation to time, place, and person. These conditions differ from "benign senescent forgetfulness," which is a mild form of memory dysfunction that generally does not become worse with time. It is essential to perform a complete diagnostic work-up of older people who have symptoms of dementia. A medical history, physical examination, assessment of medications, lab tests, psychological and cognitive testing, as well as neurological testing, will aid in distinguishing "reversible" dementias that can be treated from the "irreversible" dementias such as Alzheimer's disease that currently can be managed but not cured. Family members and service providers should be aware of changes in the older person's cognitive functioning and behavior that may signal dementia, and must avoid labeling such changes as normal aging or the catchall phrase—senility.

Although cognitive functioning cannot be restored in irreversible dementias, older persons in the early stages of these conditions often benefit from memory retraining, and from psychotherapy to cope with the changes they are experiencing. Environmental modifications that simplify tasks and aid in orienting the patient may slow the rate of deterioration and postpone institutionalization. It is also important to provide emotional and social support to family caregivers of elderly with Alzheimer's disease and other dementias. Adult day care and other such respite programs are valuable for spouses and other caregivers who assume full-time care for these patients at home, although they are limited by funding constraints.

Alcoholism and drug abuse are less common in older persons than in the young, although accurate estimates of prevalence are difficult to obtain. Physical health and cognitive function are significantly impaired in older alcoholics. Older men with a history of alcohol abuse also have a greater risk of suicides than younger men or young and old women who are alcoholics. There are few studies of the efficacy of alternative treatments for older alcoholics. Drug abuse in older persons is rarely associated with illicit drugs, but often takes the form of inappropriate use or overuse of some prescription and over-the-counter drugs. Adverse reactions are more likely to occur in older persons because of age-related physiological changes that impair the ability to metabolize many medications, and the greater likelihood of polypharmacy.

Paranoia and schizophrenia are far less common than depression and dementia in older persons. Most people with these conditions first developed them in middle-age; life changes such as relocation and confusion that result from dementia may trigger paranoid reactions in old age. Psychotherapy, especially using cognitive behavior strategies, may be effective in treating paranoia, although it is important to first determine the underlying causes of the condition and to verify these.

Many researchers have explored the feasibility of psychotherapy with older patients. Both short-term, goal-oriented therapy and long-term approaches have been advocated. Specific modes of therapy with older patients include life review and group therapy using cognitive-behavioral and supportive techniques. These interventions have been particularly effective with depressed elderly in community settings. Nursing homes are ideal settings for long-term, intense therapies using groups, but staff may not have the time or training to implement them. Behavior change and milieu therapy have resulted in significant improvements in short-term experimental interventions. Unfortunately, there are few reports on the success of such programs as part of the day-to-day activities of a nursing home.

Despite the demonstrated efficacy of many forms of psychotherapy with older persons, mental health services are significantly underutilized by them. Most treatments for mental disorders in this population take place in hospitals. Many older people prefer to seek treatment for depression and other mental disorders from a general physician. This may result in an overreliance on pharmacological treatment and an underutilization of psychotherapy in cases where the latter may be more effective. Such behavior may be attributed to reluctance among the current cohort of elderly to admit they have a psychiatric problem, a lack of knowledge about such conditions and their treatment, as well as problems with accessibility. Attitudes of mental health providers and social service providers about the value of psychotherapy for older persons, and perhaps most importantly, the lack of effective links between mental health and social services to the elderly, have been barriers in the past. As more programs evolve that integrate services, and as future cohorts become aware of mental disorders and their treatment, there will be greater acceptance and use of mental health services by older people.

References

American Psychiatric Association. *Diagnostic and statistical manual of mental disorders* (3rd ed.). Washington, D.C.: American Psychiatric Assoc., 1987.

Araki, S., and Murata, K. Factors affecting suicide in young, middle-aged and elderly men. *Journal of Biosocial Sciences*, 1986, *18*, 103–108.

Atkinson, J. H., and Schuckit, M. A. Alcoholism and over-the-counter and prescription drug misuse in the elderly. In C. Eisdorfer (Ed.), *Annual review of gerontology and geriatrics (Volume 2)*. New York: Springer, 1981.

Baltes, M., and Zerbe, M. Independence training in nursing home residents. *The Gerontologist*, 1976, *16*, 428–432.

Beck, A. T., Rush, A. J. and Emery, G. *Cognitive therapy of depression*. New York: Guilford Press, 1979.

Beck, P. Two successful interventions in nursing homes: The therapeutic effects of cognitive activity. *The Gerontologist*, 1982, *22*, 378–383.

Belsky, J. K. *The psychology of aging: Theory, research and practice.* Monterey, Calif.: Brooks-Cole, 1984.

Benson, D. M., Cameron, D., Humbach, E., Servino, L., and Gambert, S. R. Establishment and impact of a dementia unit within the nursing home. *Journal of the American Geriatrics Society,* 1987, *35,* 319–323.

Bernstein, J. C. Anorexia nervosa: 94-year-old woman treated with electroshock. *Minnesota Medicine,* 1972, *55,* 552–553.

Birren, J. E. A review of the development of the self. Paper presented at annual meetings of the Gerontological Society of America, 1982.

Blazer, D. The epidemiology of mental illness in late life. In E. Busse and D. Blazer (Eds.), *Handbook of geriatric psychiatry.* New York: Van Nostrand Reinhold, 1980.

Blazer, D. *Depression in late life.* St. Louis: Mosby, 1982.

Blazer, D., George, L., and Landerman, R. The phenomenology of late life depression. In P. E. Bebbington and R. Jacoby (Eds.), *Psychiatric disorders in the elderly.* London: Mental Health Foundation, 1986.

Blazer, D., and Williams, C. D. Epidemiology of dysphoria and depression in an elderly population. *American Journal of Psychiatry,* 1980, *137,* 439–444.

Bollerup, T. Prevalence of mental illness among 70-year-olds domiciled in nine Copenhagen suburbs. *Acta Psychiatrica Scandinavia,* 1975, *51,* 327–339.

Brink, T. L. *Geriatric psychotherapy.* New York: Human Sciences Press, 1979.

Brody, E. M., and Kleban, M. H. Day-to-day mental and physical health symptoms of older people: A report on health logs. *The Gerontologist,* 1983, *23,* 75–85.

Burger, P. C., and Vogel, F. S. The development of the pathological changes of Alzheimer's disease and senile dementia in patients with Down's syndrome. *American Journal of Pathology,* 1973, *73,* 457–476.

Busse, E. W., and Pfeiffer, E. *Behavior and adaptation in late life.* Boston: Little, Brown, 1975.

Butler, R. N. Psychiatry and the elderly: An overview. *American Journal of Psychiatry,* 1975, *132,* 893–900.

Butler, R. N., and Lewis, M. *Aging and mental health: Positive psychosocial approaches* (3rd ed.). St. Louis: C. V. Mosby, 1982.

Cadoret, R. J., Widner, R. B., and North, C. Depression in family practice: Long-term prognosis and somatic complaints. *Journal of Family Practice,* 1980, *10,* 625–629.

Chien, C. P., Townsend, E. J., and Townsend, A. R. Substance use and abuse among the community elderly: The medical aspect. *Addictive Diseases: An International Journal,* 1978, *3,* 357–372.

Coblentz, J. M., Mattis, S., Zingesser, L. H., Kasoff, S. S., Wisniewski, H. M., and Katzman, R. Presenile dementia: Clinical evaluation of cerebrospinal fluid dynamics. *Archives of Neurology,* 1973, *29,* 299–308.

Corkin, S. Acetylcholine, aging and Alzheimer's disease: Implications for treatment. *Trends in Neurosciences,* 1981, *4,* 287–291.

Crapper, D. R., Karlik, S., and de Boni, U. Aluminum and other metals in senile dementia. In R. Katzman, R. D. Terry, and K. L. Bick (Eds.), *Aging, Vol. 7: Alzheimer's disease, senile dementia and related disorders.* New York: Raven Press, 1978.

Cummings, J. H., Sladen, G. E., James, O. F. W., Sarner, M., and Misciewiz, J. J. Laxative-induced diarrhea: A continuing clinical problem. *British Medical Journal,* 1974, *1,* 537–541.

Dye, C. J. Psychologist's role in the provision of mental health care for the elderly. *Professional Psychology,* 1978, *9,* 38–49.

Eisdorfer, C., and Cohen, D. The cognitively impaired elderly: Differential diagnosis. In M. Storandt, I. Siegler and M. F. Elias (Eds.), *The clinical psychology of aging.* New York: Plenum, 1978.

Eisdorfer, C., Cohen, D., and Veith, R. The psychopathology of aging. *Current concepts.* The Upjohn Co., 1980.

Epstein, L. J. Depression in the elderly. *Journal of Gerontology,* 1976, *31,* 278–282.

Evashwick, C., Rowe, G., Diehr, P., and Branch, L. Factors explaining the use of health care services by the elderly. *Health Services Research,* 1984, *19,* 357–382.

Folsom, J. C. Reality orientation for the elderly mental patient. *Journal of Geriatric Psychiatry,* 1968, *1,* 291–307.

Folstein, M., Folstein, S., and McHugh, P. R. Mini-mental state: A practical method for grading the cognitive state of patients for the clinician. *Journal of Psychiatric Research,* 1975, *12,* 189–198.

Ford, C. V., and Sbordonne, R. J. Attitudes of psychiatrists toward elderly patients. *American Journal of Psychiatry,* 1980, *137,* 571–575.

Fraser, R. M., and Glass, I. B. Unilateral and bilateral ECT in elderly patients. *Acta Psychiatrica Scandinavia,* 1980, *52,* 13–31.

Freud, S. *Collected papers, Volume I.* London: Hogarth Press, 1924.

Gaitz, C. M., and Baer, P. E. Characteristics of elderly patients with alcoholism. *Archives of General Psychiatry,* 1971, *24,* 372–378.

Gallagher, D. Behavioral group therapy with elderly depressives: An experimental study. In D. Upper and S. Rose (Eds.), *Behavioral group therapy.* Champaign, Ill.: Research Press, 1981.

Gallagher, D. E., and Thompson, L. W. *Depression in the elderly: A behavioral treatment manual.* Los Angeles: University of Southern California Press, 1981.

Gallagher, D. E., and Thompson, L. W. Effectiveness of psychotherapy for both en-dogenous and nonendogenous depression in older adult outpatients. *Journal of Gerontology,* 1983, *38,* 707–712.

Geriscope. *Geriatrics,* 1972, *27,* 120–125.

German, P. S., Shapiro, S., and Skinner, E. A. Mental health of the elderly. *Journal of the American Geriatrics Society,* 1985, *33,* 246–252.

Gerner, R. Depression in the elderly. In O. Kaplan (Ed.), *Psychopathology of aging.* New York: Academic Press, 1979.

Gurin, G., Veroff, J., and Feld, S. *Americans view their mental health*. New York: Basic Books, 1960.

Gurland, B. J., and Cross, P. S. Epidemiology of psychopathology in old age. In L. F. Jarvik and G. W. Small (Eds.), *Psychiatric clinics of North America*. Philadelphia: W. B. Saunders, 1982.

Gurland, B., Dean, L. Cross, P., and Golden, R. The epidemiology of depression and dementia in the elderly: The use of multiple indicators of these conditions. In J. O. Cole and J. E. Barrett (Eds.), *Psychopathology in the aged*. New York: Raven Press, 1980.

Hartford, M. E. The use of group methods for work with the aged. In J. E. Birren and R. B. Sloane (Eds.), *Handbook of mental health and aging*. Englewood Cliffs, N.J.: Prentice-Hall, 1980.

Heston, L. L., Mastri, A. R., Anderson, V. E., and White, J. Dementia of the Alzheimer's type: Clinical genetics, natural history and associated conditions. *Archives of General Psychiatry*, 1981, *38*, 1085–1090.

Hiatt, L. G. Disorientation is more than a state of mind. *Nursing Homes*, 1980, *29*, 30–36.

Hirschfeld, R. M., and Klerman, G. L. Treatment of depression in the elderly. *Geriatrics*, 1979, *34*, 51–57.

Holinger, P. C., and Offer, D. Prediction of adolescent suicide: A population model. *American Journal of Psychiatry*, 1982, *139*, 302–307.

Hughston, G. A., and Merriam, S. B. Reminiscence: A nonformal technique for improving cognitive functioning in the aged. *International Journal of Aging and Human Development*, 1982, *15*, 139–149.

Ingersoll, B., and Silverman, A. Comparative group psychotherapy for the aged. *The Gerontologist*, 1978, *18*, 201–206.

Kahn, R. L. The mental health system and the future aged. *The Gerontologist*, 1975, *15*, 24–31.

Kart, C. S., and Beckham, B. L. Black-white differentials in the institutionalization of the elderly: A temporal analysis. *Social Forces*, 1976, *54*, 901–910.

Kay, D. Schizophrenia and schizophrenia-like states in the elderly. *British Journal of Hospital Medicine*, 1972, *8*, 369–376.

Kiyak, H. A. Self-monitoring in a preventive dentistry program for institutionalized elderly. Final Report, Grant No. R23DE05235, to the National Institute for Dental Research, 1980.

Kleinman, M. B., and Clemente, F. Support for the medical profession among the aged. *International Journal of Health Services*, 1976, *6*, 295–299.

Kral, V. A. Somatic therapies in older depressed patients. *Journal of Gerontology*, 1976, *31*, 311–313.

Kramer, M. The increasing prevalence of mental disorders: A pandemic threat. *Psychiatric Quarterly*, 1983, *55*, 115–145.

Kucharski, L. T., White, R. M., and Schratz, M. Age bias, referral for psychological assistance and the private physician. *Journal of Gerontology*, 1979, *34*, 423–428.

Kulka, R. A., and Tamir, L. M. Patterns of help-seeking and formal support. Paper presented at meetings of the Gerontological Society, 1978.

Langer, E. J., and Rodin, J. The effects of choices and enhanced personal responsibility for the aged: A field experiment in an institutional setting. *Journal of Personality and Social Psychology,* 1976, *34,* 191–198.

Langer, E., Rodin, J., Beck, P., Weinman, C., and Spitzer, L. Environmental determinants of memory improvement in late adulthood. *Journal of Personality and Social Psychology,* 1979, *37,* 2003–2013.

Lawton, M. P. Schizophrenia forty-five years later. *Journal of Genetic Psychology,* 1972, *121,* 133–143.

Lawton, M. P. Clinical geropsychology: Problems and prospects. In *Master lectures on the psychology of aging.* Washington, D.C.: American Psychological Association, 1979.

Lewis, M. I., and Butler, R. N. Life review therapy: Putting memories to work in individual and group psychotherapy. *Geriatrics,* 1974, *29,* 165–173.

Lipman, R., and Covi, L. Outpatient treatment of neurotic depression: Medication and group psychotherapy. In R. L. Spitzer and D. F. Klein (Eds.), *Evaluation of psychological therapies.* Baltimore: John Hopkins University Press, 1976.

McIntire, M., and Angle, C. The taxonomy of suicide and self-poisoning. In C. Wells and J. Stuart (Eds.), *Self-destructive behavior in children and adolescents.* New York: Van Nostrand Reinhold, 1981.

McIntosh, J. L. Suicide among the elderly: Levels and trends. *American Journal of Orthopsychiatry,* 1985, *55,* 288–293.

Markides, K. S. Minority status, aging, and mental health. *International Journal of Aging and Human Development,* 1986, *23,* 285–300.

Mattis, S. Mental status examination for organic mental syndrome in the elderly patient. In R. Bellack and B. Karasu (Eds.), *Geriatric psychiatry.* New York: Grune and Stratton, 1976.

Merrill, G. G. How to help patients with retirement depression. *Medical Times,* 1978, *106,* 10D–16D.

Mignogna, M. J. Integrity versus despair: The treatment of depression in the elderly. *Clinical Therapeutics,* 1986, *8,* 248–260.

Miller, M. *Suicide after sixty: The final alternative.* New York: Springer, 1979.

Mintz, J., Steuer, J., and Jarvik, L. Psychotherapy with depressed elderly patients: Research considerations. *Journal of Consulting and Clinical Psychology,* 1981, *49,* 542–548.

Mishara, B. L. Geriatric patients who improve in token economy and general milieu treatment programs: A multivariate analysis. *Journal of Consulting and Clinical Psychology,* 1978, *46,* 1340–1348.

Moore, R. A. The prevalence of alcoholism in a community general hospital. *American Journal of Psychiatry,* 1971, *128,* 638–639.

Morrant, J. C. A. Medicines and mental illness in old age. *Canadian Psychiatric Association Journal,* 1975, *20,* 309–312.

National Center for Health Statistics. Advance report of final mortality statistics: 1980. *Monthly Vital Statistics Report,* 1983, *32* (Supplement).

National Center for Health Statistics, Public Health Service. *Vital statistics of the U.S., 1979,*

(Volume II, Mortality, Part A). Washington, D.C.: U.S. Government Printing Office, DHHS Publication Number (PHS) 84-1101, 1984.

O'Shea, B., Lynch, T., Falvey, J., O'Mahoney, G. Electroconvulsive therapy and cognitive improvement in a very elderly depressed patient. *British Journal of Psychiatry*, 1987, *150*, 255–257.

Peppard, N. R. Effective design of special care units. *Provider*, 1986, 14–17.

Perl, D. P., and Brody, A. R. Alzheimer's disease: X-ray spectrometric evidence of aluminum accumulation in neurofibrillary tangle-bearing neurons. *Science*, 1980, *208*, 297–299.

Pfeiffer, E. Psychotherapy with elderly patients. *Postgraduate Medicine*, 1971, *50*, 254–258.

Pfeiffer, E., and Busse, E. W. Mental disorders in later life: Affective disorders; paranoid, neurotic, and situational reactions. In E. W. Busse and E. Pfeiffer (Eds.), *Mental illness in later life*. Washington, D.C.: American Psychiatric Association, 1973.

Post, F. The functional psychoses. In A. D. Isaacs and F. Post (Eds.), *Studies in geriatric psychiatry*. New York: John Wiley and Sons, 1978.

Rabins, P. V. Establishing Alzheimer's disease units in nursing homes: Pros and cons. *Hospital and Community Psychiatry*, 1986, *37*, 120–121.

Redick, R., and Taube, C. Demography and mental health care of the aged. In J. E. Birren and R. B. Sloane (Eds.), *Handbook of mental health and aging*. Englewood Cliffs, N.J.: Prentice-Hall, 1980.

Reisberg, B., Ferris, S. H., De Leon, M. J., and Crook, T. The Global Deterioration Scale for assessment of primary degenerative dementia. *American Journal of Psychiatry*, 1982, *139*, 1136–1139.

Rickards, L. R. Mental health services for the elderly: Block grant impact. Paper presented at meetings of the American Psychological Association, 1985.

Ringler, R. L. Aging perspectives. In N. E. Miller and G. D. Cohen (Eds.), *Clinical aspects of Alzheimer's disease and senile dementia*. New York: Raven Press, 1981.

Romaniuk, M., McAuley, W. J., and Arling, G. An examination of the prevalence of mental disorders among elderly in the community. *Journal of Abnormal Psychology*, 1983, *92*, 458–467.

Rosin, A. J., and Glatt, M. M. Alcohol excess in the elderly. *Quarterly Journal of Alcoholism*, 1971, *32*, 53–59.

Ryan, C., and Butters, N. Further evidence for a continuum of impairment encompassing male alcoholic Korsakoff patients and chronic alcoholic men. *Alcoholism: Clinical and Experimental Research*, 1980, *4*, 190–198.

Salzman, C. (Ed.). *Clinical geriatric psychopharmacology*. New York: McGraw-Hill, 1984.

Schmidt, G. L. Depression in the elderly. *Wisconsin Medical Journal*, 1983, *82*, 25–28.

Schuckit, M. A. Geriatric alcoholism and drug abuse. *Gerontologist*, 1977, *17*, 168–174.

Schuckit, M. A., and Miller, P. L. Alcoholism in elderly men: A survey of a general medical ward. *Annals of the New York Academy of Sciences*, 1976, *273*, 558–571.

Schuckit, M. A., Miller, P. L., and Berman, J. The three-year course of psychiatric problems in a geriatric population. *Journal of Clinical Psychiatry*, 1980, *41*, 27–32.

Schuckit, M. A., and Morrissey, E. R. Alcoholism in women: Some clinical and social perspectives with an emphasis on possible subtypes. In M. Greenblatt and M. A. Schuckit (Eds.), *Alcoholism problems in women and children*. New York: Grune and Stratton, 1976.

Shamoian, C. A. Assessing depression in elderly patients. *Hospital and Community Psychiatry*, 1985, *36*, 338–345.

Sholomskas, A. J., Chevron, E. S., Prusoff, B. A., and Berry, C. Short-term interpersonal therapy (IPT) with the depressed elderly: Case reports and discussion. *American Journal of Psychotherapy*, 1983, *37*, 552–560.

Siassi, I., Crocetti, G., and Spiro, H. R. Drinking patterns and alcoholism in a blue-collar population. *Quarterly Journal of Studies on Alcohol*, 1973, *34*, 917–926.

Small, G. W., Liston, E. H., and Jarvik, L. F. Diagnosis and treatment of dementia in the aged. *Western Journal of Medicine*, 1981, *135*, 469–481.

Smith-DiJulio, K., Heinemann, M. E., and Ogden, L. Diagnosis and care of the alcoholic patient during acute episodes. In N. J. Estes and M. E. Heinemann (Eds.), *Alcoholism: Development, consequences, and interventions*. St. Louis: C. V. Mosby, 1977.

Sperbeck, D. J., and Whitbourne, S. K. Dependency in the institutional setting: A behavioral training program for geriatric staff. *The Gerontologist*, 1981, *21*, 268–275.

Stenback, A. Depression and suicidal behavior in old age. In J. E. Birren and R. B. Sloane (Eds.), *Handbook of mental health and aging*. Englewood Cliffs, N.J.: Prentice-Hall, 1980.

Steuer, J. L., Mintz, J., Hammen, C. L., Hill, M. A., Jarvik, L. F., McCarley, T., Motoike, P., and Rosen, R. Cognitive-behavioral and psychodynamic group psychotherapy in treatment of geriatric depression. *Journal of Consulting and Clinical Psychology*, 1984, *52*, 180–189.

Subby, P. A community based program for the chemically dependent elderly. Paper presented at North American Congress on Alcohol and Drug Problems, San Francisco, 1975.

Talbott, J. A. A special population: The elderly deinstitutionalized chronically mentally ill patient. *Psychiatric Quarterly*, 1983, *55*, 90–105.

Terry, R. D., and Wisniewski, H. Structural aspects of aging of the brain. In C. Eisdorfer and R. O. Friedal (Eds.), *Cognitive and emotional disturbance in the elderly*. Chicago: Yearbook Medical Publishers, 1977.

Waxman, H. M., Carner, E. A., and Klein, M. Underutilization of mental health professionals by community elderly. *The Gerontologist*, 1984, *24*, 23–30.

Weeks, D., Freeman, C. P. L., and Kendall, R. E. Enduring cognitive defects. *British Journal of Psychiatry*, 1980, *137*, 26–37.

Weissman, M. M., and Myers, J. K. Rates and risks of depressive symptoms in a United States urban community. *Acta Psychiatrica Scandinavia*, 1978, *57*, 219–231.

Wells, C. E. Pseudodementia. *American Journal of Psychiatry*, 1979, *136*, 895–900.

Whitehouse, P. J., Price, D. L., Clark, A. W., Coyle, J. T., and De Long, M. R. Alzheimer's disease: Evidence for selective loss of cholinergic neurons in the nucleus basalis. *Annals of Neurology*, 1981, *10*, 122–126.

Wilsnack, R. W., Wilsnack, S. C., and Klassen, A. D. Women's drinking and drinking problems: Patterns for a 1981 national survey. *American Journal of Public Health,* 1984, *74,* 1231–1238.

Wurtman, R. J. Alzheimer's disease. *Scientific American,* 1985, *252,* 62–74.

Zarit, S. H. *Aging and mental disorders.* New York: Free Press. 1980.

Zimberg, S. The elderly alcoholic. *The Gerontologist,* 1974, *14,* 222–224.

Zung, W. W. K. Depression in the normal aged. *Psychosomatics,* 1967, *8,* 287–291.

Part IV

The Social Context of Aging

Throughout the previous three sections, we have identified how changes in the physical and psychological aspects of aging have diverse consequences for older people's cognitive and personality functioning and mental health. We have also seen how social factors (e.g., the presence of strong family and friendship ties) can affect physical changes (e.g., being at-risk for certain chronic illnesses) as well as psychological experiences (e.g., the likelihood of suicide). Within this framework of the dynamic interactions among physical, psychological, and social factors, we turn now to a more detailed discussion of the social context of aging and its congruence with older people's level of functioning.

Chapter 10 begins by examining the importance of informal social supports, particularly family, neighbors, and friends. In the Introduction, we saw how longer life expectancies, combined with earlier marriages and childbearing—which reduced the average span in years between generations—have increased the number of three- and four-generation families. The growth of the multi-generational family has numerous ramifications for relationships between spouses, between grandparents and grandchildren, between adult children and older relatives, and among siblings and other extended family members. Generally, these relationships are characterized by reciprocity, with older family members trying to remain as independent as possible. The normal physical and psychological changes of aging usually are not detrimental to family relationships, although caring for an older relative with a long-term illness can burden family members. Compared to the earlier years, late-life family relationships are more often characterized by losses that demand role shifts and adjustments. A widower may cope with the loss of his wife by remarrying, whereas a widow tends to turn to adult children and friends.

Friends and neighbors often perform family-like functions for older people. Because they are more conducive to reciprocal exchanges, they may be an even more important source of support for an older person than one's family members. As gerontologists have recognized the importance of friends, neighbors, and even acquaintances for older people's well-being, programmatic interventions have been developed specifically to strengthen these ties. Some of these, such as the use of neighborhood gatekeepers and mutual help groups, are briefly described in Chapter 10.

Where a person lives—the type of housing, age homogeneity of the neighborhood and community, and rural-urban location—affects their social interactions. Chapter 11 illustrates the importance of achieving congruence between older people's social, psychological, and physical needs and their physical environment. Relocation is an example of a disruption of this congruence or fit between the environment and the older person. Another illustration of a physical environment that no longer fits a person's social needs is when elderly in high-crime neighborhoods become so fearful of victimization that they dare not leave their homes. The extent of age homogeneity of a neighborhood can enhance older persons' social interactions and, in some instances, their feelings of safety.

Planned housing, homesharing, congregate housing, facilities with multiple levels of care, and nursing homes are ways to modify the physical environment to support older people's changing and diverse needs.

Throughout our discussion of the social context for aging, the effects of socioeconomic status on types of interactions and activities are readily apparent. Economic status is largely determined by past and current employment patterns and by the resulting retirement benefits. Chapter 12 shows how rates of labor force participation are declining among both men and women age 65 and over. These declines are due largely to the trend toward early retirement. Most people choose to retire early, provided their public or private pensions will enable them to enjoy economic security. Although most elderly apparently do not want to work full-time, many would like the option of flexible part-time jobs. For most people, retirement is not a crisis, although for people without good health, adequate finances, or prior planning, retirement can be a difficult transition. Accordingly, women, ethnic minorities, and low-status workers are most vulnerable to experiencing poverty or near-poverty in old age. The pressures on public financial assistance programs, created in part by the trend toward early retirement and the barriers to finding employment in old age, are further discussed in Chapter 18.

Chapter 13 examines how people's interactions change with age in terms of their leisure time, involvement in community, organizational and religious activities, and political participation. The extent and type of involvement is influenced not only by age, but also by gender, ethnic minority status, health, socioeconomic status, and educational level. Therefore, declines in participation may not necessarily be caused by age-related changes but instead represent the influence of other variables. Generally, involvement tends to be fairly stable across the life course; leisure and community activities and interests formed in early and middle adulthood are maintained into later life. This does not mean, however, that older people cannot develop new interests and skills. Many people form new roles and interests through senior centers, volunteering, clubs, political activism, and continuing education programs.

Chapter 14 examines attitudes toward death and dying, with an emphasis on age differences in these attitudes. The process of dying, from both a theoretical and an empirical perspective, is considered. The impact of social and cultural values, as well as individual factors such as the relationship between the dying person and caregivers, are discussed in reviewing grief and mourning. Recent trends in an individual's right to die and the debates about active and passive euthanasia also are touched upon in this chapter.

Because of the predominance of social problems faced by older women and ethnic minorities, their special needs and some practice and policy interventions are discussed in Chapters 15 and 16. Economic difficulties experienced in young and middle adulthood by these groups tend to be perpetuated in old age. These are not isolated problems, but rather of increasing concern to gerontologists and policy makers, since women over age 65 form the majority of older people, and older ethnic minorities, although a small percentage of the total older population today, are growing rapidly.

The following vignettes illustrate the diversity of social interactions experienced by older people, and set the stage for our discussion of the social context of aging.

An Older Person with Limited Social Resources

Mr. Valdres, age 73, has been separated from his wife for 20 years. He lives in a small room in an inner-city hotel. Since he worked odd jobs all his life, often performing migrant farm labor, he collects only the minimum amount of Social Security. Some months he finds it very hard to get by and has only one meal a day. Although he is not in contact with his former wife or his six children, he does have a group of buddies in the area who watch out for one another and who get together at night to have a beer and watch TV in the hotel lobby. Although he has smoked all his life and suffers from emphysema, he refuses to see a doctor or any other staff at the downtown medical clinic. He also will not apply for any public assistance, such as SSI or food stamps, in part because he does not understand what these programs are, but also because he does not want government "handouts." The hotel manager keeps track of his activities and will occasionally slip him some extra money or food.

An Older Person with Extensive Social Resources

Mrs. Howard, age 78, lives with her husband in a small town. Most of her relatives, including three of her children and eight grandchildren, live in the area, and there are large family gatherings on Sundays and holidays. She is a retired teacher; her husband was a successful local realtor until he retired. Both retired in their early seventies. They have considerable savings; in addition, they always lived simply and frugally, saving for their retirement. They have lived in the same house for the past 42 years, and their home is well maintained and recently modernized. Mrs. Howard enjoys gardening, doing housework, reading, and visiting. In addition, she is very active in her church, serves on the Advisory Board to the Area Agency on Aging, and is involved in the town's politics. She also tutors children with learning disabilities. Her days are filled with housework, talking to friends, neighbors, or relatives, or helping someone out, whether a grandchild or neighbor. Despite all her activity, she occasionally complains of being lonely and useless.

An Older Person whose Financial Resources were Depleted by a Catastrophic Illness

Mrs. Clark, age 82, spent 18 years caring for her husband, who had Alzheimer's disease. During that time, she lost contact with many of her friends, withdrew from prior participation in her church clubs, and had to quit her part-time job. Determined to care for her husband at home, she was unaware of some of the services in her community that might have assisted her. Her children lived out-of-state, and kept urging her to place Mr. Clark in a nursing home. She finally agreed to do so after she could no longer manage his daily care herself. He was moved into an excellent nursing home nearby as a private pay patient, where he died nine months later. Prior to his diagnosis of Alzheimer's, Mr. Clark had often talked about how he never wanted to be kept alive by artificial means, but he had never put his wishes into writing. In the end, when he was hospitalized with pneumonia, Mrs. Clark was faced with the painful decision about whether to keep him on a respirator. The years that Mrs. Clark had devoted to caring for her husband left her not only socially isolated, but also financially devastated after his death. She had spent nearly all their savings on his care. At the age of 82, she was faced with selling the home they had bought 54 years ago when they were first married, and applying for public assistane through Supplemental Security Income.

These vignettes illustrate the importance of informal social support networks, both for an apparently isolated person in a low-income hotel and an older person still living with a spouse. We turn now to examining the role of family, friends, neighbors, and acquaintances in older people's daily lives.

Chapter 10

The Importance of Social Supports: Family, Friends, and Neighbors

As people age, the nature of their social roles and relationships change. Earlier chapters have described and the introductory vignettes have illustrated that the way older people interact in their social world of family, friends, and neighbors is affected by physical, social, and psychological changes. For example, with children gone from the home and without daily contacts with co-workers, older people lose a critical context for social involvement. At the same time, their need for social support may increase because of changes in health, cognitive, and emotional status. Such incongruence between needs and environmental opportunities can result in stress for some older people. In previous chapters, formal support systems characteristic of the larger environment, particularly the health care system, have been described. This chapter focuses on the informal social support systems of family, friends, neighbors, and acquaintances, how these networks can reduce some of the stresses of aging, and policy and practice issues posed by the use of social networks to deliver services.

The Nature and Function of Informal Supports

The importance of informal social supports in older people's lives has been noted in numerous studies (Sussman, 1985; Shanas, 1979; Lopata, 1973; Rosow, 1967). Informal reciprocal relationships are, in fact, a crucial concomitant of an older person's well-being and autonomy. A common myth is that older people are lonely and alienated from family and friends. Yet, even the most apparently isolated and vulnerable elderly person can usually turn to some informal network for information, finances, emotional reassurance, or concrete services (Cantor, 1975). Consistent with social exchange theory discussed in Chapter 3, most older people try to maintain reciprocity in their interactions with each other and with younger people. The elderly first use informal social supports to meet their emotional needs, and move to more formal relationships only when necessary. As suggested by the person-environment model, they draw upon these informal supports as a way to enhance their competence.

With cutbacks in formal services in the 1980s, gerontologists have become more aware of the critical roles played by informal relationships. Families, friends, neighbors, and even acquaintances, such as grocery clerks and postal carriers, can be powerful antidotes to some of the negative consequences of the aging process. For example, informal networks have been found to reduce the adverse effects of illnesses and stressful life events, such as bereavement and widowhood. Alternatively, loss of social support, through divorce or death of a spouse, can contribute to health problems (Asher, 1984; Berkman and Syme, 1979; Cobb, 1976; Heller, 1979; Raphael, 1977). For older people not tied into informal networks, their use of formal services and likelihood of institutionalization is generally higher (Kammeyer and Bolton, 1968; O'Brian and Whitelaw, 1978; Vicente, Wiley, and Carrington, 1979); their personally reported well-being tends to be lower (Tannenbaum, 1975); and their burdens of adjusting to widowhood can be greater than for those with strong social supports (Lopata, 1973). Having an intimate friend, for example, has been found to be related to high morale and less likelihood of depression, even during major role losses, such as a spouse's death (Blau, 1981). Given the importance of informal social relationships, ethical and policy questions have arisen regarding how responsibility for support of the elderly should be shared between formal and informal systems.

The family—the basic unit of social relationships—is the first topic considered here. We examine the rapid growth of the multigenerational family and how relationships with spouses, adult children, parents, grandparents, siblings, and gay and lesbian partners change with age.

The Changing Concept of the Aging Family

Contrary to the myth of alienation, the family is the primary source of social support for older people. Nearly 94 percent of people over age 65, similar to Mrs. Howard in the introductory vignette, have living family members (U.S. Senate Special Committee on Aging, 1986). The immediate family tends to be the major source of help during illness, whereas the extended family ties the elderly to the community (Shanas, 1979). Even when family members live far apart, the emotional bonds between them tend to be strong, creating what has been termed "intimacy at a distance" (Rosenmayr, 1977).

Of all persons over age 75 with functional disabilities, 60 to 80 percent are assisted by their families (Comptroller General of the United States, 1977). The family not only assists directly but also provides information and advocates to assure that older members receive community services. An illustration of the importance of family support is that nearly 10 percent of older people who live in the community would require nursing home placement if family members were not providing care. For every older person in a nursing home, two or more equally impaired elderly live with and are cared for by family. If these elders were institutionalized, the number of nursing home residents would triple (Brody, 1985). The availability of family is thus often a major determinant of whether an older person lives in a nursing home or in the community (Smyer, 1980). Persons without family ties, primarily the widowed and the very old who have outlived their other family members, are those most likely to be institutionalized (Brody, Poulshock, and Masciocchi, 1978; Maddox, 1976).

THE MULTIGENERATIONAL FAMILY

As noted in Chapter 1, the rapid growth of the multigenerational family is one of the most significant demographic changes affecting family members' interactions with their older relatives. Because of the increase in life expectancy and the numbers of old-old, along with patterns of earlier marriage and childbearing in some cohorts, families frequently span three or four generations, with many individuals who have both living parents and grandchildren. Already, about 40 percent of persons age 65 and over with children (which comprises 80 percent of all people age 65 and over today) are heads of four-generation families, although very few live in the same household. Of this group of elderly, 94 percent have grandchildren; 46 percent have great-grandchildren. From the perspective of adult children, 40 percent of those in their late fifties have a surviving parent, as do 20 percent of those in their early sixties, 10 percent in their late sixties, and 3 percent in their seventies. Another way of understanding these changing family dynamics is that 10 percent of people over age 65 have a child who is also over the age of 65 (Brody, 1981; 1985). Accordingly, some adult children of the increasingly numerous persons in advanced old age are themselves in their late sixties or seventies, and experiencing their own declines in energy, health, and finances. Given continuing technological and medical advances, these trends will undoubtedly continue.

The multigenerational family is, in turn, influenced by a number of social trends that affect interactions of family members across generations. Women's labor force participation has increased. Rates of divorce and remarriage and the consequent number of "blended families" have escalated. New and diverse family structures, such as communal living, cohabitation by unmarried couples, and gay and lesbian partnerships, have grown. Whether these various family forms will result in more or less obligation, commitment, or resources to meet the needs of older dependents is still unknown.

THE ROLE OF CULTURE

Cultural values also affect family interactions. American culture places a high value on the family's privacy and independence. What occurs within it is generally viewed as its private affair, not to be interfered with by government or other outside sources. Similarly, family members' independence from each other is emphasized. Offspring are expected to move away from childhood dependency and toward the independence of adulthood. As a result of this emphasis, family members' emotional interdependence tends to be overlooked. These values affect not only commonly held views of adult child-parent relationships, but also the right of the state to intervene in high-risk family situations, for example, cases of suspected elderly abuse and/or neglect. They also partially underlie the relative infrequency of multigenerational family households in our society. This contrasts with developing countries where three- and four-generation families, although a small percentage of the total population, are more likely to live together under one roof. It is within this context—the relatively recent growth of the multigenerational family, the Western cultural emphasis on family privacy, and the major social trends affecting the aging family—that we examine the diverse types of family relationships in old age.

Older Couples

The marital relationship plays a crucial support function in most older people's lives. As parental and employment responsibilities decline, having a spouse provides built-in companionship. Of all family members, spouses are most likely to serve as confidants and to provide support. More than half of the population over age 65 is married and lives with a spouse in independent households (U.S. Senate, 1985). Significant differences exist, however, in the living arrangements of older men and women. Because of women's longer life expectancy and fewer options for remarriage, 37 percent of women age 65 and older are married, as compared to 77 percent of men (see Table 10–1). Accordingly, women represent 80 percent of the elderly who live alone (U.S. Senate Special Committee on Aging, 1986) (see Table 10–2). The proportion of elderly who are separated/ divorced/never married is approximately 4.7 percent for men, and 5.8 for women (Kaplan, 1983). There are some variations among different ethnic minority groups. For example, a larger proportion of Blacks over age 65 than whites do not live with their spouses, because of widowhood, divorce, or separation. Other ethnic minority differences are discussed in Chapter 15.

TABLE 10–1 Marital Status of Older Males and Females

	Age 65 to 74		Age 75 Plus	
Marital Status	*Males*	*Females*	*Males*	*Females*
Single	5%	5%	4%	6%
Married—spouse present	80	49	67	23
Married—spouse absent	2	2	3	1
Widowed	9	39	24	67
Divorced	4	5	2	3

Source: U.S. Bureau of the Census, *Current Population Survey,* March 1984.

TABLE 10–2 Living Arrangements of Older Males and Females

	Age 65 to 74		Age 75 Plus	
Living Arrangement	*Males*	*Females*	*Males*	*Females*
Not in household	2%	1%	8%	13%
Living alone	12	36	19	42
Living in household with someone else	7	15	8	24
Living in household with spouse present	78	49	65	21

Source: U.S. Bureau of the Census, *Current Population Survey,* March 1983.

Couples are faced with learning to adapt to changing roles and expectations throughout marriage. Family life is characterized by a continual tension between maintaining individual autonomy and negotiating issues of equitable exchange and dependence. Such tensions may be heightened in old age. As partners change roles through retirement, post-parenthood, or illness, they face the strain of relinquishing previous roles and adapting to new ones. Couples today experience a post-childrearing period of perhaps 20 to 40 years, ranging from late maturity to frailty, and must renegotiate their marital expectations and roles in light of their changed family structure. Failure to negotiate role expectations and consequent disagreements tend to be associated with feelings of inequity and depression in older spouses (Holahan, 1984). One of the most difficult transitions can be retirement, particularly when wives consider it their responsibility to plan for their husbands' retirement or when couples have difficulty working out time to be apart from one another (Keating and Cole, 1980).

Such strains tend to be heightened by the fact that long-lived relationships are a contemporary phenomenon. At the end of the nineteenth century, the average length of marriage at the time one spouse died was about 28 years; now it is over 43 years (Troll, 1986). Never before in history have the lives of so many couples remained interwoven long enough to encounter the variety of life-changing events that later stages of marriage now bring. Most older couples were not socialized for handling the associated stresses. Yet they are more likely than younger cohorts to view marriage as a lifetime commitment governed by obligation.

MARITAL SATISFACTION

Despite these potential tensions, most older partners appear satisfied, with men tending to be more satisfied with marriage and the degree to which their emotional needs are fulfilled than are women (Gilford, 1984; Rhyne, 1981). Marital satisfaction has been found to be high among those recently married, lower among those in the childrearing period—especially in middle-age—and higher in the later stages,* although spouses of the younger and older extremes of old age (ages 52–62 and 70–90) report lower satisfaction than do spouses at the mid-state of old age (age 63–69) (Gilford, 1984). Many older spouses report that their marriages improve over time (Skolnick, 1981).

Increases in marital satisfaction among the young-old may be partially due to children leaving home. Contrary to stereotypes, most women are not depressed

---

*A word of caution is necessary in interpreting data on the increase in marital satisfaction in later age. Because most studies of marital satisfaction are cross-sectional, the higher prevalence of happily married couples in later life could be a result of greater divorce or separation at earlier stages among those who are unhappily married or of older cohorts' being brought up to be satisfied with less.

when their children leave home, but rather view the "empty nest" as new-found freedom and an opportunity for new activities. In fact, rigid sex-role expectations and behaviors are often relaxed in old age, with men often more affectionate and less career-oriented and women becoming more achievement-oriented (Livson, 1983), as illustrated in the discussion of personality styles in Chapter 8. This tendency for men to turn away from occupational interests and women to focus outward on employment will probably increase in the future. Successful negotiation of such role changes appears to be related to marital satisfaction. Happy marriages have been found to be characterized by more equality, through a gradual relaxation of boundaries between sex roles, and a decreasing division of household labor according to traditional male/female sex roles, although some areas (e.g., family finances) often remain gender-differentiated (Holahan, 1984; Troll, Miller, and Atchley, 1979). Freed from issues of control over children and with more opportunities for companionship, partners may discover or develop common interests and interdependence. As a consequence, expressive aspects of the marriage—affection and companionship—may emerge more fully (Dobson, 1983).

Older partners' ability to negotiate these role transitions depends, in large part, on their prior adaptability and satisfaction in their relationship. Studies of

Marital satisfaction plays an important role in the well-being of older couples.

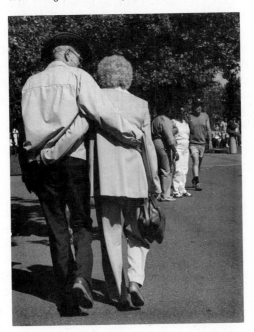

marital longevity have found that couples celebrating golden anniversaries (who form only 3 percent of all marriages) shared similar values and belief systems, were able to accommodate to one another, and viewed the spousal bond as their strongest source of companionship (Parron, 1982; Roberts, 1979–80).

For happily married older couples, their relationship is central to a "good life." Married persons appear to be happier, healthier, and to live longer than widowed or divorced persons of the same age (Brubaker, 1985; Gove, Hughes, and Style, 1983; Uhlenberg and Myers, 1981). In fact, marital satisfaction may be more important than age, health, education, or retirement in predicting life satisfaction for older women, and second only to good health for older men (Lee, 1978). These positive effects appear to emanate from three major functions that marriage performs for older couples: intimacy, interdependence, and a sense of belonging (Atchley, 1985).

Although most older couples have been together since young adulthood, a small proportion remarry after widowhood or divorce later in life. Women have fewer options to remarry, since they generally outlive their male peers, and men tend to marry women younger than themselves. Less than 25 percent of widowers aged 65 or older and less than 5 percent of widows every remarry. The divorced are more likely to remarry than are the widowed (Cleveland and Gianturco, 1976; Treas and Van Hilst, 1976). Having sufficient economic resources is an important consideration in remarrying. The major reason for remarriage for both men and women, however, is a desire for companionship. Avoiding loneliness and wanting someone to care for them are more important to men than to women (Vinick, 1978). Most older people who remarry choose someone they have previously known, with similar backgrounds and interests. Factors that appear to be related to successful late-life remarriages are: long prior friendship, family and friends' approval, adequate pooled financial resources, and personal adaptability to life changes. Remarriage is an especially complex event since both partners have a long prior family history (Brubaker, 1985). Many older couples choose to live together but not to marry, generally for economic and inheritance reasons (Sussman, 1985).

SPOUSES AS CAREGIVERS

With the increase in life expectancy, more older partners may end up caring for each other, frequently for long periods of time. A recent national survey found that 60 percent of primary caregivers to older people were wives of disabled, often older husbands. Of these caregivers, 73 percent were age 65 or older (Stone, Cafferata, and Sangl, 1986). Caregiving wives have been referred to as "hidden victims," experiencing isolation, loneliness, and role overload (Fengler and Goodrich, 1979). Older caregivers face not only the 24-hour responsibilities associated with caregiving, but also may be coping with their own aging, physical illnesses, or financial and legal burdens. These stresses may be even greater for recently married older couples who cannot draw upon a lifetime of shared experiences. In addition, few in-home services are available to support such efforts. The need for case management, education, support, and respite for older spouse caregivers has been recently recognized (Crossman, London, and Barry, 1981; Sommers, 1982). Such program needs are discussed further in Chapters 18 and 19.

DIVORCE IN OLD AGE

Although most older marriages are reasonably happy, a small percentage are not, and an increasing proportion of older couples are choosing divorce rather than tolerate an unhappy marriage. The percentage of persons age 65 and over who are divorced has doubled since 1960. In 1975, only 1 percent of all divorces involved individuals 65 years and over; in 1979, this had increased to 3.3 percent. Although late-life divorce is still relatively uncommon, 10 to 13 percent of persons age 65 and over have experienced a divorce (Brubaker, 1985; Uhlenberg and Myers, 1981), with the highest rates among Black older women.

The number of divorced older people will increase in the future; for example, it is predicted that one-third of those reaching age 65 between the years 2010 and 2014 will have been divorced at some time (Brubaker, 1985). The lifetime percentages of those who have divorced will be 15 percent for those born from 1910 to 1914, 25 percent for those born from 1930 to 1934, and 45 percent for those born from 1950 to 1954 (Cherlin, 1981). These increases may be partially explained by successive generations' acceptance of divorce as a solution to a bad marriage, and by an accompanying increase in remarriages. Remarriages, even for older couples, are themselves more likely to end in divorce than are first marriages. These trends affect the elderly's economic and social status. Being divorced in old age without remarriage often means economic hardships, especially for women, as well as diminished emotional support at a stage when other supports are also weakened. In general, divorced older persons are not as satisfied with their lives as married or widowed persons (Glick, 1984; Uhlenberg and Myers, 1981).

LESBIAN AND GAY PARTNERS

Research on gay and lesbian couples, estimated to be approximately 10 percent of the older population (Berger, 1984), is recent and limited. Generally, older lesbians have practiced serial monogamy throughout their lives, have viewed sex in terms of interpersonal relationships, and continue in later life to expect to find a new mate (Blumstein and Schwartz, 1983; Raphael and Robinson, 1980, 1981). The number of gay men with partners increases with age, peaking with 59 percent of those 46–55 years old. After age 60, gay couples decrease, because of death or the rejection of the notion of having a single, lifelong partner (Kelly, 1977). Older gay men have been found to be generally satisfied with their partners and their sex lives and report a greater sense of well-being than do younger homosexuals (Berger, 1982). For both older lesbians and gay men, sexuality apparently continues to play an important role in their lives. Both groups remain sexually active, although sexual frequency generally declines (Berger, 1982; Minnigerode and Adelman, 1978; Peplau, Cochrna, Rook, and Pedesky, 1978; Raphael and Robinson, 1980; Robinson, 1979; Wolf, 1982).

Some studies have suggested that lesbian and gay persons more easily adjust to aging than heterosexuals do, because they have coped with discrimination against sexual minorities. No one generalizable attitude toward aging among homosexuals has been found, however. Lesbian and gay partnerships tend to be characterized by more role differentiation, flexibility, and turn-taking than heterosexual relationships, characteristics which may ease their adaptation to age-related changes (Larson, 1982; Maracek, Finn, and Cardell, 1982–83; Peplau and Gordon, 1982). Older lesbians generally do not fear changes in physical appearance, loneliness, or isolation in old age as much as some heterosexual women do. Strong friendship networks of older lesbians have been found to be related to high self-esteem (Laner, 1979). Gay men, on the other hand, tend to be more concerned about age-related changes in physical appearance, although perhaps no more so than their heterosexual peers, and generally maintain positive feelings about their looks in old age (Gray and Dressel, 1985). Despite their expectations of loneliness, most gay men have closer friendship ties in old age than do heterosexual men (Friend, 1980). For many gay men, friendships may replace the family ties disrupted by declaration of their homosexuality.

A number of structural and legal barriers face homosexual couples. For example, the partners of older gays and lesbians who are hospitalized or move into a nursing home may be denied access to intensive care units and to medical records. Staff may be insensitive to and ignore their partners, even limiting their visiting. Private space for conjugal visits for gay/lesbian couples in nursing homes is virtually nonexistent. Some institutions may admit only one member of a gay couple. Families may contest a gay or lesbian partner's right to an inheritance. Although heterosexual couples may also face barriers related to conventional values in society, it is clear that a number of service and research areas specific to older homosexuals need to be addressed.

NEVER-MARRIED OLDER PEOPLE

Less than 5 percent of the elderly have never married (Troll, 1986). Professionals tend to view the never-married elderly as lonely and in need of services. In some cases, this is true. Never-married women who gave up employment to care for their parents may be without adequate income or retirement benefits after fulfilling their caregiving responsibilities. Some research, however, suggests that lifelong nonmarrieds are not especially lonely in old age (Gubrium, 1975). They may have developed extensive social networks, either through their friends or extended kin. The availability of a confidant can be a buffer against loneliness (Simons, 1983–84). Never-married people appear more likely to develop the self-reliance helpful to coping with aging.

An increasing number of organizations specifically for single people have formed, although many of these are for younger singles. Alternative living arrangements, such as share-a-home programs, may also appeal to some single elderly who choose not to continue to live alone.

SEXUAL INTIMACY

Chapter 4 reviewed the normal physical changes that affect men and women's sexual response as they age. Social factors also influence an older person's sexual behavior. Myths, stereotypes, and jokes pervade the area of sexuality in old age. Unfortunately, societal expectations of reduced sexual interest may mean that older people stop sexual activity long before they need to. Contrary to the myths, many people in their seventies and eighties participate in sexual activities. In future years, these myths may change, as the media, gerontologists, and other professionals convey the message that sex is not only permissible but desirable in old age.

Perhaps more than any other aspect of life, sexual behavior is subject to cultural regulation. Societies set standards for what is sexually desirable and undesirable, normal and abnormal. The current cohort of older people grew up in periods of restrictive guidelines regarding appropriate sexual behavior. They are now faced with new values, often dictated by the mass media, of openness and freedom of sexual expression. Older persons are told that sex is great exercise and an antidote to insomnia, depression, and loneliness! Yet this new ethic of openness can be as difficult to live with as the more restricted sexual dictates of the past. It may unduly pressure older persons, who were raised during more puritanical periods, and in whom references to sexuality may arouse feelings of shame and guilt. In dealing with older people's sexuality, practitioners need to be sensitive to their clients' values and to support their making their own choices about sexual behavior and sexuality—even if these contradict what is currently in vogue.

In professional work with older partners, definitions of sexuality need to be broadened beyond sexual intercourse. Sexuality may be defined as a deep, pervasive aspect of the total person—the sum of an individual's feelings and behaviors as male or female (Murray and Zentner, 1979). A variety of behaviors, such as touching, kissing, hugging, and lying side by side, can contribute to sexual intimacy and satisfaction, even for institutionalized older persons. Many of the current cohort of elderly grew up with taboos relating not only to intercourse, but to other forms of sexual activity, such as masturbation. Hence, older persons may need encouragement from professional counselors or others if they are to be free to affirm their sexuality and to experience intimacy with others. Professionals also need to be sensitive to the importance of touching older people—a hand clasp or back rub, for example—especially in homebound and institutional settings.

Sibling Relationships

Research on sibling relationships in later life is limited, compared to that in childhood and adolescence. The sibling relationship is generally characterized by long duration, a common heritage, and egalitarianism (Brubaker, 1985). Indeed, it is the only family relationship with the potential to last a lifetime. Most older people have siblings; the percentage identified by various studies ranges from 75 to 93 percent (Bild and Havighurst, 1976; Cicirelli, 1981; Shanas, Townsend, Wedderburn, Friis, Milhhoj, Stehouver, 1968). In one study (Cicirelli, 1982), individuals age 60–69 had a mean of 2.9 living siblings; those a decade older (70–79) had a mean of 2.2; and those over age 80, 1.1. Although the number of living siblings declines with age, even the oldest group still has an average of one living sibling.

Findings are mixed regarding the degree of closeness among siblings as they age. Studies of sibling proximity and contact have concluded that interaction decreases with age and is less common than with parent-child relations (Bild and Havighurst, 1976; Rosenberg and Anspach, 1973; Shanas et al., 1968). On the other hand, studies based on the criterion of feelings of closeness and affection suggest that with age, siblings often renew past ties and become closer, frequently through shared reminiscence. Siblings are particularly important sources of support in the lives of never-married older persons and after a spouse's death, at which time, some may share households (Shanas et al., 1968; Shanas, 1980; Ross and Milgram, 1982). Among persons with no children in Shanas's study (1980), almost 60 percent saw a sibling or other relative during the previous week, as compared to 40 percent of those with children. Contact is most frequently maintained by phone or face to face, not by letter-writing (Scott, 1983).

The strength and quality of sibling relationships also vary by socioeconomic class and sex. Frequent close companionship with siblings is more prevalent in working-class than in middle-class families (Allan, 1977). As with other kin-keeping responsibilities, women are more likely than men to maintain frequent contact with siblings. Ties of affection seem to be stronger between sisters than between brothers or cross-sex siblings. Sisters, in fact, report feeling closer in adulthood than when they were growing up (Adams, 1968; Cumming and Schneider, 1961).

Besides adult children and spouses, siblings are the most likely to provide an older person with emotional support and a permanent home (Cicirelli, 1981). The very existence of siblings as a possible source of help may be important, even if such assistance is rarely used. Siblings can also perform a socialization function in later life, acting as positive role models or as motivators to try new activities.

Current demographic trends may affect these relationships in future decades. As more couples remain childless or have only one or two children, siblings may become even more important supports. Greater longevity and better health among the current middle-aged cohort imply greater availability of living siblings in the future, with sibling relationships expected to strengthen. However, reduced fertility rates in the current period will mean that later cohorts will have fewer siblings on whom to rely.

The steadily increasing rate of divorce and remarriage will undoubtedly affect sibling relationships. With the increase in "blended" families through remarriage, there will be more half-siblings and step-siblings. For divorced older people who do not remarry, sibling interaction may become more important than when they were married. The degree of commitment to these new and varied relationships is unknown at this time.

Other Kin

Interaction with secondary kin—cousins, aunts, uncles, nieces, and nephews—appears to depend on geographic proximity, availability of closer relatives, and preference. Shanas (1980) found that about three out of every ten persons age 65 and over had seen a relative who was not a child, grandchild, brother, or sister during the previous week. Extended kin can replace or substitute for missing or lost relatives, and are important temporarily for family rituals and holidays. Personal or historical connections that allow for remembering pleasurable events may be more important than closeness of kinship in determining interactions.

Relationships with Adult Children

After spouses, adult children are the most important source of support and social contact in old age. The majority of persons age 65 and over live near their children, sharing a social life but not their homes. Most elderly state that they prefer not to live with their children, generally for reasons of privacy and a sense of autonomy. (This stated preference may, at times, represent a socially acceptable response, consistent with our cultural value of independence [Rosenthal, 1986]). Although less than 20 percent of older persons live in their children's households, this percentage increases with advancing age and for widowed, separated, and divorced elderly. Approximately 33 percent of all men, and 50 percent of all women age 65 and over who are widowed, separated, or divorced share a home with their children. However, less than 3 percent of older people live in multigenerational households composed of parents, children, and grandchildren (U.S. Senate, 1985).

Although most older parents and adult children do not live together, they nevertheless see each other frequently. Studies over the past two decades have consistently found that approximately 80 percent of older people with children live less than an hour away from at least one child; 50 percent have at least one child within ten minutes of their home; and 84 percent see an adult child at least once a week (Shanas et al., 1968; Shanas, 1979; 1980). The numbers and importance of children who live at a distance have received relatively little attention from researchers. A secondary analysis of a 1968 study found that almost 50 percent of older parents had at least one child living over 150 miles away, and 33 percent had at least one child living over 500 miles away. Those in the latter group saw each other about once a year compared to weekly visits of those within 10 miles (Schooler, 1979). More research is needed on adult children and parent interactions across a geographic distance.

Geographic separation of family members is generally due to mobility of the adult children, not of the elderly. Future cohorts of elderly may have an increasing proportion of distant children because of the growing trend toward greater residential separation between adult children and older parents (Treas, 1981). However, proximity does not appear to affect the quality of parent-child relationships (Lee and Ellithorpe, 1982). Instead, socioemotional distance seems more important than geographic distance (Shanas, 1979), and most adult children feel "close" to their older parents despite geographic distance (Cicirelli, 1981; Litwak, 1981).

In sum, studies have repeatedly found that most people over age 65 are integral members of family networks, see their adult children at least several times a week, and interact regularly by telephone or letter with relatives who live at a geographic distance. Less is known, however, about the quality of these interactions; that is, the extent to which visits are characterized by feelings of obligation rather than by genuine enjoyment and affection for the older parent. Research evidence regarding the relationship between family ties and life satisfaction is also mixed (Johnson and Bursk, 1977; Hess and Waring, 1978; Leigh, 1982).

PATTERNS OF INTERGENERATIONAL ASSISTANCE

Generally, families establish a pattern of reciprocal support between older and younger members that continues throughout an individual's lifetime. Consistent with social exchange theory discussed in Chapter 3 (Dowd, 1980; Sussman, 1985), the rule of exchange is from those with more valued resources (e.g., money, good health) to those with less. Not only concrete assistance is exchanged, but also emotional and social support (Mitchell and Register, 1984). At various points, older parents provide substantial support, especially financial assistance to their children and grandchildren, oftentimes at a geographic distance (Schorr, 1980). Parents, for example, are the most important source of support in coping with adult children's early widowhood and grief (Bankoff, 1983). In Shanas's national study (1980), 70 percent of older persons with children reported they gave help to their children, 70 percent to their grandchildren, and 50 percent to their great-grandchildren. At the same time, 70 percent reported receiving aid from their children. Older parents who are faced with chronic health conditions and thereby lose valued exchange resources are the most likely to become dependent on younger family members' help. Norms of family responsibility—that adult children should help their parents—thus become operationalized in actual caregiving behavior (Brody, 1985). As noted earlier, families provide approximately 80 percent of the in-home care for persons age 75 and over with severe chronic impairments (Comptroller General of the United States, 1977).

A common myth in our society is that families do not care for their older relatives as well as they did in the "good old days." As we saw in Chapter 2, older relatives at the turn of the century were rare and valued because of their economic contributions to the family. Yet nowadays, adult children provide more care and more difficult care to parents over much longer periods of time than they did when life expectancy was 47 years and elders comprised only 4 percent of the population. For example, five million adult children are estimated to be caring for parents—a number that does not include those who have previously provided parent care or will do so in the future (Brody, 1985). Even though caring for parents is a predictable and nearly universal experience, most people are not prepared for it (Brody, 1985).

The primary forms of assistance are emotional support, financial aid, instrumental activities inside and outside the home (e.g., transportation, meal preparation, shopping, housework), personal care (e.g., bathing, feeding, dressing), and mediating with agencies to obtain services. The type of familial assistance given is largely determined by the older member's functional level and the caregiver's gender (Spivak, Haskins, and Capitman, 1984). For example, personal care and instrumental services are most often performed by wives or daughters.

Responsibilities are usually differentiated by gender; approximately 80 percent of the family caregivers to chronically ill elderly are women (Brody, 1985). Nearly 29 percent of both primary and secondary caregivers are daughters, 23 percent wives, and 20 percent more distant female relatives or female nonrelatives, although wives and husbands constitute the majority of the sole or primary caregivers (Older Women's League, 1986; Stone, Cafferata, and Sangl, 1986). Within the female kin network, a hierarchy of preference exists, based on the centrality of the caregiver's relationship to the older person and on geographic proximity (Spivak et al., 1984). Wives are favored over all others. If the older person is unmarried, widowed, or has an ill spouse, then an adult daughter or daughter-in-law is commonly the primary caregiver. If a spouse or child is unavailable, then a sister is primarily responsible. If none of these are available, a female member of the extended family—such as a niece or a granddaughter—assumes responsibility. Even when older persons move in with the eldest son, as in East Indian and Japanese culture, the daughter-in-law is generally still the caregiver.

The prominence of women in the caregiving role should not obscure the efforts of men who are responsible relatives, or what Brody (1985) calls the "unsung heroes." But studies consistently show that men rarely provide the primary personal care; rather, they tend to assist indirectly, such as with finances. As a rule, men become involved in daily personal care and instrumental tasks only when no female relative is available. Similarly, sons in American culture are much less likely than daughters to share their household with a dependent parent (Brody and Schoonover, 1986). Even when sons are involved in similar tasks as daughters, they tend to have less stressful caregiving experiences than daughters (Horowitz, 1985).

Relationships between adult children and aging parents vary by socio-economic class. In general, middle-class adult children are more concerned with maintaining boundaries between themselves and their older parents, whereas working-class children tend to take an active role and to be more directive with their older parents (Lieberman, 1978). Likewise, middle-class adult children generally provide more emotional support and financial aid, and working-class children furnish more services (Rosenthal, 1986). Women from higher socio-economic backgrounds frequently assume a "care-manager" role, where they identify needed services and manage their provision by others, often formal service providers. Lower socioeconomic class women are more likely to be "care-providers," performing the care tasks themselves (Archbold, 1983). Usually, of course, caregivers with higher incomes have more flexible options in obtaining services for older relatives than lower income adult children.

The extent to which ethnicity rather than socioeconomic status influences intergenerational relationships is unclear. In western European cultures, both young and old view maintaining independence as a high priority. This value on individual independence is believed to underlie the lack of respect accorded to many older people of western European descent (Weeks and Cueller, 1981). In contrast, some studies have found that older Blacks and Hispanics enjoy an advantaged position in the extended family, where there is a cultural tradition of reaching out to others (Shimkin, Shimkin, and Frate, 1975; McAdoo, 1982; Dowd and Bengtson, 1978). Early studies, however, may have idealized ethnic minority families, overemphasizing the extent of support given to older parents (Rosenthal, 1983; Jackson, 1980; Nydegger, 1983). Intergenerational households among Blacks, for example, may develop from economic necessity rather than from choice, with grandparents often providing daily care and financial assistance to grandchildren. Although more caregiving exists in Black families than in white families, it is often given down the generational line, to children and grandchildren (Mutran and Skinner, 1981). In such instances where the kin network is an economic "safety net," greater interaction may not necessarily mean satisfying family life (Nydegger, 1983).

Considerable variability exists within as well as among ethnic minority groups (Nydegger, 1983). In traditional Asian-American families, the value system emphasizes the importance of the family unit rather than individual gain and independence. However, such values of family obligation are increasingly difficult to implement in a competitive, mobile society, particularly when adult children move into a higher social class than their parents (Levkoff, Pratt, Esperanza, and Tomine, 1979). Many Hispanics have developed strong inter-generational ties mandated by both their cultural heritage and economic realities (Torres-Gil, 1976). But urbanization and modernization appear to have weakened patterns of intergenerational cohesion and support characteristic of Hispanic families in the past (Maldonado, 1975).

Similarly, some studies of ethnic minority families document a growing adherence to the majority culture's norm of "mutuality at a distance" (Tobin and Kulys, 1981). In some ethnic minority groups, endorsements for norms of filial obligation and multigenerational households, for example, are stronger among young and middle-aged adults than among older adults (Hanson, Sauer and Seelbach, 1983). This suggests the tempering of idealism, as adult children and older parents face the realities of impending caregiving and dependency. The effects of changing societal conditions and of socioeconomic class on ethnic minority families are areas requiring further research (Rosenthal, 1986), and will be explored further in Chapter 15.

DEMOGRAPHIC TRENDS AND ADULT CHILD-PARENT RELATIONSHIPS

A number of social and demographic trends are affecting adult child-parent relationships, particularly caregiving. One trend is the increasing proportion of older relatives compared to younger family members. The current cohort of frail elderly, raising children during the Great Depression, had a low birth rate, which resulted in a smaller number of adult children as potential caregivers. The ratio between family caregivers and care recipients fell from 3:1 in 1910 to 1.2:1 by 1973 (Treas, 1977).

Many contemporary middle-aged individuals, described as the "sandwiched" generation (illustrated in the box on page 314), are faced with a dilemma that is a relatively new phenomenon historically—the competing responsibilities of caring for parents and children, as young adults remain economically dependent longer, and as parents live longer (Miller, 1981). The "empty nest" is frequently filled by frail elderly and by grown children who cannot afford to leave home or who return home (Brody, 1985). Women, especially, face multiple demands. More women are employed than in the past; 62 percent of women between the ages of 45 and 54, and 42 percent of women between the ages of 55 and 64 are in the workforce (U.S. Department of Labor, 1984). However, employed daughters provide nearly equal amounts of care as nonemployed daughters, either directly or through purchased services (Brody and Schoonover, 1986). In addition, 90 percent of today's middle-aged married women have children of their own to look after, compared to 66 percent of those born before the turn of the century. These

---

Women in the Middle

A woman in her mid-fifties with teenage children and a full-time job, Annette had cared for both her parents. Her mother, crippled with rheumatoid arthritis, lived with Annette's family for five years before she died. Within a year, Annette's father suffered a stroke and lived with the family for three years before his death. Annette's teenagers had resented the amount of time she gave to her parents, and her husband became impatient with how little time they had alone together. They had not had a vacation in five years. Since family and friends were not interested in helping her with the care of her parents, Annette and her husband rarely even had a night out alone together. As an employed caregiver, Annette frequently missed work and was distracted on the job whenever she had to consult doctors or take her parents for therapy during normal business hours. She felt alone, isolated, and overwhelmed by the stress. She was physically and mentally exhausted from trying to meet too many demands, not knowing that some support services were available in her community, and feeling that she had to be capable of handling these responsibilities on her own. When her mother-in-law became too frail to live alone, Annette knew her family and job would suffer once again if she tried to balance household duties, a full-time job, and the care of both older and younger relatives.

"women in the middle" (Brody, 1981), the traditional caregivers to elderly relatives, may thus be juggling extensive family responsibilities in addition to employment and their own age-related transitions. Given the increasing mobility of our society, they also may be providing care at a geographic distance. Such women generally do not reduce the amount of assistance given, but manage their multiple responsibilities by maintaining rigid schedules, negotiating caregiving tasks around their employment, and giving up their own free time (Cantor, 1983; Lang and Brody, 1983; Horowitz, Sherman, and Durmaskin, 1983). Despite the inordinate amounts of care provided, many female caregivers still feel guilty for not doing more (Brody, 1985).

Another social trend that affects the adult child-parent relationship is the growth of "reconstituted families" as a consequence of divorce and remarriage. Adult children may thus be caring not only for their biological parents and for current parents-in-law, but, if previously divorced, may be emotionally tied to their former spouse's parents, especially through their children of the earlier marriage. Such ties may lead to caregiving responsibilities for former parents-in-law as well. Difficult definitions of family membership and loyalties may complicate the distribution of time, attention, and financial resources across generations.

More elderly parents are experiencing the divorce of one of their adult children. About 25 percent of all persons who married in 1970, for example, had ended their marriages in divorce by 1977, and the phenomenon of "serial monogamy," persons having a series of divorces and remarriages throughout their lives, has also increased (Tiger, 1978). While undergoing the stresses of divorce, adult children may not have the emotional stamina nor time to assist their older parents (Smyer and Hofland, 1982). Their divorce also can affect their older parents' life satisfaction. For example, elderly parents have been found to react with feelings of loss and sadness to the stress of their adult child's divorce (Eckles, 1981; Pearson, 1986).

The Stresses of Caregiving

Most women are willing to assume primary caregiving responsibility, despite the physical, financial, and emotional costs (Cantor, 1983; Robinson and Thurnher, 1979). The caregiver's health, employment, personal freedom, privacy, and social relationships can all be negatively affected by providing care. The physical demands of providing daily personal assistance, such as changing bedding, are experienced most frequently by caregivers who live with the care recipient. Generally daughters, women comprise 74% of primary caregivers (Older Women's League, 1986).

Financial burdens include not only direct costs of medical care or hired help, but also indirect opportunity costs of lost income or missed promotions. Compared to male caregivers, women are more likely to quit their jobs or reduce their hours to provide care (Brody, 1985). As will be discussed in Chapter 16, those who interrupt employment to be caregivers generally receive fewer retirement benefits (Minkler and Stone, 1985).

The emotional burdens of feeling alone, isolated, and without time for oneself appear to be the greatest costs. Demands of elder care—in contrast to children, for example—are intensified by the lack of clear guidelines and information regarding care. Fortunately, the number of books, educational programs, and support groups for caregivers are growing (Hooyman and Lustbader, 1986; Silverstone and Hyman, 1982; Mace and Rabins, 1981; Bonjean, 1983). However, these supports cannot alter the fact that caregivers of the frail elderly, especially elderly with dementia, frequently face only increasing dependence, decline, and relentless physical care tasks, oftentimes for many years (Brody, 1985). In addition, funds for services to reduce caregivers' strains are limited. The lack of formal support resources heightens caregivers' feelings of isolation, and, in turn, of stress. In fact, feelings of burden have been found to be related primarily to the extent of social support, not to the severity of the illness (Zarit, Reever and Bach-Peterson, 1980).

In some cases, caregiving stress may become severe enough to lead to family breakdown, neglect, or abuse of the older person. Abuse can be psychological, financial, or physical. In some instances, elder abuse may be an inevitable outcome of stressful situations combined with inadequate caregiving skills (Kosberg, 1980; Quinn and Tomita, 1986). A growing number of states have passed laws requiring professionals to report familial abuse of the elderly. Unfortunately, for many older people, few community-based alternatives exist to remaining in the abusive situation. In instances of suspected abuse or neglect, the older person's right to self-determination and thus to refuse professional assistance is fundamental.

In sum, the myth of family abandonment of the elderly may be replaced by a new countermyth—that all families are able and willing to provide adequate care for older relatives (Cicirelli, 1981). This assumption has led to government policies that place greater responsibility on family caregivers, especially for the marginally poor elderly who are excluded from many low-cost or free services. In some ways, this is a return to the attitude of pre-Depression days, when families were expected to financially support aging relatives. In some cases, such as those involving elder abuse or inadequate financial and social supports, the family should not be expected to assume all caregiving functions. In most instances, the caregivers themselves are vulnerable, given that their average age is 57 years, that over 30 percent rate their own health as fair or poor, and that 30 percent have low incomes (U.S. House of Representatives, 1987). Unless family efforts are strengthened by formal support services, emotional, financial, and physical problems may be perpetuated across generations (Brody and Lang, 1982).

What Is Elder Abuse?

Five commonly defined types of maltreatment, often together referred to as abuse, are:

Physical or sexual abuse   Malnutrition or injuries such as bruises, welts, sprains, dislocations, abrasions, or lacerations

Psychological abuse   Verbal assault, threat, fear, or isolation

Exploitation   Theft or misuse of the person or the person's money or property for another person's profit or advantage

Medical abuse   Withholding or improper administration of needed medications, or withholding of aids such as false teeth, glasses, or hearing aids

Neglect   Conduct by the vulnerable adult or others resulting in the deprivation of care necessary to maintain physical and mental health.

INSTITUTIONALIZATION: A PAINFUL DECISION
FOR FAMILY MEMBERS

The strain on caregivers may cause them to seek relief through institutionalization of their older relatives. Most families first attempt to provide care on their own, without considering alternative community-based services. At the point of seeking nursing home placement, they may no longer be willing to explore community options (York and Calsyn, 1986), or the care needs have become more than the family and ancillary helpers can handle alone (Soldo and Manton, 1985). Although older persons without families are more likely to be institutionalized, 55 percent of those in institutions do have children. In most cases, children and spouses resort to institutionalization only after exhausting their own resources. In approximately 25 percent of nursing home applications, the decision to seek institutionalization has been precipitated by the family caregiver's illness or death (Teresi et al., 1980; Kraus et al., 1976). For example, the characteristics of the caregiver and of the caregiving context are better predictors of whether an Alzheimer's patient will be institutionalized than the illness characteristics or symptoms of the care receiver (Poulshock and Diemling, 1984).

Most older people and their caregivers hold negative attitudes toward nursing homes, and prefer home health care (Hatch and Franken, 1984). Placing an older relative in a nursing home is a stressful life event for the family, once referred to as the "nadir of life" for adult children (Cath, 1972). It may result in feelings of grief, guilt, shame, anxiety, fear, and hostility, and renew past familial conflicts. Most families, however, continue to visit their older relatives, and some experience an improvement in their relations with institutionalized members (Smith and Bengtson, 1979). Nursing home placement may relieve daily care tasks, but because of ambivalent feelings, may fail to reduce the perceived burden of caregiving. For instance, some wives spend almost as much time visiting their institutionalized husbands as they had devoted to caring at home. In response to such stresses, some nursing homes are developing support and educational groups for families (Richards et al., 1984; Gwyther, 1985).

Legal and Policy Questions
Regarding Caregiving

The role of adult children in caring for older relatives is an increasingly important policy and practice issue, given the trends identified earlier. The issue of family responsibility has long been a topic of debate. Many states have had filial responsibility laws that require financially able children to contribute to their aging parents' support, but the laws are rarely enforced. Social welfare policies have been organized on the premise that the family has first responsibility for dependent older persons, and that the state should intervene only after the family's resources are exhausted. For example, ours is the only industrialized society without a caregiver allowance as part of the Social Security system. Instead, many policy makers have feared that formal services to the elderly would displace families. Yet most families provide care without assistance; when they use services, it is in addition to their own care, not to replace it (Horowitz, Dono, and Brill, 1983; Weissert, 1985).

Since 1975, contrasting legislation has been introduced in Congress that either required adult children to financially support their older parents or, alternatively, supported family care through tax subsidies (Arling and McAuley, 1983). Recently, there has been increasing recognition that the costs of caregiving are too great for either the family or the state to bear alone and that policies are needed to complement family's efforts. Particularly promising is pending legislation such as the Family and Medical Leave Act. Introduced into Congress in 1987, this proposed legislation would give workers up to 18 weeks of unpaid job-guaranteed leave for the care of a dependent parent or a seriously ill or newborn child. A number of localities have initiated services to support families, either by decreasing the older person's needs for care (e.g., adult day care programs, in-home chore services), or by increasing the family's resources (e.g., educational and support groups, respite programs). Such services are described more fully in Chapters 18 and 19.

The growth of the multigenerational family and the consequent responsibilities of caregiving also have implications for practitioners. For example, family therapy has generally been based on a theoretical foundation that applies primarily to the nuclear family and considers the life cycle only through adolescence. In order to correspond to the reality that family life is no longer limited to the nuclear two-generation family, practitioners need to take account of the older person within the total family system, the effects of long-term family interactions, and each generation's developmental concerns.

Childless Elderly

Whereas the majority of older people have living children, approximately 20 percent are childless, and thus lack the natural support system of children and grandchildren. The adage that "children will take care of you in your old age" contains some degree of truth. A study of the interactions of childless older people found they had fewer social contacts than their counterparts with living children. When faced with health problems, the childless tend to become socially isolated (Beckman and Houser, 1982; Bachrach, 1980). In such instances, childless elderly turn first to their spouses for support, then to siblings, then nieces and nephews. The childless elderly also have a higher probability of living alone. Given these factors, it is not surprising that the unmarried childless utilize social services and nursing homes more than the married childless (Johnson and Catalano, 1981).

On the other hand, some childless unmarried elderly anticipate needing assistance in the future and cultivate friendships and ties with other relatives and service providers specifically for that purpose (Johnson and Catalano, 1981). If the number of childless couples continues to increase, the proportion of older people who are isolated and need formal assistance will probably grow in the future.

Grandparenthood

At the turn of the century, families with grandparents were rare. With the increase in life expectancy, more elderly are experiencing the role of grandparenthood and, increasingly, of great-grandparenthood. Of the 80 percent of older people with children, 94 percent are grandparents and 46 percent are great-grandparents. Approximately 75 percent of these grandparents see some of their grandchildren every week or two. Nearly 50 percent see a grandchild every day or so, although only about 5 percent of the households headed by older people include grandchildren (Smyer and Hofland, 1982). Geographic proximity appears to be more important than whether the grandparents get along with their own children in determining frequency of visits (Cherlin and Furstenberg, 1986).

Although the statistics convey the widespread nature of the role, comparatively little research has been conducted on the meaning and importance of grandparenthood to older persons, to grandchildren, and to the family system. The meaning and functions of grandparenthood must be viewed within the social context described above: increases in geographic mobility, divorce, reconstituted families, and employed middle-aged women who are also grandmothers.

Research findings on satisfaction derived from the grandparent role are inconsistent. Some studies have found the role to be peripheral and not a primary source of identity, interaction, or satisfaction. Instead, friendships and organizational activities appear to be related to life satisfaction more than the status of grandparenthood (Wood and Robertson, 1976). Other research has found that grandparents, especially grandmothers, derive great satisfaction from frequent interaction with their grandchildren (Kivnick, 1982).

Although most grandparents subscribe to a norm of noninterference in their grandchildren's lives, this is not necessarily detachment but rather self-reliance. In the absence of a family crisis, grandparents play a role that emphasizes emotional gratification from their grandchildren, and serves as a symbol of family continuity (Cherlin and Furstenberg, 1986). Geographic distance is not necessarily a barrier; grandparents who have close ties with their children may be important to their grandchildren even when they do not see each other often.

In a classic study by Neugarten and Weinstein (1964), elders were categorized by the meaning given to the role and by style of grandparenting. The prime significance of grandparenthood was reported to be (1) biological renewal and/or continuity (i.e., seeing oneself extended into the future); (2) emotional self-fulfillment, especially the opportunity to be a better grandparent than parent; and (3) distance from grandchildren, with little effect on the grandparents' lives. In terms of style, older grandparents were more apt to be formal or distant, whereas younger ones emphasized mutuality, informality, and playfulness. A later study identified grandparenthood as providing opportunities for feelings of immortality, for reliving one's life through grandchildren, and for indulging grandchildren (Kivnick, 1982).

The grandparenthood relationship appears to differ by sex, with grandfathers most closely linked to sons of sons, and grandmothers to daughters of daughters. Grandmothers have more influence than grandfathers on how their grandchildren relate to family and friends. However, it is unclear whether fathers who are more directly involved in parenting, rather than only as providers, will become more invested in the roles of grandfather and great-grandfather in the future.

Even less is known about how the grandparenthood role and its meaning vary by ethnic minority status. Some studies suggest greater interactions through an extended kin network and more grandparent responsibility for childrearing among ethnic minorities. When the child's mother is a single parent, the grandmother may have responsibilities essential to the child's care, especially in the Black urban community (Mutran and Skinner, 1981). Grandparent involvement in childrearing may be a consequence of teen-age pregnancy coupled with limited financial resources. It should be noted that these situations reflect differential opportunities of socioeconomic class, not ethnic minority status per se.

Rather than focusing on the role of grandparenthood as an individual attribute, recent research suggests that a systems perspective better accounts for the complexity of the grandparent-grandchild relationship. This perspective takes account of the relationships that exist between persons in a common kinship system, and recognizes that although nuclear families are becoming smaller, more members of more generations are alive at one time who share a greater part of each others' life spans (Sprey and Matthews, 1982). Although the grandparent-grandchild bond is initially mediated by parents, this bond becomes more direct as time passes, and can be substantially altered by events such as divorce. This potential for direct voluntary interaction between young adult children and their grandparents contributes not only to the individuals involved, but also to the total kinship system. As we will see in Chapter 17, direct involvement with elderly grandparents also affects attitudes toward aging and the aged.

THE EFFECTS OF DIVORCE

The growing divorce rate, discussed earlier, is a social trend that is affecting the meaning of grandparenthood. The fact that over 60 percent of divorced couples have at least one minor child (Spanier and Glick, 1981), and the phenomenon of divorce and remarriage throughout a person's lifetime clearly influence grandparenting. However, little consideration has been given to these consequences. Since the tie between young grandchildren and their grandparents is mediated by the grandchildren's parents, divorce disrupts these links, changes the balance of resources within the extended family, and requires a renegotiation of existing bonds. Who is awarded custody primarily affects the frequency of interaction with grandchildren; the grandparents whose child is awarded custody have more contact (Matthews & Sprey, 1984). Recent media coverage of grandparents' visiting rights and proposed state legislation to ensure such rights highlight the issues faced by grandparents when the in-law is awarded custody and controls the amount of child-grandparent interactions. A newly established group, Grandparents Anonymous, is pressing for grandparents' rights legislation in several states. Conversely, complex issues are also emerging concerning the liability of grandparents and step-grandparents for support of grandchildren in the absence of responsible parents. When divorce in the parent generation occurs, the norm of noninterference by grandparents generally disappears. Instead, grandparents, especially those on the side of the custodial parent, provide substantial assistance to their children and grandchildren, particularly when they live close by. Grandparents have been referred to as "the family watchdogs," who are in the background during tranquil times but are ready to step in during an emergency (Troll, 1983).

Little is known about step-grandparenting relationships. From a grandparent's perspective, the growing phenomenon of divorce-remarriage means sharing grandchildren with their newly acquired relatives under conditions in which grandchildren will be scarcer because of the declining birth rates. Grandchildren, in turn, may find themselves with four or more sets of grandparents. Kinship systems are further complicated by the fact that with the increased divorce rate, members of a grandparental couple may no longer be married to one another when they become grandparents. It is difficult to predict the magnitude of the effects—positive and negative—of these trends on intergenerational relations because of the limited research in this area.

In summary, the grandparent role is idiosyncratic and subject to negotiation (George, 1980). The role of valued grandparent is earned, and for some, it can bring considerable satisfaction (Troll, 1971). Furthermore, grandparents can play a major role within the extended family system during a family crisis such as divorce.

Friends and Neighbors as Social Supports

The estimated 5 percent of the elderly who are without family ties may nevertheless enjoy family-like relationships through contacts with friends and neighbors. Even "bag ladies" and occupants of single-room hotel-apartments, such as Mr. Valdres in our introductory vignette, generally have some friends and acquaintances to whom they can turn in emergencies. In fact, older persons who have kin may turn more to friends and neighbors for immediate assistance than to family, in part because friendship involves more voluntary and reciprocal exchanges between equals, consistent with social exchange theory described in Chapter 3 (Arling, 1976; Blau, 1981). Whether family, friends, or neighbors become involved appears to vary with the type of task to be performed as well as the helper's characteristics, such as proximity, extent of long-term commitment, and degree of interaction. Friends and neighbors may be better suited than family to perform some tasks, such as responding quickly in illness or emergencies because of their proximity and daily contacts (Litwak, 1985). Friends tend to help when it is convenient and the need for assistance is predictable (Adams, 1986). Providing transportation for an older friend is an example of a service that meets both criteria. Friends also often link the elderly to needed community services (Koser, 1981). For the most part, however, friends and neighbors play smaller roles in the long-term helping network; although they are important resources when children are absent or unavailable, their efforts usually do not approach those of family members in duration or intensity (Spivak, Haskins, and Capitman, 1984; Stoller and Stoller, 1983).

Research evidence of the contributions of friends and neighbors to morale are also mixed (Wood and Robertson, 1978; Ward, 1985). Some studies have found that friendships are associated with higher morale than are relationships with adult children. Older people who are part of well-defined friendship groups tend to have more positive self-concepts than those not part of such groups (Blau, 1981). Three explanations for these findings are: (1) people have more in common with age peers, (2) friendship is more rewarding because it is not obligatory, and (3) friendship involves older people in the larger society more than family relationships do (Adams, 1986).

Friends are often important sources of intimacy, while relatives other than marital partners usually are not (Simons, 1983–84). This is especially the case after major role transitions such as widowhood or retirement; for example, elderly widows generally prefer help from confidants because relatives may reinforce their loss of identity as "wife." Peer interaction can be an effective alternative to the marital, occupational, or grandparent role (Blau, 1981; Wood and Robertson, 1978; Rosow, 1967). The role of friend can be maintained long after the role of worker, organization member, or spouse is lost. The extent of reciprocity and quality of interaction, not the quantity, appear to be the critical factors in the maintenance of friendship networks. For instance, Lowenthal and Haven (1968) found that one intimate friendship with a confidant is as effective as several less intimate ones in preventing the demoralization often produced by widowhood and retirement.

Older people who refuse to leave their own homes and communities in order to join their adult children may recognize that friends are important sources of companionship, and that replacing lost friends can be difficult in old age. Most people experience a decline in the number of friendships over the years, although a small minority report an increase (Riley and Foner, 1968).

Types of social interaction have consistently been found to vary by sex. In general, women, such as Mrs. Howard in the introductory vignette, have more intimate, diverse, and intensive friendships than men, who tend to have more acquaintances. For many men, their wives are their only confidants, a circumstance that may make widowhood devastating for them. In contrast, women tend to satisfy their needs for intimacy throughout their lives by establishing close friendships with other women; when faced with widowhood, divorce, or separation, they can turn to other women for support (Lowenthal and Haven, 1968). Accordingly, widowed older women tend to receive more help from friends than married older women (Roberto and Scott, 1984–85). The resilience of some older women, in fact, may be rooted in their ability to form reciprocal and intimate friendships (Riley and Riley, 1986).

Both men and women tend to select friends from among people they consider their social peers—those who are similar in age, sex, marital status, sexual preference, and socioeconomic class. Most choose age peers as their friends, even though common sense would suggest that age-integrated friendship networks can reduce their vulnerability to losses as they age. A person's adult children are not likely to be chosen as confidants, primarily because of their being from different cohorts who are at different places in the life cycle and more likely to produce inequality of exchange. Age homogeneity plays a strong role in facilitating friendships in later life, in part because of shared life transitions, reduced cross-generational ties with children and work associates, and possible parity of exchange. Age as a basis for friendship may be most pronounced at those stages where the individual's ties to other networks are loosened (Hess, 1972).

Type of living environment clearly affects the quality and quantity of informal exchanges, as will be discussed in Chapter 12. Although the findings are mixed, most studies have found that age-segregated environments tend to lead to more peer group interaction, helping networks, and satisfaction with one's environment (Blau, 1981; Hochschild, 1973; Jonas and Wellin, 1980; Longino and Lipman, 1981). Age segregation, however, may not always be by choice but may result when younger people leave an area. In such cases, older people's length of residence rather than the homogeneity of the living situation may be more strongly related to extensive social ties.

INTERVENTIONS TO STRENGTHEN OR BUILD SOCIAL SUPPORTS

Because of the importance of peer group ties for the elderly's well-being, there have been an increasing number of professionally planned interventions to strengthen existing ties, or to create new ties if networks are nonexistent. Consistent with the person-environment model, such interventions are ways to alter the environment to be supportive of the older person. These interventions can be categorized as personal network building, volunteer linking, mutual help networks, and neighborhood and community development. A growing body of literature describes how to develop and implement such interventions (Hooyman, 1983; Biegel, Shore, and Gordon, 1984).

Personal network building aims to strengthen existing ties, often through "natural helpers"—people turned to because of their concern, interest, and innate understanding. Such natural helpers can provide emotional support, assist with problem solving, offer concrete services, and act as advocates. Neighbors often perform natural helping roles, and may strengthen these activities through organized block programs and block watches. Even people in service positions, often referred to as "gatekeepers," can fulfill natural helping functions, because of the visibility of their position and the regularity of their interactions with the elderly. For example, postal alert systems, whereby postal carriers observe whether an older person is taking in the mail each day, build upon routine everyday interactions. In some communities, fuel oil dealers and meter readers, who have occasional access to an older person's home, have been trained to watch

---

Gatekeepers

Mrs. Jones, 80, shuffled down the sidewalk with the aid of a cane. A boy delivering newspapers from his bicycle zoomed past, nearly hitting her. Mrs. Jones wasn't fazed. She moved on, staring straight ahead, as if she hadn't seen the youngster. Other incidents could have alerted a trained observer that Mrs. Jones was having serious trouble. She had difficulty signing her name on the back of her Social Security check when she cashed it at the bank. She couldn't count out change to pay for a cup of coffee at a local diner. When Mrs. Jones picked up her prescription at the local drug store, she had difficulty conversing with the pharmacist she had known for many years.

The Gatekeeper Project tries to address the needs of people like Mrs. Jones. The program identifies and trains Gatekeepers, people who are in contact with the public during the course of their regular work activities. In Mrs. Jones case, they could be the bank teller, the newspaper carrier, or the pharmacist. They are called Gatekeepers because they "open the gates" between isolated older people and sources of assistance, oftentimes by turning to Senior information and Assistance lines.

Washington State Aging and Adult Services Administration and Puget Sound Power and Light Company, 1986.

for signs that indicate needs for services and to refer the older person to the local information and assistance program (Washington State Aging and Adult Services Administration, 1986). Beauticians, pharmacists, ministers, bus drivers, local merchants and managers of housing for older people, as in the case of Mr. Valdres in the introductory vignette, are frequently in situations to provide companionship, advice, and referrals. In high-crime areas, local businesses, bars, and restaurants may have a "safehouse" decal in their windows, indicating where residents can go in times of danger or medical emergencies.

Churches may also serve to strengthen and build personal networks, in some cases providing a surrogate family for older people. Church members can provide help with housework, home repair, transportation, and meal preparation, as well as psychological assurance (Steinitz, 1980). In many private and public programs, volunteers are commonly used to develop family-like networks for the elderly. For example, volunteers have provided chore services in the elderly's homes, peer counseling, and senior center outreach activities.

Another approach aims to create or promote the supportive capacities of mutual help networks, which engage in joint problem solving and reciprocal exchange of resources. Mutual help efforts may occur spontaneously, as neighbors watch out for each other, or may be facilitated by professionals. They may be formed on the basis of neighborhood ties or around shared problems, such as widow-to-widow programs, stroke clubs, and Alzheimer's support groups (Gwyther and Brooks, 1984; Silverman, Brahce, and Zielinski, 1981; Mellon, 1982; Silverman, 1974). One example is the Mutual Help Model in the small town of Benton, Illinois, in which neighbors were organized to assist one another (Ehrlich, 1979). Mutual help groups can provide participants with new skills and roles, expand their social networks, and increase their problem-solving capacities.

Another approach is neighborhood and community development, which attempts to strengthen a community's self-help and problem-solving capabilities. An example is the Neighborhood Family in Miami, Florida, where older people in a low-income neighborhood worked together as a "family" to solve personal and community problems. This model combined social action with the provision of medical services (Ross, 1983). The Tenderloin Project, in a low-income area of single-room occupants in San Francisco, is another example of neighborhood development. The residents acted first on the immediate problem of crime and victimization of the elderly and then moved on to deal with issues such as nutrition and health promotion. In the process, social networks were strengthened and weekly support groups were formed (Minkler, 1986). Project LINC (Living Independently through Neighborhood Cooperation) utilized a combination of neighborhood-based intergenerational helping networks connected to the formal service system as a method to provide personal care services to the frail elderly (Pynoos, Hade-Kaplan, and Fleisher, 1984).

Relationships with Pets

For some older people, their pet may offer the most significant relationship in their lives. Many talk to their pets as if they were people, confide in them, and believe the pets are sensitive to their moods and feelings. Similarly, the loss of a pet can result in grief as intense as that precipitated by the death of a human (Carmack, 1985). The recognition that animals fulfill many human needs has led to an increase in pet-facilitated programs for older people living in senior housing and long-term care facilities. In such programs, animals have been found to evoke responses from persons who were previously nonresponsive (Robb, Boyd, and Pritash, 1980). Although a pet should never be viewed as a substitute for human relationships, gerontologists are increasingly aware that pet ownership can enhance well-being and enrich the lives of elderly in institutional environments.

Summary and Implications

The importance of informal social relationships for older people's physical and mental well-being has been widely documented. Contrary to stereotypes, very few

Pets can be an important source of comfort for many older people.

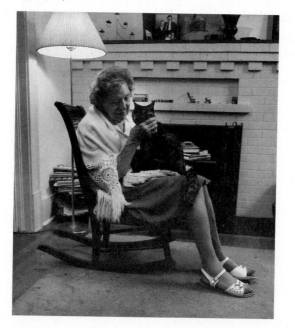

older people are socially isolated. The majority have family members with whom they are in contact, although they are unlikely to live together. Their families serve as a critical source of support, especially when older members become impaired by chronic illness or accidents. The marital relationship is most important, with more than half of all persons age 65 and over married and living with their spouse in independent households. Most older couples are satisfied with their marriages, which influences their life satisfaction generally. The older couple, freed from childrearing demands, has more opportunities to pursue new roles and types of relationships. The sexual relationship of older couples is limited less by physiological changes than by psychosocial factors, such as cultural definitions of unattractiveness and fear of failure. In general, most older people are able to enjoy sexual relationships, particularly when they are defined in terms of intimacy.

Little is known about sibling, grandparent, and other types of family interactions in old age. Comparatively little research has been conducted on lesbian and gay relationships in old age and on never-married older persons who may rely primarily on friendship networks to cope. The frequency of sibling contacts tends to decline with age, but siblings can be crucial in providing emotional support, physical care, and a home. Interaction with secondary kin tends to depend on geographic proximity and whether or not more immediate family members are available.

Contrary to the myth that adult children are alienated from their parents, the majority of older persons are in frequent contact with their children, either face to face or by phone or letter. Filial relationships are characterized by patterns of reciprocal aid throughout the life course, until the older generation becomes physically or mentally dependent. At that point, adult children—generally women—are faced with providing financial, emotional, and physical assistance to elderly relatives, oftentimes with little support from others for their caregiving responsibilities. In ethnic minority and lower socioeconomic status families, older relatives are most likely to receive daily care from younger relatives, and to be involved themselves in caring for grandchildren.

Most families, regardless of socioeconomic class or ethnic minority status, attempt to provide care for their dependent members for as long as possible, and seek institutionalization only when they have exhausted other resources. Such caregiving responsibilities are affected by a number of social trends. Most notable among these are the increasing percentage of middle-aged women—traditionally the caregivers—who are more likely to be employed, and the number of reconstituted families resulting from divorce and remarriage. The needs of caregivers are clearly a growing concern for health practitioners and policy-makers.

With the growth of three- and four-generation families, more older persons are experiencing the status of grandparenthood. Although most grandparents are in relatively frequent contact with their grandchildren, the grandparent role does not appear salient in terms of life satisfaction or identity. The demands of grandparenthood may be changing as a result of divorce and remarriages.

For many older persons, friends and neighbors can be even more critical to maintaining morale and a positive self-concept than family members. Generally, women have more interaction with friends than do men. Age-segregated settings appear to facilitate friendships, rather than isolating the elderly. In recognition of the importance of peer group interaction to physical and mental well-being, an increasing number of neighborhood and community-based interventions have been developed to strengthen friendship and neighborhood ties. In sum, the majority of older persons continue to play a variety of social roles—spouse, parent, grandparent, friend, and neighbor—and to derive feelings of satisfaction and self-worth from these interactions.

References

Adams, B. N. *Kinship in an urban setting.* Chicago: Markham, 1968.

Adams, R. G. A look at friendship and aging. *Generations,* 1986, *10,* 40–43.

Allan, G. Sibling solidarity. *Journal of Marriage and the Family,* 1977, *39,* 177–184.

Archbold, P. G. The impact of parent-caring on women. *Family Relations,* 1983, *32,* 39–45.

Arling, G. The elderly widow and her family, neighbors, and friends. *Journal of Marriage and the Family,* 1976, *38,* 757–768.

Arling, G., and McAuley, W. The feasibility of public payments for family caregiving. *The Gerontologist,* 1983, *23,* 300–306.

Asher, C. C. The impact of social support networks on adult health. *Medical Care,* 1984, *22,* 349–359.

Atchley, R. *Social forces and aging* (4th ed.). Belmont, Calif.: Wadsworth, 1985.

Bachrach, C. A. Childlessness and social isolation among the elderly. *Journal of Marriage and the Family,* 1980, *42,* 627–637.

Bankoff, E. A. Aged parents and their widowed daughters: A support relationship. *Journal of Gerontology,* 1983, *38,* 226–230.

Beckman, L. J., and Houser, B. B. The consequences of childlessness on the social and psychological well-being of older women. *Journal of Gerontology, 1982, 37,* 243–250.

Berger, R. M. *Gay and gray: The older homosexual man.* Urbana: IL: University of Illinois Press, 1982.

Berger, R. M. Realities of gay and lesbian aging. *Social Work,* 1984, *29,* 57–62.

Berkman, L. F., and Syme, S. L. Social networks, host resistance, and morality: A nine-year follow-up study of Alameda County residents. *American Journal of Epidemiology,* 1979, *109,* 186–204.

Biegel, D., Shore, B., and Gordon, E. *Building support networks for the elderly.* Beverly Hills, Calif.: Sage, 1984.

Bild, B. R., and Havighurst, R. J. Senior citizens in great cities: The case of Chicago. *Gerontologist,* 1976, *16,* Part II, 1–88.

Blau, Z. S. *Aging in a changing society* (2d ed.). New York: Franklin Watts, 1981.

Blumstein, P., and Schwartz, P. *American couples.* New York: William Morrison, 1983.

Bonjean, M. *In support of caregivers: Materials for planning and conducting educational workshops for caregivers of the elderly.* Madison: The Vocational Studies Center, School of Education, University of Wisconsin-Madison, 1983.

Brody, E. Women in the middle and family help to older people. *The Gerontologist,* 1981, *25,* 471–480.

Brody, E. Parent care as a normative family stress. *The Gerontologist,* 1985, *25,* 19–30.

Brody, E., and Lang, A. They can't do it all: Aging daughters of aged mothers. *Generations,* 1982, *7,* 18–20.

Brody, E., and Schoonover, C. Patterns of parent-care when adult children work and when they do not. *The Gerontologist,* 1986, *26,* 372–381.

Brody, S. J., Poulshock, S. W., and Masciocchi, C. F. The family caring unit: A major consideration in the long-term support system. *The Gerontologist,* 1978, *18,* 556–561.

Brubaker, T. H. *Later life families.* Bevery Hills, Calif.: Sage, 1985.

Cantor, M. Strain among caregivers: A study of experience in the United States. *The Gerontologist,* 1983, *23,* 597–604.

Cantor, M. Life space and the social support system of the inner city elderly of New York. *The Gerontologist,* 1975, *15,* 23–27.

Carmack, B. J. The effects of family members and functioning after the death of a pet. In M. B. Sussman (Ed.), *Pets and the family.* New York: Haworth Press, 1985.

Cath, S. H. The institutionalization of a parent: A nadir of life. *Journal of Geriatric Psychiatry,* 1972, *5,* 25–46.

Change. Newsletter of the National Support Center for Families of the Aging, P.O. Box 245, Swarthmore, PA 19081.

Cherlin, A. J. *Marriage, divorce, remarriage: Changing patterns in the postwar United States.* Cambridge, Mass.: Harvard University Press, 1981.

Cherlin, A. J., and Furstenberg, F. Grandparents and family crisis. *Generations,* 1986, *10,* 26–28.

Cicirelli, W. G. *Helping elderly parents: The role of adult children.* Boston: Auburn House, 1981.

Cicirelli, W. G. Sibling influence throughout the lifespan. In M. E. Lamb and B. Sutton-Smith (Eds.), *Sibling relationships: Their nature and significance across the lifespan.* Hillsdale, N.J.: Lawrence Erlbaum, 1982.

Cleveland, W. P., and Gianturco, P. T. Remarriage probability after widowhood: A retrospective method. *Journal of Gerontology,* 1976, *31,* 99–103.

Cobb, S. Social support as a moderator of life stress. *Psychosomatic Medicine,* 1976, *38,* 300–314.

Comptroller General of the United States. *Report to Congress: The well-being of older people in Cleveland, Ohio.* Washington, D.C.: United States General Accounting Office, 1977.

Crossman, L., London, C., and Barry, C. Older women caring for disabled spouses: A model for supportive services. *The Gerontologist*, 1981, *21*, 464–470.

Cumming, E., and Schneider, D. Sibling solidarity: A property of American kinship. *American Anthropologist*, 1961, *63*, 498–507.

Dobson, C. Sex-role and marital expectations. In T. H. Brubaker (Ed.), *Family relationships in later life*. Beverly Hills, Calif.: Sage, 1983.

Dowd, J. *Stratification among the aged*. Monterey, Calif.: Brooks/Cole, 1980.

Dowd, J., and Bengtson, V. C. Aging in minority populations: An examination of the double-jeopardy hypothesis. *Journal of Gerontology*, 1978, *33*, 427–436.

Eckles, E. T. Negative aspects of family relationships for older women. Paper presented at the Joint Annual Meetings of the Gerontological Society of America and the Canadian Association on Gerontology, 1986.

Ehrlich, P. *The mutual help model: Handbook for developing a neighborhood group program*. Washington, D.C.: Administration on Aging, 1979.

Fengler, A., and Goodrich, N. Wives of elderly disabled men: The hidden patients. *The Gerontologist*, 1979, *19*, 175–183.

Friend, R. A. GAYing: Adjustment and the older gay male. *Alternative Lifestyles*, 1980, *3*, 231–248.

George, L. *Role transition in later life*. Belmont, Calif.: Wadsworth, 1980.

Gilford, R. Contrasts in marital satisfaction throughout old age: An exchange theory analysis. *Journal of Gerontology*, 1984, *39*, 325–333.

Glick, P. C. Marriage, divorce, and living arrangements: Prospective changes. *Journal of Family Issues*, 1984, *5*, 7–26.

Gove, W., Hughes, M., and Style, C. Does marriage have positive effects on the psychological well-being of the individual? *Journal of Health and Social Behavior*, 1983, *24*, 122–131.

Gray, H., and Dressel, P. Alternative interpretations of aging among gay males. *The Gerontologist*, 1985, *25*, 83–87.

Gubruim, J. F. Being single in old age. *International Journal of Aging and Human Development*, 1975, *6*, 29–41.

Gwyther, L. *Care of Alzheimer's patients: A manual for nursing home staff*. Washington, D.C.: American Health Care Association and the Alzheimer's Disease and Related Disorders Assoc., 1985.

Gwyther, L., and Brooks, B. *Mobilizing networks of mutual support: How to develop Alzheimer caregivers support groups*. Duke Family Support Network Chapter, Room 153, Civitan Bldg., Duke University Medical Center, Durham, NC 27710, 1984.

Hanson, S., Sauer, W., and Seelbach, W. Racial and cohort variations in filial responsibility norms. *The Gerontologist*, 1983, *23*, 626–631.

Harris, L., and Associates. *The myth and reality of aging in America*. Washington, D.C.: The National Council on the Aging, 1975.

Hatch, R. C., and Franken, M. C. Concerns of children with parents in nursing homes. *Journal of Gerontological Social Work*, 1984, *7*, 19–30.

Heller, K. The effects of social supports: Prevention and treatment implications. In A. P. Goldstein and F. H. Kanfer (Eds.), *Maximizing treatment gains: Transfer enhancements in psychotherapy.* New York: Academic Press, 1979.

Hess, B. Friendship. In M. W. Riley, M. Johnson, and A. Foner (Eds.), *Aging and society, Vol. III: A sociology of age stratification.* New York: Russell Sage Foundation, 1972.

Hess, B., and Waring, J. M. Changing patterns of aging and family bonds in later life. *Family Coordinator,* 1978, *27,* 303–314.

Hess, B., and Waring, J. M. Divorce and the elderly: A neglected area of research. In T. Brubaker (Ed.), *Family relationships in later life.* Beverly Hills, Calif.: Sage, 1982.

Heyman, D., and Gianturco, D. Long-term adaptation by the elderly to bereavement. *Journal of Gerontology,* 1973, *28,* 359–362.

Hochschild, A. L. *The unexpected community.* Englewood Cliffs, N.J.: Prentice-Hall, 1973.

Holahan, C. Marital attitudes over 40 years: A longitudinal and cohort analysis. *Journal of Gerontology,* 1984, *39,* 49–57.

Hooyman, N. Social support networks in services to the elderly. In J. Whittaker and J. Garbarino, *Social support networks: Informational helping in the human services.* New York: Aldine, 1983.

Hooyman, N., and Lustbader, W. *Taking Care: Supporting older people and their families.* New York: The Free Press, 1986.

Horowitz, A. Sons and daughters as caregivers to older parents: Differences in role performance and consequences. *The Gerontologist,* 1985, *25,* 612–623.

Horowitz, A., Dono, J. E., and Brill, R. Continuity or change in informal support? The impact of an expanded home care program. Paper presented at meetings of the Gerontological Society of America, 1983.

Horowitz, A., Sherman, R. H., and Durmaskin, S. C. Employment and daughter caregivers: A working partnership for older people. Paper presented at meetings of the Gerontological Society of America, 1983.

Jackson, J. J. *Minorities and aging.* Belmont, Calif.: Wadsworth, 1980.

Johnson, C. C., and Catalano, D. J. A longitudinal study of family supports to impaired elderly. *The Gerontologist,* 1981, *23,* 612–618.

Johnson, E. S., and Bursk, B. J. Relationships between the elderly and their adult children. *The Gerontologist,* 1977, *17,* 90–96.

Jonas, K., and Wellin, E. Dependency and reciprocity: Home health in an elderly population. In C. Fry (Ed.), *Aging in culture and society.* New York: Bergin, 1980.

Kammeyer, K., and Bolton, C. Community and family factors related to the use of a family service agency. *Journal of Marriage and the Family,* 1968, *30,* 488–498.

Kaplan, J. Planning the future of institutional care: The true costs. *The Gerontologist,* 1983, *23,* 411–415.

Keating, N., and Cole, P. What do I do with him 24 hours a day? Changes in the housewife role after retirement. *The Gerontologist,* 1980, *20,* 84–89.

Kelly, J. The aging male homosexual: Myth and reality. *The Gerontologist,* 1977, *17,* 328–332.

Kivnick, H. *The meaning of grandparenthood.* Ann Arbor: University of Michigan Press, 1982.

Kosberg, J. Family maltreatment: Causality and practice issues. Presented at meetings of the Gerontological Society, November 1980.

Koser, G. *Enhancing and sustaining informal support networks for the elderly and disabled.* Albany: New York State Health Planning Commission, 1981.

Kraus, A. S., Spasoff, R. A., Beattie, E. J., Holden, D. E. W., Lawson, J. S., Rodenburg, M., and Woodcock, G. M. Elderly application process: Placement and care needs. *Journal of the American Geriatric Society,* 1976, *24,* 165–172.

Laner, M. Growing older female: Heterosexuality and homosexuality. *Journal of Homosexuality,* 1979, *4.*

Lang, A., and Brody, E. Characteristics of middle-aged daughters and help to their elderly mothers. *Journal of Marriage and the Family,* 1983, *45,* 193–202.

Larson, P. C. Gay male relationships. In W. Paul, J. D. Weinrich, and J. C. Gonsioreh (Eds.), *Homosexuality: Social, psychological, and biological issues.* Beverly Hills, Calif.: Sage, 1982.

Lee, G. R. Marriage and morale in later life. *Journal of Marriage and the Family,* 1978, *40,* 131–139.

Lee, G. R., and Ellithorpe, E. Intergenerational exchange and subjective well-being among the elderly. *Journal of Marriage and the Family,* 1982, *44,* 217–224.

Leigh, G. Kinship interaction over the family life span. *Journal of Marriage and the Family,* 1982, *44,* 197–208.

Levkoff, S., Pratt, C., Esperanza, R., and Tomine, S. *Minority elderly: A historical and cultural perspective.* Corvallis: Oregon State University, 1979.

Lieberman, G. L. Children of the elderly as natural helpers: Some demographic differences. *American Journal of Community Psychology,* 1978, *6,* 489–498.

Litwak, E. *The modified extended family, social networks, and research continuities in aging.* New York: Center for Social Sciences at Columbia University, 1981.

Litwak, E. *Helping the elderly.* New York: The Guilford Press, 1985.

Livson, F. B. Gender identity: A life span view of sex role development. In R. B. Weg (Ed.), *Sexuality in the later years.* New York: Academic Press, 1983.

Longino, C., and Lipman, C. Married and spouseless men and women in planned retirement communities: Support network differentials. *Journal of Marriage and the Family,* 1981, *43,* 169–177.

Lopata, H. *Widowhood in an American city.* Cambridge, Mass.: Schenkman, 1973.

Lowenthal, M. F., and Haven, C. Interaction and adaptation. *American Sociological Review,* 1968, *33,* 20–30.

Mace, N. L., and Rabins, P. *The thirty-six hour day: A family guide to caring for persons with Alzheimer's Disease, related dementing illnesses, and memory loss in later life.* Baltimore: Johns Hopkins University Press, 1981.

Maddox, G. L. Families as a context and resource in chronic illness. In S. Sherwood (Ed.), *Long term care: A handbook for researchers, planners, and providers.* New York: Spectrum, 1976.

Maldonado, D. The Chicano aged. *Social Work*, 1975, *20*, 213–216.

Maracek, J., Finn, S. E., and Cardell, M. Gender roles in the relationships of lesbians and gay men. *Journal of Homosexuality*, 1982–83, *8*, 45–50.

Matthews, D. H., and Sprey, J. The impact of divorce on grandparenthood: An exploratory study. *The Gerontologist*, 1984, *24*, 41–47.

McAdoo, H. P. Stress-absorbing systems in Black families. *Family Relations*, 1982, *31*, 479–488.

Mellon, J. *Support groups for caregivers of the aged: A training manual for facilitators.* The Natural Supports Program, Community Service Society, 105 East 22nd Street, New York, NY 10010, 1982.

Miller, D. The "Sandwich" generation: Adult children of the aging. *Social Work*, 1981, *26*, 419–423.

Minkler, M. Building support networks from social isolation. *Generations*, 1986, *10*, 46–49.

Minkler, M., and Stone, R. The feminization of poverty and older women. *The Gerontologist*, 1985, *25*, 351–357.

Minnigerode, F., and Adelman, M. Elderly homosexual women and men. *Family Coordinator*, October 1978, 451–456.

Mitchell, J., and Register, J. C. An exploration of family interaction with the elderly by race, socioeconomic status and residence. *The Gerontologist*, 1984, *24*, 48–54.

Murray, R. B., and Zentner, J. P. *Nursing assessment and health promotion through the life span* (2d ed.). Englewood Cliffs, N.J.: Prentice-Hall, 1979.

Mutran, E., and Skinner, G. Family support and the well-being of widowed: Black-white comparison. Paper presented at meetings of the Gerontological Society, 1981.

Neugarten, B., and Weinstein, K. The changing American grandparent. *Journal of Marriage and the Family*, 1964, *26*, 199–204.

Nydegger, C. N. Family ties of the aged in cross-cultural perspective. *The Gerontologist*, 1983, *23*, 26–32.

O'Brian, J., and Whitelaw, N. *Planning options for the elderly.* Portland, Ore.: Institute on Aging, Portland State University, 1978.

Older Women's League. *Report on the status of midlife and older women.* Washington, D.C., May 1986.

Parron, E. M. Golden wedding couples: Lessons in marital longevity. *Generations*, 1982, *7*, 14–16.

Pearson, J. L. *Older parents' reactions and adjustment to their child's marital separation.* Unpublished doctoral dissertation, East Lansing: Michigan State University, 1986.

Peplau, L., Cochran, S., Rook, K., and Pedesky, C. Loving women: Attachment and autonomy in Lesbian relationships. *Journal of Social Issues*, 1978, *34*, 7–27.

Peplau, L. A., and Gordon, S. L. The intimate relationships of lesbians and gay men. In E. R. Allgeirer and N. B. McCormick (Eds.), *Gender roles and sexual behavior.* Palo Alto, Calif.: Mayfield, 1982.

Poulshock, S. W., and Diemling, G. T. Families caring for elders in residence: Issues in the measurement of burden. *The Gerontologist,* 1984, *24,* 230–239.

Pynoos, J., Hade-Kaplan, B., and Fleisher, D. Intergenerational neighborhood networks: A basis for aiding the frail elderly. *The Gerontologist,* 1984, *24,* 233–237.

Quinn, M. J., and Tomita, S. K. *Elder abuse and neglect: Assessment and intervention.* New York: Springer, 1986.

Raphael, B. Preventive-intervention with the recently bereaved. *Archives of General Psychiatry,* 1977, *34,* 1450–1452.

Raphael, S., and Robinson, M. The older lesbian: Love relationships and friendship patterns. *Alternative Life Styles,* 1980, *3,* 207–229.

Raphael, S., and Robinson, M. Lesbians and gay men in later life. *Generations,* 1981, *6,* 16–18.

Rhyne, C. Bases of marital satisfaction among men and women. *Journal of Marriage and the Family,* 1981, *43,* 941–955.

Richards, M., Hooyman, N., Hansen, M., Brandts, W., Smith-DiJulio, K., and Dahm, L. *Nursing home placement: A guidebook for families.* Seattle: University of Washington Press, 1984.

Riley, M. W., and Foner, A. *Aging in society. Vol. I: An inventory of research findings.* New York: Russell Sage, 1968.

Riley, M. W., and Riley, J. Longevity and social structure: The potential of the adult years. In A. Pifer and L. Bronte (Eds.), *Our aging society.* New York: W. W. Norton, 1986.

Robb, S. S., Boyd, M., and Pritash, C. L. A wine bottle, plant, and puppy. *Journal of Gerontological Nursing,* 1980, *6,* 721–728.

Roberto, K., and Scott, J. P. Friendship patterns among older women. *International Journal of Aging and Human Development,* 1984–85, *19,* 1–11.

Roberts, W. L. Significant elements in the relationship of long-married couples. *International Journal of Aging and Human Development,* 1979–1980, 265–272.

Robinson, B., and Thurnher, M. Taking care of aged parents: A family cycle transition. *The Gerontologist,* 1979, *19,* 587–593.

Robinson, M. *The older lesbian.* Master's Thesis, California State University, Dominquez Hills, Carson, California, 1979.

Rosenberg, G. S., and Anspach, D. F. Sibling solidarity in the working class. *Journal of Marriage and the Family,* 1973, *35,* 108–113.

Rosenmayr, L. The family—A source of hope for the elderly. In E. Shanas and M. Sussman (Eds.), *Family bureaucracy and the elderly.* Durham, N.C.: Duke University Press, 1977.

Rosenthal, C. J. Aging, ethnicity and the family: Beyond modernization theory. *Canadian Ethnic Studies,* 1983, *15,* 1–16.

Rosenthal, C. J. Family supports in later life: Does ethnicity make a difference? *The Gerontologist,* 1986, *26,* 19–24.

Rosow, I. *Social integration of the aged.* New York: Free Press, 1967.

Ross, H. The neighborhood family: Community mental health for the elderly. *The Gerontologist,* 1983, *23,* 243–247.

Ross, H. G., and Milgram, J. I. Important variables in adult sibling relationships: A qualitative study. In M. E. Lamb and B. Sutton-Smith (Eds.), *Sibling relationships: Their nature and significance across the lifespan.* Hillsdale, N.J.: Lawrence Erlbaum, 1982.

Schooler, K. K. *National senior citizens survey, 1968.* Ann Arbor, Mich.: Inter-University Consortium for Political Social Research, 1979.

Schorr, A. "*. . . thy father and thy mother . . ." A second look at filial responsibility and social policy.* Social Security Administration Publication 13-11953. Washington, D.C.: U.S. Department of Health and Human Services, 1980.

Scott, J. P. Siblings and other kin. In T. H. Brubaker (Ed.), *Family relationships in later life,* Beverly Hills, Calif.: Sage, 1983.

Shanas, E. The family as social support in old age. *The Gerontologist,* 1979, *19,* 169–174.

Shanas, E. Older people and their families: The new pioneers. *Journal of Marriage and the Family,* 1980, *42,* 9–14.

Shanas, E., Townsend, P., Wedderburn, D., Friis, H., Milhhoj, P., and Stehouver, J. *Older people in three industrial societies.* New York: Atherton, 1968.

Shimkin, D. B., Shimkin, E. M., and Frate, D. A. *The extended family in Black societies.* Manton: The Hague, 1975.

Silverman, A., Brahce, C., and Zielinski, C. *As parents grow older: A manual for program replication.* Ann Arbor: Institute of Gerontology, The University of Michigan, 1981.

Silverman, P., and Associates. *Helping each other in widowhood.* New York: Health Services Press, 1974.

Silverstone, B., and Hyman, H. *You and your aging parents.* New York: Pantheon Books, 1982.

Simons, R. L. Specificity and substitution in the social networks of the elderly. *International Journal of Aging and Human Development,* 1983–84, *18,* 121–139.

Skolnick, A. Married lives: Longitudinal perspectives on marriage. In D. Eicharn, J. Clausen, N. Haan, M. Honzik, and P. Mussen (Eds.), *Present and past on middle life.* New York: Academic Press, 1981.

Smith, K. F., and Bengtson, V. L. Positive consequences of institutionalization: Solidarity between elderly parents and their middle-aged children. *The Gerontologist,* 1979, *19,* 438–447.

Smyer, M., The differential usage of services by impaired elderly. *Journal of Gerontology,* 1980, *35,* 249–255.

Smyer, M., and Hofland, B. F. Divorce and family support in later life. *Journal of Family Issues,* 1982, *3,* 61–77.

Soldo, B. J., and Manton, K. G. Health status and service needs of the oldest old: Current patterns and future trends. *Milbank Memorial Fund Quarterly,* 1985, *63,* 286–319.

Sommers, T. *Til death do us part: Caregiving wives of severely disabled husbands.* Washington, D.C.: Older Women's League, 1982.

Spanier, G. B., and Glick, P. C. Marital instability in the United States: Some correlates and recent changes. *Family Relations,* 1981, *30,* 329–338.

Spivak, S., Haskins, B., and Capitman, J. A review of research on informal support systems.

Appendix F of *Evaluation of coordinated community oriented long-term care demonstration projects.* Final Report, Contract No. 400-80-0073. Washington, D.C.: Department of Health and Human Services, 1984.

Sprey, J., and Matthews, S. Contemporary grandparenthood: A systems transition. *The Annals of the American Academy of Political and Social Science,* November 1982, 91–103.

Steinitz, L. *The church as family surrogate for the elderly.* Presented at meetings of the Gerontological Society, 1980.

Stoller, E., and Stoller, E. L. Help with activities of everyday life: Sources of support for the noninstitutionalized elderly. *The Gerontologist,* 1983, *23,* 64–70.

Stone, R., Cafferata, G., and Sangl, J. *Caregivers of the frail elderly: A national profile.* Washington, D.C.: U.S. Department of Health and Human Services, 1986.

Sussman, M. The family life of old people. In R. Binstock and E. Shanas, *Handbook of aging in the social sciences* (2d ed.). New York: Van Nostrand Reinhold, 1985.

Sussman, M. D., and Burchinol, L. Parental aid to married children: Implications for family functioning. *Marriage and Family Living,* 1962, *24,* 320–332.

Tannenbaum, D. *People with problems: Seeking help in an urban community.* Toronto: University of Toronto, Center for Women and Community Studies, 1975.

Teresi, J., Toner, J., Bennett, R., and Wilder, D. Factors related to family attitudes toward institutionalizing older relatives. Paper presented at meetings of the Gerontological Society, 1980.

Tiger, L. Omigamy: The new kinship system. *Psychology Today,* July 1978, 14–17.

Tobin, S. S., and Kulys, R. The family in the institutionalization of the elderly. *Journal of Social Issues,* 1981, *37,* 145–157.

Torres-Gil, F. M. Age, health and culture: An examination of health among Spanish-speaking elderly. Paper presented to the First National Hispanic Conference on Health and Human Services, Los Angeles, 1976.

Treas, J. Family support systems for the aged: Some social and demographic considerations. *The Gerontologist,* 1977, *17,* 486–491.

Treas, J. The great American fertility debate: Generational balance and support of the aged. *The Gerontologist,* 1981, *21,* 98–103.

Treas, J., and Van Hilst, A. Marriage and remarriage rates among older Americans. *The Gerontologist,* 1976, *16,* 132–136.

Troll, L. E. The family of later life: A decade review. *Journal of Marriage and the Family,* 1971, *33,* 263–290.

Troll, L. E. (Ed.). *Family issues in current gerontology.* New York: Springer, 1986.

Troll, L. E. Grandparents: The family watchdogs. In T. Brubaker (Ed.), *Family relationships in later life.* Beverly Hills, Calif.: Sage, 1983.

Troll, L., Miller, S., and Atchley, R. *Families in later life.* Belmont, Calif.: Wadsworth, 1979.

Uhlenberg, P., and Myers, M. A. Divorce and the elderly. *The Gerontologist,* 1981, *21,* 276–282.

U.S. Department of Labor, Bureau of Labor Statistics. *Employment and earnings: Table 3.* January 1984.

U.S. House of Representatives, Select Committee on Aging. *Exploding the myths: Caregiving in America.* Washington, D.C.: U.S. Government Printing Office, 1987.

U.S. Senate Special Committee on Aging. *Aging America: Trends and projections,* Washington, D.C.: U.S. Government Printing Office, 1986.

U.S. Senate Special Committee on Aging. *American in transition: An aging society, 1984–85 Edition.* Washington, D.C.: U.S. Government Printing Office, 1985.

U.S. Senate Special Committee on Aging. *Developments in aging: 1985.* Washington, D.C.: U.S. Government Printing Office, 1986.

Vicente, L., Wiley, J. A., and Carrington, R. A. The risk of institutionalization before death. *The Gerontologist,* 1979, *19,* 361–367.

Vinick, B. Remarriage in old age. *The Family Coordinator,* 1978, *27,* 359–365.

Ward, R. Informal networks and well-being in later life: A research agenda. *The Gerontologist,* 1985, *25,* 55–61.

Washington State Aging and Adult Services Administration and Puget Sound Power and Light Company. *Gatekeeper program.* Seattle, WA, 1986.

Weeks, J. R., and Cueller, J. B. The role of family members in the helping networks of older people. *The Gerontologist,* 1981, *21,* 388–394.

Weissert, W. G. Seven reasons why it is so difficult to make community based long-term care cost effective. *Journal of Health Services Research,* 1985, *20.*

White House Conference on Aging. *Chartbook on aging in America,* 1981.

Wolf, D. C. Growing older: Lesbians and gay men. Berkeley: University of California Press, 1982.

Wood, V., and Robertson, J. The significance of grandparenthood. In J. Gubruim (Ed.), *Time, roles and self in old age.* New York: Human Sciences Press, 1976.

Wood, V., and Robertson, J. Friendship and kinship interaction: Differential effect on the morale of the elderly. *Journal of Marriage and the Family,* 1978, 367–375.

York, J. L., and Calsyn, R. J. Family involvement in nursing homes. In L. Troll, *Family issues in current gerontology.* New York: Springer, 1986.

Zarit, S. H., Reever, K. E., and Bach-Peterson, J. Relatives of the impaired elderly: Correlates of feelings of burden. *The Gerontologist,* December 1980, *20,* 649–655.

Chapter 11

Living Arrangements and Social Interactions

As we have seen in previous chapters, successful aging depends on physical health, cognitive and emotional well-being, and a level of activity that is congruent with an individual's abilities and needs. Another important element in the aging process is the environment, both social and physical, which serves as the context for activities as well as the stimulus with which an individual interacts. According to person-environment theories of aging, an individual is more likely to experience life satisfaction in an environment that is congruent with his or her physical, cognitive, and emotional needs and abilities.

Previous chapters have examined the relationships between older persons and their social settings. In this chapter, the focus is on diverse physical environments, and their social and psychological consequences. We examine the impact of the natural and built environment on older persons' behavior, the influence of a growing older population on community planning and housing, and the interaction between older persons and their physical environments. Many of the age-related changes in physiological status, sensory function, and cognitive abilities, as well as the diseases and cognitive disorders associated with aging that have been discussed in previous chapters, are affected in important ways by the environment. These age-related changes and disease conditions make the average older person sensitive to characteristics of the setting that may have no effect on the typical younger person. They may impair the older person's ability to adapt to and interact with complex and novel environments. On the other hand, there are many older people who function as well as younger persons in a wide range of physical surroundings. Observation of these differences in individual responses has led to the concept of *congruence* or *fit* between the environment and the individual. This concept, briefly reviewed in the Introduction of this book, forms the basis of the discussion in this chapter.

Person-Environment Theories of Aging

The impact of the environment on human behavior and well-being is widely recognized in diverse disciplines. It was in the early work of psychologist Kurt Lewin and his associates (Lewin, 1935; Lewin, Lippitt and White, 1939; Barker, Dembo, and Lewin, 1941) that the environment as a complex variable entered the realm of psychology. Lewin's field theory (1935, 1951) emphasizes that any event is the result of multiple factors, individual and environmental; or more simply stated, $B = f(P,E)$ (i.e., behavior is a function of personal and environmental characteristics). A change in either the person or the environment produces a change in behavior.

Murray's theory of personality (1938), known as *personology*, provides the earliest framework for a person-environment congruence model. This theory depicts the individual in dynamic interaction with his or her setting, the type of interaction that we have portrayed throughout this book. Murray viewed humans as "motile, discriminating, valuating, assimilating, integrating beings who attempt to produce temporal unity within a changing environmental matrix" (Murray, 1938, p. 36). Thus, the individual attempts to maintain equilibrium as the environment changes. Murray's concepts of *need* and *press* are relevant for theories of person-environment congruence. In Murray's personology, need is viewed as a force in the individual that works to maintain equilibrium by attending and responding to, or avoiding certain environmental demands (e.g., the concept of press in the P-E model).

According to Murray's and other theories of person-environment congruence, the individual experiences optimal well-being when his or her needs are in equilibrium with characteristics of the environment (Kahana, 1973; Holland, 1961; Stern, 1965). Thus, for example, an older woman who has spent most of her life on a farm will adjust more readily to a small nursing home in a rural area than to a large facility in an urban center. In contrast, an older couple who have always lived in a large city may be dissatisfied if they decide to spend their retirement years on a small farm far from town; adaptation may be more difficult, and perhaps never fully achieved. To the extent that individual needs are not satisfied because of existing environmental characteristics and level of "press," it is hypothesized that the individual will experience frustration and strain.

The impact of the physical setting on the aging person, and the dynamic interaction between the two, has only recently been considered by gerontologists. Yet, the environment plays a more dominant role for the elderly than for the young, because the older person's ability to control his or her surroundings (e.g., to leave an undesirable setting) is considerably reduced. The individual's range of adaptive behaviors to a stressful environment becomes constrained because of changes in physical, social, and psychological functioning. Therefore, this perspective may be even more useful for understanding older people's behavior than for other populations.

The socioenvironmental theory, developed as a sociological perspective on aging and briefly described in Chapter 3, suggests that both the social and physical environment influence the activities of older people (Gubrium, 1973). Accordingly, social interactions occur as a function of the age homogeneity of an environment and the extent to which people are living in physical proximity to each other. Gubrium developed a matrix of social contexts that reinforce or discourage friendship formation among the elderly. (See Table 11–1.) The four environmental contexts are: (1) high age homogeneity and close proximity, (2) age homogeneity and low proximity, (3) age heterogeneity and close proximity, and (4) age heterogeneity and low proximity. The first is typical of high-rise residences for older people and generally conducive to friendship formation. The second type may be a retirement community of detached housing or townhouses that are spread out over several acres; this situation is less conducive to interactions unless the community plans activities to encourage residents to get to know each other. The third type of environment is found in apartments or urban

TABLE 11–1 Social Contexts in Aging

		Age Homogeneity	
		Homogeneous	*Heterogeneous*
Physical Proximity	*Close*	Type I	Type III
	Distant	Type II	Type IV

Source: J. Gubrium, *The Myth of the Golden Years* (Springfield, Ill.: Charles C. Thomas, 1973). Courtesy of Charles C. Thomas, Publisher, Springfield, Illinois.

housing that has residents of diverse ages living near each other, thereby encouraging facial recognition of neighbors but less chance of friendship formation than the first two types. The final category of residential environment is represented by suburban neighborhoods with housing spaced far apart and residents of diverse ages. Compared to the other types, this social context results in different activity norms and demands than the others on older people. To the extent that an older person's resources and personal needs are consistent with the needs of a given environment, a particular social context may result in greater social interaction than another one. This may be one reason why research on the impact of age-homogeneous housing on social interaction and life satisfaction among the elderly has led to mixed findings, as we will see later in this chapter.

P-E CONGRUENCE MODELS IN GERONTOLOGY

Kahana's theory of P-E fit (1973, 1975) is the first congruence model developed and empirically tested with the elderly. Kahana hypothesized that incongruence between specific individual needs and environmental press along parallel dimensions produces stress, which in turn requires adaptation, and ultimately affects the older person's well-being. For example, an older person who has a high need for privacy would experience discomfort in a nursing home that offered no opportunities for physical privacy or solitude, although, as noted below, too much privacy is not stressful. Adaptation may consist of modifying this environmental press or the individual deciding to leave the setting, if circumstances permit. Further stress and discomfort result if the individual's response does not improve the situation (Stern, 1970; French, Rodgers, and Cobb, 1974; Kahana, Liang, and Felton, 1980). Such stress is compounded for older people whose cognitive and functional capacities are severely impaired, because they are less likely to be able to modify the environment or to leave the situation.

French and colleagues (1974) suggest that a deficiency in environmental press relative to individual needs ("undersupply") has a negative effect, while an "oversupply" of press (i.e., more environmental demands than the individual prefers or is able to manage) is assumed to have no effect. Kahana's theory does not make a priori assumptions in this regard. However, empirical tests by Kahana and others (Kahana et al., 1980; Kiyak, 1977, 1978) suggest that the relative effects of undersupply and oversupply depend on the specific aspects of environmental press that are examined. For example, oversupply has been found to be as beneficial as congruence in the areas of privacy, organization, and order, whereas an undersupply of stimulation in the individual's immediate environment results in greater well-being than either congruence or an oversupply of stimulation (Kiyak, 1977). That is, older people who have as much privacy and order in their lives as they prefer, and those with more privacy and order than they prefer, are equally satisfied with their situation. In contrast, older people whose home environments are less physically stimulating (i.e., in terms of sounds, lights, and colors) than they prefer tend to be more satisfied with their environments and with their lives than elderly people whose home environments are more stimulating than they prefer.

Examples of the differential benefits of oversupply, undersupply, and congruence abound in daily situations. An older woman who lives alone and keeps her home as tidy as she likes may be experiencing more privacy and order than she would ordinarily prefer, but she is likely to be just as satisfied as if she had as much privacy and order as she wishes. If this level of homeostasis between her preference and the environment is disrupted in the direction of *less* privacy and order than this older woman prefers (e.g., grandchildren visiting for several weeks, playing with their toys in all the rooms), a situation of undersupply in these two preferences is created. Similar to the older woman in the nursing home described above, she is then likely to experience frustration, dissatisfaction, and a desire to leave the situation.

The advantage of an environment that provides less stimulation than an individual prefers is that the person can create a preferred level of stimulation; in contrast, the overly stimulating environment does not permit an individual to manipulate the situation or to impose a chosen level of stimulation on the environment. An older man who lives with his daughter and teenage grandchildren in a small home may feel overwhelmed and unable to control the high level of activity (and choice of music!) by the younger family and their friends. In contrast, an older man who lives alone in a quiet neighborhood has greater control over the level of activity in his home, even though the house may seem too quiet and unstimulating at times.

THE COMPETENCE MODEL

Another theory of person-environment transactions is Lawton and Nahemow's (1973) competence model. This approach, described briefly in this book's Introduction, assumes that the impact of the environment is mediated by the individual's competence level. Competence is defined as "the theoretical upper limit of capacity of the individual to function in areas of biological health, sensation-perception, motives, behavior and cognition" (Lawton, 1975). This definition focuses on different aspects of the individual than does Kahana's model. The competence model is more concerned with cognitive and physical capacities; Kahana's model emphasizes the individual's perceived needs and preferences. Environment is also defined somewhat differently by these theorists. In the competence model, "demand quality of the environment" refers to the potential of a given environmental feature to influence behavior (for example, the level of stimulation, physical barriers, and lack of privacy).

Lawton and Nahemow's model may be a useful one with which to follow changes in an older person's ability to negotiate the physical setting. As competence in cognition, physical strength and stamina, health and sensory functioning decline over time, the individual would be expected to experience increased problems with high environmental press. Thus, for example, grocery shopping in a large supermarket on a busy Saturday morning may become an overwhelming task for an older person who is having increasing difficulty with hearing and walking. To the extent that the aging person can reduce the level of environmental press, adaptation occurs, and the individual maintains his or her level of well-being. In this example, the older person might decide to shop in a smaller supermarket at nonpeak hours, or to avoid supermarkets altogether and use a neighborhood grocery store or order groceries by phone.

For the older person with Alzheimer's disease or other forms of dementia, it can be difficult to reestablish P-E congruence or to adapt to incongruence. This is a population that has not been examined widely within a P-E framework, but severe cognitive deterioration may result in an inability to recognize the incongruence experienced between one's needs and the external world. The dementia patient may become behaviorally disturbed unless others intervene to reestablish congruence. This may be accomplished by simplifying the environment in order to make it fit the individual's cognitive competence; for example, by providing cues and orienting devices in the home to help the individual find his or her way without becoming lost or disoriented. The ultimate goal of any modification should be to maximize the older person's ability to negotiate and control the situation, and to minimize the likelihood that the environment will overwhelm the person's competence.

Relocation

Relocation, or moving from one setting to another, represents a special case of P-E incongruence or discontinuity between the individual's physical, cognitive, and emotional competence, and the demands of the environment. Anyone who has moved from one city to another, or even from one house to another, has experienced the problems of adjusting to new surroundings, and to different orientations, floor plans, and designs of specific features in the home. A healthy person can usually adjust quite easily. An older person who has lived in his or her home for many years will require more time to adapt, even if the move is perceived as an improvement to a better, safer, more comfortable home. This is because the individual has adjusted to a particular configuration of P-E fit over a long period of time. The greater the change (e.g., moving from a private house in the suburbs to a small apartment in an urban center), the longer it will take to adapt. A relocation that entails extensive changes in lifestyle, such as a move to a retirement community or to a nursing home with its rules and policies governing the residents, requires even greater adjustments.

In general, older people are less likely to move to a different community than are younger families, but are more likely to move to a different type of housing within the same community. From 1982 to 1983, less than 5 percent of people over age 60 had relocated to a different community, compared to 34.5 percent of people aged 20 to 24. Among those who moved out of state, almost half went to Florida, California, Arizona, Texas, or New Jersey (Longino, Biggar, Flynn, and Wiseman, 1984; U.S. Bureau of the Census, 1984). This is part of a continuing trend that has resulted in a significant increase in the over age 65 population in sunbelt states. A study of more than 4,000 people over age 65 found that unmarried persons, and married couples in which both spouses retire at the same time, are more likely to move to another region than other elderly (Henretta, 1986).

The problem of relocation is compounded for the person who is experiencing multiple or severe physical disabilities and cognitive dysfunction. As we have seen in Chapter 8, these individuals have more difficulty coping with stressful life events than healthy older people. Unfortunately, these are often the very people who must relocate to hospitals and skilled nursing facilities, environments that are most incongruent with the homes of most elderly. Concern about adapting to a new setting is one reason why many frail older people who can no longer maintain their own homes are reluctant to move to congregate housing, even though they may recognize that they "should" move to a safer environment. Among 85 residents of a deteriorating neighborhood, those who were least competent in terms of psychological and social resources were least satisfied with their current housing but also were least active in attempting to find a better situation (Lawton, Kleban, and Carlson, 1973). That is, these people probably recognized that their neighborhoods no longer fit their needs, but the same characteristics that made it difficult to function independently in these settings (e.g. impaired motor and cognitive abilities, a loss of social supports) impeded them in seeking a better fit. As anyone who has searched for a new home can attest, it requires considerable stamina and determination to find housing and a neighborhood that best fits one's needs and preferences. To the extent that one is frail and unable to muster the stamina to search for such housing, it becomes even more difficult to make the transition.

For many years, gerontologists have argued about the detrimental effects of residential relocation for frail elderly. Concern has been especially great for those forced to move en masse from one nursing home to another, when, for example, a facility has to be closed for safety reasons. One of the first studies that stimulated the controversy was a longitudinal examination of older persons who had applied for admission to a nursing home (Lieberman, 1961). Death rates were higher after relocation than before the move. Subsequent studies of older people moving from one institution to another confirmed these results (Aldrich and Mendkoff, 1963; Jasnau, 1967; Bourestom, Tars, and Pastalan, 1973; Killian, 1970), and raised serious concerns about the mortality risks associated with relocating. This led to descriptions of relocation as transplantation shock, transfer trauma, and re-location stress.

More recent studies have suggested that the early studies had methodological flaws that resulted in overestimates of mortality risks (Lieberman, 1969, 1974; Wittels and Botwinick, 1974; Schulz and Brenner, 1977; Borup, Gallego, and Heffernan, 1979). Such factors as age, health status, radical versus moderate environmental change, and personal involvement in the move had not been considered by previous investigators. These variables have been noted to influence both morbidity and mortality. A recent review of 26 studies of institutional relocation concluded that relocations that disrupt an older person's perceived or actual support system are more traumatic and more likely to increase the risk of mortality than are relocations that involve intact groups of elderly or move an individual from one intact group to another (Coffman, 1981). Further-more, relocation to facilities that foster independence rather than dependency often results in improved physical and cognitive functioning (Marlowe, 1974). Positive results were also noted in a study of 78 residents of a nursing home who were transferred to a new skilled-care facility and followed for three months post-relocation. Improved morale and increased satisfaction with their living situation were found within one month among some elderly; those who had wanted to move enjoyed positive outcomes, whereas those who experienced disruption in the relocation process faced more negative outcomes (Mirotznik and Ruskin, 1985). The negative effects of relocation can generally be reduced by extensively preparing older people for a move, such as their making several visits to the new facility, seeing the rooms to which they have been assigned, and meeting the staff (Bourestom and Pastalan, 1975). Even greater involvement in the move, such as older people deciding whether to move, choosing the room or unit in the facility that best fits their needs and preferences, and deciding on the timing of the move, is beneficial to those who must relocate for any reason.

Urban-Rural Differences

With the trend toward urbanization in the Western world, a smaller proportion of all population subgroups, including those aged 65 and over, currently reside in rural farm communities. The majority of older persons (63 percent) lived in metropolitan areas (i.e., urban and suburban communities) in 1977 (U.S. Dept. of Commerce, 1978), compared with only 5 percent in communities with fewer than 2,500 residents. Ethnic minority differences are particularly pronounced in the proportion of elderly persons in urban centers. Thus, although only 29 percent of white elderly live in central cities, 55 percent of all older Blacks and 53 percent of older persons with Spanish surnames reside in these settings. Whereas 24 percent of the white population lives in medium (2,500–10,000) nonmetropolitan communities, 11 percent of Hispanics live in such settings.

There is also a "graying of the suburbs"; that is, a greater proportion of people who moved into suburban developments in the 1950s have now raised their children and have remained in these communities after retirement (Logan, 1983). Logan notes that in 1980, for the first time in U.S. history, more older people lived in the suburbs than in central cities (10.1 million versus 8.1 million, respectively). On the average, the suburbs where older people live tend to have more rental housing, lower home values, and higher population densities. These demographic changes in suburbs raise the issue of changing needs for services and businesses, as well as greater dependence on public transportation in comparison to the time when the residents were young parents.

Older persons who live in small towns have been found to have lower incomes (near the poverty level) and poorer health than those in urban areas. This is particularly true for Blacks who reside in small towns and rural areas; more than half have incomes near the poverty level (Auerbach, 1976; Lawton, 1980). Consistent with these findings, Lawton has noted that limitations in mobility and activity are greater among those in nonmetropolitan nonfarm areas and least among suburban elderly. This may be a function of income differences, but also may be related to the greater prevalence of medical and social services (e.g., hospitals, clinics, senior centers, private physicians, transportation) in urban and suburban communities. Despite attempts in the early 1970s to offset urban-rural differences in human services, significant gaps remain in terms of service delivery and availability, so that rural services for seniors do not have the quality and diversity of metropolitan areas (Taietz and Sande, 1979). Nevertheless, as noted in Chapter 6, there is little difference in health service utilization rates between rural and urban elderly, suggesting that the former do seek medical services when necessary, although they may need to travel farther to find such services.

Despite their lower income and poorer health, older persons in small communities have been found to interact more with neighbors and friends, and with people of the same and younger ages than those in urban settings (Langford, 1962; Rosencranz, Pihlblad and McNevin, 1968; Schooler, 1975). Mr. and Mrs. Howard in the introductory vignette illustrate the positive aspects of smaller communities for older people. These include factors such as the greater proximity of neighbors, stability of residents, and shared values and lifestyles. On the other hand, some researchers have found evidence to contradict the stereotype of greater family integration in rural communities. For example, in a survey of elderly in Iowa, only 19 percent of rural persons lived near their children, compared with 34 percent of urban elderly (Bultena et al., 1971). Differences were even greater in a Wisconsin survey; 26 percent and 51 percent, respectively (Bultena and Wood, 1969). Although proportionately fewer rural elderly have been found to live near their children and to receive financial and social support from them, friendship ties appear to be stronger and more numerous among rural elderly (Bultena et al., 1971; Lozier and Althouse, 1974; Lawton, Nahemow, and Teaff, 1975).

Studies of life satisfaction among older residents of small towns and metropolitan areas yield mixed reports. Metropolitan residents were found to have greater life satisfaction in two national surveys (Schooler, 1975; Hynson, 1975), but no differences emerged in an earlier study (Pihlblad and Rosencranz, 1969). When individual circumstances, such as health and income, were controlled in a reanalysis of earlier data, no significant differences emerged in life satisfaction by community size (Sauer et al., 1976).

In sum, the data suggest that older persons in rural areas and small towns are more disadvantaged in terms of income, health, and service availability than those in urban centers, who are in turn more disadvantaged than elderly in suburbs and cities. Rural elderly in general also live farther from their children than do older persons in urban settings. However, it appears that interactions with neighbors occur more frequently in smaller communities, and life satisfaction is affected less by community size than by individual differences. Based on the earlier discussion about the importance of P-E fit for older persons, we would predict that older persons who have a high need for social interaction and have lived most of their lives in rural settings would be most satisfied in such settings, and would experience severe adaptation problems in more anonymous urban environments.

The Impact of the Neighborhood

All of us live in a neighborhood, whether it is a college campus, a nursing home, a retirement park, an apartment complex, or the several blocks surrounding our homes. Because of its smaller scale, the neighborhood represents a closer level of interaction and identification than does the community. Although a neighborhood is difficult to define, Lawton (1980) points to four basic elements: (1) a geographic boundary; (2) distinguishing physical characteristics that are natural or physical, such as roads, buildings, and topography; (3) inhabitants with many characteristics in common, such as socioeconomic status and ethnic minority background; and (4) contact among inhabitants that may be merely facial recognition, or regular social interactions.

When asked to draw a neighborhood map, older persons tend to include smaller areas and more limited boundaries than younger individuals (Regnier, Eribes, and Hansen, 1973; Lee, 1970). Nearby resources such as a shopping area or park are included. In the study by Regnier and colleagues, relatively large neighborhood maps were drawn by older males, people who drove a car, those in better health, and those with higher incomes. According to P-E theories, individuals with better health and higher incomes are the most "competent" elderly.

Given these findings, it is not surprising that the closer a resource is to an individual's home (i.e., within his or her definition of neighborhood), the more likely the older person is to use it. Elderly tenants of public housing and those in neighborhoods with many older residents have been found to use proximal services (i.e., those on the housing site or within walking distance) with greater frequency than those farther away (Newcomer, 1976; Chapman and Beaudet-Walters, 1978). For example, a laundromat, grocery store, or senior center that are on-site or nearby are more popular with tenants than when these same services require the use of an automobile or bus. Older people are willing to travel farther for physician services, entertainment, family visits (although friends need to be nearby for regular visiting to occur), and club meetings, probably because these activities occur less frequently than grocery shopping and laundry. Visits to family members may occur more often, but many older persons are less concerned with proximity than with the chance to maintain family ties. Distance is less important if family members assume responsibility for driving older persons to various places, including their homes. In some cases, family members may prefer visits in the older person's home.

Proximity and frequent contact with families may not be as critical if neighbors and nearby friends can provide the necessary social support for older persons. As discussed in Chapter 10, neighbors play an important role in the elderly's social network, especially for those who have lived in the same homes for many years. Particularly for older people with children at a geographic distance, neighbors are more readily available to help in emergencies and on a short-term basis, such as contacting an ambulance when needed by the older person. It is often more convenient for neighbors than family to drive an older individual to stores and doctors' offices when they are going in that direction anyway. In addition, neighbors can provide a "security net," as partners in a "Neighborhood Watch" crime prevention program or in informally arranged systems of signaling to each other (e.g., pulling open the living room drapes everyday by 9:00 A.M. to signal that all is well). This does not mean that neighbors can or should replace family support systems because, as we have seen, families play an important role in providing emotional, physical, and financial assistance for their older members, especially for those with long-term illnesses or disabilities.

Age Homogeneity–Heterogeneity

As mentioned earlier, one factor that influences social interactions in a neighborhood is its age mix. Several studies have pointed to the greater interaction rates and satisfaction with one's neighborhood in settings that are predominantly occupied by older persons (Rosow, 1967; Bultena, 1968; Rosenberg, 1970; Teaff, Lawton, and Carlson, 1973; Hochschild, 1973). Residents of age-segregated neighborhoods, for example, often establish informational and helping networks that can compensate for weak or nonexistent family ties. Age homogeneity can facilitate friendships because of shared life situations and the parity of exchange among peers (Blau, 1981).

In contrast, another study found that older people living in areas with mixed age groups expressed *greater* satisfaction with their housing (Chapman and Beaudet-Walters, 1978). A more recent study of 232 elderly residents of mixed age communities and age-segregated housing identified no differences in life satisfaction, but those in age-segregated communities had larger and more supportive social networks (Poulin, 1984). Other studies have found little evidence of social interaction or mutual support among elderly residents of age-segregated housing (Ehrlich, Ehrlich, and Woehlke, 1982; Stephens and Bernstein, 1984; Sheehan, 1986).

Victimization and Fear of Crime

Other characteristics of residents in the neighborhood, such as socioeconomic status, may be more important determinants of social interaction than age per se. For example, age dissimilarity may be compounded by social class differences in a public housing project. Many older persons in such settings have not experienced a lifetime of poverty, whereas the youth who live in these projects often have grown up poor. Older persons in age-mixed public housing projects may be more vulnerable to victimization than those in age-homogeneous settings (Newman, 1972). This feeling of vulnerability results in fewer attempts at social interaction and more isolation on the part of older residents.

To some extent, older people's fear of youth and their unwillingness to interact with them in these settings are due to a lack of intergenerational experiences and to their stereotypes about teenagers. It is true that the perpetrators of crimes against the elderly tend to be teenage youths. This is often the case with crimes to which older people are most vulnerable: purse snatchings and pickpocketing.

A commonly held stereotype is that crime affects the elderly much more than other age groups (Ragan, 1977). In two Harris surveys (1975, 1981), most Americans, including older people, believed that crime and the fear of crime are major problems for the elderly. However, both national and local surveys (U.S. Department of Justice, 1981; Skogan and Maxfield, 1981; Russell, 1980; Goldsmith, 1977) have revealed that people over age 65 have lower rates of overall victimization than other age groups, especially when compared with the 12- to 25-year-old group. Violent crime against the older population (i.e., assault, robbery, rape) was only one-fifth the rate against younger groups between 1973 and 1980.

Older persons in urban areas have the highest rates of all age groups as victims of personal larceny with contact (i.e., purse snatchings, pickpocketing). They are just as likely as other adults to be robbed, although burglaries occur with less frequency in older households: 50 per 1000 versus 89 per 1000 in the homes of younger families. Approximately 82 percent of all personal crimes against the elderly consist of such predatory crimes as personal larceny with and without contact, and robbery with injury (Lawton, 1980–81). In general, older Blacks have a higher rate of victimization by violent crimes than older whites; older women are at greater risk of predatory crimes than older men (U.S. Department of Justice, 1981). In fact, a low actual victimization ratio occurs along with high levels of fear, creating a fear-victimization paradox (Linquist and Duke, 1982). On the other hand, the lower proportion of crimes against older people may be a fallacy, reflecting a significant underreporting of crimes by this age group (Goldsmith and Tomas, 1974). Older people may be more reluctant to report crimes than younger people because they believe it would not help solve the crime. They may also think that admitting they have been victimized reveals their vulnerability and an inability to take care of themselves.

The conditions under which crimes are committed against older people differ from those of other age groups. For example, they are more likely to be victimized during the day, by strangers, in or near their homes, and with less use of weapons (Hochstedler, 1981). This suggests that perpetrators of crimes feel they can easily overtake the older victim without a struggle. The sense of helplessness against an attacker may make many older persons more conscious of their need to protect themselves, and may produce levels of fear that are incongruent with the statistics about their relative vulnerability to violent crimes. It is true, however, that even a purse snatching can be traumatic for older women, because of the potential for injury and hip fractures during a struggle, and because of the economic consequences for women on limited incomes (O'Keefe and Reid-Nash, 1985).

A recent survey has shown that fear of crime was not much higher for the group aged 65 and older when compared with the young. But those living alone, with low income, in multiple-unit housing, and in central areas of cities expressed greater fears than other elderly respondents. Older respondents reported feeling less confident about protecting themselves against crime, and believed that they knew less than other citizens about how to make themselves and their homes less vulnerable (O'Keefe and Reid-Nash, 1985).

Variations in the levels of fear reported by the elderly may be due to residence in an urban, suburban, or rural community, to living in an age-homogeneous or age-heterogeneous neighborhood, or to personal characteristics of the older person interviewed (e.g. gender, ethnic minority status, income, previous victimization). The fear may even result from hearing about crimes perpetrated against other elderly (Yin, 1980). The media often overemphasize the level of such incidents, thereby perpetuating the myth that this age group is most vulnerable to all types of crime. As a result, fear of crime among older people is disproportionate to the actual incidence, although it may be that differences in survey methods and specific questions asked to determine level of fear are more likely to distinguish among elderly with high fear of crime from those with low fear levels (Yin, 1980). In sum, the significance of the fear of crime is not whether it is warranted or not, but the effect it has on older people's psychological well-being.

Whether or not it is based on objective grounds, fear of crime compromises satisfaction with the neighborhood (Lawton and Hoover, 1979). Annual housing surveys of older people have revealed that fear of crime is a more serious personal concern for many older people than worries about income, health, or housing (Louis Harris and Associates, 1975, 1981; Select Committee on Aging, 1977). Neighborhood attributes that were mentioned most frequently by older people dissatisfied with their housing were crime, poorly maintained housing, abandoned structures, and inadequate police protection (note that these last two variables contribute to the incidence of crime). Older persons of higher socioeconomic levels who resided in nonmetropolitan areas and owned their own homes (especially those in single-family structures) expressed greater satisfaction with their housing. All these characteristics are related to the likelihood of crime; that is, smaller communities and those with higher income residents have lower crime rates and better police protection than larger urban centers.

In response to the problems of crime, "Neighborhood Watch" and other programs have been developed to encourage neighbors to become acquainted and to look out for signs of burglaries and other crimes against neighbors and their homes. Such neighborhood crime prevention programs allow older people to have access to their neighbors; they break down the perception of neighbors as strangers and the fear of being isolated in a community, both of which foster fear of crime (Merry, 1976; Antunes, Cook, Cook, and Skogan, 1977).

Older people also have been found to be more susceptible to economically devastating crimes such as fraud, confidence games, and medical quackery (Malinchak and Wright, 1978; Elmore, 1981). Local police departments in major cities have reported higher rates of victimization against older people by con-game artists and high-pressure salesmen. Medical quackery and insurance fraud are also more common, perhaps because many older people feel desperate for quick cures or are overwhelmed by the costs of traditional medical care. They therefore become easy prey for unscrupulous people who exploit them by offering the "ultimate medical cure" or the cheapest and most comprehensive insurance coverage available. Older people are also more vulnerable to commercial fraud by funeral homes, real estate brokers, and investment salesmen. Door-to-door salesmen of hearing aids have been investigated for fraud, often because the "hearing tests" they offer are inadequate and costly. Perhaps more important than the financial consequences of fraud, such salesmen prevent the older person from seeking appropriate professional services for hearing problems, medical conditions, real estate purchases, and other transactions.

Housing Patterns of Older People

In this section, we review the residential arrangements of older persons, including private homes, planned housing and retirement communities, congregate housing and nursing homes. Older people are more likely than any other age group to occupy housing that they own free and clear of a mortgage. Almost 75 percent of all dwelling units in which elderly persons reside are owned by them; of these, 84 percent have no mortgage remaining (Lawton, 1980). This is true for single-family detached housing as well as for condominiums, mobile homes, and even for congregate facilities that offer "life care" for retired persons, but by far the greatest proportion of these (84 percent) are single-family homes. The proportion of older people owning their homes increases as one moves from urban to rural areas; the rate is 62 percent in large metropolitan areas, 74 percent in nonmetropolitan urban areas, and 90 percent on farms (Struyk, 1977). Not surprisingly, older people living alone are much less likely to own their homes than are older married couples.

INDEPENDENT HOUSING

The majority of older homeowners have occupied their homes for many years. According to the 1980 Annual Housing Survey, 40 percent of older homeowners lived in houses built before 1940; 14 percent lived in structures built between 1940 and 1949. The comparable figures for younger homeowners are 22 percent and 8 percent, respectively (Harris, 1981).

These statistics have some important implications. First, older persons who have resided in one place for many years are more likely to experience problems with deciding to move and adjusting to a new residence than those who have moved frequently throughout life and have not become attached to a particular residence. It may seem odd to family, friends, and professional service providers that an older person does not wish to leave a home that is too large and too difficult to negotiate physically, especially if he or she is frail and mobility-impaired. The problem is compounded if the home needs extensive repairs that an older person cannot afford. Despite such seemingly obvious needs for relocating, it is essential to consider older people's preferences before encouraging them to sell a home that appears to be incongruent with their needs. The emotional meaning of home, in terms of personal identity, history of family life (e.g., marriage, childrearing, grandparenting), and associations with friends and neighbors, cannot be ignored. As discussed in the section on relocation, older people who have lived in one place for many years will experience more problems adjusting to a new residence because they have adapted to a particular level of P-E fit over a long time.

At the same time, however, the older person's current level of competence may be incongruent with the physical environment, and may require a more appropriate housing situation. One solution to this dilemma is the growing number of homesharing programs around the country. These are community-based programs that are operated out of the Area Agency on Aging or other governmental or voluntary service agency. Their goal is to assist older persons who own their own homes and wish to rent rooms to others in exchange for rental income or services, such as housekeeping and assistance with other chores. The role of a homesharing agency is to serve as a "matchmaker," selecting appropriate homesharers for each older person with a home. These services have been especially popular near universities and colleges, where students can find low-cost or free living arrangements and can benefit from intergenerational contacts. The disadvantage of such programs is that, like any other living situation where dissimilar and unrelated persons share housing, differences in values and lifestyles may be too great to bridge. This is particularly true when a younger person moves into an older person's home. The success of such programs depends on appropriate matches between potential homesharers. Generally, there are more older people with homes to share than younger people wanting rooms. In some instances, such as the Miami, Florida, share-a-home program, a group of older people live together.

The second implication of prolonged home ownership among older persons is that many of these houses are old, with inadequate weatherproofing and other energy-saving features, and more deficiencies with respect to construction and maintenance. Exposed wiring, lack of sufficient outlets, and worn-out furnaces are frequent, creating fire hazards. It is not unusual to hear news stories during winter months of fires starting in older homes because of faulty wiring, overloaded circuits, and the use of space heaters because of an inadequate furnace. The latter situation is particularly troublesome for older persons who have difficulties in maintaining body heat and prefer warmer ambient temperatures (see Chapter 3). Many communities have attempted to prevent these problems by providing free or low-cost home repairs for low-income elderly and special assistance to all senior citizens to make their homes more energy efficient (for example, providing no-interest loans for weatherproofing and installing storm windows). Major cities that have experienced sudden increases in their electricity and natural gas rates have also developed programs to aid low-income people of all ages. These services can be invaluable for helping older people to maintain their independence in their own homes.

Home equity conversion mortgages, or reverse annuity mortgages, are becoming increasingly available as another means of helping elderly homeowners stay in their homes. These programs are offered by mortgage banks, with some backing from the federal government, to older people who are "house-rich but cash-poor." In effect, such programs provide a reverse mortgage, whereby the title is retained by the lender or the lender owns part of the home; the older person receives a monthly payment (or annuity) from the lender and still lives in the house. When the older person dies and the house is sold, the lender generally receives a refund on the loan, as well as a portion of the home's appreciated value.

There is some concern about the long-term risks of such mortgage plans for the lender; currently, there are no guidelines for the duration of such reverse mortgages. For example, what if the older homeowner outlives the home's equity? Lenders do not want to evict such a person, but at the same time they do not want to lose their investment. The U.S. Senate and House of Representatives are considering separate bills that would extend federal backing for these loans through the Department of Housing and Urban Development (HUD).

PLANNED HOUSING

During the past 30 years, federal and local government agencies and some private organizations (such as religious groups) have developed planned housing projects specifically for older persons, either as subsidized housing for low-income elderly or age-segregated housing for middle- and upper-income older persons. Gerontologists have attempted to understand the effects of the quality and type of housing on older persons' satisfaction level and behavior following relocation to such housing environments. In one of the first such studies, Frances Carp (1966) followed for one year 204 new occupants of a public housing project for low-income persons called Victoria Plaza, and a control sample of 148 comparable older people. (The latter had also applied to live in Victoria Plaza but were not selected to live there). Comparisons before and one year after the move revealed that the Victoria Plaza sample felt greater satisfaction with their housing and neighborhoods, and also experienced better health, improved morale, and more participation in community activities. A follow-up of surviving residents eight years later revealed continuing satisfaction and well-being. No significant changes were found among the nonmovers (Carp, 1974). A major benefit of this study is its use of a comparable control group that also desired to move. Its weakness lies in the reliance on self-report measures. One explanation for the difference is that the novelty of new and safer surroundings produced a "halo effect" for the movers; that is, they perceived all other aspects of their lives (morale, health, social participation) to have improved as a result of the new environment. This study and others that examine the impact of environmental change would be strengthened by interviewing "significant others" (e.g., spouses, roommates) to determine their evaluations of the older persons' functional and emotional status following the move.

Subsequent studies have supported the positive impact of relocation to planned housing on housing satisfaction, self-assessed health, and activity levels among low-income older people (Sherwood, Greer, Morris, and Sherwood, 1972; Lawton and Cohen, 1974). But no changes were observed by these researchers in functional health, hospitalization rates, and morale. It appears that planned housing can indeed improve the quality of life for low-income elderly, but it is difficult to generalize to other older populations, particularly those of higher income status. These research results also provide some support for the need to use objectively verifiable measures in housing studies, such as hospitalization rates and activities of daily living (which in turn is an indicator of functional health).

The problem of where to locate planned housing projects for older persons has no simple solution. As stated earlier in the discussion of neighborhood characteristics, older people are most likely to use services such as a senior center or laundromat if they are on site. Medical and meal services would also undoubtedly be more heavily utilized if they were included on the housing site. These services, however, are costly to establish and maintain. Moreover, their inclusion cuts down on the space available for residential units. As a result, planners of housing projects for senior citizens usually do not include such services in the building. Instead, they rely on existing organizations, such as local churches and Area Agencies on Aging, to provide these programs. Given the increasing tendency of planners and developers to exclude such services from housing plans, it is critical to locate housing projects for senior citizens near preexisting amenities, including supermarkets and shopping centers. In addition, public transportation should also be easily accessible. If a particular site is not already near a bus stop, this convenience should be arranged with the local public transportation authority well in advance of the completion of the housing project.

Planning must also take into account such factors as whether the area is zoned for residential, commercial, or industrial use. The topography of this site, crime rates, and security of the community are important considerations, as is the need to integrate the housing project into the neighborhood. The last item is especially crucial. In a housing project that is architecturally distinct from the rest of the neighborhood (e.g., a tall, multilevel structure in the midst of single-family homes, or a sprawling "retirement community" on the edge of an industrial area), residents are likely to experience a lack of fit with their environment and to feel isolated from the larger neighborhood. The lack of fit may also be felt by the residents of the larger neighborhood, who often reject the presence of an entire community of older people in their midst, no matter how architecturally consistent the housing project is with other neighborhood buildings. Both physical and psychological barriers are created by walls, vegetation, and architectural features that clearly distinguish a housing project from its surroundings, adding to the older residents' sense of separation from the neighborhood.

Perhaps the least desirable settings for planned housing are near an industrial area, a deteriorating urban center, or a superhighway. Unfortunately, these are the very places where public housing projects were first developed, in spite of such problems as high crime rates and inaccessibility of transportation and community services. The predictable result was tenant dissatisfaction. Useful guidelines for selecting sites for housing projects for older persons are described in a handbook developed by Green, Fedewa, Deardorff, Johnston, and Jackson (1975).

•

CONGREGATE HOUSING

Congregate housing differs from planned housing and single-family residences in its provision of communal services, at the very least a central kitchen and a dining room for all residents. Some congregate facilities also provide house-keeping, social, and health services. Others may have space for such services, but do not have established services on site, including congregate meals, home health care, and transportation services. In 1970, when the first federally supported congregate housing act was passed, these services could not be paid through HUD programs that financed the construction, but space for such services was provided. Developers and planners assumed that tenants would be charged for these additional services if they became available, or that the services would be subsidized by local agencies. Recent evidence suggests that such services have indeed become necessary, as the residents of congregate housing have reached advanced old age (Lawton, Moss, and Grimes, 1985). To the extent that a housing site has the space and resources to plan for such needs in the future, people are more likely to remain in such settings and to avoid or delay relocation to a skilled care facility.

Congregate housing is a desirable option for many older persons who do not need skilled nursing care but prefer having their meals prepared and other personal care services provided if they are to give up their homes. Probably the most important feature of congregate housing is the availability of prepared meals, which not only provide a more balanced and nutritional diet but also offer regular opportunities for socializing. Usually, residents also have the choice of eating some meals in their own units, because many congregate buildings provide each unit with a small kitchen (often a small refrigerator, a range, and a few kitchen cabinets).

The growth of congregate housing is due in great part to the interest shown by private nonprofit and profit-making corporations. However, despite their increased numbers, congregate sites are inadequate in many regions of the country and for specific segments of the aging population. Federal and local governments have significantly reduced their construction of new congregate facilities for low-income seniors since 1980. As a result, the number of congregate housing units for middle- and upper-income older persons has increased, but low-income elderly who need housing subsidies have not benefited from this increase.

There has been a growth in the number of *multilevel facilities* for older persons, that is, housing projects that offer a range from independent to congregate living arrangements, and intermediate to skilled care facilities. Such options are more widely available in housing that is purchased, less so for rental housing. As the number of oldest-old persons has increased (as noted in Chapter 1), owners and administrators of facilities that do not provide extensive nursing services have become increasingly concerned. They realize that some of their residents will eventually need to move to other facilities; they are also more aware that potential buyers of units in these facilities would prefer to have a range of services and housing options on site. Such alternatives are often of particular concern for couples, who face the likelihood that one partner will require skilled nursing care eventually. When several levels of care are available at one site, older couples can feel assured that they will be able to remain near each other, even if one becomes institutionalized.

Many housing plans for the elderly that offer options in living arrangements have *lifecare contracts, life lease contracts,* or *founders' fees.* That is, the older person must pay an initial entry fee, based on projections of life expectancy. In the case of a lifecare contract, the individual who eventually needs increased care is provided nursing home care without paying more for these services. Currently there are about 700 such retirement communities in the United States that house about 200,000 elderly (Hull, 1987). With a life lease contract or a founders' fee, the individual is guaranteed lifetime occupancy in the apartment. However, in the case of life lease contracts, if more expensive care is required, such services are generally not provided by the facility, and the older person must give up the apartment and find a nursing home. Lifecare, life lease, and founders' fees contracts also charge monthly fees, but the monthly costs are generally not as high as those charged in facilities that rely only on month-to-month payments. The advantage of lifecare contracts and founders' fees is that the individual is guaranteed lifetime care; this is important given the actuarial tables of life expectancy for those who

Multilevel housing offers a range of living arrangements.

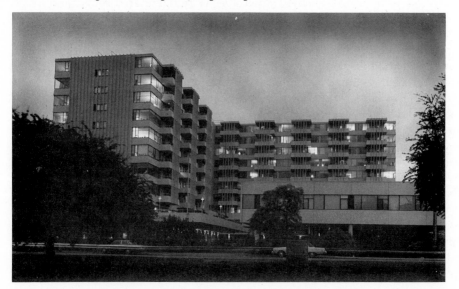

reach age 65 (another 15 years), and those who reach 70 (another 12 years). The elderly person who pays month-to-month may use up all of his or her life savings long before dying if skilled care is needed. In contrast, the option of a lifecare contract may provide a sense of security for the older person who can pay a large lump sum. The individual is taking the chance that he or she will eventually need higher levels of care, so the costs are averaged out over a long period. For those who die soon after moving in, some facilities refund part of the entry fee to the family, but in many cases there is a policy of not refunding any portion of this fee. The ability to purchase these contracts is limited to the small percentage of elderly who have considerable cash assets.

A potential risk for older people who enter into a lifecare contract is that the facility will declare bankruptcy. In an attempt to avoid this, many states that license lifecare housing projects require providers to establish a trust fund for long-term expenses.

INSTITUTIONAL LIVING FOR OLDER PEOPLE

Many people who are unfamiliar with the residential patterns of older people mistakenly assume that the majority live in nursing homes. The actual proportion of older persons living in all institutions (nursing homes, boarding homes, psychiatric hospitals) is less than 5 percent, although approximately 25 percent of all people over age 65 will spend some time in a nursing home at some point during later life (Kastenbaum and Candy, 1973). Each year more than one million older persons are discharged from long-term care institutions, almost evenly divided among discharges to the community, transfers to other health facilities, and death (NCHS, 1979). Therefore, the statistic of 5 percent is a cross-sectional snapshot of the institutional population that does not take account of movement into and out of long-term care facilities. Institutions are home for the oldest, most frail, and dependent of the aged population: for every 1,000 persons aged 65 to 74, 12 live in nursing homes. That proportion increases to 237 per 1,000 for those are aged 85 and above. The average age of nursing home residents is 82 years, and the majority (about 71 percent) are women (NCHS, 1977, 1979). As we will see in a later section on the P-E congruence approach, older people with severe physical and cognitive impairments are most likely to be stressed by high levels of environmental press. The typical nursing home resident fits this criterion and is more likely to have major long-term impairments in activities of daily living, some form of dementia, and multiple major chronic diseases.

Nursing homes are relatively new living arrangements. Until the late 1930s and early 1940s, few existed in the United States. The enactment of Medicare and Medicaid in 1965 provided the largest impetus to their development; the rate of nursing home use by the elderly has almost doubled since 1966, from 2.5 percent to 5.0 percent of the population age 65 and over (George, 1984). The growth of the nursing home industry has also been fueled by some of the trends described in

Chapters 1 and 10, specifically, declining family size, the growth in the numbers and proportion of the older population, particularly women over age 75, and the increase in employed women who were traditionally the family caregivers.

Although the majority of nursing home residents are functionally impaired and unable to live independently in the community, it is noteworthy that for every impaired older person in a long-term care facility, there are at least two—and perhaps as many as five—equally impaired older persons residing in the community (Duke Center for the Study of Aging, 1978; General Accounting Office, 1977). Poor physical health and medical need do not, by themselves, sufficiently explain institutionalization. Instead, the factor that appears to distinguish long-term nursing home residents from equally impaired older community residents is the absence of a caregiver or social support network among the institutionalized. In fact, as mentioned in Chapter 10, up to 25 percent of nursing home placements are precipitated by the caregiver's illness or death (Kraus et al., 1976).

The sex differential in nursing homes is due to women's longer life expectancy, their greater risk of multiple chronic illness, and their greater likelihood of being unmarried. The latter factor is a critical one, given that the absence of a spouse or other caregiver is a major predictor of institutionalization. For example, in 1977, 78 percent of the nursing home population was without a spouse, compared to 40 percent of the general population age 65 and older. Of these nursing home residents, 62.3 percent were widowed, 6.7 percent were divorced or separated, and 19.1 percent had never married. More than 50 percent had no close relatives, and 60 percent had no regular visitors. The widowed comprised the majority of the nursing home population (NCHS, 1977).

Over 92 percent of nursing home residents are white, compared to 6.2 percent Black, 1.1 percent Hispanic, and less than 0.5 percent each who are Native American or of Asian origin. This underrepresentation of ethnic minority groups appears to reflect cultural differences in the willingness to institutionalize older persons, greater availability of family supports, or discrimination in admission policies (generally unofficial) against minorities (NCHS, 1979).

Most nursing homes are *proprietary* or *for-profit*, and thus operate as a business that has a goal of making a profit for the owners. The number of nursing homes owned by large multifacility chains is increasing dramatically. *Nonprofit* homes are generally sponsored by religious or fraternal groups; although their goal is not to make a profit, they must be self-supporting. These are governed by a board or advisory group, rather than owners or investors as in the case of proprietary homes. Although instances of reimbursement fraud by proprietary homes have been highly publicized, the terms proprietary and nonprofit do not designate type or quality of care, but rather how the home is governed and its earnings distributed. The type of ownership affects who makes major decisions regarding the facility's staff, policies, and programs, but not necessarily the standards of care.

Nursing homes must follow a number of federal guidelines to become certified by Medicare and to meet regulations that are imposed by each state on facilities within that state. Most nursing homes are not certified for Medicare, however, primarily because this program does not reimburse for long-term care or maintenance, but only for short-term care (i.e., rehabilitation following hospitalization). Medicaid is widely applied to nursing home care, however, and pays for nearly 60 percent of all nursing home expenditures (Vladeck, 1980). Many older people with incomes below a specified level (varying across states) would not be able to afford nursing home care without Medicaid assistance. Under this program, nursing homes are reimbursed according to the level of care required by each resident. The two major levels are *skilled nursing care* and health-related or *intermediate care*. The former includes intensive round-the-clock nursing services, as well as regular medical and social services. The second option also provides round-the-clock care, but not as intensively. As a result, residents who need skilled care are billed at a higher rate. Medical personnel determine the level of care required on the basis of the older person's physical and mental status. Many who enter nursing homes at the intermediate level eventually require skilled care.

The decision to enter a nursing home is often a hurried one, in reaction to a crisis, such as the older person's imminent discharge from the hospital. Hospital staff who work with patients and families to plan the patient's discharge frequently pressure family members to make their decision after physicians and other hospital staff press them to "get those hospital beds open." This may mean that the discharge planner accepts the first available nursing home bed, rather than waiting for the best possible placement. In instances where families have more time to make a decision, it is desirable for them and their older relative to visit a number of homes. The boxed insert on page 362 offers some guidelines for selecting a nursing home.

Even when there is time to plan for placement, few older people willingly choose to live in a nursing home, and most families arrive at this decision only after exhausting their home care resources. As noted in Chapter 10, however, it is important for older people and their relatives to realize that nursing home life does offer some benefits. These include increased social contact, accessible social activities, intensive rehabilitation services, as well as relief from the stress of caregiving on family members. Although the media tend to publicize instances of abuse and violation of regulations, there are many excellent nursing homes, especially with the growing awareness of the need to improve nursing homes and the development of special units for residents with cognitive or severe physical impairments. Increasingly, residents are having more influence over their lives, through resident councils, patients' bills of rights, nursing home ombudsmen, and the advocacy of groups such as the National Citizens Coalition for Nursing Home Reform (NCCNHR). In its resident surveys, this organization has found that a major concern of residents is to be involved in decisions about their daily lives in

Guidelines for Selecting a Nursing Home

1. Is the nursing home operated as a nonprofit or a proprietary business?
   - If nonprofit, with which organization is it affiliated?
   - If proprietary, is the facility part of a chain or is it independent?

2. Does the nursing home participate in the Medicaid program?

3. What are the rates for each level of care, and what level will this particular older person require?

4. What services are included and excluded from the daily rate?

5. What types of patients are refused admission?

6. What is the staff-resident ratio during each work shift; more specifically, what is the ratio of nurses and nurses' aides to residents?

7. Does the nursing home have a rehabilitation program?
   - If yes, is there a registered physical therapist on staff, or therapy aides only?

8. What professional services besides nurses and physicians are provided? For example, is there a staff social worker? How often does a dentist, pharmacist, or member of the clergy visit the facility? What services do they provide residents?

9. Is there a residents' council in the home? If yes, what are their roles and rights?

10. What are the home's rules and regulations regarding meals, snacks, or keeping food in the room?

11. Are private rooms available for residents?
    - If yes, what is the price differential between private and shared rooms?

12. What provisions are made to assure privacy; for example, what are the rules and regulations regarding private, locked storage units? What types of personal furniture may be brought in by residents?

13. How far is the facility from the homes of family members and close friends?

Source: Adapted with permission from the authors and publisher, N. R. Hooyman and W. Lustbader, *Taking care* (New York: The Free Press, 1986.)
Note: These are guidelines only, not criteria or a prescriptive listing.

the facility. Even such basic choices as what to eat, when to wake up, and the level of privacy in their own rooms are not provided to residents of many nursing homes. Through such efforts and through increased gerontological training, health care professionals are also becoming more sensitive about ways to involve family members, friends, and members from the larger community in the care of nursing home residents.

SERVICES TO AID ELDERLY IN THE COMMUNITY

In recent years, the term *long-term care* has evolved from an emphasis on purely institutional care to a broad range of services to impaired older adults in both institutional and community settings. Under this broader definition, homemaker services, nutrition programs, congregate housing, and visiting nurse services are all part of long-term care. Nursing homes are thus only one component of a continuum of long-term care services.

Over the last decades, there has been an increase in the number of federal and local services to help older people maintain their independence for as long as possible, and in the least restrictive environment feasible. Such support services include visiting nurses, housecleaning, assistance with personal care, hot meals delivered to the home, and occasional or daily trips to an adult day health program. Some adult day centers include memory retraining programs, physical therapy, giving medications on schedule, and regular checkups by a nurse. Some centers provide intensive rehabilitative services, but most serve a social integration function. Equally important, day health programs provide respite for family members who may be caring for the older person. Clearly, such services are not suitable for the most impaired or bedbound older person, but they have been an invaluable resource for elderly with moderate levels of dementia or with serious physical impairments and chronic illnesses who can still benefit from living in more familiar noninstitutional settings. A statewide study comparing participants in adult day health centers with nursing home residents in Virginia found that the latter had more physical disabilities, more sensory impairments, and fewer social supports (Arling et al., 1984). These newly emerging community services appear to help delay institutionalization and to minimize the stress of community living for the elderly and their families.

Perhaps the greatest impetus to the development of community services to the elderly was the Older Americans Act (described in detail in Chapter 18). It was passed in 1965 and amended significantly in 1969, 1973, 1978, and 1981 to include a broader range of elderly who should receive services, and expand the types of services available. These amendments to the Older Americans Act have resulted in programs to coordinate services within the community, a special emphasis on the frail and vulnerable elderly, and efforts to maintain older persons in the "least restrictive environment" (U.S. Congress, 1982). Further amendments have been considered for 1988.

Funding to local planning units, such as Area Agencies on Aging, through this Act can be used in the following categories of preventive, supportive, and restorative services:

1. Access services: These consist of information and referral, case management, and transportation.

2. Health services: These include home health aides, physical therapists and visiting nurse services, health education, rehabilitation therapy, and specialized health services at a local center, such as foot care, dental care, and blood pressure screening.

3. Nutrition services: These can be provided at a congregate meal site such as a senior center or hot lunch program site, or in the form of home-delivered hot meals (meals-on-wheels). This category also includes nutrition education and food co-ops that purchase food at reduced prices in some senior centers.

4. Employment and volunteer services: These range from listing employment opportunities, such as through a job bank for older workers, to community and federal service employment programs aimed specifically at the elderly. The Retired Senior Volunteer Program (RSVP) emerged as an amendment to the Older Americans Act in 1969; it has since helped thousands of communities benefit from the expertise and experience of older persons while at the same time enabling older people to contribute to society.

5. Social and recreational services: The growth of senior centers in most communities has provided a significant focal point of services (e.g., social and recreational activities, education, health assessment, monitoring, and counseling) to older people, while recent developments in adult day care and respite programs for cognitively and physically impaired elderly have allowed many families to keep their older relatives at home who would have been institutionalized in the past.

6. Personal support services: These include companion services, choreworkers and homemakers, home repair services, and telephone reassurance programs. These services assist older people who cannot manage all their home maintenance or personal activities of daily living because of a short-term illness, or while recuperating from surgery or injury, and those who have become too frail to perform these tasks but are not so impaired as to move to a congregate living situation.

Medicare covers some home health care services provided by specially licensed agencies through visiting nurses, home health aides, and choreworkers, but only under specific guidelines. These include (1) the approval of a physician

Transportation and other community-based services
can enable older people to remain in their own homes.

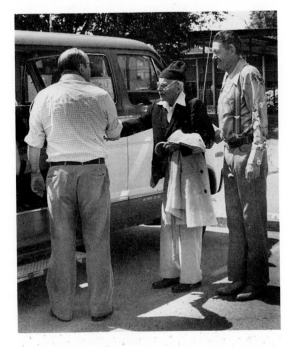

for each service to be obtained, (2) the requirement that the older person be homebound and unable to obtain services outside the home, and (3) the services must be for an acute or rehabilitative situation, not for a chronic health problem. Unfortunately, however, under current reimbursement regulations, Medicare generally cannot be used for community services such as homemaker and nutrition services without prior hospitalization or for extended periods of time. If a "continuum of long-term care" is to be successfully implemented, reimbursement regulations will have to be substantially altered from current practices that provide incentives for institutional rather than community-based care. These regulations will be discussed in more detail in Chapter 19.

A diversity of social and health services have evolved in many communities, but urban areas are more likely than rural communities to provide the variety described above. Such diversity can be a blessing for many elderly who choose to live in the community, but the lack of a coordinated service delivery system has, in the past, precluded access by those who were most in need. The recent expansion of information and referral, as well as case management programs through Area Agencies on Aging, has led to greater coordination and selection of appropriate services for the most needy elderly residing in the community.

As the number and variety of community-based services have grown, so too have questions regarding their cost-effectiveness for severely impaired older persons. That is, should such services be considered a valid alternative to institutionalization for the most vulnerable elderly, or is it more psychologically, socially, and economically advantageous for these older persons to relocate to a nursing home? Despite the loss of independence associated with institutionalization, such a move may result in a greater sense of security for the impaired older person who needs round-the-clock care.

EMERGENCY AIDS FOR INDEPENDENT ELDERLY

In recent years, several products and services have come into the marketplace to assist older people in emergency situations, especially those who are living alone. Some of these are simply pullcords in the bathroom or bedroom that are connected to a hospital or to the local emergency medical service. Others, such as the Life Safety System and Lifeline Service, are more sophisticated communication systems that use a portable medical alert device or an alarm unit connected to the phone to transmit specific signals for a fire, a medical emergency, or for "no activity" through telephone lines or computers. These systems have been found to be cost-effective in reducing the need for nursing home care and enhancing the older person's sense of security about living alone (Sherwood and Morris, 1981; Brenner, 1981; Dibner, Lowry, and Morris, 1982). Such electronic services will undoubtedly become more widely available with advances in computer technology. Indeed, computers have already been developed to turn appliances on and off; diagnose malfunctions in appliances; control light, noise, temperature and air quality; and convert information from one medium to another (e.g., sound to light). These advances in computer technology will aid older persons who choose to live independently (AARP, 1987).

Environmental Quality

Regardless of the type of housing in which older persons reside, numerous elements of environmental quality need to be taken into account. These include fire safety, security from crime, accessibility, privacy, territoriality, legibility or negotiability (i.e., the extent to which an environment is easy or difficult to orient oneself to), social activity, and stimulation. We have already reviewed security from crime in relation to specific housing types. In this section, housing characteristics that offer or fail to offer other aspects of environmental quality are discussed.

Accessibility refers to the reduction of physical barriers that impede an individual's ability to enter a building and to move from one area of a building or site to another, as well as features that enable the disabled to use buildings. We are all familiar with the international symbol of accessibility that denotes widened parking places, building entrances with ramps, and toilet stalls that are wider than average and include grab bars. These features are important for both younger and older persons who use wheelchairs. Regulations on accessible features in public buildings were established by the federal government in the early 1960s; specific standards for the slopes of ramps, width of doors, and other accessibility codes have been set by the American National Standards Institute (ANSI), and by codes established in the 1970s by many states.

These standards have made previously inaccessible facilities open to a much broader segment of the population, including the elderly. Unfortunately, however, many physical and sensory changes experienced by older persons (discussed in previous chapters) have not been considered in establishing federal or state accessibility codes. For example, older persons generally have more difficulty traversing long distances, but many congregate housing projects require long walks from individual units to the dining and recreational facilities. Older people who do not use wheelchairs may nevertheless have difficulty walking up and down stairs due to arthritis or stamina problems, but their homes may require this. Many such people "move" to the main level of their home, so that all their activities can take place on one floor. In an attempt to maximize the use of space, designers of housing and nursing homes often build cabinets and cupboards high above or below the reach of many older persons. This ignores the special problems of many older people with kyphosis or curvature of the spine, and others whose upward reach has become limited. It also creates serious difficulties for those with arthritis and other motor disorders who cannot bend down to search in floor-level cabinets. Numerous other problems are created by designers who ignore age-related changes in vision, hearing, and tactile sensations. Recommendations for designing environments to counter these problems have been offered in Chapter 5. Two excellent books on design for the aging population by Koncelik (1976, 1982) offer extensive recommendations for making nursing homes and other living environments more accessible and products easier to use by older people.

Privacy is a concept that is often ignored in designing facilities for the elderly. It is especially lacking in nursing homes, where access to residents' most personal activities (sleeping, dressing, bathing, grooming, and sexual needs) are open even to the passing stranger. Privacy is a basic need for individuals across the life span, essential for maintaining autonomy, self-reflection, and identity (Westin, 1970; Pastalan and Bourestom, 1970; Altman, 1974). Institutionalized elderly may be even more acutely aware of the need for privacy than older persons who reside in the community and college students (Kiyak, 1977). In response to a questionnaire on privacy needs, the latter two groups perceived a need for privacy along two dimensions (physical privacy, connoting physical separation from others, and solitude, the opportunity to reflect and introspect). However, elderly in institutions expressed needs for isolation as well; that is, they perceived a need for being physically distant from others and controlling others' access to themselves. It is important to return to the concept of congruence; for example, a subsequent study revealed that personal needs for privacy vary widely among elderly in nursing homes, indicating that the level of physical privacy and solitude provided must be congruent with the older person's individual needs (Kiyak, 1978). Unfortunately, most housing facilities either provide a uniform level of privacy for all residents, or offer greater privacy (e.g., single rooms) for those who can afford it.

Territoriality is a basic human need, in fact one that is shared by most animal species (Ardrey, 1966; Sommer, 1969). Individuals and social groups have a strong need to identify a given space as their own. The more a person loses control over physical space and conditions of life, the greater the need may be to identify available space as one's own. It is not uncommon for people sharing a room (e.g., college roommates, nursing home roommates, even spouses) to draw an invisible line in the middle of the room; access to the other side must be approved first by the "owner" of that side. Such behavior may include the need to ask the permission of the person who "owns" the room's only window or thermostat for access to it. Older people with dementia in institutions have been found to show less need for identifying spaces and objects as their own after being given private rooms (DeLong, 1970). Long-term care facilities that encourage older residents to furnish and decorate their rooms as they wish are more likely to reduce residents' territorial needs than those with many built-in features and predecorated units. Unfortunately, there is very little research to test the association between levels of privacy and control and the psychological well-being of older persons.

Legibility refers to the degree to which an environmental setting facilitates or impairs users' understanding and identification of a place, and the ease with which people can orient themselves in it. A home built on several levels, with a complicated system of hallways and many barriers that interfere with an understanding of the home's layout, may be interesting and challenging, but has poor legibility and makes it difficult for a newcomer or a confused resident to negotiate the environment (Lynch, 1960). This is a particularly important consideration for facilities that are designed for cognitively impaired older persons. Maps and signs, while useful, cannot make up for a poorly designed home.

The importance of environmental stimulation, or the ability of a given setting to encourage expression and activity, has long been assumed in psychology (Wohlwill, 1966; Pincus, 1968) and is implicit in the competence model. That is, environments with minimal press create a situation of stimulus deprivation and are not beneficial for even the least competent older person. Environments that stimulate the older person's cognitive, physical, and sensory capacities without overwhelming him or her can prevent an undesirable state of apathy. In the study by Kiyak (1978), described earlier, high levels of stimulation in the older person's immediate environment, together with low to moderate levels of stimulation in the larger institutional setting, resulted in greater satisfaction and improved morale. This contrasting need for high stimulation in the immediate environment and low in the larger environment may be attributable to the greater controllability of the immediate environment, where individuals can reduce the impact of high stimulation, but are helpless to control the larger institutional environment.

Summary and Implications

This chapter presented ways in which environmental factors affect the physical and psychological well-being of older people. Perhaps the most important lesson to be gained from this discussion is that a given environment is not inherently good or bad. Some environments are more conducive to the optimal functioning of *some* older people, while other people need an entirely different set of features. For example, the older person with a high need for activity and stimulation, and who has always lived in an urban setting, will be more satisfied with a large nursing home in a metropolitan center than the individual from a rural community who has always lived in a single-family dwelling. Both Lawton's competence model and Kahana's congruence model point to the necessity of examining each older person's specific needs, preferences, and abilities, and designing environments that can both meet the needs of this broad cross-section and, more importantly, flexibly respond to individual differences. To the degree that environmental press can be reduced to accommodate personal abilities and needs, the aging person can function more effectively and maintain his or her level of well-being.

Relocation represents a special case of P-E incongruence that can disturb the well-being of an impaired older person by raising the level of environmental press. Early studies emphasized the high mortality and morbidity associated with relocation of nursing home residents from one facility to another and among older people who recently moved into a nursing home. More recent studies have concluded that health status, degree of environmental change imposed by the move, and disruption of personal support systems moderate the extent of trauma produced by the relocation. Furthermore, researchers who have attempted to increase relocatees' involvement with and preparation for the move have identified beneficial effects on older people who must move.

There has been some concern with differences in housing quality and services for rural elderly. Although current cohorts are much less likely to live in farm and nonfarm rural communities than previous cohorts, those who do tend to have lower incomes and poorer health, with more limitations in activities of daily living. This is particularly true for Blacks in such communities. The recognition of these disparities has led to the growth of state and federally funded services for rural elderly, but more are needed. Older persons in rural communities appear to have more frequent social interactions with neighbors and friends than do urban elderly, but at the same time they need more formal health and social services.

The neighborhood and neighbors play a significant role in the well-being of older people. With retirement and declining health, the older person's physical lifespace becomes more constricted. The neighborhood takes on greater significance as a source of social interactions, health and social services, grocery shopping, banking, and postal services. Those who have good health and high incomes are less limited in their definition of neighborhood or lifespace. Those in public housing and especially in housing for the elderly are more likely to prefer resources in the immediate vicinity. Neighbors represent an important component of older people's social and emotional network, especially where family members are not available.

Research on older people's preferences for and ability to function in age-segregated versus age-integrated neighborhoods has yielded mixed results. Although some studies have shown greater preference for and more social interaction in the former, it appears that social class similarity and a feeling of invulnerability to victimization by teenage neighbors can improve interaction levels in age-integrated communities.

Fear of crime among older persons is widespread and is justified on the basis of victimization rates for petty larceny but not violent crimes. Older people experience one-fifth the rates that younger people do for violent crimes, but are more vulnerable to petty larceny than any other age group. The potential danger of injury and long-term disability, as well as the fear of economic loss, may contribute to this incongruity between actual victimization rates and older people's fear of crime.

The high rate of home ownership and long-term residence in their homes makes it difficult for older people to relocate to new housing, even when the new situation represents a significant improvement over the old. The poor condition of many older people's homes, and the high costs of renovating and maintaining them, sometimes makes relocation necessary, even when the older homeowner is reluctant. Better living conditions and a safer neighborhood in which several other elderly reside have been found to improve older people's morale and sense of well-being, especially following a move to planned housing projects from substandard housing. The growth of planned and congregate housing programs for seniors has raised the issue of site selection and service provision. It is especially important when designing housing for low-income older people and for those who do not drive that public transportation be located nearby and that facilities such as medical and social services, banks, and food shopping be within easy access of the housing facility. As people live longer and healthier lives beyond retirement, the need for multilevel housing (providing a range of care options) will continue to grow. Several alternative methods of purchasing such housing are available—some guarantee lifetime care, others do not provide nursing home services. Considering the high likelihood of using a nursing home facility at some time in old age, many retirees prefer to select the more comprehensive options.

The proportion of older people in a nursing home at any one time is very low, but approximately 25 percent will spend more time in such settings, especially during the last year of life. Because of the greater likelihood of physical and cognitive impairments among residents of nursing homes, it is critical to enhance the environmental quality of these facilities either at the design stage or, if the facility has already been built, by modifying features that increase privacy and control and allow for the expression of territoriality and other personal needs. Aging and institutionalization do not reduce the individual's needs for identity and self-expression.

References

Aldrich, C. K., and Mendkoff, E. Relocation of the aged and disabled: A mortality study. *Journal of the American Geriatrics Society*, 1963, *11*, 185–194.

Altman, I. *The environment and social behavior*. Monterey, Calif.: Brooks/Cole, 1975.

Altman, I. Privacy: A conceptual analysis. Paper presented at meetings of the Environmental Design Research Association, 1974.

Antunes, G. E., Cook, F. L., Cook, T. D., and Skogan, W. G. Patterns of personal crime against the elderly: Findings from a national survey. *The Gerontologist*, 1977, *17*, 321–327.

Ardrey, R. *The territorial imperative*. New York: Atheneum, 1966.

Arling, G., Harkins, E. B., and Romaniuk, M. Adult day care and the nursing home. *Research on Aging*, 1984, *6*, 225–242.

Auerbach, A. J. The elderly in rural areas. In L. H. Ginsberg (Ed.), *Social work in rural communities*. New York: Council on Social Work Education, 1976.

Barker, R. G., Dembo, T., and Lewin, K. Frustration and regression: An experiment with young children. *University of Iowa Studies in Child Welfare*, 1941, *18*.

Blau, Z. S. *Aging in a changing society* (2d ed.). New York: New Viewpoints, 1981.

Borup, J. H., Gallego, D. T., and Heffernan, P. G. Relocation and its effect on mortality. *The Gerontologist*, 1979, *19*, 135–140.

Bourestom, N., and Pastalan, L. A. Final report. Forced relocation: Setting, staff, and patient effects. Unpublished manuscript. Ann Arbor: University of Michigan, Institute of Gerontology, 1975.

American Association of Retired Persons. *The gadget book: Ingenious devices for easier living*. Washington, D.C., 1987.

Bourestom, N., Tars, S., and Pastalan, L. Alterations in life patterns following nursing home nursing home relocation. Paper presented at meetings of the Gerontological Society, 1973. Printed in *The Congressional Record—Senate*, 1974, July, 25697–25699.

Brenner, D. A Southwark community alarm partnership scheme. In A. Buter and C. Oldman (Eds.), *Alarm systems for the elderly*. Proceedings of a conference held at the University of Leeds, England, 1981.

Bultena, G. L. Age grading in the social interaction of an elderly male population. *Journal of Gerontology*, 1968, *23*, 539–543.

Bultena, G. L., Powers, E., Falkman, P., and Frederick, D. *Life after 70 in Iowa.* Sociology Report #95. Ames: Iowa State University, 1971.

Bultena, G. L., and Wood, V. The American retirement community: Bane or blessing? *Journal of Gerontology*, 1969, *24*, 209–217.

Carp, F. M. *A future for the aged: The residents of Victoria Plaza.* Austin: University of Texas Press, 1966.

Carp, F. M. Short-term and long-term prediction of adjustment to a new environment. *Journal of Gerontology*, 1974, *29*, 444–453.

Cath, S. H. The institutionalization of a parent: A nadir of life. *Journal of Geriatric Psychology*, 1972, *5*, 25–46.

Chapman, N. J., and Beaudet-Walters, M. Predictors of environmental well-being for older adults. Paper presented at meetings of the Gerontological Society, 1978.

Coffman, T. L. Relocation and survival of institutionalized aged: A re-examination of the evidence. *The Gerontologist*, 1981, *21*, 483–500.

DeLong, A. J. The microspatial structure of the older person. In L. A. Pastalan and D. H. Carson (Eds.), *The spatial behavior of older people.* Ann Arbor: Institute of Gerontology, University of Michigan, 1970.

Dibner, A. S., Lowry, L., and Morris, J. N. Usage and acceptance of an emergency alarm system by the frail elderly. *The Gerontologist*, 1982, *22*, 538–539.

Duke Center for the Study of Aging and Human Development. *Multidimensional functional assessment: The OARS methodology* (2d ed.). Durham, N.C.: Center for the Study of Aging, Human Development, 1978.

Ehrlich, P., Ehrlich, I., and Woehlke, P. Congregate housing for the elderly: Thirteen years later. *The Gerontologist*, 1982, *22*, 399–403.

Elmore, E. Consumer fraud and the elderly. In D. Lester (Ed.), *The elderly victim of crime.* Springfield, Ill.: C. C. Thomas, 1981.

French, M. P. R., Rodgers, W., and Cobb, S. Adjustment as person-environment fit. In D. Coehlo, A. Hanburg, and D. Adams (Eds.), *Coping and adaptation.* New York: Basic Books, 1974.

General Accounting Office. *The well-being of older people in Cleveland, Ohio.* Washington, D.C.: General Accounting Office, 1977.

George, L. The institutionalized. In E. Palmore (Ed.), *Handbook on the aged in the United States.* Westport, Ct.: Greenwood Press, 1984.

Goffman, E. *Asylums.* Garden City, N.Y.: Anchor Books, 1961.

Goldsmith, J. Criminal victimization of older persons. *Connecticut Law Review*, 1977, *9*, 435–449.

Goldsmith, J., and Tomas, N. E. Crime against the elderly: A continuing national crisis. *Aging*, 1974, #236–237, 10–13.

Green, I., Fedewa, B. E., Deardorff, H. L., Johnston, C. A., and Jackson, W. M. *Housing for the elderly: The development and design process.* New York: Van Nostrand, 1975.

Gubrium, J. *The myth of the golden years: A socio-environmental theory of aging.* Springfield, Ill.: Charles C. Thomas, 1973.

Harris, L. *The myth and reality of aging.* Washington, D.C.: National Council on the Aging, 1975.

Harris, L. *Aging in the eighties: America in transition.* Washington, D.C.: National Council on the Aging, 1981.

Henretta, J. C. Retirement and residential moves by elderly households. *Research on Aging,* 1986, *8,* 23–37.

Hochschild, A. L. *The unexpected community.* Englewood Cliffs, N.J.: Prentice-Hall, 1973.

Hochstedler, E. *Crime against the elderly in 26 cities.* Washington, D.C.: Bureau of Justice Statistics, 1981.

Holland, J. L. Creative and academic performance among talented adolescents. *Journal of Educational Psychology,* 1961, *52,* 136–147.

Hull, J. D. Insurance for the twilight years. *Time,* April 6, 1987, 53.

Hynson, L. M. Rural-urban differences in satisfaction among the elderly. *Rural Sociology,* 1975, *40,* 64–66.

Jasnau, K. F. Individualized versus mass transfer of nonpsychiatric geriatric patients from mental hospitals to nursing homes with special reference to the death rate. *Journal of the American Geriatrics Society,* 1967, *15,* 280–284.

Kahana, E. *Matching environments to needs of the aged.* Final Progress Report submitted to NICHD, Fall, 1973. I R01 HD 03850.

Kahana, E. F. A congruence model of person-environment interaction. In M. P. Lawton (Ed.), *Theory development in environments and aging.* New York: Wiley, 1975.

Kahana, E. F., Liang, J., and Felton, B. Alternative models of P-E fit: Prediction of morale in three homes for the aged. *Journal of Gerontology,* 1980, *35,* 584–595.

Kastenbaum, R., and Candy, S. The 4% fallacy. *International Journal of Aging and Human Development,* 1973, *4,* 15–21.

Killian, E. C. Effect of geriatric transfers on mortality rates. *Social Work,* 1970, *15,* 19–26.

Kiyak, H. A. Person-environment congruence models as determinants of environmental satisfaction and well-being. Unpublished doctoral dissertation. Wayne State University, 1977.

Kiyak, H. A. A multidimensional perspective on privacy preferences of institutionalized elderly. In W. E. Rogers and W. H. Ittelson (Eds.), *New directions in environmental design research.* Tempe: University of Arizona Press, 1978.

Koncelik, J. A. *Designing the open nursing home.* Stroudsburg, Penn.: Dowden, Hutchinson and Ross, 1976.

Koncelik, J. A. *Aging and the product environment.* Stroudsburg, Penn.: Dowden, Hutchinson and Ross, 1982.

Kraus, A. S., Spasoff, R. A., Beattie, E. J., Holden, D. E. W., Lawson, J. S., Rodenburg, M., and Woodcock, G. M. Elderly application process: Placement and care needs. *Journal of the American Geriatric Society*, 1976, 24, 165–172.

Langford, M. *Community aspects of housing for the aged*. Ithaca, N.Y.: Cornell University Center for Housing and Environmental Studies, 1962.

Lawton, M. P. Competence, environmental press, and the adaptation of older people. In P. G. Windley and G. Ernst (Eds.), *Theory development in environment and aging*. Washington, D.C.: Gerontological Society, 1975.

Lawton, M. P. *Environment and aging*. Monterey, Calif.: Brooks/Cole, 1980.

Lawton, M. P. Crime, victimization, and the fortitude of the aged. *Aged Care and Services Review*. 1980–1981, 2, 1–31.

Lawton, M. P., and Cohen, J. The generality of housing impact on the well-being of older people. *Journal of Gerontology*, 1974, 29, 194–204.

Lawton, M. P., and Hoover, S. L. *Housing and neighborhood: Objective and subjective quality*. Philadelphia: Philadelphia Geriatric Center, 1979.

Lawton, M. P., Kleban, M., and Carlson, D. The inner city resident: To move or not to move. *The Gerontologist*, 1973, 13, 443–448.

Lawton, M. P., Moss, M., and Grimes, M. The changing service needs of older tenants in planned housing. *The Gerontologist*, 1985, 25, 258–264.

Lawton, M. P., and Nahemow, L. Ecology and the aging process. In C. Eisdorfer and M. P. Lawton (Eds.), *Psychology of adult development and aging*. Washington, D.C.: American Psychological Association, 1973.

Lawton, M. P., and Nahemow, L. *Cost, structure and social aspects of housing for the aged*. Final report to the Administration on Aging. Philadelphia: Philadelphia Geriatric Center, 1975.

Lawton, M. P., Nahemow, L., and Teaff, J. Housing characteristics and the well-being of elderly tenants in federally assisted housing. *Journal of Gerontology*, 1975, 30, 601–607.

Lee, T. Urban neighborhood as socio-spatial schema. In H. M. Proshansky, W. H. Ittelson, and L. G. Rivlin (Eds.), *Environmental psychology*. New York: Holt, Rinehart and Winston, 1970.

Lewin, K. *Dynamic theory of personality*. New York: McGraw-Hill, 1935.

Lewin, K. *Field theory in social science*. New York: Harper and Row, 1951.

Lewin, K., Lippitt, R., and White, R. Patterns of aggressive behavior in experimentally created social climates. *Journal of Social Psychology*, 1939, 10, 271–299.

Lieberman, M. A. Relationship of mortality rates to entrance to a home for the aged. *Geriatrics*, 1961, 16, 515–519.

Lieberman, M. A. Institutionalization of the aged: Effects on behavior. *Journal of Gerontology*, 1969, 24, 330–340.

Lieberman, M. A. Relocation research and social policy. *The Gerontologist*, 1974, 14, 494–501.

Linquist, J. H., and Duke, J. M. The elderly victim at risk. *Criminology*, 1982, 20, 1–10.

Logan, J. R. The graying of the suburbs. *Aging*, 1983, 345, 4–8.

Longino, C., and Lipman, C. Married and spouseless men and women in planned retirement communities: Support network differential. *Journal of Marriage and the Family*, 1981, *43*, 169–177.

Longino, C. F., Biggar, J. C., Flynn, C. B., and Wiseman, R. F. The retirement migration project. Final Report to the National Institute on Aging, University of Miami, 1984.

Louis Harris and Associates. *Myth and reality of aging in America*. Washington, D.C.: National Council on Aging, 1978.

Lozier, J., and Althouse, R. Social enforcement of behavior toward elders in an Appalachian mountain settlement. *The Gerontologist*, 1974, *14*, 69–80.

Lynch, K. *The image of the city*. Cambridge, Mass.: The MIT Press, 1960.

Malinchak, A. A., and Wright, D. Older Americans and crime: The scope of elderly victimization, *Aging*, 1978, *281*, 10–16.

Marlowe, R. E. When they closed the doors at Modesto. Paper presented at NIMH conference on closure of state hospitals, Scottsdale, Arizona, February 1974.

Merry, S. The management of danger in a high crime urban neighborhood. Paper presented at meetings of the American Anthropological Association, Washington, D.C., 1976.

Mirotznik, J., and Ruskin, A. P. Inter-institutional relocation and its effects on psychosocial status. *The Gerontologist*, 1985, *25*, 265–270.

Murray, H. A. *Explorations in personality*. New York: Oxford University Press, 1938.

National Center for Health Statistics. Profile of chronic illness in nursing homes: National Health Survey, 1973–1974. *Vital and Health Statistics*, Series 13, No. 29. Washington, D.C.: 1977.

National Center for Health Statistics. The national nursing home survey: 1977 summary for the United States. *Vital and Health Statistics*, Ser. 13, No. 43, Washington, D.C.: 1979.

Neugarten, B. L., Havighurst, R. J., and Tobin, S. S. The measurement of life satisfaction. *Journal of Gerontology*, 1961, *16*, 134–143.

Newcomer, R. J. An evaluation of neighborhood service convenience for elderly housing project residents. In P. Suedfeld and J. A. Russell (Eds.), *The behavioral basis of design* (Vol. 1). Stroudsburg, Penn.: Dowden, Hutchinson and Ross, 1976.

Newman, O. *Defensible space*. New York: Macmillan, 1972.

O'Keefe, G. J., and Reid-Nash, K. Fear of crime and crime prevention competence among the elderly. Paper presented at meetings of the American Psychological Assoc., Los Angeles, 1985.

Pastalan, L., and Bourestom, N. Forced relocation: Setting, staff and patient effects. Final Report to NIMH, 1970.

Pihlblad, C. T., and Rosencranz, H. A. *Social adjustment of older people in the small town*. Columbia: University of Missouri, Department of Sociology, 1969.

Pincus, A. The definition and measurement of the institutional environment in homes for the aged. *The Gerontologist*, 1968, *8*, 207–210.

Poulin, J. E. Age segregation and the interpersonal involvement and morale of the aged. *The Gerontologist*, 1984, *24*, 266–269.

Ragan, D. K. Crimes against the elderly. Some interviews with Blacks, Mexican-Americans, and Whites. In M. D. Ragai (Ed.), *Justice in older America.* Lexington, Mass.: D.C. Heath, 1977.

Regnier, V. A., Neighborhoods as service systems. In M. P. Lawton, R. J. Newcomer, and T. O. Byerts (Eds.), *Planning for an aging society.* Stroudsburg, Penn.: Dowden, Hutchinson and Ross, 1976.

Regnier, V. A., Eribes, R. A., and Hansen, W. Cognitive mapping as a concept for establishing neighborhood service delivery locations for older people. Paper presented at the Association for Computing Machinery symposium, New York City, 1973.

Rosenberg, G. S. *The worker grows old.* San Francisco: Jossey-Bass, 1970.

Rosencranz, H. A., Pihlblad, C. T., and McNevin, T. E. *Social participation of older people in the small town.* Columbia: Department of Sociology, University of Missouri, 1968.

Rosow, I. *Social integration of the aged.* New York: The Free Press, 1967.

Russell, C. The elderly: Myths and facts. *American Demographics,* 1980, 2, 30–31.

Sauer, W. J., Shehan, C., and Boymel, C. Rural-urban differences in satisfaction among the elderly: A reconsideration. *Rural Sociology,* 1976, 41, 269–275.

Schooler, K. K. Response of the elderly to environment: A stress-theoretic perspective. In P. G. Windley and G. Ernst (Eds.), *Theory development in environment and aging.* Washington, D.C.: Gerontological Society, 1975.

Schulz, R., and Brenner, G. F. Relocation of the aged: A review and theoretical analysis. *Journal of Gerontology,* 1977, 32, 323–333.

Select Committee on Aging, U.S. Congress. *In search of security: A national perspective on elderly crime victimization.* Washington, D.C.: U.S. Government Printing Office, 1977.

Seligman, M. E. P. *Helplessness: On depression, development and death.* San Francisco: W. H. Freeman, 1975.

Sheehan, N. W. Informal support among the elderly in public senior housing. *The Gerontologist,* 1986, 26, 171–175.

Sherwood, S., Greer, D. S., Morris, J. N., and Sherwood, C. C. *The Highland Heights experiment.* Washington, D.C.: U.S. Department of Housing and Urban Development, 1972.

Sherwood, S., and Morris, J. N. A study of the effects of an emergency alarm and response system for the aged: Final report. Grant #HS01788, NCHSR, 1981.

Skogan, W. G., and Maxfield, M. E. *Coping with crime.* Beverly Hills: Sage, 1981.

Sommer, R. *Personal space.* New York: Prentice-Hall, 1969.

Stephens, M., and Bernstein, M. Social support and well-being among residents of planned housing. *The Gerontologist,* 1984, 24, 144–148.

Stern, G. Student ecology and the college environment. *Journal of Medical Education,* 1965, 40, 132–154.

Stern, G. *People in context.* New York: Wiley, 1970.

Struyk, R. J. The housing situation of elderly Americans. *The Gerontologist,* 1977, *17,* 130–139.

Taietz, P., and Sande, M. Rural-urban differences in the structure of services for the elderly in upstate New York counties. *Journal of Gerontology,* 1979, *34,* 429–437.

Teaff, J. D., Lawton, M. P., and Carlson, D. Impact of age integration of public housing projects upon elderly tenant well-being. Paper presented at meetings of the Gerontological Society, 1973.

U.S. Department of Commerce. Bureau of the Census. State population estimates, by age and components of change: 1980–1984. *Current Population Reports,* 1984 Series P-25, No. 970.

U.S. Department of Commerce. Bureau of the Census. Social and economic characteristics of the metropolitan and nonmetropolitan population: 1977 and 1970. *Current Population Reports,* Special Studies, 1978, *75,* 23.

U.S. Department of Justice. *Criminal victimization surveys in 13 American cities, 1974.* Washington, D.C.: U.S. Government Printing Office, 1975.

U.S. Department of Justice. Crime and the elderly. *Special Report, Bureau of Justice Statistics Bulletin,* December, 1981.

Vladeck, B. C. *Unloving care: The nursing home tragedy.* New York: Basic Books, 1980.

Westin, A. F. *Privacy and freedom.* New York: Atheneum, 1970.

Wittels, I., and Botwinick, J. Survival in relocation. *Journal of Gerontology,* 1974, *36,* 440–443.

Wohlwill, J. The physical environment: A problem for a psychology of stimulation. *Journal of Social Issues,* 1966, *22,* 29–38.

Yin, P. P. Fear of crime among the elderly: Some issues and suggestions. *Social Problems,* 1980, *27,* 492–504.

Chapter 12

Economic Status, Work, and Retirement

Economic status has a powerful effect on many aspects of older people's lives—their health, social relationships, living arrangements, community activities, and political participation. Patterns of employment, retirement, and income are major components of the larger environment that shape older people's daily opportunities and competence in numerous ways. Although economic resources in themselves do not guarantee satisfaction, they do determine many of the options available to older people to lead satisfying lives.

Economic status in old age is largely influenced by environmental conditions, especially past and current employment patterns and resultant retirement benefits. For many people, economic status is consistent across the life course. For example, ethnic minorities in low-paying jobs in young and middle adulthood generally face a continuation of poverty in old age. Other elderly, including widowed or divorced women who depended on their husbands' income, or retirees with only Social Security as income, may face poverty or near-poverty for the first time in their lives. This chapter begins by reviewing the employment status of the older population, and then focuses on retirement, both as a social institution and a social process. Since one of the primary consequences of retirement is reduced income, we conclude by examining the extent of poverty and near-poverty among the elderly.

Employment Status

Work and work-related values influence the life course in many ways. Men in particular, but increasingly women among younger cohorts, develop age-related expectations about the rhythm of their careers—when to start working, when to be at the peak of their careers, and when to retire; and they assess whether they are "on time" according to these socially defined schedules. In American society, the value placed on work also shapes how individuals approach employment and retirement. The current cohort of older people, in particular, was socialized to a traditional view of hard work, job loyalty, and occupational stability.

However, current demographic trends and social policies are having an impact on these values and expectations. Changing work patterns and increased longevity mean that both men and women are spending more years in employment and enjoying a longer retirement, as illustrated in Figure 12–1. As men live longer, a smaller proportion of their lifetime is devoted to paid employment, even though the number of years they work is longer. For example, a man born in 1900 could expect to live about 46 years. He would work for 32 years (70 percent of his lifetime) and be retired for about one year (6 percent of his lifetime). In contrast, if the current trends toward early retirement continue, a man born in 1981 can anticipate living about 70 years, working for 38 years (55 percent), and being retired for about 14 years (20 percent). Women, too, are living

FIGURE 12–1 Life Cycle Distribution of Education, Labor Force Participation, Retirement, and Work in the Home: 1900–1980

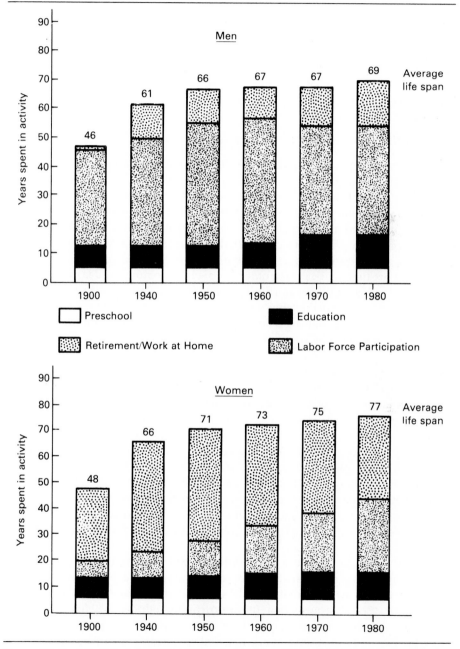

Source: "Median School Years Completed," Bicentennial Edition: Historical Statistics of the United States; Work Sharing Issues, Policy Options and Prospects, Upjohn Institute for Employment Research, 1981, Bureau of Labor Statistics Bulletin 1982. Life expectancy from U.S. Bureau of the Census.
Note: Data for 1980 is based on 1977 work life estimates.

381

longer past the age of retirement and are devoting a smaller portion of their lives to childbearing and rearing. A woman born in 1900 could expect that over 18 years of her 48-year life span (or 37 percent) she would be bearing children, whereas the comparable figure for a woman born in 1981 is 10 years of her 78-year lifespan (or 13 percent). Nowadays, adult women can also expect to devote more years to employment (Congressional Institute on the Future, 1984).

WHAT KINDS OF JOBS DO OLDER WORKERS HOLD?

Older workers are generally concentrated in jobs that initially require considerable education and a long training process (e.g., managerial and supervisory positions or self-employment) or those that have flexible retirement policies (Morse, 1979). Compared with their younger counterparts, older workers are less likely to be in jobs that are physically demanding, low or entry level, or high-tech. Those employed past age 65 tend to be married, well educated, and healthy.

Although the trend toward early retirement from full-time employment has increased, part-time work among older people has expanded and is perceived by the working public of all ages as a desirable alternative. According to a 1981 Harris poll, nearly 75 percent of the labor force prefer to continue some type of part-time work after retirement, viewing a flexible work schedule along with being able to draw partial pensions as desirable for retirees (Harris and Associates, 1981). Although the number of elderly working part-time is much smaller than the number who report that they would like to do so, the proportion of workers on part-time schedules does increase with age, as illustrated in Table 12–1.

Part-time work may reflect an attachment to working. For example, in one study, 20 percent of retirees from upper status positions continued part-time employment, 50 percent of them in the same industry, largely because of their job satisfaction and social attachment to their work (Parnes, 1981). However, part-time work more often reflects economic necessity or a high degree of felt economic deprivation. In fact, the need to supplement pension income appears to be the greatest motivation for seeking employment after retirement (Streib and Schneider, 1971), although good health, upper status occupations, and college education are the factors that generally make it possible to continue part-time work.

Barriers exist to part-time employment, however. The major obstacles are employer policies against part-time workers' drawing partial pensions, and Social Security limits on the amount that can be earned at a given age before full benefits are reduced. (Social Security benefits are currently reduced $.50 for every $1.00 earned above a fixed minimum of allowed earned income.) Employers may resist the additional administrative work entailed in hiring part-time or temporary workers, but this may be tempered by the advantage of fewer employer-paid benefits to such workers compared to full-time employees.

TABLE 12–1 Persons 45 Years and Over on Part- and Full-Time Work Schedules* (Percent Distribution)

Sex and Age	1960 Full Time	1960 Part Time	1970 Full Time	1970 Part Time	1982 Full Time	1982 Part Time	1984 Full Time	1984 Part Time
Males:								
45 to 64	94	6	96	4	93	7	94	6
65 plus	70	30	62	38	52	48	54	46
Females:								
45 to 64	78	22	77	23	76	27	75	25
65 plus	57	43	51	49	40	60	39	61

Source: U.S. Department of Labor, Bureau of Labor Statistics, Current Population Survey, 1985.

*Figures may not total 100 percent due to rounding.

DESIRE FOR EMPLOYMENT

Although more older Americans are retiring at increasingly younger ages, more are also seeking employment. According to a recent survey by the American Association of Retired Persons (AARP), 40 percent of those already retired said they would rather be working, and 70 percent of AARP's membership who were still employed said they preferred work to retirement (Yankelovich, Skelly, and White, 1986). Two factors may partially explain this apparent contradiction.

One reason is that many people choose to retire and then find they have trouble living on their retirement income. Others are forced out of work when their company closes, is taken over, or is restructured. These displaced workers, often too young to receive Social Security benefits or pensions, but too old to have many good job prospects, must continue to work to make ends meet. Of the 5.1 million workers displaced between 1979 and 1984, 20 percent were age 55 or older (U.S. Bureau of Labor Statistics, 1985).

The second reason for the stated preference to continue working after retirement is a need to feel productive and to share expertise. A job could be a new career, a continuation of earlier work, or simply a way to avoid boredom! Consider the motivation of Mr. Carlson, a 74-year-old who retired from an executive position and quickly became vice president of a newly formed, fast-growing company. In good health, he has a lot of energy, enjoys seeing things accomplished, and likes solving problems. Although most of his peers play golf daily, he maintains that he would be bored stiff, and prefers to work 50 to 60 hours a week.

UNEMPLOYMENT AMONG THE ELDERLY

Older workers who are unemployed but still seeking work, rather than voluntarily retired, stay out of work longer than younger workers, suffer a greater loss of earnings in subsequent jobs, and are more likely to become discouraged and abandon the job search (U.S. Senate Special Committee on Aging, 1986; Parnes, 1981; Rones, 1983). The unemployment rate among older workers (3.1 percent) is not large compared to some younger age groups. However, the official unemployment rate is a poor indicator of the severity of the problem, because of the long duration of unemployment among individuals over age 45 and the greater tendency of older workers to become discouraged and stop looking for work. As a result, they are not reflected in the official statistics of "workers out of work and looking." For those older persons who have to work for economic reasons or because they want to stay active, unemployment is undoubtedly a serious problem, just as it is for younger people. Those who do find jobs are likely to work at low pay or part-time or both.

Unemployed older workers have a difficult time with their job search for a number of reasons. First, they may have been in one occupation for many years and therefore lack experience in job-hunting techniques. Second, their skills may be obsolete or need to be updated. Some older job-seekers are intimidated by new technology in the workplace. To assist them, a growing number of cities are forming job referral and training services geared to older workers.

Although there has been considerable discussion about maintaining older persons in the work force, government and industry are unlikely to encourage older persons to remain in jobs or to take new jobs as long as widespread unemployment persists among the population at large (U.S. Joint Economic Committee, 1980). This view prevails, even though there is little evidence that withdrawal of older people from the labor market serves to reduce unemployment for younger populations (Crystal, 1982).

Barriers to Employment

The extent to which declining labor force participation by the elderly reflects age-based employment discrimination is a topic of considerable debate. The American public has been nearly unanimous in opposing mandatory retirement policies as discriminatory. The Age Discrimination in Employment Act (ADEA) was passed in 1967 to protect workers age 45 and over from denial of employment strictly because of age, to eliminate obstacles to prolonged employment, and thus to allow a later retirement age. This act was amended in 1978 to prohibit the use of pension plans as justification for not hiring older workers and to raise the mandatory retirement age to 70. In 1986, mandatory retirement was eliminated for businesses with more than 20 employees. (State and local public safety officers

---

Barriers to Employment

Mr. Lewis is a 60-year-old with no car, savings, or relatives nearby. He works two part-time jobs and finds it difficult to make ends meet. One of his jobs is under a government program with a local agency that signed an agreement to hire him full time when an opening arose. That was over 2½ years ago. In that time, they have hired 15 to 20 people without experience or training in the field to do the job he would like. They are all people under age 40. Mr. Lewis has a background of 20 years in large organizations, so he assumes that he has the appropriate experience.

At first, Mr. Lewis was told he had to "go through the system" to be hired full-time. Much later, after he had been through the system time and time again, it became obvious he would never be hired full-time. Eventually, he was told that "the agency feels it wants to give younger employees a chance to come up the career ladder." He is resentful at seeing these younger workers move ahead so quickly. He is beginning to wonder if he is a victim of age discrimination, but he does not know what he can do about his situation.

---

and tenured faculty members are exempt from the new provisions until 1994.) Despite such legislation, age discrimination, more than sex or race discrimination, is the fastest growing form of unfair dismissal litigation.

Although the most blatant forms of age discrimination, such as newspaper ads restricting jobs to younger people, have declined since the passage of the ADEA, more subtle forms persist. For example, the U.S. Navy recently required that their club waitresses wear mini-skirts, a requirement that was used against hiring older women. Employers can make a job situation unattractive to older workers by stopping raises and promotions and removing responsibilities to downgrade workers' jobs. In a 1981 survey of 552 employers, 20 percent admitted that workers over age 50 have fewer opportunities for promotions or training, and 12 percent stated that for older workers, pay raises are not as large as those of younger workers (Mercer, 1981). It is not surprising that eight out of ten Americans of all ages in 1981 believed that "most employers discriminate against older people and make it difficult for them to find work" (Harris and Associates, 1981).

One reason that discrimination persists is the pervasiveness of negative stereotypes about aging and productivity. (These stereotypes will be discussed further in Chapter 17.) Many employers still assume that older workers will not perform as well as younger workers because of poor health, declining energy, or diminished intellectual ability. These attitudes endure despite the growth of research findings that older workers do not differ significantly from younger workers on measures of productivity, accuracy, or absenteeism due to illness. In fact, the average number of absences among older workers in some firms is lower than that of younger workers and, in some instances, performance improves with age (Waldman and Aviolo, 1986). In a survey of 400 major U.S. corporations, older workers were perceived as loyal, dedicated, and a valuable source of information (Yankelovich, Skelly, and White, 1986). As noted in Chapter 7, older workers usually perform better than younger workers on tasks requiring experience, as contrasted with tasks depending on endurance, strength, or speed (Clark and Spengler, 1980; Foner and Schwab, 1981).

Other employment barriers that older workers face are primarily structural; skill obsolescence and age bias in the allocation of jobs are particularly significant. Shortcomings in older workers' job performance that have been identified can frequently be traced to lower levels of educational attainment and lack of technical training in earlier work experience. For example, older workers are disadvantaged in competing for jobs in the growing electronics and computer industries. A secretary who has used a typewriter for 35 years is at a real disadvantage in today's job market if she does not know how to use a word processor! Difficulties with skill obsolescence have also been aggravated by geographic shifts in industries from the mid-Atlantic and northcentral states to the southeast, southwest, and west. Since older workers with homes and family ties generally find relocating difficult, they have tended to stay in areas where finding new jobs is less likely.

Creating New Opportunities for Work

Findings about older workers' job performance have been cited by advocacy organizations for the elderly, such as the Gray Panthers, in their successful arguments for eliminating mandatory retirement. These groups maintain that judging a person's job qualifications solely on the basis of age, without regard to suitability for a job, is inequitable, and that chronological age alone is a poor predictor of job performance. Not hiring older workers deprives society of their skills and capacities. In most cases, work environments may be modified to compensate for any drawbacks associated with older workers, if employers are willing to do so.

Many ways have been suggested to restructure work to enable the elderly to have the option of longer work lives. These include federal government actions, such as modifying Social Security and pension restrictions against earnings, and giving tax credits or other tax incentives to employers who hire older workers. The private sector could create "emeritus" positions for older workers, as is already done for university professors but on a part-time paid basis; for example, a former firefighter could work as a community relations specialist and conduct information programs in schools. Some companies, such as the Travelers

Insurance Corporation, allow employees to return as consultants, and retrain older workers to enter jobs on a part-time basis where there is a shortage of workers. Flexibility for older workers can also be created through job sharing, allowing some work to be done at home, and individualizing working hours. Some European countries have "gliding out" plans of staged retirement that permit a gradual shift to a part-time schedule for older workers. Older people in less industrialized societies, for example, tend to withdraw gradually from physically demanding or time-consuming tasks, rather than face retirement at a predetermined age (Foner and Schwab, 1981).

The need for new opportunities for older workers will increase by the year 2000, when a majority of the older population is expected to choose employment, a trend counter to the current situation where most older people are retired. Reasons for this shift include a decreasing pool of younger workers, increasingly expensive health and social services for the elderly, a lifelong career orientation, and economic expectations to continue a similar lifestyle (Pifer and Bronte, 1986). Already, older people are moving into jobs traditionally filled by youth (e.g., providing service at fast-food restaurants), largely because of the decline among young people willing to work in such positions. By 1995, the median age of the work force is expected to be 37.3 years, compared to 34.8 years in 1982 (Rosen and Jerdee, 1985). The aging of the "baby boomers" will undoubtedly create a new image of older workers!

Retirement

With increased longevity and changing work patterns, retirement has become as much an expected part of the life course as having a family, completing school, or working. This is a relatively recent phenomenon in Western society, however. Retirement developed as a twentieth-century social institution, along with industrialization, surplus labor, and a rising standard of living. Social Security legislation, passed in 1935, established the right to financial protection in old age and thus served to institutionalize retirement. Based on income deferred during the worker's years of employment, Social Security was viewed as a reward for past economic contributions to society, which entitled the worker to a share of the country's wealth.

Retirement serves a variety of functions in an industrialized society. It can stimulate and reward worker loyalty. In addition, it is a way to remove older, presumably more expensive, workers, and replace them with younger employees, assumed to be more productive. It thereby serves as a way to reduce the number of people holding or seeking jobs.

Although Social Security was presented to the public as a means to support people physically unable to maintain jobs, retirement has become associated in the public mind with the chronological age of 65 (the age of eligibility for full

Social Security benefits) and, in turn, with being old, physically disabled and no longer capable of full-time employment—an association that has had long-run deleterious consequences for older people.

TREND TOWARD EARLY RETIREMENT

Despite our society's work-oriented values and the importance of income derived from work, employment and retirement policies since the 1900s have been directed toward encouraging early retirement. For example, nine out of ten pension plans, particularly for white-collar workers, provide financial incentives for early retirement. Even employees who were not planning on retirement often feel they cannot turn down attractive retirement benefits. These programs, combined with mandatory retirement policies that were in effect until 1987, a highly competitive work force, and rapidly changing technologies, result in few older persons being employed, as illustrated in Table 12–2. This trend may be compounded by a growing emphasis on leisure as an alternative to the work ethic, particularly among the middle-aged and young-old. Furthermore, many older persons retire early because of poor health, even though they may wish to continue working. (These issues will be discussed in more detail later in this chapter.) Today, only 16.3 percent of men age 65 and over and 7.5 percent of their female counterparts are in the labor force (U.S. Special Committee on Aging, 1985–86). These figures represent a decline from 1950, when 46 percent of older men and 10 percent of older women were employed. This phenomenon of low employment is described as the "graying of America's population, but not of its work force" (McConnell, 1983).

The trend toward early retirement has also extended down to the preretirement age among men but not among women. Between 1970 and 1985, the labor force participation rate among males aged 55 to 64 declined from 83 percent to 67.9 percent. In contrast, women in the 55 to 64 age group have increasingly joined the work force. The percentage of women in this age category who were employed increased from a low of 27 percent in 1950 to 43 percent in 1970, then declined slightly to 42 percent in 1985 (U.S. Senate Special Committee on Aging, 1985–86). Despite the increase in labor force participation among women, most women still retire by age 65. The declining labor force participation rates of the older population are consistent with patterns in most other industrialized countries, reflecting the increased availability of retirement pensions.

THE TIMING OF RETIREMENT

The arbitrary nature of any particular age for retirement is shown by the fact that most people retire between the ages of 62 and 64, and very few continue to work past age 70, even though 1978 legislation changed the mandatory retirement age to 70. In fact, it can hardly be said that age 65 is the "normal" retirement age.

TABLE 12–2 Labor Force Status by Age, Sex, and Ethnic Minority Status: Third Quarter 1984 (Not Seasonally Adjusted)

	Age					
	50 to 54	*55 to 59*	*60 to 61*	*62 to 64*	*65 to 69*	*70 plus*
Percent in labor force:						
Total male	89.4	80.2	68.0	47.7	24.7	11.6
Total female	59.0	49.3	39.5	28.8	13.9	4.3
White male	90.5	81.6	68.7	48.7	25.0	11.9
White female	59.0	48.7	39.0	28.3	13.8	4.3
Black male	81.3	68.9	62.0	38.1	21.6	9.5
Black male	59.0	53.9	33.3	32.8	14.9	4.6

Source: U.S. Department of Labor, Bureau of Labor Statistics, 1985.

Instead, 60.6 years is the median age for retirement. Three-quarters of all new Social Security beneficiaries each year retire before their sixty-fifth birthday, and most begin collecting reduced benefits at age 62, the minimum age for eligibility (U.S. Senate Special Committee on Aging, 1985). Federal workers retire at an average age of 61, even though there has not been a mandatory retirement age for federal employees (Crystal, 1982).

The average retirement age in heavy industries, such as steel and auto manufacturing, is even lower than age 62, because of private pension inducements. These plans provide supplemental pension payments at an adequate level, thereby allowing employees to retire before the age of Social Security eligibility. The "30 years and out" pension provisions of labor contracts in the auto industry have been widely supported by union members. Those who retire from the military after the minimum required 20 years often move on to other careers that enable them to draw double pensions after age 65. With longer life expectancies, some may even move into a third career during their post-military years.

The timing of retirement is influenced by several factors. Certainly, one element is the minimum age of eligibility for an adequate retirement income, provided either through Social Security or a private pension. Economic factors (e.g., expected level of pensions, income and net assets) are central, inasmuch as they directly influence decisions about the feasibility of retirement and indirectly contribute to worker health and job satisfaction. Another factor has been mandatory retirement age in one's job, (although this will no longer be a salient factor with the elimination of mandatory retirement in 1986). Clearly, however, these are not the only issues. In one study, 80 percent of retirees surveyed would not accept a job even if it were offered to them (Parnes, 1981). Other studies have found, however, that most retirees would continue to work if they were physically able or had an appropriate and flexible job (McConnell, Fleisher, Usher, and

Kaplan, 1980). Most retirees seem not to want the constraints inherent in full-time employment; rather, they want the option of retiring early from regular employment, as well as opportunities for new career directions or for part-time and other flexible work to meet their economic and social needs. Some researchers have suggested that even delays in Social Security benefits and reductions in the early retirement benefits of private pensions would have little effect on delaying the retirement age. In addition, the elimination of mandatory retirement laws may not discourage early retirement, since only a small percentage of retirees have been forced to leave their jobs because of such requirements (Rosen and Jerdee, 1985).

In addition to income, the timing of retirement may be determined by health, families' preferences, informal norms of the work situation, and long-range plans. Some workers retire to escape boring, repetitive jobs, such as assembly line and office work. Workers who have a positive attitude toward retirement but a negative view of their jobs, often because of undesirable and stressful working conditions, are likely to retire early. In contrast, workers with high satisfaction in interesting jobs are less likely to retire early. Higher status professional or managerial workers and those who are self-employed tend to be highly committed to their work and to want to remain employed for as long as possible. Well-educated employees are less likely to retire early than those with a high-school education or less, as illustrated by Mrs. and Mrs. Howard in the introductory vignette (Foner and Schwab, 1981).

The effects of gender on the retirement decision are not clear-cut. In general, women of retirement age have been found to be more interested in working longer and in alternatives such as part-time work than are men (Usher, 1981). Women who want to continue working may be late-career starters who enjoy work or who fear early widowhood, or they may be financially insecure because of divorce and a short or discontinuous work career. In general, degree of satisfaction in retirement for both men and women appears to be related to similar factors, particularly income and health. The slightly lower levels of retirement satisfaction found among women seem to be due primarily to their lower retirement incomes (Seccombe and Lee, 1986).

The most important factors for the timing of retirement appear to be income and health. One-third of the retirees in a 1981 Harris survey reported that they were forced to retire; of these, almost two-thirds claimed disability or poor health as the reason (Harris and Associates, 1981). Self-reports of poor health as the motivation for retirement need to be interpreted cautiously, however. Retirees may report poor health as the reason, despite their actual health status, because they perceive this to be a socially acceptable response. Two categories of people who retire early have been identified: those with good health and adequate financial resources who desire additional leisure time, and those with low incomes and health problems that make their work burdensome (Clark and Spengler, 1980; Morgan, 1980). Poor health, when combined with an adequate retirement income, usually results in early retirement. In contrast, poor health and an inadequate income generally delay retirement by reason of necessity. The extent to which poor health influences retirement also varies with the job, with health problems being a greater motivation for retirement from physically demanding jobs than from office work, for example.

The complexity of variables discussed thus far, in terms of the causes, timing, and consequences of retirement, suggest several distinct types of retirement situations. These can be summarized as follows:

- Strong preference for retirement as soon as financially feasible
- Retirement following unemployment
- Retirement due to health problems
- Compulsory retirement and willingness to take it
- Compulsory retirement and reluctance to take it (Atchley, 1979).

These various circumstances of retirement have different consequences for satisfaction with retirement.

SATISFACTION WITH RETIREMENT

The importance of factors other than policies that set retirement age and benefits suggests the value of examining retirement as a *process* that affects people's lives in multiple ways. This concept encompasses not only the timing and type of retirement situation, but also the phases after the event of retirement. Atchley (1976) has suggested that an initial euphoric, busy, honeymoon phase is followed by a letdown or disenchantment phase, followed by a reorientation to the realities of retired life. This sequence leads to a subsequent stable phase, when the retiree has settled into a predictable and satisfying routine. These phases are presented as a "typical progression of processes" (Atchley, 1976), although not every individual will experience all the phases or in the order described. Although Atchley did not offer empirical evidence to support his framework, a recent study found the immediate postretirement period to be characterized by enthusiasm, with some degree of temporary letdown during the second year of retirement (Ekerdt, Bosse, and Levkoff, 1985).

The early gerontological literature emphasized retirement as a life crisis (Atchley, 1976; Streib and Schneider, 1971). As described in Chapter 8, it is included in many lists of major life events that require some adjustment. Although it *is* a major transition, most retirees adjust well and are relatively satisfied with their life circumstances. For most American workers, retirement is desired, and their decision is not *whether* to retire but *when*. A variety of factors affect the degree of satisfaction. Retirement in itself does not directly affect levels of social activity, life satisfaction, morale, or self-esteem (Palmore, Fillenbaum, and George, 1984). Rather, satisfaction in retirement depends more on factors such as health, the voluntary nature of retirement, income, family situation, type of occupation, work values, job history, and perceptions of daily activities as useful. Not unexpectedly, those who retire willingly are more satisfied than those who feel forced to retire, either because of mandatory retirement policies or health problems (Parnes, 1981; Streib and Schneider, 1971). Those who retire early because of poor health or lack of job opportunities are less satisfied with being retired, but they are also less pleased with other aspects of their lives, such as their housing, standard of living, and leisure (Parnes and Nestel, 1981). In general, however, early retirement has more negative effects than later retirement (Palmore et al., 1984).

Occupational status is also an important predictor of the likelihood of retirement satisfaction, with lower status workers having more health and financial problems, and therefore less satisfaction, than higher level white-collar workers. The more meaningful work characteristics of higher status occupations may "spill over" into a greater variety of satisfying nonwork pursuits throughout life, which are conducive to more social contacts and more structured opportunities during retirement (Kohn and Schooler, 1982). For example, a college professor may have a work and social routine that is more readily transferable to retirement than does a construction worker. Recent research suggests that retirees with strong traditional work values are not as satisfied as retirees with weaker work values (Hooker and Ventis, 1984). This is consistent with an earlier finding that retirees who are not work-oriented adjust to retirement more easily than "workaholics" (Streib and Schneider, 1971). Differences between retirees in upper and lower status occupations, however, do not develop with retirement, but rather reflect variations in social and personal resources throughout the life course (Ward, 1982). Less is known about the effect of occupational status on retirement satisfaction among ethnic minorities (Atchley, 1979), or about sex differences in the antecedents, consequences, and decision-making processes of retirement (George, Fillenbaum, and Palmore, 1984). For Blacks and low-income males, the negative economic impact of retirement can be somewhat ameliorated by income maintenance subsidies and programs for the elderly (Fillenbaum, George, and Palmore, 1984). Women's retirement plans, like men's, appear to be strongly influenced by their own pension and Social Security eligibility, not by their husbands' situations (Shaw, 1984).

In general, health and financial security appear to be the major determinants of retirees' satisfaction with life, rather than retirement status per se (George and Maddox, 1977; Streib and Schneider, 1971). Retirement does not *cause* poor health, as is commonly assumed (Palmore et al., 1984). Although health does deteriorate after retirement for some people, other people's health improves after retirement because they are no longer subject to stressful, unhealthy, or dangerous work conditions (Minkler, 1981). Contrary to stereotypes about the negative health effects of retirement, people who die shortly after retirement were probably in poor health before they retired (George and Maddox, 1977). In fact, deterioration in health is more likely to cause the retirement than vice versa (Palmore et al., 1984). Studies that have found that retirees have more physical and mental illness than nonretirees have relied on cross-sectional data, so that it remains uncertain whether retirees had these disabilities prior to retirement. The misconception that people become ill and die as a consequence of retirement undoubtedly persists on the basis of findings from cross-sectional data, as well as reports of isolated instances of such deaths. In addition, the traditional American ideology that life's meaning is derived from work may reinforce the stereotype that retirement has negative consequences. Another factor is that retirees may be motivated to exaggerate their health limitations in order to justify their retirement. Leaving the labor force because of health problems, however, may later be associated with dissatisfaction in retirement.

Leisure Activities and the Importance of Planning

Community involvement is another important predictor of well-being in retirement. Most retirees do not miss their jobs per se, but rather the income, associations with fellow employees, and activity levels related to work (NCOA, 1981). Retirement affects identity, self-esteem, and feelings of competence to the extent that it influences such involvement. As we will see in Chapter 13, leisure and community activities during retirement vary by economic status, but do not differ significantly between retirees and workers of the same age. Retirement tends to be characterized by a continuity of preretirement activities, with little or no change in social interactions, church attendance, or community participation (Foner and Schwab, 1981; Mutran and Reitzes, 1981; Streib and Schneider, 1971).

The continuity of leisure activities from working years through retirement suggests the importance of preparation and planning prior to retirement. In fact, preparation has been found to be associated with a more positive retirement experience. People who have focused only on work all their lives cannot expect suddenly to develop leisure interests and skills upon their retirement. Most pre-retirees weave fantasies about the trips they will take or the household projects they will complete. After a "honeymoon period" of enjoying new pursuits for about six months, they often find that these activities will not meaningfully fill every day for the next 20 or 30 years. As will be discussed in Chapter 13, if nonwork interests are not developed prior to retirement, they are unlikely to be cultivated after retirement. Instead, people need to develop activities outside of the worker role during their employed lives.

Comprehensive retirement planning programs that address social activities, health promotion, and family relationships are one way of encouraging this development. Unfortunately, existing retirement preparation programs often include only information about pension benefits, not health and lifestyle planning. Because such programs are not widespread, only about 10 percent of the labor force benefits from any kind of retirement planning. Older men with more years of education, higher occupational status, and private pensions have greater access to these programs, as do government employees. Accordingly, the group of older workers who would benefit most from retirement preparation—those with less education, lower occupational status, no pension coverage, and consequently lower retirement income—are the least likely to have access to such services (Beck, 1984). Another approach to preparation is to restructure work patterns, gradually allowing longer vacations, shorter work days, and more opportunities for community involvement during the preretirement working years, thereby easing the transition to more leisure time.

In sum, most people do not have a problem with retirement as a transition, provided they have sufficient preparation for it and an adequate income, enjoy good health, were not forced to retire, and were not wedded to their work. When people are unhappy in retirement, it is more often because of health or income problems than because of the loss of the worker role per se. Retirement policies, labor market conditions, and individual characteristics all converge on the decision to retire. Collectively, these individual decisions translate into a rate of retirement for our society. The rate or level of retirement, in turn, has an impact on businesses, communities, and society at large. Thus, while the individual's experience of retirement as a process is not necessarily painful, our society is increasingly confronting the problem of retirement as a complex social institution, in which longer life expectancies and earlier retirement have resulted in prolonged dependence on Social Security and other retirement benefits as well as loss of older worker's skills. These institutional difficulties are discussed further in Chapter 18.

Sources of Income in Retirement

Sources of income for the older population include savings, assets and investments, Social Security, private pensions, and, for a small percentage, a salary. The distribution of these income sources is illustrated in Figure 12–2. Mr. Valdres and Mrs. Howard in the introductory vignettes demonstrate the diversity among older people in their reliance on these various income sources.

SOCIAL SECURITY

Social Security remains the heart of the retirement income system. The elderly depend more heavily on Social Security for their income than on any other source. In 1982, 40 percent of all income received by elderly units (i.e., a married couple with one or both members aged 65 or older and living together, or a person

FIGURE 12–2 Income Sources, Aged Units 65 and Older, 1982

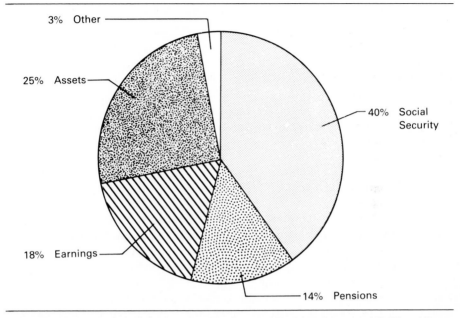

Source: Susan Grad, *Income of the population 55 and over, 1982.* U.S. Department of Health and Human Services, Social Security Administration, 1984.

aged 65 or older not living with a spouse) was from Social Security. Of all older persons, 90 percent received Social Security income, and 15 percent derived all their income from Social Security. In all, more than one-third of elderly household units depended on Social Security for 80 percent or more of their income (Bureau of Labor Statistics, 1983).

Yet Social Security was never intended to provide an adequate retirement income, but rather a floor of protection or the first tier of support. It was assumed that pensions and individual savings would also help support people in their later years. This assumption has not been borne out, as reflected in the proportionately lower income received by retirees from savings and private pensions. It has been estimated that, without Social Security, poverty rates among the elderly would increase from 12.4 percent to about 50 percent (U.S. Senate, 1986). Not surprisingly, the elderly with the lowest incomes have Social Security as their sole source. In 1982, for example, 80 percent of aggregate income received by elderly units with incomes under $5,000 came from Social Security benefits (Grad, 1984a).

The Social Security system is based on the concept of earned rights, rather than universal eligibility for all older persons. In order to be insured, a worker retiring now must be age 62 or more and must be employed consecutively for at

---

Older Person Living on Social Security

As an example of the difficulty of living on Social Security, a New York city woman wrote to the Older Women's League, "I will be 65 in February, but cannot afford to retire since my $500 a month Social Security income (which is all I will have in this world) will pay for rent, utilities and nothing else. It is not possible to move to cheaper quarters. . . . I receive no assistance in paying for utilities. . . . I have severe physical problems which preclude my being able to work for too much longer. I am an unmonied city dweller, but cannot even qualify for Medicaid."

Source: The OWL Observer, From the Mailbag, July/August 1984, p. 10.

least eight years or 34 quarters. The level of benefits received is based on a percentage of the retired worker's average monthly earnings that were subject to Social Security tax. Insured persons are eligible for full benefits at age 65; if they choose to retire at age 62, their monthly benefits are permanently reduced and are not increased when they reach age 65. Approximately 60 percent of all recipients currently receive such reduced benefits because they have retired even before the age of 62. As noted earlier, Social Security benefits are also reduced for those who work after age 65. This "earnings test" has been strongly criticized as an unfair deterrent to older people's labor force participation. Limited income exceptions now exist (Crystal, 1982).

The pattern of early retirement has created public concern about the financial strain on Social Security, federal pensions, and other income programs for the elderly. Such concern has increased with the decline in the number of workers paying into the Social Security system for every 100 persons drawing benefits; this ratio dropped from 410 to 320 between 1970 and 1980, and may fall to as low as 200 by the year 2025 (Parnes, 1983). As a result, some policymakers have advocated policies to discourage early retirement; for example, the age of Social Security eligibility is to be increased from age 62 to 67 by the year 2027, as specified by the 1983 amendments. Despite concerns in the early 1980s that the fund might go bankrupt, the U.S. Senate Special Committee on Aging (1986) has concluded that trust funds will be solvent for the next 75 years. This is because the Social Security trust fund takes in more money than it pays out. For example, by 1990, it is projected to have an annual surplus of $50.7 billion (Kingson, Hirshorn, and Harootyan, 1986; U.S. Senate, 1986). If this continues to be the case, the Social Security "crisis" of the 1980s appears to be resolved. The extent to which concern about shifting dependency ratios has fueled public perceptions of intergenerational inequity is discussed further in Chapter 18.

Since June 1975, Social Security benefits have been automatically increased annually whenever the Consumer Price Index increases by 3 percent or more.

This is known as the *cost of living adjustment,* or COLA. Social Security benefits have thus been protected from inflation. The average monthly benefits for an individual and couple in 1987 were about $639 and $877, respectively. Since benefits are related to a worker's wage and employment history, women and ethnic minorities, with their history of intermittent or part-time work, tend to receive less than this average.

Women's Social Security payments may also be sharply reduced by widowhood or divorce. A widow may start to collect surviving dependents' benefits when she reaches age 60; however, she will lose 28.5 percent of what she would receive if she waited until age 65. Widows and divorcees under age 60 who are not disabled and who do not have children under age 18 entitled to Social Security or who are not responsible for disabled persons cannot receive Social Security benefits. This group of women, who generally do not have a paid work history and do not qualify for any public benefits, are often referred to as *displaced homemakers.* Since the average age at widowhood is 56 years, many women face this "widow's gap." A woman who is divorced after at least 10 years of marriage and who reaches retirement age may collect up to 50 percent of her ex-husband's retirement benefits, but only when he retires and if she remains single. Because many widows or divorced women do not meet these criteria, a large percentage of single older women live in poverty or near-poverty conditions. These gender inequities will be discussed further in Chapter 16.

Social Security is a regressive tax (i.e., having the same effect on both the rich and the poor), which means that low-income workers, many of whom are women and ethnic minorities, pay a larger percentage of their monthly salary to taxes. For example, an employee earning $12,000 in 1983 paid 6.7 percent of his or her wages in Social Security, whereas an executive earning $200,000 paid only 1.2 percent (Olson, 1984). Some minority advocates contend that Social Security is discriminatory because ethnic minorities, as a group, pay more Social Security tax on the basis of low income and also have reduced total benefits because of lower average life expectancy than that of the general population. (In fact, because of this difference in life expectancy, many ethnic minorities do not live long enough to collect their first Social Security check!) On the other hand, Social Security's benefit structure is least generous to high-income contributors, who receive a

---

Displaced Homemaker

Mrs. Kelly lost her husband over a year ago at the age of 56. Her daughter was 15 years old at the time. When she turned 16, Mrs. Kelly's Social Security check stopped. Mrs. Kelly has no health insurance; she cannot work because she is caring for her 90-year-old mother. Nevertheless, she is too young for Social Security and Medicare benefits.

smaller percentage of what their income was prior to retirement and who must now pay income tax on 50 percent of their Social Security benefits. Generally, however, high income contributors do not need the floor of support provided by Social Security because they are covered by pensions and assets.

ASSETS

Income from assets (e.g., savings, home equity, personal property) comprised 25 percent of all income received by older people in 1982, and was the second most important source. However, it was unevenly distributed, with nearly 33 percent of the elderly units reporting no asset income, and 33 percent of those with asset income reporting less than $500 a year. In fact, only 28 percent of those with such income received more than $5,000 a year from this source (Grad, 1984b). The assets that the elderly hold exist primarily as home equity. (In 1980, nearly 75 percent of older people owned their homes [U.S. Senate Special Committee on Aging, 1986].) Home equity, however, does not represent liquid wealth and therefore cannot be relied on to cover daily expenses. Thus, most elderly cannot depend on financial assets as a substantial source of income.

EARNINGS

Earnings were an important income source to the young-old in 1982, but declined in importance with age. Thus, individuals age 65 to 67 received 35 percent of their income from earnings, compared with only 4 percent for those 80 years and older. Overall, current job earnings formed 18 percent of the income of elderly units (Grad, 1984a). This low percentage is consistent with the declining labor force participation among people age 65 and over.

PENSIONS

While most jobholders are covered by Social Security, which is a *general public pension,* some employees are covered by *job-specific pensions.* These are available only through a specific position of employment and are administered by a work organization, union, or private insurance company. Job-specific pensions include *public employee pensions* (for those who work for federal, state, or local governments) and *private pensions.* Most private pensions, which developed after the passage of Social Security, are intended to supplement Social Security retirement benefits. Employee pensions provided only 14 percent of the older population's aggregate 1982 income; overall, one in three elderly units received some income from public and/or private pension benefits; one in four had income from private pensions only (Crystal, 1982). Job-related pensions are generally intended to be supplements to Social Security, so that average benefits tend to be relatively low. In a survey of 977 pension plans, the average annual pension for a worker employed for 30 years was $2,720, the equivalent, on the average, of 22 percent of employment income (Schulz, Leavitt, and Kelby, 1979).

Pension benefits are generally based on earnings or a combination of earnings and years of service. Eligibility age is usually between ages 60 and 65, although it ranges from ages 50 to 70. Only about 3 percent of pension plans provide for cost-of-living increases. Yet an annual inflation rate of 5 percent for 15 years can erode the real value of benefits by about one-half, making inflation the greatest threat to those dependent on private pensions. Federal policies support private pension programs by postponing taxation of pension benefits, allowing benefits to be invested and to generate earnings which are not taxed. Only when the pension is drawn is tax paid, after the money has produced many years of earnings (Parnes, 1983).

Private pensions go to workers with long, continuous service in jobs that have such coverage. In general, these are higher income, relatively skilled positions concentrated among large, unionized, and/or industrial employers. As a result, employees who benefit from private pensions tend to be in the middle and upper income brackets. Pension coverage varies dramatically by class, race, and gender, being relatively low for women, ethnic minorities, and lower income workers in small, nonunion plants and low-wage industries, such as retail sales and services. These problems are compounded for women, who are more likely than men to be "in and out" of the labor force and therefore less likely to achieve the required length of service for vesting. Nonemployed women face an additional problem: Most pension plans reduce benefits for those who elect to protect their spouses through survivors' benefits. In the past, many men have chosen higher monthly benefits rather than survivors' benefits; when they died, their wives were left without adequate financial protection.

The Employment Retirement Income Security Act (ERISA), enacted in 1974 to strengthen private pension systems, was the first major effort to regulate them. As a result, private pension plans must *vest* benefits (vesting refers to the amount of time a person must work on a job in order to acquire rights to the pension) in such a way that all covered workers are guaranteed a full pension upon retirement after 10 or 15 years with the company, regardless of whether or not they remain with that organization until retirement. This means that a person could work for one firm for 12 years, move to a second company until retirement at age 65, and then receive pensions from both based on years of service. Although vesting options increased under ERISA, portability (whereby pension contributions and rights with one organization can be transferred to another) remains low. This has been criticized for penalizing worker mobility and career changes. For example, an individual who serves 40 years with one company will receive a higher pension than one who spent 20 years with one firm and 20 with another.

ERISA also strengthened standards for financing, administering, and protecting pension plans. Tax-exempt individual retirement accounts (IRAs) were created for workers with pension coverage, and were made available to all workers in 1981, in an effort to increase personal savings for retirement. (Under the 1986 tax reform plan, employees with other private pensions will no longer be able to use an IRA as a tax deduction.) Yet IRAs are not an option for most workers; they are used primarily by those earning $50,000 or more who have disposable income (Schulz, 1985). Lower income workers generally cannot spare the money, and the tax benefit is considerably less for them. (This tax benefit is greatest at higher incomes because it is based on a tax deduction.) Ironically, the people who need retirement income the most generally cannot take advantage of IRAs. As with employer pension plans, the tax deferral of IRAs provides the equivalent of a long-term interest-free loan (e.g., tax shelter) to the predominantly high-income taxpayers who use IRAs.

Poverty Among Old and Young

The economic position of older people has improved since the 1960s. In 1959, 35.2 percent of the population aged 65 and over fell below the official poverty line, compared to 12.6 percent in 1985 (Uhlenberg and Salmon, 1986). In contrast, the poverty rate was 11.7 percent of those aged 18 to 64, and 14.1 percent of all persons under age 65 in 1985 (U.S. Bureau of the Census, 1986).* (The poverty level for a single adult younger than age 65 was then $5,593, compared to $5,156 for an elderly individual.) The U.S. Census Bureau has assumed that the costs of food and other necessities are lower for the elderly—an assumption that is not valid. If the same poverty standard were applied to the elderly as to the other age groups, the poverty rate for the elderly would increase to 15.2 percent (Villers, 1987). At the other extreme, 5.6 percent of all households headed by an older person have incomes exceeding $50,000 in 1985. This translates into 27 percent of households headed by Americans over the age of 65 having an annual income in excess (averaging $5,533) of what they need in order to live comfortably. On a per capita basis, this amount is higher than well-off American households in any other age group. Another indicator of the older population's improved economic status is that people aged 50 and over hold one out of every two discretionary dollars, a fact that has particular relevance for marketing products to this segment of the population (U.S. Bureau of the Census, 1986).

The primary factors underlying these gains are improved and longer coverage by pensions, the 1972 increases in Social Security benefits, the 1975

---

*Poverty is a measure of the adequacy of money income in relation to a minimal level of consumption—the poverty level. This level is fixed in real terms and adjusted for family size. The dollar values of the poverty levels are adjusted each year to reflect changes in the Consumer Price Index. In 1985, the official poverty line for an elderly individual was $5,156 and for an older couple, $6,503. This means that an individual whose weekly income fell below $99 was classified as officially poor, and *not* poor if that income were greater, even by only one dollar!

automatic annual cost of living adjustments (COLAs) in Social Security, and implementation of the Supplemental Security Income program. As a result of these policy changes, a widely held public perception is that the elderly are better off financially than other age groups—a perception based, to some extent, on the reality of their improved condition. This perception is also fueled by the increase of poverty among children under age 18, making them the poorest age group. (In 1985, this rate was 20.7 percent [U.S. Bureau of the Census, 1986].)

It is true that when all sources of income are considered (including tax and in-kind benefits), fewer older families have subpoverty resources than younger families, but the distribution of income among the elderly is extremely diverse (see Table 12–3). For instance, in 1984, approximately 20 percent of older families reported incomes under $10,000, whereas 25 percent had incomes of $30,000 or above. Among elderly individuals, 25 percent had incomes under $5,000; about 11 percent had incomes of $20,000 or above (Kingson, Hirshorn, and Harootyan, 1986). Similarly, a larger percentage of older families have economic resources just above the poverty line, and thus are *at-risk* of poverty or economically vulnerable, as illustrated in Table 12–3. More likely than other age groups to be among the "near-poor," over one-third of the elderly have incomes below 150 percent of the poverty line (Cook and Kramek, 1986). In 1984, the incomes of 21.2 percent of the elderly were below the near-poverty thresholds of $6,624 for a single older person and $7,853 for an older couple (U.S. Bureau of the Census, 1984). Similarly, 16.7 percent of persons aged 65 and over were in families with incomes just between the poverty level and 1½ times that level, compared to less than 10 percent of those under age 65 (U.S. Bureau of the Census, 1984). Furthermore, cohorts continue to experience income loss as they enter old age and therefore economic deprivation relative to younger cohorts because the elderly have fewer chances to increase their incomes (Schulz, 1985).

The group just above the poverty level may be especially hard hit by the economic problems that accompany retirement, because their income may be too high to allow them to qualify for public financial assistance (e.g., Supplemental Security Income), but too low to ensure an adequate standard of living. Even

TABLE 12–3 Percent of Elderly and Nonelderly Persons by Ratio of Income to Poverty, 1984

	Age	
Ratio of Income to Poverty Level	*Under 65*	*65 and Older*
Below poverty	14.7	12.4
100 to 124 percent poverty	4.5	8.8
125 to 150 percent poverty	5.1	7.9
Total below 150 percent	24.3	29.1

Source: Special tabulation of March 1985 Current Population Survey, U.S. Bureau of the Census.

those with pensions may have marginal levels of income. It is generally agreed that retirees must receive 60 to 90 percent of their preretirement income in order to maintain an adequate standard of living. Yet it has been estimated that in some industries, as few as 13 percent of married workers with 30 years employment were enrolled in private pension programs that provided this replacement rate (Schulz, Leavitt, and Kelby, 1979). Instead, 24 percent of older people rely on Social Security or SSI checks of $300 to $400 a month for 80 percent or more of their income (Kingson, Hirshorn, and Cornman, 1986). In addition, about 1 in 10 older persons never qualify for Social Security benefits because they were employed in occupations such as domestic work not covered by the system. Since retirement from the labor force can reduce individual incomes by one-third to one-half, most retirees must adjust their standard of living downward, at the same time as their out-of-pocket spending for health care needs may increase (Estes, Gerard, and Clarke, 1984). Chapters 18 and 19 address this matter further.

The stereotype of the static nature of poverty, suggested by cross-sectional information, must be altered to take account of the fact that many older people move in and out of poverty over time (Holden, Burkhauser, and Myers, 1986). When such individual movements are identified, the risk of falling below the poverty line *at some time* during a specified period is more than double the highest average risk among older couples, and is raised by almost 30 percent for widows. For example, many women become poor for the first time in their lives after spending down resources in order to qualify for the needs-based Medicaid program. There are also many "hidden poor" among the elderly, who are either institutionalized or living with relatives and thus not counted in official census statistics. Including these people in the total count would significantly raise the poverty rate among older people. In sum, more older people are at marginal levels of income and at greater risk of poverty than younger people; they are also more likely to be trapped in long-term poverty (Duncan, 1984).

Economic marginality is more pronounced among older women, those who live alone, ethnic minorities, and the old-old. Their economic hardships are often compounded by a lifetime of discrimination, by historical factors such as working at jobs with no pension or inadequate health insurance, and by recent stressful events, such as loss of spouse or declining health. Mr. Valdres and Mrs. Clark in the introductory vignettes illustrate these elderly. Mr. Valdres worked as a migrant farm laborer and therefore relies on the minimum Social Security level for his income. Mrs. Clark, on the other hand, thought her savings would be adequate for her old age, but the cost of caring for her ill husband for 18 years left her penniless. Elderly singles living alone are nearly five times as likely to be poor as elderly couples. The poverty rate among elderly singles is 19 percent. Of those who live alone, over 50 percent are over age 75 (Commonwealth Fund Commission, 1987). In 1985, about 18.7 percent of all persons 85 years or older were poor—a rate comparable to that among children under age 18 (U.S. Bureau of the Census, 1986).

As will be discussed in detail in Chapter 16, older women are among the poorest group in our society, particularly women living alone and those aged 85 and older. The risk of poverty among couples and single men has sharply fallen, leaving poverty in old age a characteristic primarily of single, frail women. This is consistent with the feminization of poverty in general. Although women accounted for more than half (59 percent) of the older population in 1985, they comprised nearly three-quarters (72.4 percent) of the elderly poor. Over 15 percent of older women were poor, compared to 8.5 percent of elderly men; this rate increases to 19.7 percent among women age 85 and over (U.S. Bureau of Census, 1986). Widows had the lowest median income of women living alone ($6,568). In 1983, widows accounted for 48 percent of all elderly poor, reflecting the loss of pension income and earnings often associated with the death of a wage-earner spouse (U.S. Bureau of the Census, 1985). The median income of widowed women was four-fifths that of widowed men ($7,936), since men are more likely to have retained pensions or earned income after a spouse's death (U.S. Senate Special Committee on Aging, 1986). Even though there has been some decline in poverty among older women over the past 20 years (consistent with the improvement of the economic status of elderly generally), the position of older women relative to middle-aged women has still not improved (Uhlenberg and Salmon, 1986). In 1980, the average female wage earner who spent her career employed in manufacturing received a retirement income less than two-thirds that of her male counterpart. The primary reasons for these gaps are women's interrupted work histories related to family responsibilities and their resultant lower Social Security benefits, less likelihood of private pensions to supplement Social Security, lower wages, and fewer part-time work options. The gaps between older men's and women's incomes actually increased between 1960 (when older women's average earnings were 67 percent of men's) and 1980 (when they were only 61 percent). This trend, particularly perplexing since women's average wage rose at a faster rate than men's over the same time period, can be attributed to the formulas used to calculate men and women's pension benefits (Tracy and Ward, 1986).

Black and Hispanic elderly of both sexes have substantially lower incomes than their white counterparts, as shown in Table 12–4. In 1985, the median income of older Black and Hispanic men was about half that of white men aged 65 and older. Although the differences were less pronounced among women, the median incomes of elderly Black and Hispanic women were generally two-thirds to three-quarters those of white women. Minority women's slight economic advantage relative to that of their male peers stems from the higher rates of unemployment and unsteady work histories among minority males. Not surprisingly, the poverty rates among minority elderly are higher than among whites. In 1985, the poverty rate among Black elderly was triple—and among Hispanic elderly, double—the rate among white elderly; over 30 percent of older Blacks and nearly 24 percent of elderly Hispanics were poor, compared to 11

TABLE 12–4 Median Income of Persons Age 65 and Older by Age, Race, and Sex, 1984

Race	Both sexes		Male		Female	
	65 to 69	70 plus	65 to 69	70 plus	65 to 69	70 plus
All races	$8,250	$6,556	$11,837	$8,663	$5,782	$5,540
White	8,655	6,889	12,180	9,109	5,966	5,765
Black	5,431	4,217	7,097	5,114	4,477	3,850
Hispanic	5,033	4,754	6,551	5,289	4,289	4,346

Source: U.S. Bureau of the Census, unpublished data from the March 1984 Current Population Survey.

percent of elderly whites. (U.S. Bureau of the Census, 1986). Poverty rates were the highest among minority women living alone. In 1984, nearly three out of every five older Black women not living with family had incomes below the poverty line, making them the most economically deprived group in our society (U.S. Senate Special Committee on Aging, 1985). Disparities between ethnic minority groups are discussed further in Chapter 15. In sum, despite the improved financial situation of the elderly generally, large pockets of poverty and near-poverty exist among the older population, particularly among women, ethnic minorities, those over age 75, and those who live alone.

Public Assistance

Of the older population, 11 percent receives some type of public assistance, primarily in the form of Supplemental Security Income (SSI) and Medicaid (health insurance for the poor, regardless of age). The proportions are higher among ethnic minority elderly women. For example, 37 percent of Black females and 22 percent of Black males received assistance in 1980 (Marsh, 1981).

SSI was established in 1974 to provide a minimum income for older Americans living on the margin of poverty. In contrast to Social Security, SSI does not require a history of covered employment contributions. Instead, eligibility is determined by a categorical requirement that the recipient be 65 years of age, blind, or disabled, and demonstrate need based on assets and income. (The current limit on cash assets is $1,800 for individuals and $2,700 for couples). SSI provides a subsistence income to over four million needy persons, 75 percent of whom are women age 75 and over. In 1987, the maximum federal SSI benefit was $340 a month for an individual and $510 for a couple, or about 90 percent of the poverty line in 1987. Older people whose Social Security income is less than that amount can apply for a monthly SSI payment to bring them up to that income level. Nevertheless, the federal SSI benefits fall substantially below the poverty line. Even when states supplement federal benefits (the median state supplement is $36 a month), benefit levels remain low.

Thus, despite the increased reliance on public assistance programs and the growing public perception that the elderly are no longer needy, low income is a substantial problem for older people, many of whom become "poor" or "near-poor" for the first time in their lives in old age. The distribution of income and assets among the elderly is highly skewed, with the bottom group getting a small share of both total income and government benefits (Crystal, 1982). Although some older people are financially quite comfortable, many are not, particularly since reduced income is not necessarily accompanied by reduced needs or desires for goods and services. An additional problem is that older people spend a greater share of their income than younger people on the basic necessities of food, housing, and health care—areas particularly hard hit by inflation.* The elderly are also less likely to have reserve funds to cover emergencies, such as catastrophic medical expenses. As a result, low-income elderly are at risk of malnutrition, poorly heated and inadequate housing, neglect of medical needs, and increasing isolation.

Summary and Implications

Although it is a relatively new phenomenon, retirement has become a normative expectation of old age in this country. Increasingly, Americans are leaving work in their early sixties and looking forward to a decade or more of leisure time in relatively good health. Not all retirement is desired; many older people would prefer the opportunity for part-time work. However, although flexible work opportunities for older people could be created, they rarely are, and the employment rate among older Americans is very low. In some cases, this is due to age discrimination; in other cases, it is due to mandatory retirement in the past and other public policies. Health status, the availability of pensions, and attitudes toward the job also influence the decision about when to retire.

Most retirees adjust well to this important transition, and are relatively satisfied with their lives. Those with good health, higher status jobs, adequate income, and previously developed social networks and leisure interests are most likely to be satisfied. Preparation for the retirement transition is beneficial, but planning assistance is generally not available to those who need it most—workers who have less education, lower job status, and lower retirement incomes.

---

*On the other hand, Social Security benefits, the primary source of income for low-income elderly, have been protected from inflation. Since over 90 percent of persons aged 65 and over are receiving Social Security benefits, this implies that virtually all older persons have at least one source of income that rises at a rate equal to that of price increases (Clark and Sumner, 1985).

Retirement preparation programs that do exist often address only financial needs, not health and lifestyle issues. Retirement by itself does not cause poor health or loss of identity and self-esteem. Unhappiness in this stage of life is more often due to poor health and low income.

Although a smaller percentage of elderly have incomes below the poverty line than they did in the past, more older people than younger people live at marginal economic levels. Social Security is the major source of retirement income for a large proportion of the older population, but it was never intended to be the only source. Those who depend on Social Security alone are the poorest elderly group. Private pensions tend to be small in relation to previous earnings, to be subject to attrition through inflation, and to go only to workers in large, unionized or industrialized settings. Recent federal legislation has protected pension rights to some extent. Income from assets is distributed unequally among the older population, with a small number of elderly receiving sizable amounts from savings and investments, whereas the most common asset of older people is their home, which provides no immediate income. In addition to those elderly who are officially counted as living below the poverty line, many others live near this level, and many are "hidden" poor who live in nursing homes or with their families. Frail, unmarried women—and ethnic minority women especially—are the most likely to live in or near poverty. Public assistance programs, such as SSI and Medicaid, have not removed the very serious financial problems of the elderly poor.

The trends toward greater longevity, early retirement, low rates of labor force participation, and pockets of poverty among older women, ethnic minorities, and the old-old suggest that a growing problem for the United States is the increase in the relative size of an older population encouraged not to work. The increased segmentation of life into a period of full-time work and one of total or partial retirement is, to a great extent, a product of our present pension systems. The ending of mandatory retirement laws is a first step to a smoother mix of labor and leisure across life. But this does not address the underlying economic incentives for retirement inherent in U.S. pension systems. More basic and far-reaching changes are needed, including greater flexibility in the workplace—opportunities for part-time work and a gradual transition from full-time productive work to leisure activities and retirement—and policies to address levels of unemployment in the general population.

References

Atchley, R. *The sociology of retirement.* New York: Wiley/Schenkman, 1976.

Atchley, R. Issues in retirement research. *The Gerontologist,* 1979, *19,* 44–45.

Atchley, R. Retirement as a social institution. In R. H. Turner and J. F. Short (Eds.), *Annual Review of Sociology* (Volume 8). Palo Alto, Calif.: Annual Reviews, 1982.

Beck, S. Retirement preparation programs: Differentials in opportunity and use. *Journal of Gerontology*, 1984, *39*, 596–602.

Bureau of Labor Statistics. *Handbook of labor statistics*. Washington, D.C.: U.S. Government Printing Office, 1983.

Clark, R., and Spengler, J. *The economics of individual and population aging*. Cambridge, Mass.: Harvard University Press, 1980.

Clark, R., and Sumner, D. Inflation and the real income of the elderly: Recent evidence and expectations for the future. *The Gerontologist*, 1985, *25*, 146–152.

Commonwealth Fund Commission. *Old, alone and poor. A plan for reducing poverty among elderly people living alone*. Baltimore, Md., 1987.

Congressional Institute for the Future. *Tomorrow's elderly*. 1984.

Cook, F. L., and Kramek, L. Measuring economic hardship among older Americans. *The Gerontologist*, 1986, *26*, 38–48.

Crystal, S. *America's old age crisis: Public policy and the two worlds of aging*. New York: Basic Books, 1982.

Duncan, G. *Years of poverty, years of plenty: The changing economic fortunes of American workers and families*. University of Michigan: Institute for Social Research, 1984.

Ekerdt, D., Bosse, R., and Levkoff, S. An empirical test for phases of retirement: Findings from the Normative Aging Study. *Journal of Gerontology*, 1985, *40*, 95–101.

Estes, C., Gerard, L., and Clarke, A. Women and the economics of aging. *International Journal of Health Services*, 1984, *14*, 55–68.

Fillenbaum, G., George, L., and Palmore, E. Determinants and consequences of retirement among men of different races and economic levels. *Journal of Gerontology*, 1984, *40*, 85–94.

Foner, A., and Schwab, K. *Aging and retirement*. Monterey, Calif.: Brooks/Cole, 1981.

Fox, A. Income changes at and after Social Security benefit receipt: Evidence from the Retirement History Study. *Social Security Bulletin*, 1984, *47*, 3–23.

George, L., Fillenbaum, G., and Palmore, E. Sex differences in the antecedents and consequences of retirement. *Journal of Gerontology*, 1984, *39*, 364–371.

George, L., and Maddox, G. Subjective adaptation to the loss of work role: A longitudinal study. *Journal of Gerontology*, 1977, *32*, 456–462.

Grad, S. Income of the aged and nonaged, 1950–1982. *Social Security Bulletin*, 1984a, *47*, 3–17.

Grad, S. *Income of the Population 65 and Over, 1982*. U.S. Dept. of Health and Human Services, Social Security Administration, 1984b.

Harris, L., and Associates. *Aging in the eighties: America in transition*. Washington, D.C.: National Council on the Aging, 1981.

Holden, K., Burkhauser, R., and Myers, D. Income transitions of older stages of life: The dynamics of poverty. *The Gerontologist*, 1986, *26*, 292–297.

Hooker, K., and Ventis, D. Work ethic, daily activities, and retirement satisfaction. *Journal of Gerontology*, 1984, *39*, 478–484.

Kingson, E., Hirshorn, B., and Cornman, J. *Ties that bind: The interdependence of generations*. Washington, D.C.: Seven Locks Press, 1986.

Kingson, E., Hirshorn, B., and Harootyan, L. *The common stake: The interdependence of generations.* The Gerontological Society of America, 1986.

Kohn, M., and Schooler, C. Job conditions and personality: A longitudinal assessment of their reciprocal effects. *American Journal of Sociology,* 1982, *87,* 1257–1286.

Marsh, R. The income and resources of the elderly in 1978. *Social Security Bulletin,* 1981, *44,* 3–11.

McConnell, S. Retirement and employment. In D. Woodruff and J. Birren (Eds.), *Aging: Scientific perspectives and social issues* (2d ed.). Monterey, Calif.: Brooks/Cole, 1983.

McConnell, S., Fleisher, D., Usher, C., and Kaplan, B. *Alternative work options for older workers: A feasibility study.* Los Angeles: Ethel Percy Andrus Gerontology Center, 1980.

Mercer, W. M. *Employer attitudes: Implications of an aging work force.* New York: William M. Mercer, 1981.

Minkler, M. Research on the health effects of retirement. *Journal of Health and Social Behavior,* 1981, *22,* 117–130.

Morgan, J. Economic realities of aging. Paper presented at the Convocation on Work and Retirement, University of Southern California, 1980.

Morse, D. *The utilization of older workers* (Special Report #33). Washington, D.C.: National Commission for Manpower Policy, 1979.

Mutran, E., and Reitzes, D. Retirement identity and well-being: Realignment and role relationships. *Journal of Gerontology,* 1981, *36,* 733–740.

National Council on the Aging. *Aging in the eighties: America in transition.* Washington, D.C., 1981.

Olson, L. K. Aging policy: Who benefits? *Generations,* Fall 1984, 10–14.

Palmore, E., Fillenbaum, G., and George, L. Consequences of retirement. *Journal of Gerontology,* 1984, *39,* 109–116.

Parnes, H. *Work and retirement: A longitudinal study of men.* Cambridge, Mass.: MIT Press, 1981.

Parnes, H. Health, pension policy and retirement. *Aging and work,* 1983, *6,* 93–103.

Parnes, H., and Nestel, G. The retirement experience. In H. Parnes (Ed.), *Work and retirement: A longitudinal study of men.* Cambridge, Mass.: MIT Press, 1981.

Pifer, A., and Bronte, L. *Our aging society: Paradox and promise.* New York: W. W. Norton, 1986.

Rones, P. Labor market problems of older workers. *Monthly Labor Review,* May 1983.

Rosen, B., and Jerdee, T. Postponing retirement: Can government and organizations make it attractive. *Business Horizons,* Nov.-Dec. 1985, 72–77.

Schulz, J. H. *The economics of aging* (3d ed.). Belmont, Calif.: Wadsworth, 1985.

Schulz, J. H., Leavitt, T. D., and Kelby, L. Private pensions fall far short of preretirement income levels. *Monthly Labor Review,* 1979, *102,* 28–31.

Seccombe, K., and Lee, G. Gender differences in retirement satisfaction and its antecedents. *Research on Aging,* 1986, *8,* 426–440.

Shaw, L. Retirement plans of middle-aged married women. *The Gerontologist*, 1984, *24*, 154–159.

Soldo, B. America's elderly in the 1980s. *Population Bulletin*, 1980, *35*, 1–47.

Streib, G., and Schneider, C. J. *Retirement in American society: Impact and process.* Ithaca, N.Y.: Cornell University Press, 1971.

Tracy, M., and Ward, R. Trends in old-age pensions for women: Benefit levels in ten nations, 1960–1980. *The Gerontologist*, 1986, *26*, 286–291.

Uhlenberg, P., and Salmon, M. G. Change in relative income of older women, 1960–1980. *The Gerontologist*, 1986, *26*, 164–170.

Usher, C. E. Alternative work options for older workers: Part I—Employees' interest. *Aging and Work*, 1981, *4*, 74–81.

U.S. Bureau of the Census. *Money income and poverty status of families and persons in the United States.* Washington, D.C., 1984.

U.S. Bureau of the Census. *Current population survey.* Washington, D.C., 1985.

U.S. Bureau of the Census. *A marketers' guide to discretionary income.* Washington, D.C., 1986.

U.S. Bureau of the Census. Money income and poverty status of families and persons in the United States: 1985 (Advance Data from the March 1986 Current Population Survey), Series P-60, No. 154, August 1986.

U.S. Joint Economic Committee, Special Study on Economic Change. *Social Security and pensions: Programs of equity and security.* Washington, D.C.: U.S. Government Printing Office, 1980.

U.S. Senate Special Committee on Aging. *Aging America: Trends and projections (1985–86 ed.).* Washington, D.C.: U.S. Department of Health and Human Services, 1986.

U.S. Senate Special Committee on Aging. *America in transition: An aging society* (1984–85 ed.). Washington, D.C.: U.S. Government Printing Office, 1985.

U.S. Senate Special Committee on Aging. *Developments in aging: 1984* (Volume I). Washington, D.C.: U.S. Government Printing Office, 1985.

Villers Foundation. *On the other side of easy street: Myths and facts about the economics of old age.* Washington, D.C., 1987.

Waldman, D. A., and Aviolo, B. J. A meta-analysis of age differences in job performance. *Journal of Applied Psychology*, 1986, *71*, 33–38.

Ward, R. Occupational variation in the life course: Implications for later life. In N. Osgood (Ed.), *Life after work: Retirement, leisure, recreation and elderly.* New York: Praeger, 1982.

Yankelovich, Skelly and White, Inc. *Workers over 50: Old myths, new realities.* American Association of Retired Persons, 1986.

Chapter 13

Changing Roles:
Community,
Organizational,
and Political

The living arrangements, neighborhoods, and socioeconomic status of adults, as well as their physical capacities, attitudes, skills, and values all influence their social activity patterns. People's use of time and arenas of involvement vary with the opportunities provided by the environment and with each developmental stage in the life cycle. Young and middle-aged adults may feel that there is not enough time for all they want to do. Their days are crowded with task-oriented activities—employment, child care, and household maintenance. During middle-age, people may idealize the free time of retirement, postponing travel or classes until they are retired and have "time for things like that." With retirement, the departure of children, and other role changes, most older adults experience discretion over their use of time, perhaps more than at any other point in their adult lives (Rosow, 1985). The reality of nonwork time for retirees, however, may be quite different from their middle-age fantasies of "if only we had the time." For example, a longitudinal study of retirees found that they had overestimated the extent and variety of activities they would pursue upon retirement (Bosse and Ekerdt, 1981). Poor health, reduced income, transportation difficulties, isolated living arrangements, and role changes all may disrupt and reduce anticipated activities in old age.

This chapter focuses on the activity patterns most common among older people in American society, including leisure pursuits, membership in community and interest associations, volunteering, religious participation and meaning, and political involvement. Even with changes in their competence in physical health and physiological functioning, as described in earlier chapters, older people can stay active by modifying their level and type of involvement in community and organizational activities, thereby reestablishing congruence between their needs and abilities and the demands of the social environment. For each of these forms of community and organizational involvement, the factors that influence the rates and patterns of participation, the functions of such participation, and gender and ethnic minority variations in activities are considered.

Variations in Activities in Old Age

As described in Chapter 3, there are widely different perspectives on participation in old age—from activity theory, which stresses the beneficial effects of continued involvement, to disengagement theory, which argues the appropriateness of withdrawal. These and other theoretical perspectives have addressed the questions: Does age bring a desire for increased social autonomy? Are older people content to disengage from society? Is daily activity essential to successful adjustment to aging? How is use of time related to life satisfaction and to feelings of competence toward the larger environment? These questions have long been topics of research and debate, and still are today.

Although time is less fragmented upon retirement than it is at earlier life stages, there still are numerous constraints on how people choose to become involved in different social arenas. As identified in earlier chapters, the normal physical and psychological changes of aging, and any diseases that affect older persons, may limit their capacities to engage in certain activities and to maintain competence in relation to environmental demands. Cohort experiences and socialization to certain activities and values, gender and ethnic minority group memberships, and type of living arrangements (e.g., a retirement community or nursing home) may interact and result in certain activities being stratified by age. Some older individuals may not undertake particular activities because they feel they lack the skills, physical strength, or knowledge to do them, or that they are too old to undertake such activities. Atchley (1971) has suggested that if "activity competence" is not learned by middle-age, it never will be. This implies that active and creative use of free time in youth is necessary to assume it in the later years.

Past activity patterns and personality dynamics also clearly shape the use of time. There appears to be continuity between leisure pursuits enjoyed at earlier and later stages of life, consistent with continuity theory (discussed in Chapter 3). Adults have been found to have a core of leisure activities that persists across the life course, although the specific means of carrying out such patterns may alter with age (Kelly, 1982; Kelly, Steinkamp and Kelly, 1986; Bosse and Ekerdt, 1981; Teague, 1980). As people's interests crystallize over the life span, they generally become more selective about how they invest their time and energy.

Leisure Pursuits

The term *leisure* evokes different reactions in people. For some, it signifies wasting time. For others, it is only the frenzied pursuit of "leisure activities" on the weekends that sustains them through the work week. People's reactions to the concept of leisure are clearly influenced by cultural values attached to work. In American culture, the Puritan work ethic has tended to instill a mistrust of nonproductive uses of time. Some implicit assumptions in our society have been that work is better than leisure; group activities are better than solitary ones; and active pursuits, such as sports, are better than contemplation or meditation. Because of American cultural values of productivity and hard work—values that are particularly strong for the current generation of older persons but that may be changing for future cohorts—many older people lack experience in satisfying nonwork activities at earlier stages in their lives (Neulinger, 1974).

Societal values regarding leisure are changing, however, with more legitimacy given to leisure throughout the life cycle, as evidenced by the growing number of classes and therapists that specialize in this area. For low-income or ethnic minority elderly or for older people in developing countries, however, leisure may be a meaningless concept, if they have had to continue working or lack the resources for satisfying recreational time.

Independent of such social norms, leisure can be defined as any activity characterized by the absence of obligation that is inherently satisfying and has intrinsic meaning. Accordingly, leisure implies feelings of freedom and pleasure. People who engage in sports, travel, or visits to museums and do not experience such feelings may still be at "work" rather than at "leisure" (Kelly, 1982; Kleiber and Kelly, 1980; Gordon, Gaitz, and Scott, 1976).

Disagreement regarding the value of leisure pursuits for older people is reflected in the gerontological literature. An early perspective was that leisure roles cannot substitute for work roles, because they are not legitimated by societal norms. Since work is a dominant value in American society, it was argued that individuals cannot derive self-respect from leisure. It was also observed that older individuals, fearing the embarrassment of failing in a leisure activity, avoid leisure pursuits that are common to younger people (Miller, 1965).

The counterargument is that leisure is neither demoralizing nor traumatizing to most older people. It is argued that leisure can replace the work role and provide personal satisfaction in later life, especially when the retired person has good health and an adequate income, and when retirement activities build upon preretirement skills and interests (Atchley, 1971). Other studies have concluded that when income is secure, leisure roles can generally substitute for employment-related roles (Thompson, 1973). For people who find greater satisfaction in employment than in family, participating in instrumental activities or in organizations where they can exert control may be necessary during retirement (Keith, Goudy, and Powers, 1984).

Another perspective is that retirement is legitimated in our work-oriented society by an ethic that esteems leisure that is earnest, occupied, and filled with activity—a "busy" ethic, which is consistent with the activity theory of aging (Ekerdt, 1986). For those with strong work values, work-like activities are probably important for achieving satisfaction in retirement (Hooker and Ventes, 1984). The prevalence of the "busy" ethic is reflected in the question commonly asked of retirees: What do you do to keep busy? "Keeping busy" and engaging in activities analogous to work are presumed to ease the adjustment to retirement by adapting retired life to prevailing societal norms, although the "busy" ethic is contrary to our definition of leisure as intrinsically satisfying. In fact, activity has been found in many instances to be positively related to life satisfaction in retirement (Lawton, 1978; O'Brien, 1981; Hooker and Ventes, 1984).

Although there are wide variations among older individuals, patterns of activity have been identified. Most leisure time is not spent in public recreation programs developed specially for the elderly. The proportion of persons engaged in community organizations, sports, exercise, and outdoor recreation declines consistently by age, with the activities of those of age 75 and older becoming more home-based (Kelly, Steinkamp, and Kelly, 1986). Compared to younger people, older people are more likely to engage in solitary and sedentary pursuits, such as watching television, visiting with family and friends, and reading; they are also less likely to participate in active sports, attend cultural events, travel, or visit theaters, parks, and libraries (Bosse and Ekerdt, 1981; Kaplan, 1979; Lawton, 1978; Moss and Lawton, 1982). Although the amount of time spent watching television is only slightly more than for younger groups, viewing habits differ. The elderly are more likely than younger people to watch programs with serious informational content, including news programs, documentaries, and travelogues, and to prefer nonfiction programs (e.g., variety and quiz shows) to drama (Gordon et al., 1976).

Leisure activities also vary by gender and socioeconomic status. Older men are more likely to participate in sports, fishing, travel, and gardening, while women, such as Mrs. Howard in the introductory vignette, tend to pursue handiwork and crafts, watch television, socialize, and read (Payne and Whittington, 1976). The activities of lower income older persons commonly include watching television, family socializing, hunting, fishing, and hobbies, often with same sex companions, whereas higher income individuals generally prefer activities that emphasize creativity and personal development, such as work with clubs and organizations, participation in cultural events, traveling, and entertaining guests at private parties (Kelly et al., 1986; Gordon et al., 1976). These differences in activities are attributable primarily to the costs of pursuing them, not necessarily to inherent differences in people of low and high socioeconomic status. Less is known about how leisure pursuits vary among ethnic minority groups.

All older people spend considerable time in obligatory activities, such as housework, shopping, and personal care. As their health declines, they may devote even more time to these routine pursuits, and become less involved in externally oriented activities such as community organizations, exercise, and travel (Kelly et al., 1986; Lawton, 1978). For low-income elderly, these routines may be their only options. When judged by younger persons or by middle-class standards, these obligatory activities may be viewed as "boring" or "nonproductive." Yet the ability to perform these more mundane activities—personal care, cooking, tinkering and puttering around the house—can be critical to maintaining competence levels. Furthermore, these routines may represent realistic adjustments to declining energy levels. In fact, such leisure pursuits may reflect rational choices to develop ways of coping that are consistent with changes in environments.

The Meaning and Functions of Leisure for Older People

Leisure activities have been classified in terms of the following psychological benefits perceived by elderly participants: companionship (e.g., playing cards or going dancing); compensation for past activities (e.g., picknicking instead of hiking); temporary disengagement (e.g., watching TV); comfortable solitude (e.g., reading); expressive solitude (e.g., knitting and crocheting); and expressive service (e.g., volunteer service, attending meetings of social groups) (Tinsley, Teaff, Colbs, and Kaufman, 1985). Leisure activities also serve to help maintain ties with others and to provide new sources of personal meaning and competence to replace earlier sources that have been lost (Kelly et al., 1986; Newman and Newman, 1979). A positive association has been found between leisure activities and feelings of well-being among older people (Foner and Schwab, 1981). This relationship does not mean, however, that leisure activity itself creates well-being, since older people who are active also tend to be healthier and of higher socioeconomic status. In fact, it appears that the quality of interactions with others in leisure pursuits may be more salient than the number of interactions for life satisfaction and morale (Larson, Zuzanek, and Mannell, 1985).

Even when income and health are limited, routine leisure pursuits, such as shopping, housework, and sitting quietly in reflection, can all be critical to maintaining an older person's sense of competence, self-esteem, and social relationships, as suggested by Butler and Gleason's (1985) definition of productivity to include more than work (Lawton, 1978). Similarly, meditation and contemplation may not be "wasting time," but can be personally satisfying. In fact, older people may need to accept less externally oriented activities in order to attain a sense of "ego integrity," as defined by Erikson (Kleiber and Kelly, 1980). In sum, older people need not be actively and creatively involved every moment to experience personal satisfaction from leisure (Kelly et al., 1986).

A challenge for those working with older people is to create leisure opportunities that participants perceive as meaningful and as contributing to their sense of satisfaction and well-being. Structured opportunities also need to maximize older people's skills and interests, and be broadly inclusive, serving an ethnically and economically diverse population. Such options may be especially important for single older persons who lack daily companionship (Larson, Zuzanek, and Mannell, 1985).

Senior centers are one mechanism to provide such opportunities. These vary greatly in the type and quality of activities offered, ranging from purely social events, to social action, to the delivery of services. However, less than 25 percent of older persons participate in senior centers for several reasons (Harris and Associates, 1981; Foner and Schwab, 1983). Individuals may be busy elsewhere, uninterested in the center's activities, in poor health, or lack the necessary transportation. As noted in Chapter 11, people are more likely to participate in senior centers that are physically close to their homes. Some elderly refuse to participate in senior centers because they will be with other older persons only. The low proportion of men in most centers may deter other men from participating. Furthermore, most centers draw from a relatively narrow population, reaching primarily healthy, middle-income older people with "a life history of joining clubs" (Trela, 1976; Ward, 1979), and who are attracted by recreational

Many senior centers offer classes on diverse topics.

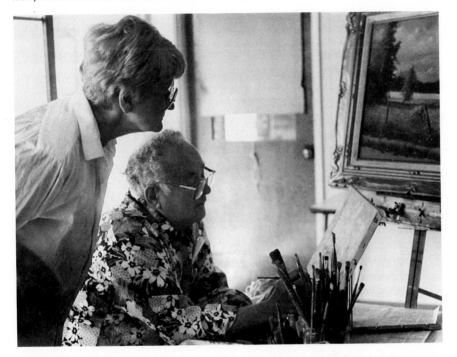

programs that are consistent with their lifestyles (Hanssen, Nichols, Buckspan, Henderson, Helbig and Zarit, 1978; Kaplan, 1979). Senior center arts projects, for example, may involve participants in art classes, tours to operas, symphonies, ballet, and stage productions, thus satisfying the needs of some older people, but failing to reach out to those who lack the income to take advantage of such activities.

Membership in Voluntary Associations

Given the emphasis in our society on being active, productive, and a joiner, voluntary association membership is often assumed to be "good" for older people. Based on such assumptions, well-meaning professionals may go to considerable lengths to try to recruit older people to such associations, oftentimes without success. Overall, older people are less likely to belong to organizations than are younger people, but their reduced membership does not necessarily indicate a slackening of interest with age. Rather, membership is most closely tied to social class and is more characteristic of our society than of most other cultures. When socioeconomic status is taken into account, older people show considerable stability in their general level of voluntary association participation from middle-age until their sixties (Cutler, 1977).

The kind of organizations in which older people participate varies by gender and ethnic minority status. Older women are more likely to belong to religious and cultural organizations, whereas older men tend to be members of unions, service clubs, and fraternal organizations (Cutler, 1976). Older Blacks have higher rates of organizational membership than older whites or members of other ethnic minority groups, although for both Blacks and whites, membership is most frequent among those with better health, greater income, and higher education levels (Babchuk, Peters, Hoyt, and Kaiser, 1979; Ward, 1979). Black and white elderly differ in the types of associations they join; older Blacks are especially likely to belong to church-related groups and social and recreational clubs; older whites generally belong to nationality organizations and senior citizen clubs (Clemente, Rexroad, and Hirsch, 1975). Some of these memberships are related to historical circumstances rather than to age or ethnic minority status per se.

Older persons who are active in community and interest organizations derive a variety of benefits. Socializing appears to be the primary reward, especially for people like Mrs. Howard in the introductory vignette. Because many organizations are age-graded, people interact with others similar in age and interests. These interactions often result in friendships, support, and mutual exchanges of resources.

Voluntary associations can also serve to maintain the social integration of older people, countering losses in roles and in interactions with others (Cutler, 1977). Older people in voluntary organizations have been found to have higher morale than nonmembers, although this may be attributed to their higher levels of health, income, and education, factors which themselves have been found to contribute to well-being. When these other characteristics are taken into account, organizational membership is apparently unrelated to overall life satisfaction (Ward, 1979). When people join organizations primarily to "make the time pass," their membership is generally not central to their sense of well-being. In contrast, the most satisfied members of organizations are those who become involved in order to have new experiences, achieve something, be creative, and help others (Ward, 1979). Such members, in turn, participate actively through planning and leadership. Their responsibilities yield them more novel experiences and greater feelings of competence and creativity than is the case with those who participate in only social and recreational activities, such as card playing for pleasure and "passing the time" (Babchuk, Peters, Hoyt, and Kaiser, 1979). Opportunities for more active participation are found in advocacy groups composed primarily of older people, or in organizations such as advisory boards to Area Agencies on Aging where older people must, by charter, be in leadership roles. Thus, voluntary association membership appears to be more satisfying when it provides opportunities for active, intense involvement and significant leadership roles (Ward, 1979).

Volunteer Work

Many community and interest organizations exist to serve others; the volunteers, in turn, are assumed to benefit from their participation in service functions. Older persons have long played a critical role as volunteers in hospitals, senior centers, and institutions such as children's homes and schools. This kind of volunteering, similar to participation in voluntary associations, is more characteristic of American society than others.

Within the past ten years, a number of national organizations composed entirely of senior volunteers have formed. One of the best known is the Foster Grandparent Program, which pairs seniors with disabled children; it has been found to be mutually beneficial to both. This mutual aid concept was extended to the Senior Companion Program, in which able-bodied seniors serve disabled older people. The Peace Corps has also increased its recruitment of older volunteers; approximately 4 percent of its volunteers in developing countries today are seniors. The Older American Volunteer Program of ACTION recruits older people to work with disadvantaged groups. The International Executive Services Corps of Retired Executives (SCORE) permits retired executives to use their technical and financial experience in a consultant-type arrangement to companies in the United States and abroad. Largest of the volunteer networks is the Retired Senior Volunteer Program (RSVP), which is part of the National Older American's Volunteer Program, authorized by the 1969 Amendments to the Older Americans Act. RSVP has over 700 projects in schools, hospitals, adult and child day centers, and nursing homes, involving over 300,000 older volunteers (Pepper, 1981).

In spite of these extensive senior volunteer networks, the elderly actually volunteer less than other age groups.* Of persons aged 65 and over, approximately 10 percent are volunteers, compared to about 23 percent of Americans generally (Harris and Associates, 1981; ACTION, 1975; Chambré, 1984). However, when volunteering is broadly defined to include informal activities, 37 percent of the elderly had volunteered during 1980–81 (Gallup, 1981). Among the older population, rates of volunteering are highest among whites who are in their sixties, are employed, have higher incomes, and are better educated. The young-

---

*Rates of volunteering measured are obviously affected by how volunteering is defined. One approach has defined it in a restricted manner, as unpaid work within the context of an organization (e.g., a friendly visitor to nursing homes). A second approach includes informal activities as well (e.g., a friend who regularly visits is a volunteer) (Chambré, 1984).

old, and those still employed, are more likely to volunteer than the old-old. One reason for this is the greater incidence of illness among the latter that reduces opportunities to volunteer. Those who have a broad range of social interests and believe they can make a valuable contribution are also more likely to volunteer (Monk and Cyrns, 1974; Harris and Associates, 1982).

As is the case generally in voluntary activities, women (especially widows) are more likely to volunteer than men, and they have different reasons for doing so. Although women generally view volunteering as a way to help others, men more frequently define it as a substitute for the worker role (Payne and Whittington, 1976). Differences have also been noted among ethnic minorities. Volunteering as a way to help others through informal networks is frequent in ethnic minority communities, primarily through the Black churches. Mutual aid (e.g., providing food and lodging to older persons) is common in Native American communities. Volunteer activities among Pacific/Asian elderly are ethnically specific and reinforce the continuation of Pacific/Asian value systems. Older Chinese, for example, often work through family associations or benevolent societies. Some Japanese elders participate in clubs, which are an extension of the "family helping itself" concept that is rooted in traditional Japanese culture. The Hispanic community has been found to emphasize self-help, mutual aid, neighborhood assistance, and advocacy for their older members (Height, Toya, Kamekawa, and Maldonado, 1981).

Volunteer programs serve two major beneficial functions: They provide individuals with meaningful leisure activities, and they furnish organizations with experienced, reliable workers at no cost. The research literature emphasizes that volunteering can compensate for changes in work and family roles in old age. An underlying assumption of the activity theory of aging is that when older people can maintain previous levels of activity, they enhance their well-being; this goal can presumably be achieved through volunteering by substituting one role for another (Swartz, 1978). As noted previously, however, retirement is not associated with a greater tendency to volunteer (Harris and Associates, 1982), and volunteering is apparently not a work-substitute for retirees (Chambré, 1984).

The continuity theory of aging is a better explanation of volunteer involvement: Older persons who volunteer are primarily volunteers who have grown older. Their long-standing involvement either remains constant or expands as they age (Atchley, 1971; Chambré, 1984; Dye, Goodman, Roth, and Jensen, 1973). Since volunteering appears to be a pattern established relatively early in life, it is probably too late to make new recruits among previously uninvolved persons when they retire. Other elderly may be recruited but, because they have not previously been volunteers, they may drop out as the novelty of volunteering wears off. From the point of view of those who run programs dependent on volunteers, recruitment needs to occur during the individual's work life (e.g., through expanded released time or loaned personnel programs by employers). Even so, there will be many "middle-aged dropouts" from such programs, especially among those whose voluntary work has centered largely on their children's activities or as part of their jobs.

Although the activity theory of aging does not fully explain volunteerism, many older individuals personally benefit from their volunteer activity. For example, volunteers at a Veterans Administration hospital were found to have a greater "will to live" and higher life satisfaction, as well as less anxiety and depression, than a comparison group of nonvolunteers (Hunter and Linn, 1981). Similarly, participants in a Senior Companion Program scored higher on social resources and mental and physical health than nonvolunteers, even though they were not necessarily better off economically. Volunteers were found to be less lonely and to perceive their help as vital to others (Fogelman, 1981). From the perspective of social exchange theory, volunteering may ensure valued resources as a basis of exchange, primarily by assisting others rather than being perceived as dependent.

On the other hand, older volunteers may not be placed in responsible, ongoing positions, and may feel frustrated by what they perceive to be a lack of respect for their "free" labor. Voluntary work is often defined as menial work perceived to be "below the dignity" of professionals. In such instances, when older volunteers' resources are not valued, they do not experience privilege or prestige (Dowd, 1980).

Volunteers clearly make a major social and financial contribution to communities and to the economy. Since volunteers often save human service agencies substantial money, there is an ongoing debate about whether volunteers are exploited as a means of cutting costs. Such debate is heightened when social services are reduced, and volunteers, frequently women, are expected to fill gaps in programs. For low-income older persons in particular, volunteering can be an unaffordable luxury. The National Council of Senior Citizens contends that many older volunteers need additional income and would prefer part-time paid work. The Council has taken a position against any program that asks older people to perform, on a volunteer basis, community service work for which younger people are paid.

A number of trends will influence the meaning and functions of voluntarism for older persons. Changing economic conditions, particularly inflation, may mean that fewer individuals can afford the additional costs of transportation, meals, and out-of-pocket expenses. With the increasing emphasis nationally on self-help and mutual aid, people may choose instead to become more active in neighborhood and community advocacy organizations that seek to empower individuals through solving problems. In the future, the elderly are likely to be more involved in advisory councils and commissions, in lobbying efforts, as legislative aides and interns, and in national senior organizations, such as those described later in this chapter. These volunteer and advocacy efforts will continue to face the challenge of developing new ways to involve low-income, ethnic minorities, and frail/disabled older persons (Allen, 1981).

Religious Participation and Religiousness

Of the various options for organizational participation, the most common choice for older persons is a religious affiliation.* Across the life span, church and synagogue attendance is lowest among those in their thirties, peaks in the late fifties to early sixties (with approximately 60 percent of this age group attending), and begins to decline in the late sixties or early seventies. Despite this slight decline, the rate of church or synagogue attendance for older people exceeds that of other age groups, with 49 percent of persons over age 65 attending church or synagogue in an average week and many more attending less frequently (Mindel and Vaughan, 1978; Princeton Religion Research Center, 1982). Furthermore, people age 65 and over are the most likely of any age group to belong to church-affiliated groups and fraternal associations (Cutler, 1976). In contrast to other types of voluntary organizations, leadership positions in churches and synagogues tend to be concentrated among older people.

One reason for inconsistent empirical findings regarding the relationship between aging and religion is that rates of church attendance in themselves do not indicate the extent of religiosity among older persons (Hunsberger, 1985). Religious behaviors can be examined in terms of three factors: (1) participation in religious organizations, (2) the personal meaning of religion and religious activities within the home, and (3) the contribution of religion to individuals' adjustment to the aging process and their confrontation with death and dying. Declines in rates of religious participation after age 70 may reflect health and transportation difficulties more than lack of religiousness. In fact, while attendance at formal services declines with age, older individuals apparently compensate by an increase in internal religious practices through reading the Bible, listening to religious broadcasts, praying, or studying religion (Gray and Moberg, 1977). Thus, some older people who appear to be disengaged from religious organizations may be fully engaged nonorganizationally, experiencing a strong and meaningful subjective relationship to religion (Ainlay and Smith, 1984; Mindel and Vaughan, 1978).

Religion appears to be more important in older people's lives than for younger people. In a 1982 national survey, 75 percent of persons age 65 and over stated that God was very influential in their lives, and more than 80 percent claimed their religious faith as the most important influence. Some 67 percent rate themselves in the three highest categories for leading a religious life, yet 84 percent wished that their religious faith were stronger (Princeton Religion

---

*This discussion of religion and the elderly is limited to the broad cultural mainstream of American society. A multinational, multicultural review of religion is beyond the scope of this book. Since world religions differ greatly, the religious values, attitudes, and practices discussed here may have little generalization beyond our society to other major segments of the world.

Research Center, 1982). Older people adhere to more orthodox or conservative religious viewpoints than do younger people; belief in immortality and literal interpretations of the scripture are more prevalent than among younger persons (Kalish, 1976; Moberg, 1970), although this may shift with the growing numbers of younger people currently attracted to fundamentalist religions.

Although religion appears to be very important to many older people, they probably also valued it when they were young. That is, contrary to popular stereotypes, we do not become more religious as we age. Researchers who broadly conceptualize the religious practices of the elderly to include patterns of belief, religious orientation, and stability of religious attitudes, rather than only activities within the formal association of the church, have found that the importance of religion remains stable over time (Blazer and Palmore, 1976). Religious *beliefs,* as contrasted with church attendance, appear to be relatively stable from the late teens until age 60, and to *increase* thereafter (Argle and Beit-Hallahmi, 1975).

Most surveys on religiousness share the limitations of cross-sectional research, as discussed in Chapter 1. That is, they do not attempt to measure the individual's past religious values and behaviors. The few longitudinal studies available suggest that historical trends may be more important than the effects of age (Hunsberger, 1985). Thus, although religious convictions appear to become more salient over the years, this may be a generational phenomenon captured by the cross-sectional nature of most of the research. The current cohort of older persons, raised during a time of more widespread religious involvement, had their peak rates of attendance in the 1950s, when this country experienced a church revival. All cohorts, not only the elderly, have shown a decline in church or synagogue attendance since 1965, although this may be changing in the 1980s. There are also other possible effects of selective survival. Orthodox religious persons are less likely to smoke, drink alcohol excessively, and participate in other behaviors that have been linked to early death. The survival of the more religious may make the older population as a whole appear to be more orthodox in their beliefs than younger age groups.

Studies of religious activity have found both gender and ethnic minority differences. Consistent with patterns of involvement in other organizations, women, particularly Black women, have higher rates of church membership than do men. Religion also appears to be central to the lives of most older Blacks of both sexes and to be related to their life satisfaction. In a study of four ethnic groups, older Blacks revealed the greatest sense of personal well-being; religion with shared weekly church activity was a factor three times more important than all others in predicting happiness among older Blacks (Reynolds and Kalish, 1974). A more recent study found that religiosity among Blacks was positively related to life satisfaction and to frequency of church attendance, regardless of age and sex (Heisel and Faulkner, 1982). The high esteem afforded Black elderly in the church may partially underlie these positive associations. In a study comparing Mexican-

Americans and whites for two time periods (1976 and 1980), Mexican-Americans were found to be more religious as measured by church attendance, self-rated religiousness, and private prayer. Furthermore, these three factors were positively related to their life satisfaction (Markides, 1983).

Although the relationship between religious involvement and life satisfaction is not clear-cut (Steinitz, 1980), religious activities and attitudes have generally been found to be positively associated with happiness, a sense of usefulness, and adjustment to old age. The strength of these relationships increases over time (Blazer and Palmore, 1976; Hadaway, 1978; Hunsberger, 1985; Kivett, 1979). Holding conservative religious beliefs has been found to be related to greater serenity and less fear of death (Moberg, 1965). Individuals for whom faith provides meaning experienced greater feelings of internal control and a more positive self-concept (Kivett, 1979). It is unclear, however, whether religiousness itself is beneficial, or if the sense of belonging is the determinant, since religious participation is associated with other types of group involvement (Pieper, 1981). Satisfaction, serenity, or acceptance of death may result not from faith per se, but rather from participation in social networks and reference groups that offer support and security. Older people themselves list among the benefits of religion both the meaning it gives to life and the social interaction it affords (Pieper, 1981).

THE VALUE OF SPIRITUAL WELL-BEING

Recent literature differentiates spiritual well-being from organized religion. Spiritual well-being is defined by the National Interfaith Coalition of Aging as the "affirmation of life in a relationship with God, self, community and environment that nourishes and celebrates wholeness" (Delloff, 1983). According to this perspective, people can be very religious without being spiritual and vice versa (Fischer, 1985). Listening to music, viewing a sunset or a painting, loving, and being loved can all be profound spiritual activities. It is believed that people can only be fully spiritual human beings if they find meaning in life generally, or in specific daily events, such as working on a project (Missine, 1986). High levels of spirituality have been found to be associated with mental health indicators, such as purpose in life, self-esteem, and social skills (Paloutzian and Ellison, 1982). Spirituality has been identified as an important factor in an individual's perception of quality of life (irrespective of age or socioeconomic status) and in maintaining a healthy lifestyle (Levine, 1983). Spiritual well-being is related not only to the quality of life, but also to the will to live. Some gerontologists and theologians maintain that the person who aims to enhance spiritual well-being and to find meaning in life will have a reason to live, despite losses associated with aging (Thorson, 1983). In fact, dealing with loss has been viewed as one of the great spiritual challenges of aging (Fischer, 1985).

The spiritual dimensions of health care have been examined. Practitioners who view spiritual well-being as important to the elderly's physical and mental health have attempted to develop instruments to profile an individual's spiritual interests and resources. For example, the Personal Life Events Inventory (Westberg, 1979), which is an adaptation of the Social Readjustment Rating scale (Holmes and Masuda, 1974), described in Chapter 8, contains a section on philosophical-spiritual dimensions. (See box.) Some health promotion screening tools include questions on the individual's spiritual or philosophic values, life goal-setting, and approach to answering questions, such as: What is the meaning of my life? How can I increase the quality of my life? (Institute of Lifestyle Improvements, 1978). Proponents of this approach advocate training health care providers to be sensitive to, and to ask questions about, spiritual well-being in order to respond to older people's total needs (McSherry, 1983).

MEETING OLDER PEOPLE'S NEEDS

The increasing recognition of the elderly's spiritual well-being among those who work with older people may be in part a reaction to organized religion's limited outreach and programming for older parishioners. In the past, most churches have been oriented to serving relatively youthful families, through programs for children, teens, and young adults. The elderly were assumed to benefit from the same programs that serve the rest of the church membership. Only in recent years have churches begun to recognize their older members' special needs and to develop ministries specifically to serve them (Palmore, 1980).

Measuring Spiritual Well-Being

The Personal Life Events Inventory asks whether older respondents have experienced the following:

Lack of meaningfulness in life

Lack of strong purpose in life

A major change in one's world view or philosophy

A new set of values or priorities in one's life

Change in relationship with God

Change in church activity or prayer life

A significant spiritual experience

Spiritual emptiness

Constant feelings of guilt

Reprinted with permission from G. Westberg, "Multiplying Wholistic Health Centers," in *Increasing the Impact.* Battle Creek, Mich.: Kellogg Foundation, 1979.

As an indicator of the growth of church programs for older members, over 50 specific services have been identified at the national, regional, and local levels. These include counseling, adult day care, advocacy, education, income maintenance, in-home services, nutrition services, retirement training, and transportation (Steinitz, 1981; Cook, 1976). A growing number of churches are developing housing programs, such as retirement homes and congregate care facilities, described in the previous chapter. Churches and synagogues are increasingly aware that ministry to the elderly must involve more than prayer; church-based advocacy and organizing are needed as well. With cutbacks in government services, churches are often faced with filling service gaps through volunteer chore programs, nutrition sites, and meals and home care for the homebound. Although churches and synagogues are increasingly responding to the elderly's daily care needs, they generally have not co-sponsored programs with other religious organizations or with public agencies, although they are beginning to do so in some communities (Tobin and Ellor, 1983).

The 1971 White House Conference on Aging provided the impetus for deliberately coordinating the religious and voluntary sectors through two new organizations: the National Voluntary Organizations for Independent Living for the Aging (NVOILA) and the National Interfaith Coalition on Aging (NICA). NVOILA focuses on coordinating services to enable older people to remain in their homes. The primary objective of NICA is to vitalize the role of the church and synagogue with respect to their responsibilities in improving the quality of life for the aging (Letzig, 1983).

Political Participation

Another major arena of participation in American society is political life. Political acts range from voting to participation in a political party or a political action group (e.g., organizations seeking to forward the interests of the elderly) to running for or holding elective office. In examining older people's political behavior, three factors make any interpretation of the relationship between age and political behavior complex. These factors are *stages in the life cycle, cohort effects,* and *historical* or *period effects* (Foner, 1972), as discussed in Chapter 1.

Historical effects have influenced interpretations of the elderly's political behavior, particularly analyses of the extent of conservatism. Some early studies of political participation found older people to be more conservative than younger people (Campbell, 1962). Older people's apparent conservatism partially reflects the fact that people born and raised in different historical periods tend to have perspectives reflecting those times, in this instance, the historical effect of party realignments in the late 1920s and 1930s. Before the New Deal of the 1930s and 40s, people entering the electorate identified with the Republican party to a disproportionate extent; they have voted Republican ever since, and form the majority of the population over age 65 (Cigler and Swanson, 1981; Hudson and Strate, 1985). The apparent association of Republicanism with age thus reflects generational differences, not the effects of aging per se (Dobson, 1983; Glenn and Hefner, 1972). Age differences in conservatism/liberalism are less a matter of people becoming more conservative than of their remaining the same, whereas successive generations entering the electorate since World War II have become comparatively more liberal. (However, this pattern may be shifting in the 1980s, with the predominance of younger conservatives in the Republican party.) Older persons are generally stable in their political orientations, or change their beliefs slowly. For all age groups, political behavior is often a habit, with most people retaining the political opinions formed when they were younger (Holloway and George, 1979).

As seen in earlier discussions of cross-sectional samples, it is misleading to look once at a group of individuals of various ages, compare their attitudes and reported behaviors, and maintain that differences based on age alone have been isolated. Conclusions about older people's political behavior and attitudes are thus limited by the cross-sectional nature of most research on these variables, which has not taken account of historical and cohort effects. In short, how a person thinks politically can be traced largely to environmental and historical factors, not to that person's age.

Given these methodological limitations and the multifaceted nature of political relationships to age, what is known about older people's political behavior and attitudes? In general, greater conservatism, as measured by preference for a conservative party and voting behavior, does exist among older people. For example, older people have been found to identify with the Republican party more than younger people (Dobson, 1983; Hudson and Binstock, 1976). A Los Angeles Times exit poll in the 1984 presidential election concluded that persons 60 years and older accounted for 17 percent of all voters, with 60 percent voting Republican and 40 percent voting Democratic. The New York Times found a similar Republican to Democratic split: 63 percent to 36 percent (U.S. Senate Special Committee on Aging, 1986). Older people tend to be more conservative on "new politics" issues (e.g., nuclear disarmament, women's rights, abortion, homosexual rights, and relations with foreign countries), issues of "law and order," and racial issues (Hudson and Strate, 1985).

The elderly are not necessarily conservative on all issues, however. In recent elections, many low-income and retired blue-collar elderly have opposed the fiscal conservatism of the Republican party. On government policies related to pensions and health care, older people are less conservative and more likely to favor a national health insurance than younger people, in part reflecting their recognition of the benefits of Medicare and Medicaid (Campbell and Strate, 1981). Overall, individuals of all ages are not ideologically consistent in their issue-specific preferences (Hudson and Strate, 1985). Rather, age differences on particular issues may reflect the closeness of issues to people's lives; the further removed a political issue, the less age appears to affect attitudes toward them (Douglass, Cleveland, and Maddox, 1974). Furthermore, both older and younger people may hold beliefs on specific issues that contradict their views on more general principles. Within a heterogenous group such as the elderly—not only between younger and older generations—differences of opinion on any political issue are likely to equal or exceed variations between age groups (Hudson and Strate, 1985).

VOTING BEHAVIOR

Older Americans are somewhat more likely than younger adults to vote in both presidential and nonpresidential elections. They currently make up 15 percent of the general electorate and 20 percent of those who vote, and these percentages are growing. Early studies of voting behavior in the 1960s and the 1970s found that voting rates peaked in the age range of 40 to 50 years old, then declined after age 60 (Hudson and Binstock, 1976). In more recent elections, however, declines in voting among those over age 65 have not been as sharp, and voting participation for those 75 years and over has been found to be comparable to that for the entire population age 25 and over (59 percent in 1980) (U.S. Senate Special Committee on Aging, 1985). According to 1980 and 1982 census data, rates of voting increased steadily with age until age 75 or 80. In the November 1980 election, voters age 55 to 64 had the highest participation rate (71 percent); the 65- to 74-year-old group had the next highest (69 percent). In the 1982 congressional elections, 65 percent of those aged 65 through 74 voted, which was the highest percentage of any age groups. Older voters also tend to be well informed, even though most never finished high school (Ragan and Davis, 1982).

In instances where there has been a lower voter turnout among older people, factors other than aging are probably the cause, including gender, ethnic minority, education, and generational factors (Cutler, Pierce, and Steckenrider, 1982). For example, the voter turnout of ethnic minority groups is consistently lower than that of whites. Only 55 percent of Black elderly vote in Presidential election years, 46 percent in Congressional elections, and less than 33 percent of Hispanic elderly regularly vote (Cuellar, 1978). The political acculturation of ethnic minority groups also influences their participation. For example, Mexican-American elders, historically fearful of deportation, have an overriding respect and fear of authority figures, creating a "politics of deference," and a cautious, conservative approach to political involvement (Torres-Gil, 1976). Again, these differences do not reflect age or ethnic identity per se, but rather lower educational levels, feelings of powerlessness, cohort experiences, and real or perceived barriers to voting and other political activities.

Voting does *not* decline among older individuals who are better educated, actively involved, and in good health. Thus, declines in voting found in elections prior to the 1980s were probably not due to age per se, but rather to such factors as the lower educational level of this current cohort of older people, and the fact that women, who predominate numerically among the elderly, have historically participated less than men in voting, regardless of their educational, income, and age levels (Dobson, 1983).

In fact, when education, sex, and ethnic minority status are taken into account, interest in politics actually *increases* with age (Glenn, 1974). Older members of political parties tend to have more influence than younger members because of their years of party involvement and their overrepresentation at nominating conventions and in public offices. Older persons are nearly as active as younger adults in local political activities, such as working for the party in a local election (Hudson and Strate, 1985). The older electorate therefore has the potential to exert political influence substantially beyond what their numbers might suggest (Cutler, Pierce, and Steckenrider, 1984).

SENIOR POWER

What are the prospects that the elderly as a group will come to exercise significant political power? Research on "senior power" reflects an ongoing debate about whether age can serve as a catalyst for a viable political movement. In the model of interest group politics, social policy arises from the conflicts and accommodations of organized groups, each seeking to fulfill their interests (Lowi, 1969). It is contended that older people can be a powerful political constituency in this process, because of the relatively high rates of voting and political party leadership mentioned earlier. In addition, older people's consciousness of their potential to influence policies to respond to their interests is presumed to be growing. Consistent with the subculture theory of aging, discussed in Chapter 3, this political consciousness is assumed to develop from shared values and common experiences with discrimination (Anderson and Anderson, 1978; Rose, 1965). Since future cohorts of older people will be better educated and healthier, and will retire earlier with higher incomes, it is argued that they will have more resources essential to political power. Future cohorts are also presumed to experience increasing pride, dignity, and shared consciousness in old age. As the older population increases and our society becomes more aware of the social, economic, and political issues created by the "graying" of the population, older persons will identify more with their peers and define problems collectively (Cutler, 1982). Thus, age will become a more salient aspect of politics, even if all older persons and organized groups of seniors do not speak (or vote) with a unified political voice. Neil Cutler (1983), for example, argues persuasively that heterogeneity does not preclude age—like gender and ethnic minority status— from exerting political influence.

The alternative argument, that older people do not constitute a significant age-based political force, has been advanced primarily by Hudson and Binstock (Binstock, 1972; Hudson and Binstock, 1976; Hudson and Strate, 1985). Their first point is that older people do not form a distinct subculture; in fact, the diversity of the older population precludes their having shared interests around which to coalesce. Most older people, especially the young-old in their early sixties, do not identify themselves as "aged," nor do they perceive their problems as stemming from their age. They may be more likely to identify themselves on the basis of other status distinctions, such as ethnic minority status, religion, or social class. This suggests that the elderly are not the captive of any single political philosophy, party, or mass organization. Therefore, according to this alternate position, age alone is not a relevant factor in predicting political behavior or age group consciousness based on differential access to resources (Streib, 1965). Because aged-based consciousness is lacking and older people are stable in their partisan attachments, the elderly are unlikely to be swayed by politicians' appeals to the age vote, nor can they substantially influence social policy development (Binstock, 1972; Hudson and Strate, 1985).

The number and variety of age-based national organizations nevertheless appear to support the viewpoint that older people are a powerful political force. Conscious organizing of the elderly is not without historical precedent in this country. The first age-based politically oriented interest group grew out of the social and economic dislocations of the Depression. Called the Townsend Movement, after its founder, Dr. Francis E. Townsend, it began in California in 1933 and reached its peak in 1936, with 1½ million members nationally. It proposed a tax on all business transactions to finance a $200/month pension for every pensioner over age 60. However, passage of the Social Security Act, in which groups of older people played a supporting but not a leading role, took away its momentum, and the organization died out in the 1940s. Most political divisions during the turbulent period of the Depression were class- and labor-based, rather than age-based; the Townsend Movement did demonstrate, however, that old age could be a short-term basis for organizing (Vinyard, 1982; Fischer, 1978).

The McClain Movement, another early age-based organization, was initially part of the Ham and Eggs movement, which aimed to establish financial benefits for older persons through a referendum in the 1938 California elections. George McClain formed this group to exert political pressure on local legislatures to improve conditions for older people. McClain lost many of his followers after economic conditions improved in the 1940s (Hudson and Binstock, 1976).

Over 1,000 separately organized senior citizens groups currently exist at the local, state, and national levels, with at least 10 major national organizations involved in political action for older persons (Pratt, 1983). Three of these are mass membership organizations: the National Council of Senior Citizens (NCSC), the National Association of Retired Federal Employees (NARFE), and the American Association of Retired Persons together with the National Retired Teacher's Association (AARP). These organizations have a combined membership of approximately 17 million, a figure that represents a significant political force (Pratt, 1983).

The National Council of Senior Citizens (NCSC) was developed by organized labor in the early 1960s with the objective of passing Medicare. Although anyone may join, most members of NCSC are former blue-collar workers who receive insurance and other tangible membership benefits. The National Association of Retired Federal Employees (NARFE) was also formed for a specific political purpose—the passage of the Federal Employees Pension Act in the 1920s. It has since concentrated on bread and butter issues for federal employees, such as labor/management relations, rather than broader political issues affecting older persons generally. NARFE is the smallest of these three national organizations, with its membership primarily in the Washington, D.C., area. The best known and largest of these organizations is the American Association of Retired Persons–National Retired Teacher's Association (AARP), with a membership of over 13 million. A major function has been to offer benefits to its primarily middle-class, professional membership, although it has become increasingly active in the national political process since the late 1960s (Vinyard, 1982).

Four trade associations, one professional society, a confederation of social welfare agencies, and other organizations concerned with aging issues also exist at the national level. The trade associations are the American Association of Homes for the Aged, the American Nursing Home Association, the National Council of Health Care Services (consisting of commercial enterprises in the long-term care business, such as the nursing home subsidiary of Holiday Inns), and the National Association of State Units in Aging (NASUA), which is composed of administrators of state area agencies on aging. The emphasis of these associations is on obtaining federal funds and influencing the development of regulations for long-term care facilities and the delivery of public services. The professional association most active in aging policy issues, the Gerontological Society of America (GSA), is composed of professionals from many disciplines. The GSA has become active in public policy issues since the 1960s, primarily in efforts to influence the allocation of research and education funds.

The major confederation of social welfare agencies concerned with aging is the National Council on the Aging (NCOA), which encompasses almost 2,000 organized affiliates, including public and private health, social work, and community action agencies. It serves as technical consultant to organizations addressing problems facing older people. The National Caucus for the Black Aged is relatively new; its membership is primarily professional (both minority and nonminority), and concerned with increasing the responsiveness of aging programs to Blacks. Although it is one of the newer organizations advocating for the elderly, the National Caucus for the Black Aged is one of the most politically active associations working on their behalf.

Political momentum is also building in several organizations that began at the grass-roots level and now have a nationwide membership and enjoy national recognition. The Older Women's League (OWL), founded in 1981, brings

---

Political Activism and Older Women

Tish Sommers is an example of the increasing political activism of older women. Sommers, a long-time homemaker, learned about the vulnerability of older women when she was divorced at age 57. She found that newly single homemakers her age had a hard time getting benefits that people who have been employed take for granted. She coined the term *displaced homemaker* and built a force of women. They successfully lobbied for centers where displaced homemakers had job training during the late 1970s. In 1980, she and Laurie Shields founded the Older Women's League, a national organization that has grown to over 14,000 members and over 100 chapters. Her maxim has always been "Don't agonize, organize." During the six years of organizing OWL, Sommers also fought a battle with cancer. Even at her death in 1986, she was still fighting, organizing groups nationally around the right to maintain control over the conditions of one's death.

---

together people concerned about issues affecting older women, especially health care and health insurance, Social Security, and pensions. The Older Women's League has advocated for older women both in the federal policy-making process and within the programs of national associations, such as the GSA. Women activists within OWL may represent a trend away from the comparatively lower rates of past political participation among older women.

The Gray Panthers aims to form grass-roots intergenerational alliances around issues affecting all ages, but emphasizes social action to solve problems faced by older people. The Gray Panthers is the most radical of these national organizations, emphasizing social change and "transcending" existing social values and structures. More than any other present-day senior group, the Gray Panthers has been the outgrowth of one person, its founding leader Maggie Kuhn (Pratt, 1983).

The existence of these national organizations has been interpreted by some political observers as an indication of the elderly's political power. In contrast, Binstock (1972) argues that these groups were organized on a short-term basis to promote specific pieces of legislation, not to intervene continually in the political process on issues affecting older people. Critics contend that the electoral potency and representativeness of these organizations have not yet been tested (Binstock, 1972; Pratt, 1983, 1976). With a few exceptions, the major legislative breakthroughs in the field of aging in the past 20 years have been engineered by presidents and members of Congress, not by age-based organizations. For example, the Age Discrimination in Employment Act of 1967 was an outgrowth of presidential initiative, with strong backing from labor (Pratt, 1983). Even when age-based organizations were influential in the passage of aging policy in the 1970s, they played a supportive, not determining role (Pratt, 1976; Hudson and Strate, 1985). Such legislative successes have been due not to the elderly's political power, but rather to legislators' beliefs that older people are worse off than other groups (Hudson, 1981). Binstock views age-based organizations as only an implicit electoral force that politicians are eager not to offend. But legislators who sit on broadly based committees (e.g., the House Ways and Means) frequently betray a less than total commitment to age-based issues when support for them would offend other politically powerful constituencies. An example is the 1981 passage of the Omnibus Budget Reconciliation Act, which restricted Old Age Insurance benefits (Binstock, 1984).

National age-based organizations have been subject to other criticisms. Binstock sees them as primarily concerned with "middle man programs," (e.g., grants and contracts) in which they serve as intermediaries between funding organizations and older people. For example, trade associations, such as the American Nursing Home Association, are concerned with the conditions surrounding the payment of funds to older people, since these affect their ability to sustain their organizations. Professional associations, such as the Gerontological Society of America, concentrate their lobbying efforts on ensuring a fair share of research and educational funds. Critics argue that these organizations do not evaluate policies in terms of their impact on older people generally, but rather by the likely effect on their own members (Vinyard, 1982; Binstock, 1972).

Another criticism is that these organizations are reformist, using fairly conventional lobbying methods toward noncontroversial, piecemeal adjustments, rather than advocating major new policies to redistribute income (Harootyan, 1981; Vinyard, 1982). For example, although the National Council of Senior Citizens has actively support Medicare and income tax reform, most national organizations have not been concerned with policies that most affect low-income older persons, such as Supplemental Security Income and Medicaid. In the 1960s, AARP did not lobby for Medicare, and NARFE has rarely taken a stand on issues other than improvements in retired federal employee benefits. One reason for this is that the membership of these associations is primarily middle class and higher income working class (Pratt, 1983). The poorest of the older population lack many of the resources necessary to advance their interests (Ragan and Davis, 1982). In fact, the pressure group system is biased toward the most advantaged who are organized to press their claims (Vinyard, 1982).

Critics also maintain that members of these national organizations tend to be apathetic, largely because of a lack of an age-based consciousness (Pratt, 1983). In fact, some associations such as AARP recruit members primarily on the basis of direct member services (e.g., insurance, drug discounts, travel, etc.), not by appeals to change existing policies (Pratt, 1983; Hudson and Strate, 1985). Rather than collaborate on common concerns, these organizations have, in the past, tended to compete for their share of incentives offered through the political system, according to Binstock (1972). In recent years, however, more collaborative efforts have been initiated, as evidenced by the Leadership Council of Aging Organizations, formed in 1976. This Leadership Council, composed of representatives of over 20 national organizations, has analyzed how the federal budget affects older people, taken stands against reductions in programs serving the elderly, and helped to ensure the continuation of the Senate Special Committee on Aging. Age-based organizations are obtaining greater access to government officials at various stages of policy development, and have influenced specific issues, particularly at the local level (Hudson and Strate, 1985).

Organized political activity at the state and local levels has grown recently, particularly through the formation of Silver Haired Legislatures (SHLs) in 23 states. SHLs, which are modeled after state legislatures, provide seniors with sophisticated knowledge of legislative lobbying through training and direct experience; in some states, they have had a major influence on the legislative process. Elected SHL representatives also serve to hear concerns and spread information to local elders. Other states have a Senior Citizens Lobby to coordinate the advocacy work of different senior groups and develop a unified legislative package (National Council of Silver Haired Legislatures, 1986).

In sum, national organizations of elderly people have influenced social and health policies, even though they have not functioned consistently to deliver a unified bloc of votes, nor to change significantly the social and economic conditions faced by the most disadvantaged segments of the elderly. Age-based organizations, however, may have more influence in the future, especially as more politically astute and active older persons are drawn into their ranks at the local and state levels.

Summary and Implications

As earlier chapters have documented, changes in employment and parenting roles, income, and physical and sensory capacities often have detrimental social consequences for the elderly. Nevertheless, there are arenas in which older people may still experience meaningful involvement and develop new opportunities and skills. This chapter has considered five of these arenas: leisure time pursuits, voluntary association membership, volunteering, religious involvement, and political activity. The meaning and functions of participation in these arenas are obviously highly individualized. Participation may be a means to strengthen and build informal social networks, influence wider social policies, serve other persons, and substitute for role changes. The extent of involvement is influenced not by age alone, but also by a variety of other salient factors, including gender, ethnic minority status, health, socioeconomic status, and educational level. Because of the number of interacting variables, age-related patterns in participation are not clearly defined.

In general, there are some age-related differences in types of leisure pursuits; with increasing age, people tend to engage in more sedentary, inner-directed, and routine pursuits in their homes than social activities or obligations outside the home. Changes in organizational participation and volunteering are less clearly age-related. Participation in voluntary associations stabilizes or declines only slightly with old age. Declines that do occur are likely to be associated with poor health, inadequate income, and transportation problems. Volunteering tends to represent a life-long pattern of community service.

Past research on religious and political participation by the elderly has pointed inaccurately to declines in old age. Although formal religious participation, such as church or synagogue attendance, appears to diminish, other kinds of religious behavior, such as reading religious texts or listening to religious broadcasts, increase. Spirituality has been differentiated from religion as a positive factor in older people's physical and mental well being.

In the 1980s, voting by older people has generally increased. Declines in voting and political participation in the past may have been functions of low educational status or physical limitations, not of age per se. In fact, older persons' skills and experiences may be more valued in the political arena than in other spheres.

Most forms of organizational involvement appear to represent stability across the life course; the knowledge and skills necessary for a varied set of activities in old age are generally developed in early or middle adulthood and maintained into later life. On the other hand, preretirement patterns are not fixed; individuals can develop new interests and activities in later life, often with the assistance of senior centers, continuing education programs, or community or special interest organizations.

References

ACTION. *American Volunteer, 1974.* Washington, D.C.: U.S. Government Printing Office, 1975.

Ainlay, S. C., and Smith, D. R. Aging and religious participation. *Journal of Gerontology,* 1984, *39,* 357–564.

Allen, K. K. The challenge facing senior volunteering. *Generations,* 1981, *4,* 8–9.

Anderson, W. C., and Anderson, N. The politics of age exclusion: The Adults Only Movement in Arizona. *The Gerontologist,* 1978, *18,* 6–12.

Argle, M., and Beit-Hallahmi, B. *The social psychology of religion.* Boston: Routledge and Kegan Paul, 1975.

Atchley, R. Retirement and leisure participation: Continuity or crisis? *The Gerontologist,* 1971, *11,* 13–17.

Babchuk, N., Peters, G., Hoyt, D., and Kaiser, M. The voluntary associations of the aged. *Journal of Gerontology*, 1979, 34, 579–587.

Binstock, R. H. Interest-group liberalism and the politics of aging. *The Gerontologist*, 1972, 12, 265–280.

Binstock, R. H. Reframing the agenda of policies on aging. In M. Minkler and C. Estes (Eds.), *Readings in the political economy of aging*. Farmingdale, N.Y.: Baywood, 1984.

Binstock, R. H., Levin, M. A., and Weatherly, R. The political dilemmas of social intervention. In R. H. Binstock and E. Shanas (Eds.), *Handbook of aging and the social sciences* (2d ed.). New York: Van Nostrand Reinhold, 1985.

Blazer, D., and Palmore, E. Religion and aging in a longitudinal panel. *The Gerontologist*, 1976, 16, 82–85.

Bosse, R., and Ekerdt, D. Change in self-perception of leisure activities with retirement. *The Gerontologist*, 1981, 21, 650–654.

Butler, R., and Gleason, H. *Productive aging: Enhancing vitality in later life*. New York: Springer, 1985.

Campbell, A. Social and psychological determinants of voting behavior. In W. Donohue and C. Tibbits (Eds.), *Politics of age*. Ann Arbor: University of Michigan, 1962.

Campbell, J. C., and Strate, J. Are old people conservative? *The Gerontologist*. 1981, 21, 580–591.

Chambré, S. M. Is volunteering a substitute for role loss in old age? An empirical test of activity theory. *The Gerontologist*, 1984, 23, 292–299.

Cigler, A. J., and Swanson, C. Politics and older Americans. In F. J. Berghorn, C. E. Schafer and Associates (Eds.), *The dynamics of aging*. Boulder, Colo.: Westview Press, 1981.

Clemente, J., Rexroad, D., and Hirsch, C. The participation of the Black aged in voluntary associations. *Journal of Gerontology*, 1975, 30, 469–476.

Cook, Jr., T. C. *The religious sector explores its mission in aging*. Athens, Ga.: National Interfaith Coalition on Aging, 1976.

Cuellar, J. B. El Senior Citizens Club: The older Mexican American in the voluntary association. In B. G. Myerhoff and A. Bimic (Eds.), *Life's career—aging: Cultural variations on growing old*. Beverly Hills: Sage Publications, 1978.

Cutler, N. Subjective age identification. In D. Mangen and W. Peterson (Eds.), *Research instruments in social gerontology*. Minneapolis: University of Minnesota Press, 1982.

Cutler, N. Age and political behavior. In D. Woodruff and J. Birren (Eds.), *Aging: Scientific perspectives and social issues* (2d ed.). New York: D. Van Nostrand, 1983.

Cutler, N., Pierce, R., and Steckenrider, J. How golden is the future? *Generations*, Fall, 1982, 38–43.

Cutler, S. J. Age profiles of membership in sixteen types of voluntary associations. *Journal of Gerontology*, 1976, 31, 462–470.

Cutler, S. J. Aging and voluntary association participation. *Journal of Gerontology*, 1977, 32, 470–479.

Delloff, L. The WHCOA and WAA: Spiritual well-being gets lost. *Generations,* 1983, *8,* 8–10.

Dobson, D. The elderly as a political force. In W. Browne and L. K. Olson (Eds.), *Aging and public policy.* Westport, Conn.: Greenwood Press, 1983.

Douglass, E. B., Cleveland, W. P., and Maddox, G. (1974). Political attitudes, age and aging: A cohort analysis of archival data. *Journal of Gerontology,* 1974, *29,* 666–675.

Dowd, J. *Stratification among the aged.* Monterey, Calif.: Brooks/Cole, 1980.

Dye, D., Goodman, M., Roth, M., and Jensen, K. The older adult volunteer compared to the non-volunteer. *The Gerontologist,* 1973, *13,* 215–218.

Ekerdt, D. J. The busy ethic: Moral continuity between work and retirement. *The Gerontologist,* 1986, *26,* 239–244.

Fischer, D. H. *Growing old in America.* Oxford, England: Oxford University Press, 1978.

Fischer, K. *Winter grace. Spirituality for the later years.* New York: Paulist Press, 1985.

Fogelman, C. Being a volunteer: Some effects on older people, *Generations,* 1981, *4,* pp. 24–25.

Foner, A. The polity. In M. W. Riley, M. Johnson, and A. Foner (Eds.), *Aging and society.* New York: Russell Sage Foundation, 1972.

Foner, A., and Schwab, L. *Aging and retirement.* Monterey, Calif.: Brooks/Cole, 1981.

Foner, A., and Schwab, K. Work and retirement in a changing society. In M. W. Riley, B. Hess, and K. Bond (Eds.), *Aging and society: Selected reviews of recent research.* Hillsdale, N.J.: Lawrence Erlbaum Assoc., 1983.

Gallup Organization, Inc. *Americans volunteer—1981.* Princeton, N.J.: The Gallup Organization, Inc., 1981.

Glenn, N. A. Aging and conservatism. *The Annals of the American Academy of Political and Social Science,* 1974, *CDXV,* 176–186.

Glenn, N., and Hefner, T. Further evidence on aging and party identification. *Public Opinion Quarterly,* 1972, *36,* 31–47.

Gordon, D., Gaitz, C. M., and Scott, J. Leisure and lives: Personal expressivity across the life span. In R. Binstock and E. Shanas (Eds.), *Handbook of aging and the social sciences.* New York: D. Van Nostrand, 1976.

Gray, R. M., and Moberg, D. O. *The church and the older person.* Grand Rapids, Mich.: Erdmans, 1977.

Hadaway, C. K. Life satisfaction and religion: A reanalysis. *Social Forces,* 1978, *57,* 636–643.

Hanssen, A., Nichols, M., Buckspan, L., Henderson, B., Helbig, T., and Zarit, S. Correlates of senior center participation. *The Gerontologist,* 1978, *18,* 193–200.

Harootyan, R. G. Interest groups and aging policy. In R. Hudson (Ed.), *The aging in politics: Process and policy.* Springfield, Ill.: Charles C. Thomas, 1980.

Harris and Associates. *The myth and reality of aging in America.* Washington, D.C.: National Council on the Aging, 1974.

Harris and Associates. *Aging in the eighties: American in transition.* Washington, D.C.: National Council on the Aging, 1981.

Height, D., Toya, J., Kamekawa, L., and Maldonaldo, D. Senior volunteering in minority communities. *Generations,* 1981, *5,* 14–18.

Heisel, M. A., and Faulkner, A. O. Religiosity in an older Black population. *The Gerontologist,* 1982, *22,* 354–368.

Holloway, H., and George, J. *Public opinion: Coalitions, elites, and masses.* New York: St. Martin's Press, 1979.

Holmes, T. H., and Masuda, M. Life change and illness susceptibility. In B. S. Dohrenwend and B. P. Dohrenwend (Eds.), *Stressful life events: Their nature and effects.* New York: Wiley, 1974.

Hooker, K., and Ventes, D. Work ethic, daily activities and retirement satisfaction. *Journal of Gerontology,* 1984, *39,* 478–484.

Hudson, R. B. The graying of the federal budget and its consequences for old-age policy. In R. B. Hudson (Ed.), *The aging in politics: Process and policy.* Springfield, Ill.: Charles C. Thomas, 1981.

Hudson, R. B., and Binstock, R. Political systems and aging. In R. Binstock and E. Shanas (Eds.), *Handbook of aging and the social sciences.* New York: D. Van Nostrand, 1976.

Hudson, R., and Strate, J. Aging and political systems. In R. Binstock and E. Shanas (Eds.), *Handbook of aging and the social sciences* (2d ed.). New York: D. Van Nostrand Reinhold, 1985.

Hunsberger, B. Religion, age, life satisfaction, and perceived sources of religiousness: A study of older persons. *Journal of Gerontology,* 1985, *40,* 615–620.

Hunter, K., and Linn, M. Psychosocial differences between elderly volunteers and non-volunteers. *Aging and Human Development,* 1981, *12,* 205–213.

Institute of Lifestyle Improvements. Minnesota Self-Health Assessment Screen. Stevens Pt.: University of Wisconsin/Stevens Creek Foundation, 1978.

Kalish, R. Death and dying in a social context. In R. Binstock and E. Shanas (Eds.), *Handbook of aging and the social sciences.* New York: D. Van Nostrand, 1976.

Kaplan, M. *Leisure: Lifestyle and lifespan.* Philadelphia: W. B. Saunders, 1979.

Keith, P., Goudy, W., and Powers, E. Salience of life areas among older men: Implications for practice. *Journal of Gerontological Social Work,* 1984, *8,* 67–82.

Kelly, J. R. *Leisure.* Englewood Cliffs, N.J.: Prentice-Hall, 1982.

Kelly, J. R., Steinkamp, M., and Kelly, J. Later life leisure: How they play in Peoria. *The Gerontologist,* 1986, *26,* 531–537.

Kivett, V. Religious motivation in middle age: Correlates and implications. *Journal of Gerontology,* 1979, *34,* 106–115.

Kleiber, D., and Kelly, J. Leisure, socialization and the life cycle. In Seppo Iso-Anola (Ed.), *Social psychological perspectives on leisure and recreation.* Springfield, Ill.: Charles C. Thomas, 1980.

Larson, R., Zuzanek, J., and Mannell, R. Being alone versus being with people: Disengagement in the daily experience of older adults. *Journal of Gerontology,* 1985, *40,* 375–381.

Lawton, M. P. Leisure activities for the aged. In M. Wolfgang (Ed.), *Planning for the elderly: Special Issue of the Annals of the American Academy of Political and Social Sciences,* July 1978, pp. 71–80.

Letzig, B. Aging: A common denominator for interfaith action. *Generations,* 1983, *8,* 15–17.

Levine, S. The hidden health care system. *Medical Care,* March 21, 1983, 378.

Lowi, T. J. *The end of liberalism.* New York: W. W. Norton, 1969.

Markides, K. S. Aging, religiosity and adjustment: A longitudinal analysis. *Journal of Gerontology,* 1983, *38,* 621–626.

McSherry, E. The spiritual dimension of elder health care. *Generations,* 1983, *8,* 13–21.

Miller, S. The social dilemmas of the aging leisure participant. In A. Rose and W. Peterson (Eds.), *Older people and their social world.* Philadelphia: F. A. Davis, 1965.

Mindel, C., and Vaughan, C. E. A multidimensional approach to religiosity and disengagement. *Journal of Gerontology,* 1978, *33,* 103–108.

Missine, L. Keynote presentation from the Conference on Religion, Spirituality, and Aging. American Society on Aging, 1986.

Moberg, D. Religiosity in old age. *The Gerontologist,* 1965, *5,* 78–87.

Moberg, D. Religion in the later years. In A. M. Hoffman (Ed.), *The daily needs and interests of older people.* Springfield, Ill.: Charles C. Thomas, 1970.

Moberg, D. O. Subjective measures of spiritual well-being. Presented at the Baltimore Meeting of SSSR, *Abstracts,* October 31, 1981, 12.

Monk, A., and Cryns, A. Predictors of voluntaristic intent among the aged: An area study. *The Gerontologist,* 1974, *14,* 425–429.

Moss, M., and Lawton, M. P. Time budgets of older people: A window on four lifestyles. *Journal of Gerontology,* 1982, *37,* 115–123.

National Council of Silver Haired Legislatures. Newsletter, 1986. P. O. Box 1060, Hallendale, Fl., 33009.

Neulinger, J. *The psychology of leisure: Recent approaches to the study of leisure.* Springfield, Ill.: Charles C. Thomas, 1974.

Newman, B., and Newman, P. *Development through life: A psycho-social approach.* Homewood, Ill.: Dorsey, 1979.

O'Brien, G. E. Leisure attributes and retirement satisfaction. *Journal of Applied Psychology,* 1981, *66,* 371–384.

Palmore, E. The social factors in aging. In E. Busse and D. Blazer (Eds.), *Handbook of geriatric psychiatry.* New York: Van Nostrand Reinhold, 1980.

Paloutzian, R. F., and Ellison, C. W. Loneliness and quality of life measures: Measuring loneliness, spiritual well-being and their social and emotional correlates. In L. A. Peplau and D. Perlman (Eds.), *Loneliness: A sourcebook of current theory, research and therapy.* New York: Wiley InterScience, 1982.

Payne, B., and Whittington, F. Older women: An examination of popular stereotypes and research evidence. *Social Problems,* 1976, *23,* 488–504.

Pepper, C. Senior volunteerism: Alive and well in the 80's. *Generations,* 1981, *4,* 6–7.

Pieper, H. Church membership and participation in church activities among the elderly. *Activities, Adaptation and Aging,* 1981, *1,* 23–29.

Pratt, H. J. *The gray lobby: Politics of old age.* Chicago: University of Chicago Press, 1976.

Pratt, H. J. National interest groups among the elderly: Consolidation and constraint. In W. P. Browne and L. K. Olson (Eds.), *Aging and public policy.* Westport, Conn.: Greenwood Press, 1983.

Princeton Religion Research Center. *Religion in America.* Princeton, N.J.: The Gallup Poll, 1982.

Ragan, P., and Davis, W. The diversity of older voters. In B. Hess (Ed.). *Growing old in America* (2d ed.). New Brunswick, N.J.: Transaction Books, 1982.

Reynolds, D., and Kalish, R. Anticipation of futurity as a foundation of ethnicity and aging. *Journal of Gerontology,* 1974, *29,* 224–231.

Rose, A. M. The subculture of the aging: A framework for research in social gerontology. In A. M. Rose and W. A. Peterson (Eds.), *Older people and their social world.* Philadelphia: F. A. Davis, 1965.

Rosow, I. Status and role change through the life cycle. In R. Binstock and E. Shanas (Eds.), *Handbook of aging and the social sciences* (2d ed.). New York: Van Nostrand Reinhold, 1985.

Steinitz, L. Y. Religiosity, well-being and Weltanschauung change among the elderly. *Journal for the Scientific Study of Religion,* 1980, *19,* 60–67.

Steinitz, L. Y. The local church as support for the elderly. *Journal of Gerontological Social Work,* 1981, 42–53.

Streib, G. F. Are the aged a minority group? In A. W. Gouldner and S. M. Miller (Eds.), *Applied sociology.* New York: Free Press, 1965.

Swartz, E. I. The older adult: Creative use of leisure time. *The Journal of Geriatric Psychiatry,* 1978, *11,* 85–87.

Teague, M. Aging and leisure: A social psychological perspective. In Seppo Iso-Ahola (Ed.), *Social psychological perspectives on leisure and recreation.* Springfield, Ill.: Charles C. Thomas, 1980.

Thompson, G. B. (1973). Work versus leisure roles: An investigation of morale among employed and retired men. *Journal of Gerontology,* 1973, *28,* 339–344.

Thorson, J. Spiritual well-being in the secular society. *Generations,* Fall 1983, *8,* 10–11.

Tinsley, H., Teaff, J., Colbs, S., and Kaufman, N. A system of classifying leisure activities in terms of the psychological benefits of participation reported by older persons. *Journal of Gerontology,* 1985, *40,* 172–178.

Tobin, S. S., and Ellor, J. W. The church and the aging network: More interaction needed. *Generations,* Fall 1983, *8,* 26–28.

Torres-Gil, F. Political behavior: A study of political attitudes and political participation among older Mexican Americans. Unpublished dissertation, Heller School, Brandeis University, 1976.

Trela, J. Social class and association membership: An analysis of age-graded and non-age-graded voluntary participation. *Journal of Gerontology,* 1976, *31,* 198–203.

U.S. Senate Special Committee on Aging. *Aging America: Trends and projections, 1985–86 Edition.* Washington, D.C.: U.S. Government Printing Office, 1986.

Vinyard, D. The rediscovery of the elderly. In B. Hess (Ed.), *Growing old in America* (2d ed.). New Brunswick, N.J.: Transaction Books, 1982.

Ward, R. The meaning of voluntary association participation to older people. *Journal of Gerontology,* 1979, *34,* 438–445.

Weiner, A. I., and Hunt, S. C. Retirees' perception of work and leisure meanings. *The Gerontologist,* 1981, *21,* 444–448.

Westberg, G. Multiplying wholistic health centers. In *Increasing the impact.* Battle Creek, Mich.: Kellogg Foundation, 1979.

Chapter 14

Death, Dying, Bereavement, and Widowhood

You have probably heard of people who "lost their will to live" or "died when they were ready." Such ideas are not simply superstitions. Similar to other topics addressed throughout this book, death involves an interaction of physiological, social, and psychological factors. The social context is illustrated by the fact that all cultures develop beliefs and practices regarding death in order to minimize its disruptive effects on the social structure. These cultural practices influence how members of society react to their own death and that of others. Although measures of death are physical, such as the absence of heart beat or brain waves, psychosocial factors can influence the biological event. For instance, terminally ill people have been found to die shortly after an important engagement, such as a child's wedding, a family reunion, or holiday, suggesting that their "will to live" prolonged life to that point (Kalish, 1984). How people approach their own death and that of others is closely related to personality styles, sense of competence, coping skills, and social supports, as discussed in Chapter 8.

This chapter examines age-related attitudes toward death in our culture; the dying process and its meaning to the dying person; the conditions for care of the dying; the concept of the right to die; the rituals of bereavement, grief, and mourning; and the experience of widowhood. Research on death and dying and professional interventions to support dying persons and their families are relatively recent and are a significant and growing area for gerontological research and practice; these interventions are discussed briefly in this chapter.

The Changing Context of Dying

In our culture, dying is associated primarily with old age. Although, as we have seen, aging does not cause death, and younger people also die, there are a number of reasons for this association. The major factors are medical advances and the increase in life expectancy. In preindustrial societies, death rates were high in childhood and youth, and parents could expect that one-third to one-half of their children would die before the age of ten (Marshall, 1980). Now it is increasingly the old who die, making death predictable as a function of age. Death has thus come to be viewed as a timely event, the completion of the life cycle in old age. Others view death not only as the province of the old, but also as an unnatural event that is to be fought off as long as medically possible. At the end of prolonged chronic illness, when medicine may care for but not cure the patient, dying may seem more unnatural than if the person had been allowed to die earlier in the progression of the illness. With expanded technological mastery over the conditions of dying, chronically ill people have often been kept alive long past the point at which they might have died naturally in the past.

The surroundings in which death occurs have also changed with increased medical interventions. In preindustrial society, most people died at home, with the entire community often involved in rituals surrounding the death. Now over two-thirds of all deaths occur in institutions, generally in hospitals and nursing homes (Amenta, 1985), with only small groups of relatives and friends present. This is the case even though most people express a preference to die at home surrounded by friends and family (Kalish and Reynolds, 1976; DuBois, 1980).

ATTITUDES TOWARD DEATH

More insulated from death than in the past, most people are uncomfortable with talking about it, especially the prospect of their own death. Freud, in fact, recognized that although death was natural, undeniable, and unavoidable, people behaved as though it would occur only to others; that is, *they* will die, but not *me* (Kastenbaum, 1977). Fear and denial are natural and comforting responses to being unable to comprehend our own death and nonexistence (Becker, 1973). Such fear has tended to make death a taboo topic in our society. Although in recent years death has become a more legitimate topic for scientific and social discussion, most people are more likely to talk about it on a rational, intellectual level than to discuss their own death.

Whether people's fear of death is natural or learned is unclear. When asked what they fear most about death, respondents mention suffering and pain, loss of their body, punishment, loss of self-control, the unknown, loneliness, the effect on survivors, and the destruction of the personality (Schultz, 1978; Pattison, 1977; Kalish and Reynolds, 1976; Kastenbaum and Aisenberg, 1976). In general, people fear the process of dying, particularly the prospect of dying slowly and in pain, more than death itself. Yet, when questioned directly, people are more concerned with the death of close friends and family than their own, and generally express an acceptance of death (Kalish and Reynolds, 1976, Kastenbaum and Aisenberg, 1976; Bengtson, Cuellar, and Ragan, 1977). For example, 89 percent of a national sample agreed that death can "sometimes be a blessing," and 80 percent felt it was better to make plans concerning death than to ignore or deny it (Riley, 1970). In a sample of persons aged 45 to 74, 66 percent replied they were "not at all afraid of death" (Bengtson et al., 1977). Although the validity of responses to questions about one's own death is difficult to ascertain, it appears that most people both deny and accept the reality of dying. These ambivalent views reflect the basic paradox surrounding death, in which we recognize its universality, but cannot comprehend or imagine our own dying (Weisman, 1972).

VARIATION BY AGE AND SEX

Studies of variables, such as education, marital, and health status that are related to anxiety about death, have produced conflicting results (Wagner and Lorion, 1984). Attitudes toward death and dying do appear to differ by sex and age. In research utilizing metaphors for death, women fear death but are also more accepting of their own death, viewing it as peaceful, like a "compassionate

mother" or an "understanding doctor." Men tend to perceive death as antagonis-
tic, a "grinning butcher" or a "hangman with bloody hands" (Back, 1971; Keith,
1979). Compared to older men, older women are less negative about death
(Kalish and Reynolds, 1976; Keith, 1979). In general, older people think and talk
more about death and appear to be less afraid of it than younger people (Stillion,
1985; Cole, 1978–79; Martin and Wrightsman, 1965). A number of factors may
explain this apparent paradox of a lessened fear of death in the face of its
proximity. Having internalized society's views, older people may see their lives as
having ever-decreasing social value, thereby lowering their own positive expectation of the future (Stillion, 1985). If they have lived past the age they
expected, they may view themselves as living on "borrowed time" (Kalish, 1985).
A painless death tends to be viewed as preferable to deteriorating physically and
mentally and being socially useless or a burden on family (Marshall, 1980). In
addition, dealing with their friends' deaths, especially in age-segregated retirement communities or nursing homes, can help socialize older people toward an
acceptance of their own death. Experiencing deaths more frequently, they are
more likely to think and talk about death on a regular basis than are younger
people (Kalish, 1976). If they achieve the developmental stage of ego integrity,
as described in our discussion of Erikson in Chapter 8, they tend to be more
accepting of death as fair.

Death fears do not increase among older people with terminal conditions,
although depression may be a frequent response (Kalish and Reynolds, 1976;
Kalish, 1982; Marshall, 1980). People who have solved problems effectively
throughout their lives, viewed their lives as satisfying, and related well to others
tend to adjust best to terminal illness (Hinton, 1975; Weisman and Warden, 1975).
On the other hand, older people who live alone, have worse self-rated health, and
are chronically depressed and isolated tend to be more preoccupied with and
fearful of death than accepting of it (Lesnoff-Caravaglia, 1985; Wass, Christian,
Myers, Murphy, 1979; Bengtson et al., 1977). Differences among ethnic minority
and religious groups also have been found, but comparatively little research has
been conducted on these variations within our society.

It is unclear whether variability in the acceptance of death is due to age or
cohort differences. For example, the current cohort of older people has fewer
years of formal schooling than younger generations, a factor that affects attitudes
toward death. The interactive effects of other variables with age need to be further
probed. For instance, in all age groups the most religious persons have less
anxiety about dying (Feifel and Nagy, 1986). For the religious, death is the
doorway to a better life. Similarly, people who are most confirmed in their lack of
religious belief also express less fear about death. Those most fearful about death
are the irregular church-goers, or those intermediate in their religiosity whose
belief systems may be confused and uncertain (Downey, 1984; Marshall, 1980;
Kalish, 1976). Religion apparently can either comfort or create anxiety about an
afterlife, but it provides some individuals with one way to try to make sense of

death (Marshall, 1980). More recent data from a national hospice study suggest that few older people facing death draw strength from the prospect of an afterlife (Kastenbaum, Kastenbaum, and Morris, in preparation).

Age is also a factor in how survivors react to death. Because the death of older people is often anticipated, it may be viewed as a "blessing" for someone whose "time has come" rather than as a tragic experience. In some instances, hospital emergency room personnel have been found to be less likely to administer life-saving procedures to an older person than to a younger person with the same life-threatening condition (Sudnow, 1967). Young people are expected to fight death, whereas older people are assumed to accept dying passively.

The elderly have also been found to react differently to perceptions of limited remaining time, and thus to death as an *organizer of time*. Compared to youth, older people confronting death may conclude that nothing meaningful can be accomplished because all activities will be short-lived and unfinished. Accordingly, many older people whose death is imminent make less effort than younger people to alter their way of life or to attempt to complete projects. Instead, they are more likely to turn inward to contemplation, reading, or spiritual activities (Kalish and Reynolds, 1976). The awareness of one's mortality can stimulate a need for the "legitimization of biography," to make sense of one's life and one's death. People who successfully achieve such legitimation experience a new freedom and relaxation about the future (Marshall, 1980). Many older people consider a sudden death to be more tragic than a slow one, desiring time to see loved ones, settle their affairs, and reminisce.

DEATH AS LOSS

Researchers have also defined death as loss—loss of self, of all forms of sensory awareness, and of loved ones. Seven values lost through death have been identified:

1. Loss of ability to have experiences
2. Loss of ability to predict subsequent events
3. Loss of body (and fear of what will happen to the body)
4. Loss of ability to care for dependents
5. Loss suffered by friends and family (e.g., causing grief to others)
6. Loss of opportunity to continue and plan projects
7. Loss of being in a relatively painless state.

Of 563 respondents, those between 15 and 39 years of age cited causing grief to friends as their major anticipated concern, whereas those over age 40 chose the inability to care for dependents as a primary loss through death (Diggory and

Rothman, 1961). In a later survey of a somewhat older and lower income sample, older respondents were less concerned about caring for dependents and causing grief to friends and relatives than were younger respondents (Kalish and Reynolds, 1976). One reason for this difference may be that older people are already experiencing "bereavement overload" through the increased frequency of family and friends' deaths, and thus are more aware of the reduced impact of their death on others (Kastenbaum and Aisenberg, 1976). Loss of the ability to retain self-control can be an especially poignant loss for a dying person. It is important to recognize that the meaning to an older person of loss of the physical body may be very different from the loss of self-control over how they die.

The Dying Process

One of the most widely known frameworks for understanding the stages of the dying process has been advanced by Kübler-Ross (1969), described briefly in Chapter 8. According to Kübler-Ross, dying persons experience five stages in reaction to their death: (1) denial and isolation, (2) anger and resentment, (3) bargaining and an attempt to postpone, (4) depression and sense of loss, and (5) acceptance. As discussed in Chapter 8, each of these stages represents a form of coping with the process of death.

Denial is initially a healthy buffer, but it can prevent dying persons from moving to subsequent stages if others are unwilling to talk with them about their concerns. In the second stage, anger ("Why me?") may be displaced on family or medical staff and can lead to withdrawal and avoidance. This stage may be the most difficult for caregivers to tolerate. In the bargaining stage, the dying person may try to make a deal with God to live long enough to attain some goal or to postpone death as a reward for good behavior. The fourth stage is depression, which represents a natural grieving process over the final separation of death. The dying person may withdraw from loved ones as a way to prepare for this separation. The final stage, acceptance, is achieved only if the dying person is able or allowed to express and deal with earlier feelings, such as anger and depression. The dying person thereby achieves a sense that personal tasks have been accomplished and the struggle is over. Rather than a happy stage, the acceptance phase is almost devoid of feelings, and should not be confused with wishing to die. Although Kübler-Ross cautioned that these stages were not invariant, immutable, or universal, she nevertheless implied that progression from one to the other is normal and adaptive; she encouraged health care providers to help their patients to advance through them; and she depicted the final stage as consummatory.

Kübler-Ross (1975) emphasizes that dying can be a time of growth. By accepting death's inevitability, dying persons can use life meaningfully and productively and come to terms with who they really are. Since the dying are "our best teachers," those who work with them can learn from them and emerge from such experiences with fewer anxieties about their own dying (Kübler-Ross, 1969). The religious assumptions and allegations about life after death that are embedded in Kübler-Ross's writings, however, have evoked scientific and theological criticism, and have often detracted from the importance of her work with dying patients (Fox, 1981).

Although her work is controversial, Kübler-Ross has been a pioneering catalyst, increasing public awareness of death and the needs of the dying and their caregivers. Her framework should be viewed as a helpful cognitive grid or guideline of possible moods and ways of coping with death, not as a fixed sequence that determines a "good death." Empirical testing of the stage theory has produced mixed findings. Apathy, apprehension, and anticipation have been found as well as acceptance of death (Weissman and Kastenbaum, 1968). Any of these feelings and behaviors may occur at any time during the dying process, and the person may move back and forth between them, displaying several of the feelings simultaneously. Family members and health care providers must be cautious about implying that the dying person must follow these stages, and thus creating the illusion of control by naming phases. Instead, they should be open to the dying person's choice of whether and how to move through these stages (Kalish and Reynolds, 1976). In sum, subsequent studies have found that there is no "typical," unidirectional way to die through progressive stages (Fox, 1981, Schneidman, 1980, Kastenbaum, 1977). Instead, there may be an alternation between acceptance and denial, between understanding what is happening and magically disbelieving its reality (Schneidman, 1980). Consistent with the framework of dynamic interactions discussed throughout this book, the dying process is shaped by an individual's own personality and philosophy of life, by the specific illness, and by the social context (e.g., whether at home surrounded by family who encourage the expression of feelings, or isolated in a hospital).

AN APPROPRIATE DEATH

Questions have also been raised about whether acceptance of death should be the goal of dying. The concept of an *appropriate death* has been suggested as an alternative goal for those working with the dying. An appropriate death means that the person has died as he or she wished to do, which generally is consistent with past personality patterns. Dying people can sustain hope if they maintain their belief in "significant survival,"—the belief in our lives that we have done "something worth doing and that others think so too" (Weisman, 1972). Another hopeful perspective is to view death as a healthy companion to life (Kastenbaum, 1977). Most people try to maintain as much control over their dying as possible in order to render it meaningful (Marshall, 1980). Although an appropriate death is usually only partially obtained, those working with the dying can help them to exert such control.

The Dying Trajectory Framework

An alternative to the framework of stage theories is the concept of *dying trajectory*, or the perceived course of dying and expected time of death. The pace of a dying trajectory can be sudden or slow, regular or erratic, and it is usually shaped by the condition causing death (e.g., dying from lung cancer versus a heart attack) (Pattison, 1977; Glaser and Strauss, 1968). Most people with terminal conditions have an idea of how much longer they will live, and plan their lives within that interval. Difficulties for the patient can arise when health care professionals or family members perceive a different course of dying. For example, with expected, lingering death, hospital staff may treat patients as if they were socially dead and may withdraw from them prior to their biological death (Glaser and Strauss, 1968). The process whereby professional support is withdrawn after it is decided that a person's illness cannot be reversed has been called *regressive intervention,* and is more likely to occur when the patient is old (Watson and Maxwell, 1977).

A *death crisis* in the dying trajectory is an unanticipated change in the amount of time remaining to live. The living-dying interval, which occurs between the death crisis and the actual time of death, is characterized by three phases. During the *acute phase,* the dying person expresses maximum anxiety or fear. At the *chronic phase* of dying, anxiety declines as the person faces death's reality, confronts questions about the dying process and the future, and enacts necessary rituals and preparations. The *terminal phase* is characterized by the dying person's withdrawal (Glaser and Strauss, 1968).

CARE OF THE DYING

Both frameworks—the stages of dying and dying trajectories—highlight the importance of giving attention to the ways in which care is provided to the dying. Although most dying people prefer to die at home, the common practice has been to hospitalize them, with most deaths occurring in nursing homes or hospitals (Amenta, 1985). In the past, medical personnel have tended to be uncomfortable with dying patients. As death approached, they may have interacted less with the dying person, oftentimes isolating them by moving them to a private room, pulling the curtains around their bed, and speaking about them as if they were unfeeling objects and socially dead (Glasser and Strauss, 1968). Nursing homes have often tried to prevent upsetting other residents by hiding a fellow resident's death and thereby avoiding reminders of their mortality (Haber, Tuttle, and Rogers, 1981). As a result, many dying people may feel abandoned, humiliated, and lonely at the end of their lives (Kalish and Reynolds, 1976; Weisman, 1972).

These conditions have begun to change, with more training provided to health care providers who work with the dying. Medical professionals have become more open in talking about death with their patients as well as among themselves. This breaking of "professional silence" is in part a reaction to external pressures, including the growth of death education programs, patients who insist on being informed about their illnesses, and current public affirmations about the "right to know" and the "right to die" (Fox, 1981). In the past 20 years, for example, nurses' interest in the humane care of terminally ill patients and their families has dramatically increased. Dissatisfied with prior patterns of care, nurses have advocated a supportive, holistic, and egalitarian collaboration among health care providers, which more compassionately responds to dying patients and their caregivers (Germain, 1980). Some health care professionals have also given more recognition to spiritual support for the dying (Conrad, 1985).

The Dying Person's Bill of Rights states that individuals have rights to treatment as living persons until death, to participate in decisions about their care, to be free from pain, to maintain their individuality, and to be cared for by sensitive and knowledgeable people (Barbou, 1975). Assuring relief from physical pain is essential to humane care. In addition, dying persons should be provided with opportunities to make the circumstances of their dying consistent with their preferences and lifestyle. It is critical to establish conditions in which dying persons can be open about their concerns and reassured by others for expressing feelings, without necessarily being forced to be expressive. Individual needs and preferences for privacy, making decisions, and saying good-byes should be supported. The social support of friends and family, more than other interventions, has been identified as a major source of strength for older dying people (Kastenbaum et al., in preparation).

Hospice Care   Another trend toward being more responsive to dying patients and their families has been the expansion of the hospice model of caring for the terminally ill. Hospice is a philosophy of caring and an array of services that can best be implemented through the home, although its principles can also be enacted as inpatient services for the terminally ill (Koff, 1981). It is dedicated to helping individuals who are beyond the curative power of medicine to remain in familiar environments that minimize pain, and to maintain personal dignity and control over the dying process. Assessment and coordination of the physical, psycho-social, and spiritual needs of patient and family are fundamental to the hospice approach. St. Christopher's Hospice, started by Dr. Cicely Saunders in Great Britain in 1977, was the first hospice, and is a self-contained facility with its own home-residential care.

The first hospice in the United States was developed in 1974 in New Haven, Connecticut, and now over 1,600 hospices exist in our country. The majority of these provide in-home services for cancer patients (McCann and Enck, 1984). In 1986, Congress passed legislation making hospice a permanent Medicare benefit, and granting a modest increase in reimbursement rates, although funding regulations are restrictive. Even though older people have been both providers and recipients of hospice care (Kastenbaum et al., in preparation), there is some evidence that hospices underserve the older population compared to other age groups (Kalish, 1985).

Both professional and lay providers contribute as an interdisciplinary team to hospice goals. For example, hospice workers advocate for providing dying persons with full and accurate information about their condition. Another important function is to develop supportive environments in which people can tell their life stories and find meaning in their deaths. Listening, touching the dying person, and family involvement are all emphasized by the staff. In addition, hospice staff work directly with family and friends to help them resolve their feelings, clarify expectations, and relate most effectively to the dying patient. Hospice workers also recognize the importance of bereavement counseling after the death, generally following up with support to grieving family members. Unfortunately, hospice models of care are still unavailable to most terminally ill persons, because of restrictive Medicare reimbursement mechanisms for inpatient care, and lack of Medicaid funding for hospice benefits.

Despite its many benefits, hospice is not always the best approach, since caring for a dying person at home can severely strain the resources of family and friends (Parkes, 1980). Such burdens on families, discussed further in Chapter 19, have intensified with restrictions in funding for home health care. A danger is that cost-containment objectives may take priority over the goals of quality care for the dying and their families (Aroskar, 1985). If the preference of most people to die at home is to be realized, more community-based programs to ease the strain on family caregivers must be developed.

Psychotherapeutic Approaches   Due largely to Kübler-Ross's work, increased recognition has been given to the value of psychotherapy with dying persons. Until recently, psychotherapists have generally preferred to work with people presumed able to return to productive life, as discussed in Chapter 8. The focus of most psychotherapy with dying persons is to support the process of working through their denial and despair, thereby enabling them to live out their remaining months as fully as their disease allows. Even in the first interview, a therapist should strive to open the door for the dying person to communicate without fear and anxiety (Kübler-Ross, 1975). The process and satisfaction of personal growth, not a sense of accomplishment, are believed to be of therapeutic value in themselves (LeShan, 1969; Becker, 1973). Caring relationships with health care providers may also have therapeutic effects, even though formal psychotherapy is not involved (Kalish, 1982).

Although traditional medical treatments are generally used with dying patients, other more controversial approaches include faith-healing, acupuncture, meditation, and treatment of cancer by laetrile. Each of these treatments has its adherents and detractors, even within the medical profession. One controversial treatment that claims effectiveness, especially in healing cancer patients defined as terminally ill by their physicians, is the combined imagery, relaxation, and psychotherapy program developed by physician Carl Simonton (Simonton, Matthews-Simonton, and Creighton, 1978). The Simonton approach maintains that cancer patients have the power to get rid of the cancer; this emphasis on self-responsibility is assumed to marshall whatever will to live exists (Kalish, 1982). We have probably all heard anecdotes of cancer patients who practiced meditation and relaxation and lived well beyond their prognosis, again suggesting the complex interaction of psychological, social, and medical aspects of living and dying. Adherents of approaches that emphasize patient responsibility also recognize that when people have decided they are ready to die, they should be supported in that decision.

The Right to Die

Along with the increased attention to the ways in which people choose to die and the meanings they assign to their deaths, the right-to-die movement has grown in recent years. It has given rise to new discussions of *euthanasia*, or elective death. Whether others have a right to help people die, and under what conditions, has been debated throughout history. But recent debates about the complex philosophical, social, and legal issues raised by euthanasia have intensified with increased medical advances used to prolong life. These issues revolve around three different types of patients: the terminally ill who are conscious, the irreversibly comatose, and the brain-damaged or severely debilitated who have good chances for survival but are at a low level of existence (e.g., Alzheimer's patients) (Creine, 1975). The most recurrent and widely publicized cases have involved the question of withholding life-sustaining treatment from patients who are unable or incompetent to make this decision for themselves (Fox, 1981).

Euthanasia can be *passive* (allowing death) or *active* (causing death). In passive euthanasia, treatment is terminated, and nothing is done to prolong the patient's life artificially. Clear legal or medical standards do not exist regarding whether treatment must be continued in hopeless cases. Omitting life-saving procedures is risky for medical professionals, even in the final stages of irreversible dementing illness, when older people sometimes refuse to accept food and water by mouth. The risk is that physicians who withhold treatment may potentially be liable to prosecution for murder or manslaughter.

In 1982, a team of prominent physicians concluded that it is ethically permissible to withhold artificially administered food and water, and that patients with an irreversible illness need only be made comfortable (Wanzer et al., 1984). Despite clear directives from these and other medical professionals, court decisions have not supported such actions consistently enough to establish the protection of legal precedent. As a result, considerable disagreement exists within the medical community about how to handle the dilemmas created by "elective death" (Robertson, 1983). The courts have become a major forum for deliberating questions about the proper definition of life and death, the "right to die," and the right to decline and discontinue potentially life-prolonging treatment.

PASSIVE EUTHANASIA (VOLUNTARY ELECTIVE DEATH)

The act of elective death may take many forms, generally classified as *direct* or *indirect.* For example, an older person may choose active suicide by deliberately taking an overdose of sleeping medications. In passive suicide, a patient might omit vital medications or fail to comply with dietary restrictions; the effects of the patient's decision may be subtle and gradual. For instance, older people may make decisions that are equivalent to choosing to die by refusing extra help at home or by insisting on hospital discharge directly to their home, in spite of their need for skilled nursing care. When older people neglect their care needs or choose an inappropriate living situation because of impaired judgment, involuntary treatment laws can sometimes be used to move them to protected settings. If their "failure to care" is not immediately life-threatening, however, they usually have to be allowed to deteriorate to that point before being legally compelled to comply with treatment. In most cases, older people who commit suicide through the gradual process of self-neglect do not fall within the narrow confines of involuntary treatment laws. All of these are *direct*; the patients involved have voluntarily carried out their own death.

Voluntary *indirect* forms of elective death highlight the issue of the right to refuse treatment. In such cases, patients have specified in advance the conditions under which their lives should be ended, granting discretion to others to cease "heroic" or "extraordinary" treatment to maintain life. In 36 states and the District of Columbia, Natural Death legislation has provided for the right of patients and/or their families to refuse treatment in the final stages of terminal illness. Through a document called a *Living Will*, patients in states with such laws can direct physicians at hospitals to withhold life-sustaining procedures in the event of an irreversible terminal illness. A Living Will thus provides some measure of protection against unwanted medical measures, even in states that have not passed legislation through Natural Death Acts; it is also crucial in helping family members make decisions when they are unable to consult a comatose or mentally incompetent relative. Two national organizations—Concern for Dying and the Society for the Right to Die—support passive euthanasia and publish information and examples of Living Wills.

One limitation of a Living Will is that persons faced with imminent death may feel differently about their desires for extraordinary measures than they had anticipated when their death was further removed in time. The individual's condition, however, may prohibit him or her from changing the document. Family members who initially agreed to a Living Will may later be unwilling to allow the person to die without some intervention. A Living Will usually applies only in cases of terminal illness when death is imminent, and may contain ambiguous language. In most cases, it applies only to refusal of treatment, not to removal of life-sustaining procedures (Older Women's League, 1986).

Because of these ambiguities, hospitals and doctors, fearing later law suits, may not adhere to a Living Will. For example, as a result of a complaint by a nurse in a recent California case, two doctors were charged with murder for removing the feeding tube from an irreversibly comatose patient, even though the patient's desire not to have life-prolonging treatment was known (Older Women's League, 1986). For the medical profession, there are few liabilities for continuing to treat a patient, but there may be grave dangers in stopping treatment.

Therefore, despite natural death legislation, physicians tend to be cautious when it comes to withholding life-sustaining procedures. Because of numerous "gray areas," particularly in interpreting key words such as *terminal* and *imminent*, individual cases are brought to court for judicial rulings to resolve ambiguities in the laws. In one California case, a mentally competent 70-year-old man completed the legal documents needed to have his respirator turned off. The state Court of Appeals ruled unanimously that his wish was a "constitutional, guaranteed right which must not be abridged" (*Bartling* v. *Superior Court,* 1984). The hospital refused, claiming that his medical condition did not fit the state's legal standard of "terminally ill with death imminent." He tried several times to remove ventilator tubes, but hospital officials put restraints on his wrists. A Superior Court judge upheld the view that the man's condition was not "terminal," because death was not imminent. The patient eventually won the case, but died, with the tube still in, in the course of litigation (Older Women's League, 1986). This case highlights the gap between legal theory and medical practice.

ACTIVE EUTHANASIA (INVOLUNTARY ELECTIVE DEATH)

"Direct involuntary elective death" refers to actions deliberately taken to end a person's life without her or his permission, in contrast with allowing the natural process of dying. Such active euthanasia, closest to the idea of mercy killing, is a form of criminal homicide and excluded from Living Will legislation. States vary widely on whether cases are prosecuted and juries are willing to convict. For example, in a recent California case, an older woman who had cared for her bed-bound husband for years and strangled him with a nylon stocking to end his suffering was not prosecuted. In contrast, a 75-year-old Florida man who shot his wife, as the only solution to terminate her suffering from Alzheimer's disease and osteoporosis, was sentenced to 25 years in prison without parole (Sommers, 1985).

Ethical and legal problems become even more complex regarding suicide, and in providing assistance to someone committing suicide. Should persons who are terminally ill, such as cancer patients, be allowed to shorten their own lives? Is

Living Will Declaration

INSTRUCTIONS
Consult this column for help and guidance.

To My Family, Doctors, and All Those Concerned with My Care

This declaration sets forth your directions regarding medical treatment.

I, _____, being of sound mind, make this statement as a directive to be followed if I become unable to participate in decisions regarding my medical care.

If I should be in an incurable or irreversible mental or physical condition with no reasonable expectation of recovery, I direct my attending physician to withhold or withdraw treatment that merely prolongs my dying. I further direct that treatment be limited to measures to keep me comfortable and to relieve pain.

You have the right to refuse treatment you do not want, and you may request the care you do want.

These directions express my legal right to refuse treatment. Therefore I expect my family, doctors, and everyone concerned with my care to regard themselves as legally and morally bound to act in accord with my wishes, and in so doing to be free of any legal liability for having followed my directions.

You may list specific treatment you do not want. For example:

Cardiac resuscitation
Mechanical respiration
Artificial feeding/
  fluids by tubes

Otherwise, your general statement, top right, will stand for your wishes.

I especially do not want: _____

_____

_____

_____

_____

_____

_____

You may want to add instructions for care you do want—for example, pain medication; or that you prefer to die at home if possible.

Other instructions/comments: _____

_____

_____

_____

	Proxy Designation Clause: Should I become unable to communicate my instructions as stated above, I designate the following person to act in my behalf:
If you want, you can name someone to see that your wishes are carried out, but you do not have to do this.	Name _____
	Address _____
	If the person I have named above is unable to act in my behalf, I authorize the following person to do so:
	Name _____
	Address _____
Sign and date here in the presence of two adult witnesses, who should also sign.	Signed: _____ Date: _____
	Witness:_____ Witness:_____
	Keep the signed original with your personal papers at home.
	Give signed copies to your doctors, family, and to your proxy.

Source: Reprinted by permission of the Society for the Right to Die, 250 W. 57th St., New York, N.Y. 10107.

Issues Raised by the Right to Die

Consider the case of a California couple, both home-bound and under the care of round-the-clock nurses. The wife had emphysema and was unable to walk, talk, or stand up straight without severe breathing difficulties. She was attached 24 hours a day to a machine that delivered oxygen to her through two nasal prongs. The husband, in the final stages of congestive heart disease, was subject to hallucinations and could not walk, read, hear clearly, get dressed, bathe himself, or control his bladder. If they had waited four months, they could have celebrated their fiftieth wedding anniversary, but instead they chose, as they put it in their letters to their children, to "terminate their terminal illnesses." During the last year of their lives, they had discussed their plans with their children and grandchildren, written detailed letters describing their intentions and philosophies, and carefully studied manuals published by Right to Die societies. Their adult children believed that their parents, perceiving a painful and narrowed future, had availed themselves of their right to choose the dignity of death over the sanctity of life (Fadiman, 1984).

it suicide to refuse treatment if the result of refusal is death, or is it letting the disease take its course? The Hemlock Society distinguishes between "rational suicide" (i.e., the option of ending one's life for good and valid reasons) and suicide that is caused by a rejection of life because of emotional disturbance. The Hemlock Society not only promotes the right of mature terminally ill persons to determine for themselves the time, place, and circumstances of their death, but also calls for decriminalization of assistance to a person who has made that decision. The Hemlock Society maintains that their manuals on nonviolent methods to commit suicide with prescription barbiturates can assure a gentle, peaceful death.

HOW DO PEOPLE VIEW EUTHANASIA?

Reactions to the practice of euthanasia are colored by a combination of professional belief, the patient's belief, and perceptions of societal benefits and costs. Those who support a policy of euthanasia maintain it promotes a "good" or dignified death through allowing choice and being compassionate to the dying person's suffering. Remote chances for recovery are not believed to justify treatment that would only prolong suffering. In response, opponents of euthanasia argue that medical diagnosis and prognosis are not infallible, that a "hopeless" patient may survive to lead a meaningful life, and that relevant new medical discoveries may be made that would save their lives. Their fundamental objection is that euthanasia cheapens life, ultimately being used as a "solution" to remove those whom society considers burdensome. Some opponents maintain that euthanasia, or even the concept of a natural death, can lead to premature rejection of the right to life of the "useless" elderly, and is tantamount to a form of "gerontocide" (Kastenbaum and Aisenberg, 1976).

Despite these objections, physicians, clergy, and the public are becoming more accepting of euthanasia. Public acceptance, measured by national surveys in 1950, 1973, 1977, and 1985 (Ostheimer and Ritt, 1976; Sommers, 1985; Ward, 1984; Gallup, 1985) has grown, with eight in ten Americans in the most recent survey believing that ill patients should be able to ask doctors to stop life-supporting medical treatments. The public is more tolerant of passive euthanasia (e.g., "letting him die"), however, than of active euthanasia (e.g., "putting him out of his misery").

Perhaps somewhat surprisingly, the current generation of older people appears to be the least supportive of euthanasia. They are less likely than younger people to agree that patients should be allowed to die, even if they or their families request it (Kalish and Reynolds, 1976; Ostheimer and Ritt, 1976; Haug, 1978; Ward, 1984). This has been attributed to cohort effects, particularly to lower education levels and greater religiousness among older cohorts. One predictor of favorable attitudes toward euthanasia is the belief that people have a right to make their own health decisions without relying on a physician's advice (Haug, 1978).

Thus, resistance to euthanasia by the current generation of older people may also be due to their greater acceptance of a physician's authority.

Physicians do not easily accept the concept that it may be best to do less, not more, for a patient. Coupled with traditional pressures for aggressive treatment is the tendency for medical professionals to equate a patient's death with professional failure (Creine, 1975). Nevertheless, passive euthanasia to alleviate suffering is becoming a widely accepted part of medical practice (Williams, 1973; Creine, 1975). The 1984 statement on euthanasia by physicians presented two fundamental guidelines: The patient's role in decision making is paramount, and a decrease in aggressive treatment of the hopelessly ill patient is advisable when treatment would only prolong a difficult and uncomfortable process of dying (Wanzer et al., 1984).

Societal cost-benefit criteria come into play in discussions of euthanasia, given the reality of limited resources. As society tries to contain soaring health care costs, physicians are subject to demands for financial restraint. The majority of the money spent on medical care in a person's lifetime goes to services received during the last years and months of life (Scitovsky, 1984). Nearly 25 percent of Medicare expenditures cover costs in the last year of life (Older Women's League, 1986). For example, a study of Medicare enrollees in Colorado who had died in 1978 found that 60 percent of all health care expenditures were in the last three months of life, with more hospital days and more intensive hospital ancillary services (McCall, 1984). On the societal level, huge expenditures to keep a comparatively small number of people alive take resources away from other medical needs, and may indirectly contribute to deaths among other groups (Callahan, 1986; Fuchs, 1974). Issues of this kind are clearly illustrated in decisions involving organ transplants and, most recently, in the controversy surrounding artificial mechanical hearts: Should money be spent on organ transplants to benefit a relatively few people, or should these people be permitted to die and our health resources focused on prevention and outreach? Rapid improvements in medical technology have not been matched by refinements in the law and the ethics of using those therapies. Euthanasia thus raises not only difficult moral and legal dilemmas but resource allocation issues that cannot be ignored. Because these issues will become more critical in the future as medical technology develops even more, they will be discussed further in our Epilogue. On a personal level, many dying people find that the medical technology that prolongs their lives cannot make their lives pleasurable or meaningful, and it may financially ruin their families.

Bereavement, Grief, and Mourning Rituals

Death affects the social structure through the person's survivors, who have social and emotional needs resulting from that death. Some studies have found that the intensity of these needs is reflected in the higher rates of suicide, hospitalization for psychiatric disorders, visits to physicians, and somatic complaints (Schultz, 1978; Marshall, 1980; Kalish, 1982). Numerous epidemiological studies over the past 20 years reveal an excess mortality in the newly widowed, particularly among younger white male widowers (Jacobs and Ostfeld, 1977; Parkes, Murray, and Fitzgerald, 1969). However, these studies have failed to take account of other factors that may influence mortality in bereavement, such as length of illness in the deceased spouse, preexisting illness in the survivor, and socioeconomic and ethnic minority status (Jacobs and Ostfeld, 1977). High mortality rates may also reflect fatigue, self-neglect, or stress resulting both from caring for the dying person and from mourning (Kalish, 1982). Although findings on mortality are inconsistent, the first six months of widowhood appear to be the most stressful, especially for older men who are more at risk of poor health and death. To minimize these disruptive effects, survivors need help in dealing with their grief. Such support is especially critical for older persons, who, as we have seen in earlier chapters, generally face multiple losses (Freeman, 1984). The relationship between bereavement and suicide in both males and females in older groups also requires further investigation.

Bereavement refers to the state of being deprived of a loved one by death. *Grief* is the emotional response to bereavement. Grief reactions to bereavement are complex, with most survivors experiencing some adjustment problems for a year or more following the loss. *Mourning* signifies culturally patterned expectations about the expression of grief. These expectations form a continuum, with one end indicating normal grief and the other end indicating pathological grief reactions of physical and mental illness.

Grief reactions can include shock and disbelief, guilt, psychological numbness, depression, loneliness, fatigue, loss of appetite, sleeplessness, and anxiety about one's ability to reorganize and carry on with life (Martocchio, 1985; Parkes, 1970; Parkes and Brown, 1972; Glick, Weiss, and Parkes, 1974; Kalish and Reynolds, 1976; Kalish, 1982; Schulz, 1978). There appear to be clusters or phases of grief. The initial response is generally shock, numbness, and disbelief, followed by all-encompassing sorrow, which tends to last for a few weeks. In the elderly, somatic illnesses tend to be associated with and intensify the reaction to loss at these early stages (Gromlich, 1968). Not only do recently bereaved elderly report more illnesses and increased use of new medications, but they also usually rate their overall health more poorly (Thompson, Breckenridge, Gallagher, and Peterson, 1984; Lindemann, 1979).

An intermediate stage of grief often involves an idealization and searching for the presence of the deceased person, as well as an obsessional review in an attempt to find meaning for the death. Anger toward the deceased, toward God, and toward caregivers may also be experienced. When the permanence of the loss is accepted and yearning ceases, anguish, disorganization, and despair often result. The grieving person tends to experience a sense of confusion, a feeling of aimlessness, a loss of motivation, confidence, and interest, and an inability to make decisions. Grieving persons gradually readjust and begin to reorganize their behavior through new activities and relationships. The final stage—recovery—is usually required for the expression of feelings, and may occur from six months to several years after death (Schulz, 1978; Parkes, 1970). Some people never fully cease grieving (Kalish, 1982). For most people, some of the pain of loss remains for a lifetime. The elderly's experiences with grief may be even more complex than other age groups for several reasons. As noted in Chapter 8, they are more likely to experience unrelated, multiple losses over relatively brief periods, at a time when their coping capacities and environmental resources are often diminished. The cumulative effects of losses may be greater, especially if the older person has not resolved earlier losses, or interprets current losses as evidence of an inevitable continuing process (Freeman, 1984).

Bereavement does not follow a fixed or universal sequence, but rather is a process characterized by overlapping responses and individual variability (Kalish, 1982; Marshall, 1980). To expect grieving persons to progress in some specified fashion is inappropriate, and it can be potentially harmful to them (Martocchio, 1985). Adjustment to bereavement may be more difficult when death is sudden or unexpected (Glick et al., 1974; Schulz, 1978; Kalish, 1982). As noted in Chapter 8 in the discussion of anticipatory coping, an expected death allows survivors to prepare for the changes through "anticipatory grief," but it does not necessarily minimize the grief and the emotional strain. Some studies indicate that longer periods of anticipatory grief are associated with post-mortem depression and high medical risk, in part because of the stress of the long anticipation and of caring for the dying person (Fulton and Gattesma, 1980; Clayton, Halikas, Maurice, and Robins, 1973; Gerber, Rusalem, Hannon, Battin, and Atkin, 1975). The high medical risks faced by survivors who had cared for a dying spouse suggest that interventions should be directed at those who are experiencing anticipatory grief, that is, during the spouse's illness (Herriott and Kiyak, 1981).

Factors that have been found to help minimize grief are whether the death is viewed as natural, the degree to which relationships seem complete, and the presence of surviving confidants to provide emotional support (Carey, 1979–80). To work through grief successfully requires facing the pain and fully expressing the related feelings (Martocchio, 1985). In recent years, health care providers have recognized the importance of grief work, and view grieving as a natural healing process (Benoliel, 1985; Martocchio, 1985). Because of the cumulative impact of multiple losses, the elderly especially may need assistance in grief resolution, perhaps through life review and encouragement of new risk-taking (Freeman, 1984). Unfortunately, most studies of bereavement have been based on case studies or retrospective studies during the early phase of grief. There are few well-controlled longitudinal studies of the bereavement process. An additional limitation is that few researchers have controlled for the effects of variables such as sex, ethnic minority status, age, social class, and education. Our understanding of the emotional components of bereavement is based largely on middle-aged, middle-class Caucasians.

Mourning involves cultural assumptions about appropriate behavior during bereavement. Mourning rituals develop in every culture as a way to channel the normal expression of grief, to define the appropriate timing of bereavement, and to encourage support for the bereaved among family and friends. Professionals need to be sensitive to cultural and ethnic differences regarding the meaning of death and the burial of the dead. As Kastenbaum (1977) notes, the "death system" of cultural groups involves people (e.g., funeral directors, florists, life insurance agents in Western society), places (funeral homes), objects (tombstones), times (Memorial Day), and symbols (black dress, funeral music). The major function of the death system is to help both the individual and society deal with the problems created by death.

The funeral, for example, serves as a rite of passage for the deceased and a focal point for the expression of the survivors' grief. Funerals also allow the family to demonstrate cohesion through sharing ritual, food, and drink, and thus minimize the disruptive effects of the death. Funerals and associated customs are more important in societies with a high mortality throughout the life cycle than in modern society, where death is predominantly confined to the old. Money donations instead of flowers, and cremations instead of land burial signal the development of new kinds of death rituals today. Contemporary funerals have been criticized for being costly, for exploiting people at a time when they are vulnerable, and for elaborate cosmetic restorations of the body (Kastenbaum and Aisenberg, 1976). Legislation has been enacted recently to control some of the excesses of the funeral industry. Despite such criticisms, however, most people approve of traditional funerals; and some type of ceremony appears to make the death more real to the survivors and to offer a meaningful way to cope with the initial grief.

Widowhood

A spouse's death requires more readjustment on the part of the bereaved than any other stressful life event (Gallagher, Thompson, and Peterson, 1981–82; Owen, Fulton, and Markuson, 1982–83), and is faced by many older people—especially women. As we have seen in Chapter 1, most older women by age 70 are widows; but most older men do not become widowers until after age 85. By age 75 or older, 67 percent of women are widows, compared to 34 percent of males. With the average age of widowhood at 56 years and the average life expectancy approaching 80, many women face over 20 years of widowhood. The proportion of widows among nonwhites is twice that among white women; nonwhite women are also widowed earlier (U.S. Senate Special Committee on Aging, 1986). This is a reflection of the shorter life expectancy of nonwhite men in our society, as discussed in Chapter 1.

The impact of widowhood can be attenuated through a number of complex socio-psychological variables. These include the adequacy of the social support network, the individual's characteristic way of coping with stress, and religious commitment (Gallagher et al., 1981–82). Other variables that appear to affect the degree of stress of widowhood are age and gender.

It is unclear whether the stress of bereavement is greater for the young than for the old. Although younger spouses have been found initially to manifest more intense grief, a reverse trend has been noted after 18 months, with older spouses showing exacerbated grief reactions. As noted earlier, the elderly are more likely to experience other losses simultaneously, which may intensify and prolong their grief. In a study of the relationship between widowhood and physical health, younger widows presented psychological complaints (such as anxiety and depression), whereas older women reported an increase in physical symptoms and somatic illness (Parkes, 1964; Parkes and Brown, 1972).

Findings are mixed regarding the association between age and psychological response to bereavement. Some studies have found that older widows experience less psychological distress (for example, restlessness, sleep disturbance, and irritability) than younger widows (Maddison and Viola, 1968; Parkes, 1964). Conflicting results have also been found regarding the value of anticipatory grieving in helping individuals adjust to a loss (Marshall, 1980). For younger widowers, anticipatory grief tended to reduce the intensity of their bereavement (Rando, 1986; Ball, 1977; Carey, 1979–80). As noted arlier, this was not always the case among older widowers studied, largely because of the lengthy chronic illness preceding the spouse's death (Gerber, Rusalem, Hannon, Battin, and Atkin, 1975).

GENDER DIFFERENCES IN WIDOWHOOD

Whether widowhood is more difficult for women or men is unclear. Certainly, coping or adaptation to widowhood is related to income. Adequate financial resources are necessary to maintain a sense of self-sufficiency and to continue participation in meaningful activities. Older widows are generally worse off than widowers in terms of finances, legal problems, and prospects for remarriage. Women who have been economically dependent on their husbands often find their incomes drastically reduced, especially if they do not yet qualify for Social Security or if their husbands had not chosen survivors' pension benefits. Insurance benefits, when they exist, tend to be exhausted within two years of the husband's death.

Financial hardships may be especially great for women who have been caring for a spouse during a long chronic illness or who have depleted their joint resources during the spouse's institutionalization. Furthermore, many older widows have few opportunities to augment their income through paid employment. As noted earlier, older women have limited chances of remarrying into an economically desirable situation. Consequently, 60 percent of all widows age 65 and over live alone or with nonrelatives, and only 25 percent of older widows report living reasonably free of financial worries. An estimated 40 percent of older widows live near or below the poverty line (Rix, 1984). Although finding jobs for older widows has been suggested as a way to meet their economic needs, employment is not necessarily an appropriate adaptive strategy for them (Morgan, 1984).

Some women, however, do not depend on a man for economic or social support. Because women generally have more diverse, extensive friendship networks than men do, and because widowhood is prevalent in later life, many women form strong support networks with other widows. These friendship groups can compensate for the loss of a husband's companionship, and ease the adjustment to living alone. Friends are of greatest support when they accept the widow's emotional ambivalence, do not offer advice, and respond to what she defines as her needs (Lopata, 1973). Among women over age 70, two-thirds of whom are widowed, the married person is the unusual case, and the married individual has fewer friends than does the widow in the same age group (Blau, 1981).

Many widows have no interest in remarriage. Even among Lopata's (1973) study of widows with happy prior marriages, 36 percent said they would not marry again. Although many persons feel great loss with a spouse's death, for some who have been restricted in their marriage or who faced long-term caregiving responsibilities, widowhood can bring relief and opportunities to develop new interests. In fact, for those in unhappy marriages who feel they cannot divorce, death may be the only acceptable separation.

Adjusting to the loss of a spouse is likely to be most difficult for women who have had few economic and social resources throughout their lives, and when the identity of wife is lost without the substitution of other viable roles (Carey, 1979–80; Lopata, 1975). For example, Lopata (1973) found that widows who did not have their own friends or who had only couple-based friendships before their husband's death generally had difficulty forming new friendships and were left without satisfying roles. They also tended not to have access to social services. In our couples-oriented society, such women were lonely and isolated, and turned primarily to their children for emotional support. Friendships were thus the least frequent and the least deeply involving among the most disadvantaged, uneducated of the urban widows studied by Lopata. Blau (1981) also found that lower-class women who did not share social activities with other women, outside of neighboring, were less likely to have a reserve of social options upon which to draw in widowhood. Whether widows have strong friendship networks thus appears to vary with socioeconomic class, with whether they had a social network and satisfying roles before their husband's death, and with the prevalence of widowhood among a person's own age, sex, and class peers (Blau, 1981).

A woman's change in status inevitably affects her relationship with her children and other relatives. Most widows move in with their children only as a "last resort," although their children may view them as "helpless" and urge them to make the move. Older widows tend to grow closer to their daughters through patterns of mutual assistance, but more distant from their sons (Adams, 1968). The extent to which children serve to reduce their widowed parents' loneliness is unclear (Shanas, Townsend, Wedderburn, Friis, Milhoj, Stehouwer, 1968; Blau, 1981), and friends may be more important sources of emotional support than adult children (Blau, 1981; Lopata, 1979).

Most research on widowhood has focused on women, inasmuch as there are five widows to every widower in our society. Less is known about the effects of widowhood on older men. Men more often complain of loneliness, and appear to make slower emotional recoveries, than do women. They may have more difficulty expressing their grief and adjusting to the loss than women do, because of their lower degree of involvement in family and friendship roles throughout life, their life-long patterns of restraining emotions, their limited prior house-keeping and cooking, and the greater likelihood of a double role loss of worker and spouse (Berardo, 1970). Many men have depended on their wives for emotional support, household maintenance, and planning their social lives. Given these factors, men appear to "need" remarriage more than women do, and perhaps have been socialized to move more quickly into restructuring their lives through remarriage. Other studies have concluded that the impact of bereavement on older people's mental health is comparable for both men and women (Gallagher et al., 1981–82; Heyman and Gianturco, 1973). Men, however, have been found to experience more medical problems (as measured by increased physicians' visits and use of medications) during the six months following their wife's death (Gerber et al., 1975). Although widowhood may significantly impair older men's emotional and medical well-being, it is less likely to place men at an economic disadvantage. More research is needed on how men cope with the loss of their wives. Even less is known about how older men's experience of widowhood varies by social class or ethnic minority status.

Generally, widowhood increases social isolation for both men and women, with loneliness perceived as a major problem. In fact, for widowed persons generally, mental and physical impairments are higher than those for married persons of the same age (Barrett, 1978). Rates of chronic illness, suicide, and death tend to be even higher for those widowed persons without additional support systems, especially a confidant.

In order to provide such support for persons coping with loneliness and isolation, mutual help groups and bereavement centers have been developed by both mental health professionals and lay organizations. Women are the most frequent participants. These widow-to-widow groups are based on the principle of bringing together people who have the common experience of widowhood and who can help each other identify solutions to shared concerns. They recognize that a widowed person generally accepts help from other widowed people more readily than from professionals or family members. Support groups thus can provide widows with effective role models and can help integrate them into a social network and enhance their sense of competence toward the environment (Silverman and Cooperband, 1975; Silverman, 1980). Unfortunately, these groups are limited, and few controlled outcome studies have been conducted on the effectiveness of such innovative programs.

Summary and Implications

Although death and dying have been taboo topics for many people in our society, they have become more legitimate issues for scientific and social discussion in recent years. At the same time, there has been a growing emphasis on how professionals should work with the dying and their families, as well as a movement to permit death with dignity.

Two major frameworks have been advanced for understanding the dying process: the concept of stages of dying and the formulation of a dying trajectory. Both frameworks are only an inventory of possible sequences, not fixed steps.

Most people appear both to deny and to accept death, being better able to discuss others' deaths than their own and fearing a painful dying process more than the event of death itself. Different attitudes toward dying have been noted among the elderly and the young. Older people are less fearful and anxious about their death than younger people and would prefer a slow death which allows them time to prepare. Likewise, survivors tend to view an older person's death as less tragic than a younger individual's.

Professionals and family members can address the dying person's fears, minimize the pain of the dying process, and help the individual to attain a "good death." One of the major developments in this regard has been hospice care, a philosophy of caring that can be implemented in both home and institutional settings, and provides people with more control over how they die.

The movement for a right to a dignified death has prompted new debates about euthanasia. Both passive and active euthanasia raise complex moral and legal questions that have been only partially addressed by the passage of Living Will legislation and a growing number of judicial decisions. Economic issues are also at stake; as resources for health care become more scarce, questions about how much public money should be spent on maintaining chronically ill people are likely to intensify.

Regardless of how individuals die, their survivors experience grief and mourning. The intensity and duration of grief appears to vary by age and sex, although more research is needed regarding sex differences in reaction to loss of spouse and adjustment to widowhood.

By age 70, the majority of older women are widows; a much smaller number of older men become widowers, generally not until after age 85. The status of widowhood has negative consequences for many women in terms of increased legal difficulties, reduced finances, and few remarriage prospects. Although men are less economically disadvantaged by widowhood, they may be lonelier and have more difficulty adjusting than women do. For both men and women, social supports, particularly close friends or confidants, are important to physical and mental well-being during widowhood. In addition to mourning rituals to help widows and widowers cope with their grief, more support services, such as widows' support groups, are needed. Health and social service professionals can play a crucial role in developing services for the dying and their survivors that are sensitive to cultural, ethnic minority, and sex differences.

References

Adams, B. N. *Kinship in an urban setting.* Chicago: Markham, 1968.

Amenta, M. Hospice in the United States: Multiple models, and varied programs. *Nursing Clinics of North America,* 1985, *20,* 269–279.

Aroskar, M. Access to hospice: Ethical dimensions. *Nursing Clinics of North America,* 1985, *20,* 299–309.

Back, K. W. Metaphors as a test of personal philosophy of aging. *Sociological Focus,* 1971, *5,* 1–8.

Ball, J. F. Widows' grief: The impact of age and mode of death. *Omega,* 1977, *7,* 307–333.

Barbou, J. The dying person's Bill of Rights. *American Journal of Nursing,* 1975, *75,* 99.

Barrett, C. Sex differences in the experience of widowhood. Paper presented at the meetings of the American Psychological Association, 1978.

Bartling v. *Superior Court,* 163 Cal. App. 3d 186 (1984).

Becker, E. *The denial of death.* New York: The Free Press, 1973.

Bengtson, V., Cuellar, J., and Ragan, P. Stratum contrasts and similarities in attitudes toward death. *Journal of Gerontology,* 1977, *32,* 76–88.

Benoliel, J. Loss and terminal illness. *Nursing Clinics of North America,* 1985, *20,* 439–448.

Berardo, F. M. Survivorship and social isolation: The case of the aged widower. *Family Coordinator,* 1970, *19,* 11–25.

Blau, Z. S. *Aging in a changing society.* New York: Franklin Watts, 1981.

Callahan, D. Health care in the aging society: A moral dilemma. In A. Pifer and L. Bronte, (Eds.), *Our aging society: Paradox and promise.* New York: W. W. Norton, 1986.

Carey, R. Weathering widowhood: Problems and adjustments of the widowed during the first year. *Omega,* 1979–80, *10,* 163–174.

Clayton, P., Halikas, J., Maurice, W. L., and Robins, E. Anticipating grief and widowhood. *American Journal of Psychiatry* 1973, *122,* 47–51.

Cole, M. A. Sex and mental status differences in death anxiety. *Omega,* 1978–79, *9,* 139–142.

Conrad, N. Spiritual Support for the Dying. *Nursing Clinics of North America,* 1985, *20,* 415–425.

Creine, D. *The sanctity of social life: Physicians' treatment of critically ill patients.* New York: Russell Sage, 1975.

Diggory, J. C., and Rothman, D. Z. Values destroyed by death. *Journal of Abnormal and Social Psychology,* 1961, *30,* 11–17.

Downey, A. Relationship of religiosity to death anxiety of middle-aged males. *Psychological Reports,* 1984, *54,* 811–822.

DuBois, P. *The hospice way of death.* New York: Human Sciences Press, 1980.

Fadiman, A. The liberation of Lolly and Gronky. *Life Magazine,* 1984, 71–94.

Feifel, H., and Nagy, W. T. Another look at fear of death. *Journal of Consulting and Clinical Psychology,* 1981, 278–286.

Fletcher, J. Elective death. In E. Fuller Torrey (Ed.), *Ethical issues in medicine.* Boston: Little Brown, 1968.

Fox, R. The sting of death in American society. *Social Service Review,* 1981, 42–59.

Freeman, E. Multiple losses in the elderly: An ecological approach. *Social Casework,* 1984, 287–296.

Fuchs, V. *Who shall live? Health, economics, and social choice.* New York: Basic Books, 1974.

Fulton, R., and Gattesma, D. G. Anticipatory grief: A psychosocial concept reconsidered. *British Journal of Psychiatry,* 1980, *137,* 45–54.

Gallagher, D., Thompson, L., and Peterson, J. Psychosocial factors affecting adaptation to bereavement in the elderly. *International Journal of Aging and Human Development,* 1981–82, *14,* 79–95.

The Gallup Report. No. 235, April 1985, p. 29.

Gerber, I., Rusalem, R., Hannon, N., Battin, D., and Atkin, A. Anticipatory grief in aged widows and widowers. *Journal of Gerontology,* 1975, *30,* 225–229.

Germain, C. Nursing the dying: Implications of Kübler-Ross' stage theory. In R. Fox (Ed.), The social meaning of death. Special issue of *The Annals of the American Academy of Political and Social Science,* 1980, *447,* 89–99.

Glaser, B., and Strauss, A. *Time for dying.* Chicago: Aldine, 1968.

Glick, I., Weiss, R., and Parkes, C. M. *The first year of bereavement.* New York: Wiley–Interscience, 1974.

Gromlich, E. Recognition and management of grief in elderly patients. *Geriatrics,* 1968, *23,* 87–92.

Haber, D., Tuttle, J., and Rogers, M. Attitudes about death in the nursing home: A research note. *Death Education,* 1981, *5,* 25–28.

Haug, M. Aging and the right to terminate medical treatment. *Journal of Gerontology,* 1978, *33,* 586–591.

Herriott, M., and Kiyak, H. A. Bereavement in old age: Implication for therapy and research. *Journal of Gerontological Social Work,* 1981, *3,* 15–43.

Heyman, D., and Gianturco, D. Long term adaptation by elderly to bereavement. *Journal of Gerontology,* 1973, *28,* 359–362.

Hinton, J. The influence of previous personality on reactions to having terminal cancer. *Omega,* 1975, *6,* 95–112.

Jacobs, S., and Ostfeld, A. An epidemiological review of the mortality of bereavement. *Journal of Gerontology,* 1977, *28,* 359–362.

Kalish, R. Death and survivorship: The final transition. *The Annals of the American Academy of Political and Social Sciences,* 1982, *464,* 163–173.

Kalish, R. *Death, grief, and caring relationships* (2d ed.). Monterey, Calif.: Brooks/Cole, 1984.

Kalish, R. The social context of death and dying. In R. Binstock and E. Shanas (Eds.), *Handbook of aging and the social sciences* (2d ed.). New York: D. Van Nostrand Reinhold, 1985.

Kalish, R., and Reynolds, D. *Death and ethnicity: A psychocultural study.* Los Angeles: University of Southern California Press, 1976.

Kastenbaum, R. *Death, society, and human experience.* St. Louis: C. V. Mosby, 1977.

Kastenbaum, R. Dying and death: A life-span approach. In J. Birren and K. W. Schaie (Eds.), *Handbook of the psychology of aging.* New York: Van Nostrand Reinhold, 1985.

Kastenbaum, R., and Aisenberg, R. *The psychology of death: Concise edition.* New York: Springer, 1976.

Kastenbaum, R., Kastenbaum, B. K., and Morris, J. *Strengths and preferences of the terminally ill.* Data from the National Hospice Demonstration Study, in preparation.

Keith, P. Life changes and perceptions of life and death among older men and women. *Journal of Gerontology,* 1979, *34,* 870–878.

Koff, T. H. *Hospice: A caring community.* Cambridge, Mass.: Winthrop Publishers, 1981.

Kübler-Ross, E. *On death and dying.* New York: Macmillan, 1969.

Kübler-Ross, E. (Ed.). *Death: The final stage of growth.* Englewood Cliffs, N.J.: Prentice-Hall, 1975.

Lerner, M. When, why, and where people die. In O. Brimm et al. (Eds.), *The dying patient.* New York: Russell Sage, 1970.

LeShan, L. Mobilizing the life force. *Annals of the New York Academy of Science,* 1969, *164,* 847–861.

Lesnoff-Caravaglia, G. *Values, ethics and aging.* New York: Human Sciences Press, 1985.

Lindemann, E. *Beyond grief: Studies in crisis intervention.* New York: Jason Aronson, 1979.

Lopata, H. Z. *Widowhood in an American city.* Cambridge, Mass.: Schenkman, 1973.

Lopata, H. Z. Widowhood: Societal factors in life-span disruptions and alternatives. In N. Datan and L. Ginsberg (Eds.), *Life-span developmental psychology: Normative life crises.* New York: Academic Press, 1975.

Lopata, H. Z. *Women and widows.* New York: Elsevier, 1979.

Maddison, D., and Viola, A. The health of widows in the year following bereavement. *Journal of Psychosomatic Research,* 1968, *12,* 297–306.

Malcolm, A. Plaintiff in death, but suit goes on. *New York Times,* November 8, 1984.

Marshall, V. *Last chapters: A sociology of aging and dying.* Monterey, Calif.: Brooks/Cole, 1980.

Martin, D., and Wrightsman, L. S. The relationship between religious behavior and concern about death. *Journal of Social Psychology,* 1965, *45,* 317–323.

Martocchio, B. Grief and bereavement. *Nursing Clinics of North America,* 1985, *20,* 327–346.

McCall, N. Utilization and costs of Medicare services by beneficiaries in their last year of life. *Medical Care,* 1984.

McCann, B., and Enck, R. Standards for hospice care: A JCAH hospice project overview. *Progress in Clinical and Biological Research,* 1984, *156,* 431–449.

Morgan, C. Continuity and change in the labor force activity of recently widowed women. *The Gerontologist,* 1984, *24,* 530–535.

Moseley, J. Alterations in Comfort. *Nursing Clinics of North America,* 1985, *20,* 427–437.

Older Women's League. *Death and dying: Staying in control to the end of our lives.* Washington, D.C.: 1986.

Ostheimer, J., and Ritt, L. Life and death: Current public attitudes. In N. Ostheimer and J. Ostheimer (Eds.), *Life or death—Who controls?* New York: Springer, 1976.

Owen, G., Fulton, R., and Markuson, E. Death at a distance: A study of family survivors. *Omega,* 1982–83, *13,* 191–225.

Parkes, C. M. Effects of bereavement on physical and mental health: A study of the medical records of widows. *British Medical Journal,* 1964, *2,* 274–279.

Parkes, C. M. 'Seeking' and 'finding' a lost object. *Social Science and Medicine,* 1970, *4,* 187–201.

Parkes, C. M. The first year of bereavement. *Psychiatry,* 1970, *33,* 444–467.

Parkes, C. M. Terminal care: Evaluation of an advisory domicilliary service at St. Christopher's House. *Postgraduate Medical Journal,* 1980, *56,* 685–689.

Parkes, C. M., and Brown, R. J. Health after bereavement: A controlled study of young Boston widows and widowers. *Psychosomatic Medicine,* 1972, *34,* 449–461.

Parkes, C. M., Murray, B. B., and Fitzgerald, R. G. Broken heart: A statistical study of increased mortality among widows. *British Medical Journal,* 1969, *1,* 740–743.

Pattison, E. M. *The experience of dying.* Englewood Cliffs, N.J.: Prentice-Hall, 1977.

Rando, T. A. A comprehensive analysis of anticipatory grief: Perspectives, processes, promises and problems. In T. A. Rando (Ed.), *Loss and anticipatory grief.* Lexington, Mass.: D. C. Heath, 1986.

Riley, J. What people think about death. In O. Brim et al. (Eds.), *The dying patient.* New York: Russell Sage, 1970.

Rix, S. *Older women: The economics of aging.* Washington, D.C.: Women's Research and Education Institute, 1984.

Robertson, J. *The rights of the critically ill.* Cambridge, Mass.: Ballinger, 1983.

Rowland, K. F. Environmental events predicting death for elderly. *Psychological Bulletin,* 1977, *84,* 349–372.

Schneidman, E. Death work and stages of dying. In E. Schneidman (Ed.), *Death: Current perspectives.* Palo Alto, Calif.: Mayfield, 1980.

Schulz, R. *The psychology of death, dying, and bereavement.* Reading, Mass.: Addison-Wesley, 1978.

Schwab, J. J., Chalmers, J. M., Conroy, S. J., Farris, P. B., and Markush, R. E. Studies in grief: A preliminary report. In B. Shoenberg, I. Gerber, A. Wiener, A. H. Kutscher, D. Peretz, and A. Carr (Eds.), *Psychosocial aspects of bereavement.* New York: Columbia University Press, 1975.

Scitovsky, A. A. The 'high cost of dying': What do the data show? *Health and Society,* 1984, *66,* 591–608.

Shanas, E., Townsend, P., Wedderburn, D., Friis, H., Milhoj, P., and Stehouwer, J. *Older people in three industrial societies.* New York: Atherton Press, 1968.

Silverman, P. *Helping each other in widowhood.* New York: Health Sciences Pub. Corp., 1974.

Silverman, P. *Mutual help groups: Organization and development,* Beverly Hills, Calif.: Sage, 1980.

Silverman, P., and Cooperband, A. "On widowhood: Mutual help in the elderly widow." *Journal of Geriatric Psychiatry,* 1975, *8,* 9–27.

Simonton, O. C., Matthews-Simonton, S., and Creighton, J. *Getting well again.* Los Angeles: Tercher, 1978.

Sommers, T. On matters of life and death. *Gray Panther Network.* Summer 1985, 12.

Stillion, J. *Death and the sexes.* Washington, D.C.: Hemisphere Publishing, 1985.

Sudnow, D. *Passing on: The social organization of dying.* Englewood Cliffs, N.J.: Prentice-Hall, 1967.

Thompson, L., Breckenridge, J., Gallagher, D., and Peterson, J. "Effects of bereavement on self-perspections of physical health in elderly widows and widowers. *Journal of Gerontology,* 1984, *39,* 309–314.

U.S. Senate Special Committee on Aging. *Aging America: Trends and projections, 1985–86.* U.S. Department of Health and Human Services, 1986.

Wagner, K., and Lorion, R. Correlates of death anxiety in elderly persons. *Journal of Clinical Psychology,* 1984, *40,* 1235–1241.

Wanzer, S., Adelstein, J., Cranford, R., Federman, D., Hook, E., Moertel, C., Sofar, P., Stone, A., Taussig, H., and Vey Eys, J. The physician's responsibility toward hopelessly ill patients. *New England Journal of Medicine,* 1984, *310,* 955–959.

Ward, R. *The aging experience: An introduction to social gerontology.* New York: Harper and Row, 1984.

Wass, H., Christian, M., Myers, J., and Murphy, M., Jr. Similarities and dissimilarities in attitudes toward death in a population of older persons. *Omega,* 1979, *9,* 337–354.

Watson, W. H., and Maxwell, R. J. *Human aging and dying.* New York: St. Martin's Press, 1977.

Weisman, A. D. *On dying and denying.* New York: Behavioral Publications, 1972.

Weisman, A. D., and Kastenbaum, R. The psychological autopsy: A study of the terminal phase of life. *Community Mental Health Journal Monograph No. 4.* New York: Behavioral Publications, 1968.

Weisman, A. D., and Warden, J. W. Psychosocial analysis of cancer deaths. *Omega,* 1975, *6,* 61–75.

Williams, R. Propagation, modification, and termination of life: Contraception, abortion, suicide, euthanasia. In R. Williams (Ed.), *To Live and to Die: When, why, and how.* New York: Springer, 1973.

Chapter 15

Populations at Risk: Older Ethnic Minorities

When discussing the physiological, psychological, and social changes experienced by older people, there is a tendency to speak about the elderly as if they were a homogeneous group. Yet, as illustrated throughout this book, the older population is more heterogeneous than any other. Two primary variables in this differentiation are *gender* and *ethnic minority status*. To be old and a member of an ethnic minority group, or to be an older woman, is to experience environments substantially different from those of a white male. It also means a higher risk of being unhealthy, poor, alone, and inadequately housed.

Whereas relevant differences among older people arising from their gender and their ethnic minority status have been noted throughout this text, the next two chapters focus specifically on these factors because of their interactive effects with age and the resulting higher incidence of social problems. This chapter examines demographic changes and variations in socioeconomic status, health, and living arrangements among older ethnic minorities. The next chapter discusses similar variables among older women. In this sense, both older women and ethnic minorities are affected by changes in the environment that are not always congruent with their needs as they age. Each chapter begins by examining the relatively limited research on these groups, as compared with that on older white males, and concludes with a brief discussion of implications for the development of public policies and services for older ethnic minorities and women.

Defining Ethnicity

Ethnicity as discussed here involves three components: culture, social status, and support systems. These components influence the way people feel about themselves and how they interact with their environments, resulting in particular patterns of adjustment to the experience of aging. Thus, ethnicity may produce differing responses to aging, even among older Americans who share common experiences with poverty and discrimination. By identifying the culturally conditioned beliefs and values in an older person's heritage, we can gain a better understanding of that person's attitudes and behaviors in the face of their own aging. For example, many Japanese-American elderly emigrated from small farming villages where ancestor worship was practiced, reflecting the respect traditionally accorded older people. They have grown old in a country where youth is more highly valued than age, and thus may experience conflicts between the views they hold and those of their children.

Ethnicity may or may not encompass minority status, since there are older people in the United States who belong to white ethnic groups that are not necessarily "minorities," as defined by the U.S. Congress as federally protected groups (Holzberg, 1982). Gutmann's (1979) work on immigrants from eastern, central, and southern Europe demonstrates that white ethnics may preserve their traditional cultural practices and homogeneity, and remain essentially segregated within their own ethnic communities, but not necessarily experience prejudice, discrimination, or oppression.

WHO ARE THE ETHNIC MINORITY ELDERLY?

For purposes of this chapter, ethnic minority elderly includes older people belonging to groups whose language and/or physical and cultural characteristics make them visible and identifiable, who have experienced differential and unequal treatment, and who regard themselves as objects of collective discrimination by reason of their social class or race (Manuel, 1982; Wirth, 1945). Specifically, we examine the life conditions and adaptation to aging among people of color—Blacks, Hispanic-Americans (including Mexican-Americans/Chicanos, Puerto Ricans, Cubans, and Latin Americans), Native Americans, and Pacific-Asians (including Japanese, Chinese, Filipino, Korean, Guamanian, Samoan, other Pacific Islanders, and the newer immigrants from Southeast Asia).

Although our focus is on people of color who have experienced economic and racial discrimination, we also consider how ethnicity or cultural homogeneity influences the aging process. Hence, we use the term *ethnic minority elderly* throughout this book. Characteristics of *ethnic minorities* relevant to aging (Wirth, 1945; Moore, 1971a; Manuel, 1982) include:

- Each group has a special history.
- The special history has been accompanied by discrimination, resulting in fewer power resources.
- A subculture has formed, along with a social consciousness conducive to marital and social endogamy, or inbreeding.
- Coping structures have developed.

Based on its unique history, each ethnic minority population developed its own methods of coping with the inevitable conflicts between traditional and adopted ways of life, leading to both vulnerabilities and strengths in the ways they adjust to aging.

Ethnic minorities form a small percentage of the older U.S. population; approximately 89 percent of the population age 65 and over is white, 11 percent is nonwhite (U.S. Bureau of the Census, 1980). Within each ethnic minority group, older people form a smaller percentage of the total ethnic minority population, as compared to the percentage of people age 65 and over within the white population, as illustrated in Table 15–1. The different age distributions of these groups reflect variations in their fertility, morality, and immigration rates. A general trend is the growing presence of females in each of these ethnic minority populations, with older men more likely than older women to be married, and less

Group activities offer opportunities for interaction among ethnic minorities.

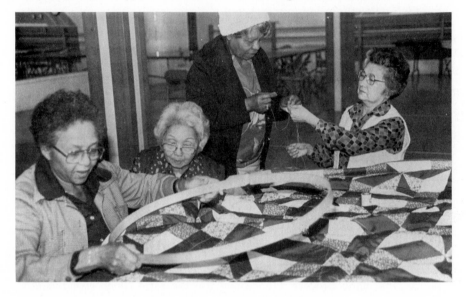

TABLE 15–1 Distribution of the Elderly Population

	% of Total Population, 65+	% of the Ethnic Minority Population, 65+	Median Age
Whites	89.8	12.2	31.3
Blacks	8.2	7.9	24.9
Asian-Americans	0.6	5.9	28.7
Native Americans	0.3	5.2	22.8
Hispanic-Americans	2.8*	4.9	23.2

Source: U.S. Bureau of the Census, 1980 Census of Population, Supplementary Reports, 1980.

*The sum of the specific percentages reported above will never round off to approximately 100 percent if a Hispanic percentage is included. The reason for this anomaly is that the U.S. Bureau of the Census does not treat the Hispanic category (which includes Mexicans, Venezuelans, and Latinos who self-designate themselves as being white) as one that is mutually exclusive from the racial categories. Thus, the Hispanic data are also included within each of the racial categories.

likely to be widowed or divorced—a pattern similar to that found among the older white population (Jackson, 1985).

Although small in size, ethnic minority populations are of increasing concern to gerontologists because of the disproportionately greater number of problem conditions they face, relative to whites. In addition, they are expected to increase at a proportionately higher rate than whites, as discussed in Chapter 1. For example, it has been predicted that the immigrant groups of the twentieth century—Hispanics, Asians, and Pacific Islanders—will redefine American culture in the twenty-first century (Torres-Gil, 1986). During that transition, an aging society will need to grapple with the cultural homogeneity of an elderly minority population and the cultural diversity of its younger minority populations, who will not form a significant portion of the older population until after the year 2015.

RESEARCH HISTORY

Ethnogerontology is the newest and perhaps most underdeveloped field of social gerontology (Jackson, 1985). It is the study of the causes, processes, and consequences of race, national origin, and culture on individual and population aging. A predominant concern has been the documentation of social inequities between dominant and minority aged.

From 1940 to 1970, when both scholarly and political concern with the elderly grew, little was written about the special circumstances of ethnic minority elderly. In 1956, Tally and Kaplan first raised the question: Are the Black aged doubly jeopardized relative to their white counterparts? That is, do lifetime factors of economic and racial discrimination make adjusting to old age more difficult for Blacks (and other minorities) than for whites? As a result of such double jeopardy, do ethnic minorities experience lower life satisfaction (Cuellar and Weeks, 1980)? The *double jeopardy* hypothesis also raises the policy question of whether ethnic minority status alone constitutes a sufficient basis for targeting special services and policies.

A second but related position asserts that patterns of racial stratification and inequalities have changed recently, and that Blacks' opportunities throughout their lives are related to their economic class position rather than to their minority group status. Social class rather than minority membership jeopardizes them (Wilson, 1978). Debates about double jeopardy, whether it exists and is related to socioeconomic status or to race per se have been central in research and policy discussions in ethnogerontology. More recently, however, ethnogerontologists have argued that double jeopardy should not be a central concept, because empirical tests of it have rarely produced useful information about age changes as opposed to age differences (Jackson, 1985). They suggest that double jeopardy may be time-bound, resulting largely from major social and political changes in the status of minorities, not from racial differences. The effects of ethnic minority group status on age changes in the later years thus remain an open question.

The counterargument to the double jeopardy hypothesis is that age is a leveler of differences in income and life expectancy (Dowd and Bengtson, 1978). As an illustration, racial differences in health and income that are typical in younger populations often narrow with age (Markides, 1983). In fact, after age 75, the probabilities of death for nonwhites actually fall approximately 10 percent below those for whites, due to a combination of genetic and socioenvironmental factors. After age 80, minority women and men, who are the hardiest of their race, can expect to outlive their nonminority counterparts. For instance, the death rate for Blacks age 85 and over is lower than for whites, although the rate of chronic illness is higher (Jackson, 1983). This is known as the *white/nonwhite mortality crossover*, and is cited as an indicator that nonwhite elderly do not face a double jeopardy in terms of health (Manton, 1982). However, it has been suggested that the apparent racial crossover is due to enumerative errors, not to health differences (Manton, 1982). To date, the relative health status of whites and nonwhites is not well understood, and even the most basic age patterns of mortality risks are debated (Manton, 1982: Jackson, 1985). The need for more research on both the double jeopardy hypothesis and the apparent racial crossover in life expectancy is reflected in much of the literature on the ethnic minority elderly. What is conclusive is that tremendous variation occurs both across and within ethnic minority categories (Dowd and Bengtson, 1978).

The year 1971 marked a turning point in the recognition of the ethnic minority elderly as a special area of study within gerontology. In that year, the National Caucus on the Black Aged was formed (later becoming the National Center and Caucus of the Black Aged), and a session on "Aging and the Aged Black" was held at the White House Conference on Aging. This conference was especially important from a policy perspective, because reports showed that twice as many of the ethnic minority elderly live below the poverty level relative to white elderly. Therefore, the session highlighted the need for income and health care supports. Since 1971, the National Association for Spanish-speaking Elderly, the National Indian Council on Aging, and the National Pacific/Asian Resource Center on Aging have been established. The National Center and Caucus on the Black Aged is the most influential minority organization. Each of these associations functions as an advocacy group, and as a research and academic center.

The census has been the primary source of information for these organizations involved in planning services for ethnic minority elderly. Census data, however, are criticized for undercounting minority subgroups, misclassifying individuals, or merging data about various nonwhite groups (Rogers and Gallion, 1978; Jackson, 1980; 1985). For example, the census data have often grouped people by race as "white," "black" or "other."

Despite the recent growth and diversity of research on ethnic minority elderly, there are few definitive conclusions about this segment of society. It is a segment made up of many subgroups exhibiting a diversity of cultural patterns. Consequently, few generalizations can be made that are valid for this population as a whole. We turn next to a brief review of the life conditions of each of the four major ethnic minority groups.

Black Elderly

Although the Black older population is growing at a faster rate than either the general Black population or the white elderly population, the percentage of elderly among the Black population is still smaller than among its nonminority counterpart. That is, 7.9 percent of the Black population is over 65 years of age, compared to 12.2 percent of the white population. The young outnumber the old in the Black population, due primarily to the higher fertility of Black women and Blacks' higher mortality at midlife. The median age of Blacks, 24.9 years, is almost seven years younger than the median age for whites (U.S. Bureau of the Census, 1980). In 1980, the life expectancy for Black men and women was 65.5 and 74.5 years, respectively, compared with the life expectancy of 70.3 years for white men and 76.8 years for white women (U.S. Senate Special Committee on Aging, 1986). The leading causes of death among Blacks are hypertension, heart disease, and diabetes. On the other hand, the Black population is expected to increase by 45.6 percent by 2020. This will raise the older proportion of the total Black population from less than 8 percent to 9.3 percent by the year 2020 (Manuel and Reid, 1982).

The ratio of Black men to Black women age 65 and over is 68.3 males for every 100 females, similar to the ratio of 67.2 males for every 100 females among the nonminority population (U.S. Department of Health and Human Services, 1980). The slight relative favorability for males among Blacks compared to whites may be related to the "crossover effect" mentioned earlier, where the mortality differentials between the oldest-old Black men and women are less pronounced than among whites (Jackson, 1982). The Black male aged 85 and over is more "advantaged" in terms of health than his white counterpart, relative to the oldest-old Black females. Despite this relative advantage, women age 80 and over are the most rapidly growing group of Black elderly, and they have the longest average remaining lifetime. On the other hand, older Black males have a greater probability of being widowed and less chance of being married than their white counterparts (U.S. Department of Health and Human Services, 1980).

Although Blacks form only about 8 percent of the population age 65 and over, they represented nearly 32 percent of the low-income elderly in 1984 (U.S. Senate Special Committee on Aging, 1986). Approximately 36 percent of Black families headed by persons age 65 and over in 1984 were estimated to be below the poverty line, three times the proportion of white families who were poor. The incidence of poverty increases dramatically among households composed of unrelated Black individuals, especially females, age 65 and over (Jackson, 1985). Differences in education do not explain this gap. For example, poverty is almost as high among Black women who attended high school as among those with less than six years of schooling (Jackson, 1985). This gap in income level between white and Black elderly has not changed substantially in the past 10 years. The short-term trend, however, is toward a growing gap, as public income supports (e.g., Supplemental Security Income) are reduced. In addition, the proportion of older Black female-headed families in poverty has been increasing.

As noted in Chapter 12, the primary reason for the lower socioeconomic status of older Blacks is their pattern of limited employment opportunities throughout their lives and their concentration in low-paying, sporadic jobs, often not covered by Social Security prior to the 1950s. This reduces not only their lifetime earnings, but also their Social Security and pension benefits. In 1980, approximately 60 percent of Black men and 90 percent of Black women received only the minimum Social Security benefits (Watson, 1983). In addition, older Blacks are less likely to receive pension income than are whites. Accordingly, more Black than white elderly rely on Supplemental Security Income (SSI). In 1977, for example, the proportion of Black families with heads 65 years old or over receiving SSI was four times greater than the corresponding percentage of white families. Some advocates have argued that Blacks should be eligible for Social Security earlier than whites because of their lifetime experiences with racism and their resultant lower life expectancy (Jackson, 1977).

The incidence of chronic diseases has been estimated to be twice as high among Blacks as among whites, and Blacks more often perceive themselves as being in poor health than do their white counterparts (Manual and Reid, 1982). For example, older Blacks experience hypertension more frequently than their white peers. They also experience more days of functional disability (i.e., substantially reduced daily activities) and bed disability (i.e., being confined to bed for at least half of the day) and at earlier ages than whites. Proportionately more Blacks are completely incapacitated and unable to carry on any major activity (e.g., paid employment, keeping house), although still residing in community-based households (Soldo and DaVita, 1977).

The disproportionate concentration of Black elderly at the lower end of the socioeconomic scale appears to explain much of the variance in their health status and utilization of health care services. As discussed in Chapter 6, numerous studies have found that the lower an individual's socioeconomic status, the higher the prevalence of disease and the age-specific death rate (Cantor and Meyer, 1974; Dowd and Bengtson, 1978; Shanas and Maddox, 1985). As noted earlier, mortality is generally higher among Blacks than among whites, except for those age 80 and over, at which point the mortality rate of Blacks becomes lower.

Despite their poor economic and health conditions, many elderly Blacks appear to have a greater sense of satisfaction in their lives than do their white counterparts, who have better living conditions (Bild and Havighurst, 1976). This difference has been explained in terms of the spiritual orientation of many Black people and the support of their extended families. Patterns of help-seeking may also underlie Black elderly's relatively high morale. Older Blacks tend to draw from a more varied pool of informal helpers and are more likely to use them interchangeably than their white counterparts (Gibson, 1986). Another surprising difference is that Blacks are more likely than whites to say that they expect to have long lives, even though they define themselves as old at an earlier chronological age than whites (Reynolds and Kalish, 1974; Bengtson, Kasschau and Ragan, 1977).

The extent to which elderly Blacks are at the center of an extended family network has been the focus of considerable research (Mitchell and Register, 1984; Taylor, 1985). Almost 50 percent of Black women live alone, a higher proportion than their white counterparts. One reason for this is that widowhood is more prevalent among older Blacks and is more likely to have occurred at an earlier age (Jackson, 1983). Although most older Blacks do not live in extended families, approximately 20 percent of them, compared to 12 percent of their white counterparts, live with some family member other than their spouse. Among older Black women aged 65 to 74, 19 percent have family living with them in *their* homes, compared to 7.4 percent of white women (Manuel and Reid, 1982). Most often, these are three-generation households, with older Black women providing financial assistance and care for grandchildren, as well as children of other family members and friends (Jackson, 1980; Shimkin, Shimkin and Frate, 1978). Although Blacks are more likely to receive help from children and grandchildren, and to take children into their homes, giving help to children and grandchildren is a function of age, marital and socioeconomic status, and health, not just of race (Mitchell and Register, 1984). In addition, as mentioned in Chapter 10, these intergenerational housing arrangements may be overcrowded and develop out of economic necessity rather than choice, suggesting that the close, loving Black extended family may be a myth (Jackson, 1977). Similar to whites, however, adult children remain a primary source of assistance and an integral part of the support networks of elderly Blacks (Taylor, 1985).

In 1980, only 3 percent of Blacks age 65 and older were institutionalized (U.S. Bureau of the Census, 1980). However, these statistics may reflect the lack of nursing homes in Black communities, inadequate income to pay for private nursing home care, and the greater probability that an older Black person, dependent upon Medicaid, has fewer institutional options (Morrison, 1983). Lower rates of nursing home placement may also be due to present or historical acts of racism by medical providers and nursing home staff.

Hispanic-American Elderly

Following Blacks, Hispanic-Americans are the largest ethnic minority population, with over 85 percent concentrated in metropolitan areas. They are also the fastest-growing population group in the United States (Torres-Gil, 1986). As stated earlier, Hispanic-Americans include many groups, each with its own distinct national/cultural heritage: Puerto Ricans, Cubans, Central or South Americans, Mexicans, and the native Mexican-American, or Chicano population whose history in the United States predates settlement by English-speaking groups. Although bonded by a common language, these groups differ substantially in terms of geographic concentration, income, and education. Mexican-Americans are the largest but poorest group, constituting 60 percent of the Hispanic population and concentrated in five, primarily rural, southwestern states. The largest populations of Puerto Ricans and Cubans are in New York City, New Jersey, and Florida. However, those patterns are changing as more Hispanics move to the Midwest.

Compared to whites and to other ethnic minorities, the Spanish-speaking population is a youthful group, with a median age of 23.2 years, seven years younger than the norm in the United States (Lacayo, 1984). Less than 5 percent of this population is 65 years of age and over, a figure which has been stable over the past decade. A number of factors underlie the relative youthfulness of the Hispanic-American population. One variable is its lower average life expectancy. The most important contributing factor, however, is the generally high fertility rate. The number of children born and the average family size exceed the national average. Immigration and repatriation patterns are secondary factors, with the youngest (and often poorest) people most likely to move to a new country, and some middle-aged and older Mexicans moving back to Mexico (Moore, 1971b; Markides and Martin, 1983; Torres-Gil, 1986). Despite its current relative youthfulness, the Hispanic population has experienced the greatest rate of increase in median age of all ethnic groups from 1960 to 1980. This suggests that the percentage of older Hispanic-Americans may rise steeply in the future, as younger cohorts reach old age (Torres-Gil, 1986). Nevertheless, given the high fertility rate, the proportion of elderly among Hispanic-Americans will remain well below that of the total U.S. population.

Gender patterns of Hispanic-Americans are similar to those of other groups of elderly. Women live longer and outnumber men, more often remaining widowed and living alone than men do. In fact, older Hispanic-American men marry or remarry more often than men in other ethnic minority groups; 83 percent of older Hispanic-American males are married, but only 33 percent of older Hispanic women live with a spouse (Lacayo, 1984).

Two sociocultural factors are significant in considering the economic and health status of older Hispanic-Americans. More than any other ethnic minority group, they have retained their native language, partially because of geographic proximity to their home country, combined with the availability of mass communication systems (Torres-Gil, 1986). Although serving to preserve their cultural identity, their inability to speak English has been a major barrier to their education, employment, and utilization of social and health services. Another barrier has been encountered by those who entered the country illegally and thus have been unable to apply for Social Security, Medicare, or Medicaid. This legal barrier to eligibility, however, has recently been altered by changes in immigration laws for those who entered prior to 1982. On the other hand, the peak arrival of Latin Americans has taken place in the 1980s; immigrants are arriving at a time when the United States is undergoing major economic and political changes and is less tolerant toward noncitizens. All these factors may partially explain why such large numbers of Hispanic elderly have minimal education and work in unskilled, low-paying jobs with few benefits, particularly retirement pension benefits (Torres-Gil, 1986). Hispanic-Americans are the most educationally deprived group in our society, with 45 percent of their elderly having less than five years of school, and 66 percent less than eight years (Lacayo, 1980). In addition, they are the least likely of any older minority group members to be in the paid workforce. Many aged 55 and over, for example, have had to leave the paid workforce because of poor health.

The foregoing employment and educational conditions contribute to the high rate of poverty among older Hispanic Americans. In 1984, up to 21.5 percent were estimated to live below the poverty level (of $4,979 for an individual), compared to 10.7 percent for older whites; up to 42 percent hovered just above the "near poverty" threshold (U.S. Bureau of the Census, 1984). The poverty rate for older Hispanics is about twice the level for older non-Hispanics. Despite their pressing economic needs, however, these elderly appear to underutilize public social services. For example, in a 1980 study in San Diego, 92 percent of the Hispanic respondents met the criterion for SSI, but only 42 percent received SSI assistance. Only 62 percent of the Hispanic elderly in one study were aware of more than two social services available to them (Lacayo, 1980). This gap between eligibility and receipt of benefits has been partially attributed to service providers' cultural and linguistic insensitivity (Cuellar and Weeks, 1980).

The poverty of Hispanic-Americans is undoubtedly a major factor in their generally poor health, as illustrated by a survey of low-income Hispanics in Los Angeles where 30 percent had major health problems (Young, 1982). Physiological aging tends to precede chronological aging, with those in their late forties experiencing health disabilities typical of 65-year-old whites. Arthritis, high blood pressure, circulatory disorders, diabetes, cataracts, glaucoma, and heart disease have been identified as the most common health problems (Lacayo, 1984; Asociacion Nacional Pro Personas Mayores, 1980). On two indicators of health status—days of restricted activity and days of bed disability per person per year—Hispanic-Americans are in an intermediate position between Caucasian and Black elderly (Markides and Martin, 1983). In addition, older Hispanics use hospitals less frequently than other older people, and have the highest unattended need for dental care (Lacayo, 1984). Social and cultural barriers to health care, such as mistrust of white medical providers, and political factors, such as less health insurance coverage and greater dissatisfaction with services, may partially underlie their low utilization of services (Torres-Gil, 1976; Andersen, 1981). About 3 percent are in nursing homes, with 10 percent of those over age 85 institutionalized, compared to 23 percent of oldest-old whites (U.S. Bureau of the Census, 1980).

In terms of life expectancy, Hispanics appear to be in an intermediate position between whites and Blacks. For example, a study conducted in San Antonio, Texas, showed life expectancies at birth of 66.9 years and 74.1 years for Hispanic males and females, respectively (Bradshaw and Fonner, 1979).

Historically, the extended family has been a major support to older Hispanics, especially in rural areas. A study of informal support networks found that Hispanic elderly had consistently higher levels of interaction and a greater potential for support from children than either white or Black elderly, even controlling for gender, social class, and levels of functional ability (Cantor, 1979). Approximately 9.7 percent of Hispanic elderly live in extended families, 60 percent with spouses, and 30 percent alone (U.S. Bureau of the Census, 1980). There is some evidence that Hispanics, more than other ethnic minority groups, live with friends and neighbors (Jaco, 1957; Rubel, 1966). Those who live alone are generally inadequately housed, with the incidence of substandard housing two to three times greater among Hispanics than among whites (Bell and Zellman, 1976). In contrast to early research that emphasized the supportive qualities of the Hispanic family, more recent studies have suggested that intergenerational sharing in such families—as among Blacks—is a social myth or stereotype (Maldonado, 1980). Maldonado (1980), in particular, has been critical of the concept that the extended family confers high status on the elderly. He maintains that the caring extended family no longer fits the reality of most elderly Hispanics, and is used to justify the lack of services to Hispanic communities. With the urbanization of the Hispanic population, younger Hispanics are increasingly unable to support an extended family, with a commensurate increase in tension between generations (Maldonado, 1980). Jackson (1980) attempts to resolve the contradictory evidence on family relations by concluding that the strength of family ties for the elderly within each minority group represents a continuum ranging from nonexistent to extremely strong; one cannot categorize one ethnic group as having uniformly stronger ties than another.

Native American Elderly

Except for very general trends, less systematic data are available for Native Americans than for the other ethnic minority groups discussed thus far. The two federal agencies responsible for collecting data, the Bureau of Indian Affairs and the Census Bureau, frequently disagree on their estimates, making it difficult to generalize about Native American elderly. An additional complication in generalizing findings is that this population includes Indians, Eskimos, and Aleuts; there are over 400 different tribal groups, which speak over 200 distinct languages (National Indian Council on Aging, 1984).

As is the case with other ethnic minorities, the Native American population is younger than the white population. With a median age of 22.8 years, only 5.2 percent of this population is 65 years of age and older (U.S. Bureau of the Census, 1980). The current life expectancy at birth is 65 years, approximately seven years less than for the white population, and it tends to be even lower in nonreservation areas (U.S. Bureau of the Census, 1980; Butler and Lewis, 1982). With a sex ratio of approximately 64.5 men to every 100 women age 65 and over, more than 75 percent of Native American men, but less than 50 percent of their female counterparts, are married (National Indian Council on Aging, 1984).

The first research effort to document the conditions faced by older Native

Americans nationwide was completed by the National Indian Council on Aging in 1980. Compared with a similar survey of all persons aged 60 and over in Cleveland, Ohio, older Native Americans were found to be poorer, less skilled, and more often seeking work; 12 percent had no formal education, and only 22 percent graduated from high school. The average income of older Native Americans is approximately 75 percent that of all other elderly groups (National Indian Council on Aging, 1984).

Similar to other ethnic minority populations, the poverty of older Native Americans tends to reflect lifelong patterns of unemployment, employment in jobs not covered by Social Security, especially those on reservations, and poor working conditions. The median income for this group is barely above the poverty threshold; less than 2 percent earn incomes in excess of $15,000 annually. In some areas, as many as 75 percent of all Native Americans are unemployed, with 33 percent having incomes below federal poverty levels, compared with less than 13 percent of whites (Williams, 1980; U.S. Bureau of the Census, 1984; Murdock and Schwartz, 1978). Only 40 percent of Indians over age 60 receive Social Security, a lower rate than among other ethnic minority groups (Raisz, 1986). By age 45, incomes have usually peaked among male Native Americans, and decline thereafter. Native American women are generally less educated than the men, and seldom earn even half the income of the men, putting them in a severely disadvantaged position. Another factor negatively affecting the socioeconomic and living conditions of Native American women is that over 55 percent of those age 60 and over are widowed. High unemployment and low income levels tend to result in the necessity of intergenerational living arrangements among the Native American elderly, with nearly 66 percent of them supporting other family members with their inadequate incomes (National Indian Council on Aging, 1984). Without government-sponsored social and health services, many older Native Americans could not survive.

Older Native Americans have a higher incidence of accidents, tuberculosis, diabetes, liver and kidney disease, influenza, pneumonia, hearing and sight impairments, and problems stemming from obesity, gall bladder, or arthritic ailments than whites (National Indian Council on Aging, 1984). Although liver and kidney problems often result from lifelong problems with drinking, alcoholism generally takes its toll before old age (Rhoades, Marshall, Attneave, Bjork, and Beiser, 1980). Many Indian elderly prefer traditional health care from their own tribal medicine people and resist using non-Indian medical resources. The Indian Health Service provides health care to those on reservations, but very few urban elderly seek out such care, generally because of the cost, transportation difficulties, or professionals' lack of sensitivity to Indians' ritual folk healing or cultural definitions of disease. Only 3 percent of the 200 reservations have nursing homes. Accordingly, among those over 85 years of age, only 13 percent are in nursing homes, compared to 23 percent of whites (U.S. Bureau of the Census, 1980).

Native Americans perceive their physical and mental health to be poorer than white elderly do, and some studies have documented a higher incidence of alcoholism and suicide (National Indian Council on Aging, 1984). Research findings regarding the mental health of older Native Americans are mixed, with some studies suggesting that those who maintain a tribal identity experience less stress than their white counterparts. As they grow older, they appear to shift to a more passive relationship with their world, accepting age-related changes as a natural part of life (Goldstine and Gutmann, 1972). This movement from active mastery to passive accommodative styles is consistent with Gutmann's findings for diverse cultures, described in Chapter 8. It is also an adaptation to the decreasing P-E congruence experienced by many ethnic minorities as they age. Native Americans' low utilization of mental health services is not necessarily a reflection of fewer mental health problems, but may represent greater barriers to treatment (Markides, 1986).

A factor that often creates adjustment problems is the degree to which older Native Americans' lives are dictated by government bureaucratic policies. The Bureau of Indian Affairs largely determines daily practices on the reservations. Although the Bureau's regulations are intended to ensure basic support, they have been criticized for their inflexibility and for denying traditional cultural values. As an example, land-grazing privileges were historically extended to all tribal members for as long as they desired; today, older Indians must transfer their grazing rights to their heirs before they qualify for supplemental financial assistance. Although extra income may be welcome, the program serves to deprive the old of their traditional position within the tribal structure (Jeffries, 1972). The history of older Native Americans and their relationship with the federal bureaucracy must be considered in efforts to develop culturally appropriate social and health services.

Historical factors also strongly influence the family relationships of Native Americans. Historically, the old were accorded respect and fulfilled specified useful tribal roles, including that of the "wise elder" who instructs the young and assists with child care, especially for foster children and grandchildren (National Indian Council on Aging, 1984). They also maintained responsibility for remembering and relating tribal philosophies, myths, and traditions, and served as religious and political advisors to tribal leaders. These relationships have changed, however, with the restructuring of Native American life by the Bureau of Indian Affairs and by the increasing urbanization of native populations.

Despite these changes, many Native American elderly, particularly in rural settings, continue to live in an extended family. Approximately 60 percent of all Native American households live with family members (e.g., spouse, children, grandchildren, and foster children). Some 25 percent of Indian elderly care for at least one grandchild, and 67 percent live within five miles of relatives (National Indian Council on Aging, 1984). This pattern of helping family members, combined with deep mistrust of governmental programs, underlies Native Americans' comparatively low utilization of social and health services.

Pacific-Asian Elderly

Pacific-Asian elderly are perhaps more diverse than any other ethnic minority, given the varied historical and cultural experiences of the Japanese, Filipino, Chinese, and other more recent refugees. They include people aged 65 and over who have immigrated from an Asian country (Asian-Americans, as classified by the Bureau of Census) and those who became Americans by virtue of territorial expansion and political annexation (Pacific Islanders). Among the Asian-Americans are the Burmese, Cambodians, Chinese, East Indians, Indonesians, Japanese, Koreans, Laotians, Malayans, Filipinos, Thais, and Vietnamese. The Pacific Islanders include the Fijians, Guamanians, Hawaiians, Micronesians, Samoans, and Tongans. At minimum, there are 18 Pacific Island and Asian-American groups, each having its own distinct language and culture. Therefore, it is necessary to avoid assuming that all Pacific-Asian elderly have similar socioeconomic characteristics, language, culture, or immigration histories. Almost 60 percent of Pacific-Asian Americans reside in three western states—California, Hawaii, and Washington.

Slightly over 5.9 percent of the Pacific-Asian population is 65 years of age and over, with the total Asian population in the United States increasing rapidly since the 1970s, due to the 1965 repeal of quotas based on race and nationality (U.S. Bureau of the Census, 1980). The percent of the total population, age 65 and older, within specific groups among the Asian-American population is reported in Table 15–2.

In contrast to other ethnic minority groups and to the white elderly, men living alone constitute a larger percentage of the older Pacific-Asian population. This reflects the continuing influence of disproportionate male immigration in the early part of the century and past restrictions on female immigration rather than a higher life expectancy for men among Pacific-Asians. The overall sex ratio of Pacific-Asian elderly was 96 males to 100 females in 1980, whereas the ratio was 68 males to 100 females in the general elderly population (Kii, 1984). In contrast to other subgroups of elderly, the ratio of men to women *increases* with age,

TABLE 15–2 Distribution of the Older Pacific-Asian Population

	% of the Population, 65+
Chinese	6.2
Hawaiian	4.0
Japanese	8.0
Korean	3.3
Filipino	6.3

Source: U.S. Bureau of the Census, 1980 Census of Population, Supplementary Reports, 1980.

particularly for Filipino and Chinese elderly. These sex ratios are reflected in current patterns of living arrangements and marriage. For example, a high proportion of elderly Filipino men have remained single: 28.1 percent compared to 7.5 percent for men in the total older population in 1970. In 1970, over 26 percent of Chinese elderly men lived alone, in contrast to 16 percent for the general older population (Pacific-Asian Elderly Research Project, 1978).

Compared to the national average, Pacific-Asian groups show higher proportions of extended family arrangements. Some 18 percent of all Chinese families, 16 percent of Japanese families, and 23 percent of Filipino families are extended (Ignacio, 1976), in contrast to the national average of 12 percent in 1970. The majority of Pacific-Asian elderly, however, live by themselves or with a spouse, not with children. Some 2 percent over 65 years, and 10 percent over age 85 are in nursing homes. One of the major reasons for a relative decline in intergenerational living arrangements is acculturation of the elderly's offspring into the larger society. For example, many Chinese elderly prefer to remain in their ethnic communities rather than live with children who have moved to the suburbs or across the country. Both geographic distance and language barriers can isolate older Pacific-Asians from their children and grandchildren.

The Pacific-Asian elderly who were born in this country around the turn of the century or who came to the United States during the early 1900s share the experience of discrimination and isolation. Laws discriminating against Asians are numerous, ranging from the Chinese Exclusion Act of 1882, the Japanese Alien Land Law of 1913, the Executive Order of 1942 for the internment of 110,000 persons of Japanese ancestry, denial of citizenship to first-generation Asians in 1922, the anti-miscegenation statute of 1935, and more recently, Public Law 95-507, excluding Asians as a protected minority under the definition of "socially and economically disadvantaged" (U.S. Commission on Civil Rights, 1979). Such legislation has contributed to feelings of mistrust, powerlessness, and fear of government among many Pacific-Asian elderly.

The elderly Asians who immigrated prior to 1924 generally differ substantially in their occupational and educational background from those who came later. As a result of denial of property rights and discrimination against them for public jobs, most Asian elderly who immigrated in the early part of the century are less educated and more economically deprived than many of their white counterparts. Older Pacific-Asians have, on the average, 6 years of school, with the exception of the Japanese, who average 8.5 years. Many still speak only their native language. For example, only 1.4 percent of the foreign-born Chinese elderly and less than 1 percent of the Japanese elderly speak English (Kim, 1983). Their social worlds, therefore, have been limited to ethnic enclaves, where they have developed small retail and service businesses and entertainment that cater to their own ethnic groups. While representing segregation from the general society, these ethnic enclaves are a center for leisure activities and for the delivery of services to Pacific-

Asian elderly. These functions served by the closely knit community, however, will probably not exist for future generations of Pacific-Asians, who have been more geographically and socially mobile.

Although Japanese-American elderly tend to be economically better off than other ethnic minority groups, 14 percent of Pacific-Asian elderly live below the poverty level (U.S. Bureau of the Census, 1980). The poverty figures are even higher among female heads of households over age 75, ranging from 31.1 percent to 40.4 percent (Kim, 1983). Many older Chinese and Filipinos have experienced a lifetime of low-paying jobs, often in self-employment, garment factories, service or farming work not covered by Social Security or other pensions. Filipino males, in particular, were concentrated in live-in domestic, migrant agricultural, or other unsettled work, often living in homogeneous male camps and failing both to gain an insured work history and to develop close ties with family and neighborhood.

As is the case with elderly Hispanics, many older Pacific-Asians qualify for public financial supports, such as Supplemental Security Income, but do not apply. After years of living under discrimination and fear of deportation, they resist seeking help from a government bureaucracy. Their reluctance to seek nonfamilial assistance is also influenced by cultural and linguistic traditions emphasizing personal status and self-restraint. When unsure of others' social status, some older Pacific-Asians avoid interaction with them. In the past, they turned to the benevolent societies and clubs in their tightly knit communities, as well as to their families. Yet many are caught between their cultural traditions of group and familial honor, and the values of their adopted culture which stress independence and self-sufficiency, making them loath to turn to others for support.

Traditional values also underlie this population's comparative underutilization of Medicare and Medicaid, and their reliance on non-Western medicine or family and friends to assist them with their health problems. It has been estimated that 33 percent of Pacific-Asian elderly have never seen a doctor or a dentist (Kim, 1983). What is unclear is whether this low utilization of health services is due to their having fewer chronic diseases than their majority group peers, or to their reluctance to use formal Western health services. Some studies point to a sense of shame, particularly among the Japanese-American elderly, about the use of public services as an indicator of dependency and inability to care for oneself (Ishizuka, 1978). When bilingual and bicultural personnel are used within service programs, some of this resistance to the use of services has been overcome (Pacific-Asian Elderly Research Project, 1978; Yip, 1981). Another barrier has been the myth held by some service providers that Pacific-Asian elderly do not have problems and "take care of their own."

Health statistics for Pacific-Asian elderly are very limited. In Hawaii and California, life expectancies for older Japanese and Chinese are longer than those for the white elderly population age 65 and over (Kii, 1984). Other studies have found poor health to be a major problem among the Chinese elderly (Carp and

Kataoka, 1976; Lyman, 1976). Health status and behaviors are areas requiring additional comparative research.

The impact of the larger environment on physical well-being is illustrated by the fact that the incidence of cardiovascular disease among Japanese-Americans approximates that found in the general population of the United States rather than that found in their country of origin (Kim, 1983). The suicide rate among Chinese elderly is three times as high as among their white peers; this has been attributed to the incongruities between the Chinese elderly's values and the reality of their lives in an alien culture (Lyman, 1976). Older Japanese males in California have been found to be hospitalized for schizophrenia more frequently than their white counterparts. However, since cultural factors influence the diagnosis of mental health problems (Hendricks and Hendricks, 1981), this finding may not necessarily reflect the mental health status of this population.

Implications for Service Delivery

Because it is important that gerontologists develop services responsive to ethnic minority elderly, we will briefly consider the implications of sociocultural factors for the delivery of social and health services. Several studies point to under-utilization of services by ethnic minority elderly and by the poor in locations with concentrations of ethnic minorities (Cueller, 1980; Gutmann, 1980). For example, Medicaid is not fully used by potentially eligible minority elderly. Among the older Japanese in San Diego, slightly more than 50 percent were familiar with Medi-Cal (the term for Medicaid in California), but only 7 percent used it (Ishizuka, 1978). Some 68 percent of rural Native American elderly were aware of Medi-Cal, but only 17 percent utilized it (National Indian Council on Aging). Underutilization of Medicaid has been attributed to lack of knowledge about the program, difficulties in applying, and an aversion to accepting publicly funded benefits. Other barriers to service utilization include:

- Nonminority staff who are not bilingual, who are insensitive to ethnic differences, and who serve meals that conflict with customary dietary preferences
- Lack of transportation to services
- Ethnic minority elderly's fear of doctors and hospitals, which may be related to present or historical acts of racism by medical providers
- Lack of faith in the efficacy of health and social service professionals

Pacific-Asian elderly, followed by Hispanic-Americans, tend to be least knowledgeable about social services (Ishizuka, 1978).

Although some service providers have rationalized that the ethnic minority elderly do not utilize formal services because they have their families' assistance, underutilization of services cannot be explained in terms of strong family support. In fact, a study of Black elderly found that those who received aid from their families were also those who needed and used the greatest number of social services, which suggests their need for a variety of formal and informal supports (Mindel and Wright, 1982).

The implication for practice is not whether ethnic minority elderly need services, but rather how services can be designed to take account of inter- and intracultural and geographic differences. From this perspective, *preferential* consideration is needed to reduce social inequities between the elderly of dominant and minority groups, along with *differential* consideration to take account of the diversity of needs and to increase the participation of various ethnic minority groups (McCaslin and Calvert, 1975). According to several researchers (Cuellar, 1980; Moriwaki, 1981; Colen and Soto, 1979; Cuellar and Weeks, 1980; Colen, 1983; National Pacific-Asian Resource Center on Aging, 1981), services are most likely to be used by ethnic minority elderly under the following conditions:

1. Services should be located in the ethnic minority community, easily accessible, near complementary supports, and transportation should be provided.

2. Services should adhere to the cultural integrity of the ethnic minority group's lifestyle; for example, nutrition programs should include appropriate ethnic foods.

3. The organizational climate should be informal and personalized.

4. Staff should include bilingual and/or indigenous workers, who are culturally sensitive and who use personalized outreach methods to establish trust and rapport.

5. Ethnic minorities should be involved in both the planning and the delivery of services.

6. Services should be advertised in ways to reach ethnic minorities, such as through minority-oriented television and radio programs and newspapers, and announcements made through churches, neighborhood organizations, and civic and social clubs.

The assumptions underlying such strategies are that the needs of ethnic minority elderly are best understood by members of their own groups, that these elderly should be treated as distinct populations, and that ethnic minorities should concentrate on the welfare of their own elderly, rather than on the well-being of older people in general. These assumptions have led to demands by advocates for the minority aged that separate indigenous services be developed, that research and training programs give special attention to ethnic minorities, that ethnic minority practitioners be employed as service providers, and that federal regulations for aging programs include minority-specific statutes. These demands have been met in many communities, such as in Seattle with a special Asian Health Program that has both community-based and nursing home care, and in San Francisco with the On Lok program that provides comprehensive care for older Chinese.

Recently, however, the premises and strategies used by these minority advocates have been challenged (Torres-Gil, 1982). The extent to which ethnic minority professionals reflect the needs of their older members has been questioned, as well as whether ethnic minority issues are overemphasized. Critics of separate strategies advocate that ethnic minorities become involved in larger issues that affect all older persons, and that programs should be developed on the basis of need, regardless of ethnic minority status (Lambrinos and Torres-Gil, 1980; Torres-Gil, 1982). This argument is supported by data that show the increased mobility and economic independence of younger minorities and their consequent upward and outward movement from formerly insulated ethnic communities. As younger members of ethnic minority groups move into the mainstream culture, the need for preferential services is assumed to decrease.

Others would argue, however, that even greater attention needs to be given to ethnic minorities in a period of growing competition for scarce resources. Two recent policy directions, decentralization and targeting services to the old-old, may, in fact, serve to exclude older members of minorities, who are less able to influence decentralized decision making and less likely to reach advanced age. The persistent high unemployment among nonwhites, which will perpetuate major gaps in earnings, Social Security, and pension coverage in old age, suggests that strategies targeted to ethnic minority elderly will continue to be necessary in the near future. During the current period of scarce resources, advocacy efforts are required to sustain the economic and social position of both minority and nonminority aged, suggesting the importance of collaborative efforts to ensure that low-income white and ethnic minority elderly do not fall below the presumed "safety net" of services. In addition, more consideration needs to be given to improving the circumstance under which younger ethnic minorities will age, especially employment conditions, so that they will be better off when old. Such a perspective recognizes the need for cross-generational approaches to addressing environmental inequities.

Summary and Implications

Although age is sometimes called the great equalizer, today's elderly are a highly diverse group. As we have seen throughout this book, differences in income, health, and social supports significantly affect the elderly's quality of life. An important source of this diversity is ethnic minority status. Ethnogerontology, or the study of the causes, processes, and consequences of race, national origin, and culture on individual and population aging, is the newest field of gerontology. One of the earliest debates in that field continues: whether ethnic minorities experience double jeopardy because of their race or whether age is a leveler of differences in income and life expectancy.

This chapter has reviewed the life situations of Blacks, Hispanic Americans, Native Americans, and Pacific-Asian elderly. Although there are variations among these groups, several common themes also emerge. For most ethnic minority elderly, their resources and status reflect social and economic discrimination experienced earlier in life. Many, especially those who migrated to the United States, experience cultural and language differences as well. They face shorter life expectancy and increased risks of poverty, malnutrition, substandard housing, and poor health. Social and health care assistance is of particular concern to ethnic minority elderly. Cultural and language difficulties, physical isolation, and lower income, along with problems of service accessibility, underlie their underutilization of health and social services. Efforts must continue to modify such services to be more responsive to the particular needs of ethnic minority elderly.

In recent years, the older population has been growing faster among ethnic minorities than among whites—a trend that is expected to continue. Still, white elderly outnumber their ethnic minority peers. The status of ethnic minority elderly is not likely to improve greatly in the immediate future. The factors that largely determine the older population's quality of life—education, employment, income, and health—will not vary considerably among the ethnic minority population now approaching retirement age. This trend suggests the importance of targeting services to meet the needs of ethnic minority elderly, although some minority aging advocates maintain that policies and programs should be directed toward improving the status of all older people. Efforts to increase opportunities for education and employment among younger minorities will be necessary to assure that the next generation will enjoy a higher quality of life than their predecessors.

References

American Indian elderly: A national profile. Albuquerque, N.M.: National Indian Council on Aging, 1981.

Andersen, R. Access to medical care among the Hispanic population of the southwestern United States. *Journal of Health and Social Behavior,* 1981, 22, 78–79.

Asociacion Nacional Pro Personas Mayores (ANPPM). A national study to assess the service needs of the Hispanic elderly. Los Angeles: Asociacion Nacional Pro Personas Mayores, 1980.

Beard, V. Health status of a successful Black aged population related to life satisfaction and self-concept. In W. Watson and Associates (Eds.), *Health in the Black aged.* Washington, D.C.: National Center on Black Aged, 1977.

Bell, D., and Zellman, G. *Issues in service delivery to ethnic elderly.* Santa Monica, Calif.: Rand Corp., 1976.

Bengtson, V., Kasschau, P., and Ragan, P. The impact of social structure on aging individuals. In J. Birren and K. W. Schaie, (Eds.), *Handbook of the psychology of aging.* New York: Van Nostrand Reinhold, 1977.

Bild, B., and Havighurst, R. The life of the elderly in large cities. *The Gerontologist,* 1976, 16, Part II, 5–10.

Bradshaw, B., and Fonner, E. The mortality of Spanish-surnamed persons in Texas: 1969–1971. In F. D. Bean and W. P. Frisbie (Eds.), *The demography of racial and ethnic groups.* New York: Academic Press, 1979.

Butler, R., and Lewis, M. *Aging and mental health.* St. Louis: Mosby, 1982.

Cantor, M. H. The informal support system of New York's inner city elderly: Is ethnicity a factor? In D. E. Gelfand and A. J. Kutzik (Eds.), *Ethnicity and aging: Theory, research and policy.* New York: Springer, 1979.

Cantor, M., and Meyer, M. Health and the inner city elderly. Paper presented at the meetings of the Gerontological Society, 1974.

Cantor, M., Rosenthal, K., and Wilken, L. Social and family relationships of Black aged women in New York City. *Journal of Minority Aging,* 1979, 4, 50–61.

Carp. F. M., and Kataoka, E. Health problems of the elderly in San Francisco's Chinatown. *The Gerontologist,* 1976, 16, 30–38.

Colen, J. Facilitating service delivery to the minority aged. In R. McNeely and J. Colen (Eds.), *Aging in minority groups.* Beverly Hills: Sage, 1983.

Colen, J. N., and Soto, D. *Service delivery to aged minorities: Techniques of successful programs.* Sacramento: California State University, 1979.

Cuellar, J. *Minority elderly Americans: A prototype for area agencies on aging.* San Diego: Allied Home Health Association, 1980.

Cuellar, J., and Weeks, J. Minority elderly Americans: The assessment of needs and equitable receipt of public benefits as a prototype in area agencies on aging. Final Report. San Diego: Allied Home Health Association, Grant AOA/DHHS 90-A-1667(01), 1980.

Davis, D. Growing old Black. In J. S. Quodogne (Ed.), *Aging, the individual and society.* New York: St. Martins Press, 1980.

Dowd, J., and Bengtson, V. Aging in minority populations: An examination of the double jeopardy hypothesis. *Journal of Gerontology,* 1978, 33, 427–436.

Employment and the elderly. *National Indian Council on Aging Quarterly,* Winter 1981, 1, 2–4.

Gibson, R. Outlook for the Black family. In A. Pifer and L. Bronte (Eds.), *Our aging society.* New York: W. W. Norton, 1986.

Goldstine, T., and Gutmann, D. A TAT study of Navajo aging. *Psychiatry*, 1972, *35*, 373–384.

Gutmann, D. Use of informal and formal supports by white ethnic aged. In D. E. Gelfand and A. J. Kutzik (Eds.), *Ethnicity and aging: Theory, research and policy.* New York: Springer, 1979.

Gutmann, D. *Perspective on equitable share in public benefits by minority elderly.* Washington, D.C.: Catholic University of America, Administration on Aging, Grant 90-A-1617, 1980.

Harper, B. C. Some snapshots of death and dying among ethnic minorities. In R. C. Manuel (Ed.), *Minority aging: Sociological and social psychological issues.* Westport, Conn.: Greenwood Press, 1982.

Hendricks, J., and Hendricks, C. D. *Aging in mass society: Myths and realities* (2d ed.). Cambridge, Mass.: Winthrop Publishers, 1981.

Holzberg, C. Ethnicity and aging: Anthropological perspectives on more than just the minority elderly. *The Gerontologist*, 1982, *22*, 249–257.

Ignacio, L. F. *Asian American and Pacific islanders.* Philipino Development Associations, San Jose, Calif., 1976.

Ishizuka, K. C. *The elder Japanese.* San Diego: Campanile Press, 1978.

Ishikawa, W. *Pacific Asian elderly.* San Francisco: Hurron Resources Corp., 1978.

Jackson, J. The Black aging: A demographic overview. In R. Kalish (Ed.), *The later years.* Monterey, Calif.: Brooks/Cole, 1977.

Jackson, J. *Minorities and aging.* Belmont, Calif.: Wadsworth, 1980.

Jackson, J. Death rates of aged Blacks and Whites, 1964–1978. *The Black Scholar*, 1982, *13*, 36–48.

Jackson, J. J. The politicization of aged Blacks. In W. Browne and L. K. Olson (Eds.), *Aging and public policy.* Westport, Conn.: Greenwood Press, 1983.

Jackson, J. J. Race, national origin, ethnicity and aging. In. E. Shanas and R. Binstock (Eds.), *Handbook of aging and the social sciences.* New York: Van Nostrand Reinhold, 1985.

Jaco, E. Social factors in mental disorders in Texas. *Social Problems*, 1957, *4*, 320–328.

Jeffries, W. L. Our aged Indians. *Triple jeopardy—Myth or reality.* Washington, D.C.: National Council on Aging, 1972.

Kii, T. Asians. In E. Palmore (Ed.), *Handbook on the aged in the United States.* Westport, Conn.: Greenwood Press, 1984.

Kim, P. Demography of the Asian-Pacific elderly: Selected problems and implications. In R. L. McNeely and J. L. Colen (Eds.), *Aging in minority groups.* Beverly Hills: Sage, 1983.

Lacayo, C. Hispanics. In E. Palmore (Ed.), *Handbook on the aged in the United States.* Westport, Conn.: Greenwood Press, 1984.

Lacayo, C. G. *A national study to assess the service needs of the Hispanic elderly.* Los Angeles: Asociacion Nacional Pro Personal Mayores, 1980.

Lambrinos, J., and Torres-Gil, F. Policymakers historically ignore minorities. *Generations*, 1980, *4*, 24, 72.

Levkoff, S., Pratt, C., Esperanza, R., and Tomina, S. *Minority elderly: A historical and cultural perspective.* Corvallis: Oregon State University, 1979.

Lyman, S. M. *Chinese Americans.* New York: Random House, 1976.

Maldonado, D. The Chicano aged. In J. S. Quodagne (Ed.), *Aging, the individual and society.* New York: St. Martin's Press, 1980.

Manton, K. Differential life expectancy: Possible explanations during the later years. In R. C. Manuel (Ed.), *Minority aging: Sociological and social psychological issues.* Westport, Conn.: Greenwood Press, 1982.

Manuel, R. C. *Minority aging: Sociological and social psychological issues.* Westport, Conn.: Greenwood Press, 1982.

Manuel, R. C. The study of the minority aged in historical perspective. In R. C. Manuel (Ed.), *Minority aging: Sociological and social psychological issues.* Westport, Conn.: Greenwood Press, 1982.

Manuel, R., and Reid, J. A comparative demographic profile of the minority and nonminority aged. In R. C. Manuel (Ed.), *Minority aging: Sociological and social psychological issues.* Westport, Conn.: Greenwood Press, 1982.

Markides, K. Minority aging. In M. W. Riley, B. Hess, and K. Bond (Eds.), *Aging and society.* Hillsdale, N.J.: Lawrence Erlbaum, 1983.

Markides, K. S. Minority status, aging and marital health. *International Journal of Aging in Human Development,* 1986, *23,* 285–300.

Markides, K., and Martin, H. *Older Mexican Americans.* Austin: University of Texas at Austin, Center for Mexican American Studies, 1983.

McCaslin, R., and Calvert, W. R. Social indicators in Black and White: Some ethnic considerations in delivery of services to the elderly. *Journal of Gerontology,* 1975, *30,* 60–66.

McNeely, R. L., and Colen, J. L. *Aging in minority groups.* Beverly Hills: Sage, 1983.

Mindel, C., and Wright, R. The use of health and social services by the minority elderly: The role of social support systems. *Journal of Gerontological Social Work,* 1982, *4,* 3–4.

Mitchell, J., and Register, J. An exploration of family interaction with the elderly by race, socioeconomic status and residence. *The Gerontologist,* 1984, *24,* 48–54.

Montiel, M. The social science myth of the Mexican-American family. *El Grito,* 1970, *2,* 56–63.

Moore, J. W. Situational factors affecting minority aging. *The Gerontologist,* 1971a, *11,* 88–93.

Moore, J. W. Mexican Americans. *The Gerontologist,* 1971b, *11,* 30–35.

Moriwaki, S. Y. Ethnicity and aging. In I. M. Burnside (Ed.), *Nursing and the aged* (2d ed.). New York: McGraw Hill, 1981.

Morrison, B. J. Physical health and the minority aged. In R. C. McNeely and J. C. Colen (Eds.), *Aging in minority groups.* Beverly Hills: Sage, 1983.

Murdock, S. H., and Schwartz, D. F. Family structure and the use of agency services: An examination of patterns among Native Americans. *The Gerontologist,* 1978, *18,* 475–481.

National Indian Council on Aging. Indians and Alaskan natives. In E. Palmore, *Handbook on the aged in the United States*. Westport, Conn.: Greenwood Press, 1984.

National Pacific-Asian Resource Center on Aging. *Pacific/Asians: The wisdom of age*. National Mini-Conference on the Pacific-Asian Elderly, White House Conference on Aging, 1981.

Pacific-Asian Elderly Research Project. *Understanding the Pacific Asian elderly census and baseline data: A detailed report*. Los Angeles, 1978.

Palmore, E. *Handbook on the aged in the United States*. Westport, Conn.: Greenwood Press, 1984.

Raisz, H. Our Native American sisters. *Hotflash* (Newsletter of the National Action Forum for Older Women), 1986, 5, 1–7.

Reynolds, D., and Kalish, R. Anticipation of futurity as a function of ethnicity and age. *Journal of Gerontology*, 1974, 29, 224–231.

Rhoades, E., Marshall, M., Attneave, C., Bjork, J., and Beiser, M. Impact of mental disorders upon elderly American Indians as reflected in visits to ambulatory care facilities. *Journal of the American Geriatric Society*, 1980, 28, 33–39.

Rogers, E. J., and Gallion, T. E. Characteristics of elderly public Indians in New Mexico. *The Gerontologist*, 1978, 18, 482–487.

Rubel, A. *Across the tracks: Mexican Americans in a Texas city*. Austin: University of Texas Press, 1966.

Shanas, E., and Maddox, L. Health, health resources and the utilization of care. In R. Binstock and E. Shanas (Eds.), *Handbook of aging and the social sciences*. New York: Van Nostrand Reinhold, 1985.

Shimkin, D., Shimkin, E., and Frate, D. *The extended family in Black societies*. Chicago: Aldine Publishing, 1978.

Slaughter, O., and Mignon, B. Service delivery and the Black aged: Identifying barriers to utilization of mental health services. In R. C. Manuel (Ed.), *Minority aging: Sociological and social psychological issues*. Westport, Conn.: Greenwood Press, 1982.

Soldo, B. J., and DaVita, C. *Profiles of the Black aged*. Washington, D.C.: Georgetown University Center for Population Studies, 1977.

Tally, T., and Kaplan, J. The Negro aged. *Gerontological Society Newsletter*, 1956, 3 (4).

Taylor, R. The extended family as a source of support to elderly Blacks. *The Gerontologist*, 1985, 25, 488–495.

Torres-Gil, F. Age, health and culture: An examination of health among Spanish-speaking elderly. Presented at the First National Hispanic Conference on Health and Human Services, Los Angeles, September 22, 1976.

Torres-Gil, F. The special interest concerns of the minority professional: An evolutionary process in affecting social policies for the minority aged. In R. C. Manuel (Ed.), *Minority aging: Sociological and social psychological issues*. Westport, Conn.: Greenwood Press, 1982.

Torres-Gil, F. Hispanics: A special challenge. In A. Pifer and L. Bronte (Eds.), *Our aging society*. New York: W. W. Norton, 1986.

U.S. Bureau of the Census. *1980 Census of Population.* General Population Characteristics, Chapter B, 1980.

U.S. Bureau of the Census. *Supplementary Reports, 1980 Census of Population.* Age, sex, race and Spanish origin of the population by regions, divisions and states, 1980. PC80-S1-1, Washington, D.C.: USGPO, 1980.

U.S. Bureau of the Census. *Current Population Reports,* 1984.

U.S. Commission on Civil Rights. *Civil rights issues of Asia and Pacific Americans: Myths and realities.* Washington, D.C., 1979.

U.S. Department of Health and Human Services. *Characteristics of the Black elderly—1980.* Administration on Aging, 1980.

U.S. Senate Special Committee on Aging. *Aging America: Trends and projections.* U.S. Department of Health and Human Services, 1986.

Valle, R. The demography of Mexican-American aging. In R. L. McNeely and J. L. Colen (Eds.), *Aging in minority groups.* Beverly Hills: Sage, 1983.

Watson, W. Mental health of the minority aged: Selected correlates. In R. C. Manuel (Ed.), *Minority aging: Sociological and social psychological issues.* Westport, Conn.: Greenwood Press, 1982.

Watson, W. Selected demographics and social aspects of older Blacks. In R. L. McNeely and J. L. Colen (Eds.), *Aging in minority groups.* Beverly Hills: Sage, 1983.

Wesly-King, S. Service utilization and the minority elderly: A review. In R. L. McNeely and J. L. Colen (Eds.), *Aging in minority groups.* Beverly Hills: Sage, 1983.

1981 White House Conference. Aging: The Indian issue. *National Indian Council on Aging Quarterly,* Autumn 1981, *1* (4).

Williams, G. C. Warriors no more: A study of the American Indian elderly. In C. L. Fry (Ed.), *Aging in culture and society.* New York: J. E. Bergin Publishers, 1980.

Wilson, W. J. *The declining significance of race: Blacks and changing American institutions.* Chicago: University of Chicago Press, 1978.

Wirth, L. The problem of minority groups. In R. Linton (Ed.), *The science of man in the world crises.* New York: Columbia University Press, 1945.

Yip, B. Accessibility to services for Pan-Asian elderly: Fact or fiction? In E. P. Stanford (Ed.), *Minority aging: Policy issues for the 80s.* San Diego: Campanile Press, 1981.

Young, J. *Aging in Los Angeles County: A needs assessment of service to older persons in planning service area 19 California.* Los Angeles County Department of Senior Citizen Affairs and Clairmont Graduate School, Center for Applied Social Research, 1982.

Chapter 16

Populations at Risk:
Older Women

Previous chapters have illustrated numerous areas in which women's experiences with aging differs from men's: in patterns of health and life expectancy, marital opportunities, social supports, employment, and retirement. We have devoted a separate chapter to elaborate on those differences, with attention to how personal and environmental factors interact vis-à-vis the special problems facing women in old age. The impact of social factors, particularly economic ones, on physiological and psychological variables is vividly illustrated in terms of women's daily lives. This chapter first reviews the economic conditions faced by older women, then their health and social status, and how these factors interact. The chapter concludes with a brief discussion of program and policy options to reduce older women's vulnerability to poverty, poor health, and social isolation, primarily through changes affecting their socioeconomic conditions.

Concern for Older Women's Needs

A major reason for gerontological research and practice to take account of older women's special needs is that they form the fastest growing segment of our population. The aging society is primarily a female society. In 1980, women represented 60 percent of the population 65 years and over, and 74 percent of those over age 75 (Markson, 1983). As noted in Chapter 1, there are 80 men between ages 65 and 69 for every 100 women in the same age group. Among those age 85 and over, there are only 40 men for every 100 women (U.S. Senate Special Committee on Aging, 1986), with differences in this ratio among ethnic minorities, as noted in Chapter 15. As described in Chapter 1, these dispropor-tionate ratios result from differences in life expectancy between women and men, which are due to a combination of biological and lifestyle factors, such as women's greater likelihood of consulting doctors, and their lower rates of smoking, problem drinking, and risk-taking. At age 65, women can expect to live about 18 more years, compared to 14 years for men at the same age. At age 75, the comparable figures are 12 more years for women, and 9 more years for men. Even at age 85, the life expectancy for males is 1½ years less than that for females (Verbrugge, 1985).

Not only do demographic factors shape the context of older women's lives, but the problems of aging are increasingly women's problems. Older women are more likely than older men to be poor; to have inadequate retirement income; to be widowed, divorced, and alone; and to be caregivers to other relatives.

Despite their greater problems, many older women display resilience and innovativeness in the face of adversity (Riley and Riley, 1986). For example, women who live alone are not necessarily unhappy. On the average, women are less likely than men to die following a spouse's death (Helsing and Szklo, 1981). Many older women are remarkable survivors, having developed skills to cope with discontinuities and losses throughout their lives. There is growing awareness of middle-aged and older women's capacity to move in new directions—to advance their education, to enter new occupations, and to combine marriage and care for dependents with employment and volunteer roles. The impact of advocacy groups, such as the Older Women's League, on federal legislation clearly illustrates older women's power as activists. It is predicted that today's middle-aged women, who are enacting more diverse roles than past cohorts, will reach old age with even greater role flexibility and skills in coping with complex, changing life experiences (Riley and Riley, 1986).

Given the predominance of older women, it might be supposed that women, rather than men, would be the major focus of social gerontology. Yet, older women were nearly invisible in social gerontological research until the mid-1970s. For example, women were not added to the Baltimore Longitudinal Study (one of the major studies described in Chapters 1 and 5) until 1978. It was not until 1975 that the first older women's caucus met at the Annual Meetings of the Gerontological Society of America. The 1981 White House Conference on Aging was the first to sponsor a special committee on older women's concerns. Research on issues specific to women, such as menopause, estrogen replacement therapy, and osteoporosis, has been relatively limited until the 1980s.

In recent years, however, older women's resilience as well as their vulnerability to social, economic, and health problems have been increasingly recognized, primarily as the result of the educational and advocacy efforts of such interest groups as the Older Women's League (OWL). Although the women's movement of the 1970s tended to focus on issues specific to younger women, recently younger feminists have aligned themselves with efforts to influence older women's economic and social situations. Women of all ages have become more aware of their interdependence as both the primary recipients and providers of social and health services, and of the potential power of age-integrated women's organizations. Younger and older women are beginning to unite around issues of caregiving, for example, pressing for unpaid, job-guaranteed leave for the care of both dependent parents and newborn children through the Family and Medical Leave Act currently before Congress. Women are caregivers throughout their lives, whether as daughters, daughters-in-law, wives, mothers, or staff members within public social service agencies, nursing homes, and hospitals. Their role as unpaid caregivers and as underpaid employees are interconnected, and influence all aspects of their lives. Women's unpaid and undervalued work as family caregivers, along with their employment in low-status, low-paid jobs, result in economic insecurity in old age, with consequent negative effects on their health status and health care options.

Older Women's Economic Status

As described in Chapter 12, women age 65 and over account for nearly 71 percent of the older poor population (Minkler and Stone, 1985). They thus form one of the poorest groups in our society, with almost 16 percent of them living in poverty, compared to 8.5 percent for men. (*Older Women's League Observer*, 1983; U.S. Bureau of the Census, 1980). In 1985, the median annual income of older women was $6,300, compared with a median income of $10,900 for men. Nearly 50 percent of all older women had incomes below $5,000 in 1984, compared with only 20 percent of their male peers. Furthermore, older men were three times as likely as older women to be financially well-off, with incomes of $20,000 or more (Older Women's League, 1986).

Unmarried women living alone, ethnic minority women, and those aged 75 and over are especially likely to be poor. For example, the poverty rate among unmarried older women living alone in 1985 was 26.8. Seven out of ten poor elderly women live alone (U.S. Bureau of the Census, 1986). As we have seen in Chapter 15, the poverty rate of Black and Hispanic older women is more than double that of white older women, and increases for ethnic minority women living alone. In 1985, nearly 55 percent of older Black women not living with family had incomes below the poverty level (U.S. Bureau of the Census, 1986). The rate also increases with age for all women, to nearly 25 percent among women age 85 and over (Coalition on Women and the Budget, 1984; U.S. Senate Special Committee on Aging, 1985). These figures may not reveal the extent of poverty among single older women, primarily widows, who are not counted as poor despite their low income, because they may live in a household headed by a younger person whose income is above the poverty line. When these hidden poor are taken into account, up to 55 percent of older women have been estimated to be poor (Estes, 1985).

A primary reason for their economic vulnerability is that most women of this current cohort aged 65 and over did not work consistently for pay, largely because they were socialized to marry, have children, and depend on their husbands for economic support. Their labor force participation rate was 9.7 percent in 1950, rose slightly in the 1950s, and then dropped to 7.8 percent in 1983. When they did work, women tended to be concentrated in low-paying positions without adequate pensions. Although older Black women were more likely to have worked during their youth than their white counterparts, their rates of labor force participation throughout their lives were not significantly higher; and they were most likely to work in low-paying jobs (Rix, 1984). Generally dependent on men for both their income and their retirement benefits, most women of previous generations lacked the means to build up their economic security for old age.

A deleterious consequence of such dependency is that when women have become widowed or divorced, they have frequently lost their primary source of income. This vulnerability, resulting from the close interconnection between marital status and income level, has been described as being "only one man away from poverty" (Friends of the San Francisco Commission on the Status of Women, 1980). With nearly 63 percent of older women living without a spouse, many women face old age without pension income, particularly if their husbands did not select survivors' benefits. (In fact, only about 2 percent of widows receive survivors' benefits from a husband's pension [Bernstein, 1980]). The total average death benefits left by husbands to widows was approximately $12,000 in 1979, including all income from life insurance, Social Security, and other pensions. Of those eligible for benefits, only 25 percent of widows receive them in full, primarily because of misinformation about how to access these funds (Bernstein, 1980). Income level and marital status are thus inextricably linked, especially for older women without spouses (O'Rand, 1984).

At age 65, widows can receive full Social Security benefits based on their husband's earnings or their own, whichever is larger. However, because most women aged 60 and over are unemployed, the majority opt for reduced benefits at age 62, which then do not increase when they reach age 65. This monthly income is barely adequate, even for women who support only themselves and their homes. As noted by Tish Sommers, former President of the Older Women's League, "Motherhood and apple pie may be sacred, but neither guarantees economic security in old age" (1975, p. 11).

Older women are also not immune to the increasing divorce rate; recent statistics indicate that 16 percent of divorces occur among women age 45 and over, a rate that is increasing (Lesnoff-Caravaglia, 1984; Warlick, 1983). Older divorced women are even more economically vulnerable than are widows, with the majority lacking alimony payments and less than 50 percent receiving property settlements (U.S. Bureau of the Census, 1980). Further compounding the problem for divorced women is the Social Security regulation that a marriage of less than nine years' duration does not allow for the payment of a divorced spouse's Social Security benefits. Upon retirement, divorced wives married for at least ten years are entitled to a benefit amount of 50 percent of their ex-husband's benefits. If the former husband continues to work, they are not eligible for benefits until the husband retires. The average monthly Social Security benefit for divorced wives of retired workers in 1980 was $177 (Rix, 1984). Women who in their youth cared for husbands and children thus frequently find themselves alone and with less than subsistence income in old age. These dire economic conditions have prompted a number of proposals to ensure homemakers' economic security in old age, such as paying them Social Security or some other form of income, but none of these proposals has received widespread Congressional support. The likelihood of such endorsement in the future is small, considering current legislative efforts to reduce federal spending.

Although not all older women are poor, those who rely primarily on their own resources are likely to have fewer assets such as savings, to have lower lifetime earnings, to depend on Social Security as their sole source of income, and to receive low benefits as retirees or disabled workers. Even though they form 63 percent of Social Security beneficiaries, older women are three times more likely than their male peers to receive only the minimum benefits. Yet, a person who receives only Social Security income is seven times more likely to be poor than one who also has wage and salary income (Older Women's League, 1986). In

1982, 66 percent of women received Social Security benefits that placed them below the poverty level (Rix, 1984). Monthly benefits averaged $399 for women, and $521 for men in 1985 (Older Women's League, 1986).

A number of political, social, and economic factors underlie these low benefit levels. One factor that affects both men and women age 70 and over is that the Social Security program was not established until 1935; thus, there are relatively fewer years upon which to base benefits for the cohort of elderly today. An additional handicap for women is that they are more likely than men to have interrupted their work for marriage and childrearing. Women of the current elderly cohort generally worked until marriage or the birth of children, and then withdrew from the paid labor force, either permanently or until their children were grown. They often assumed their first full-time job on the average of five years later than male workers. The disadvantage of this pattern is that Social Security benefits are averaged over the number of years that a person is in the salaried work force and has paid into the system. Even though five years of no or low work benefits can be dropped from this average in computing Social Security benefits, most women have taken off more than five years from employment to devote to childrearing and homemaking. It is not surprising that only 37 percent of the women applying for Social Security benefits based on their own earnings in 1980 had a continuous earnings record since 1937 (Rix, 1984). Homemakers have no individual eligibility and no credits to add to their employment credits and cannot receive disability supports on their own, despite the economic value of their household labor to their families.

Another factor affecting Social Security benefits for women is that those who are employed tend to be concentrated in part-time, short-term, or irregular and poorly paid jobs. Even when they have been employed throughout their lives, most women have received inadequate salaries, generally in low-status service and clerical jobs. As a result, they frequently find that their husband's Social Security benefits are higher than benefits based on their own work records. In such instances, women who have worked all their lives in low-paying jobs are not much better off at retirement than women who have never worked for pay outside the home.

Women are also less likely to have private pensions than men, both because of their concentration in low-paying positions and their shorter work careers, and because mandatory pension laws were not in effect when many women of this cohort were employed (i.e., in their twenties and thirties). As discussed in Chapter 12, pension plans reward the long-term steady worker with high earnings and job stability, a pattern that tends to be more characteristic of men than of women who have interrupted their careers to marry and rear children. This continues to be the trend even among the current cohort of working women. In 1984, approximately 44 percent of men were covered by private pensions, compared with fewer than 20 percent of women who had been employed. Those women with pensions receive approximately half the benefit incomes of men because of salary differentials during their working years. A woman whose family role resulted in economic dependence on her husband can benefit from his private pension only if he is covered by one, does not die before retirement age, stays married to her, and is willing to reduce his monthly benefits in order to provide her with a survivor annuity (O'Rand, 1984). Given the economic vicissitudes of aging, most older men choose higher monthly benefits rather than survivors' benefits. Such a choice can be detrimental to older women, since, as noted earlier, most wives outlive their husbands by an average of eight years. Fortunately, pension provisions enacted by Congress in 1980 will benefit older women by shortening the time it takes to earn a pension and improving coverage for lower income workers, for those who begin work after age 60 and those who continue to work after age 65. However, most of these provisions become effective for pension plans beginning in January 1989, and thus do not affect the current cohort of older women.

Older women without private pensions and whose Social Security income falls below the poverty line must rely on Supplemental Security Income (SSI). In 1982, women comprised nearly 75 percent of older SSI recipients, receiving an average monthly benefit of only $284 in addition to Social Security (O'Rand, 1984). For women who value economic self-sufficiency, dependency on the government for such support can be stigmatizing.

In summary, traditional family roles of women tend to result in discontinuous work histories. This pattern, combined with limited pension opportunities and lower Social Security benefits, produces a double jeopardy for women's economic status in old age. As discussed in the following section, the disadvantaged economic position of older women also increases their health risks.

Older Women's Health Status

As noted in Chapter 6, older people who are poor, represented primarily by women and ethnic minorities, tend to be less healthy than higher income elderly. Their living conditions are not conducive to good health. Compared to their wealthier peers, they are more likely to be living alone, to have inadequate diets, to have less access to information about how to maintain their health, and to have fewer dental visits and physician contacts per year (Filner and Williams, 1979; Van Mering and O'Rand, 1981). Since older women, especially the never-married and widowed, predominate among the elderly poor, women's health status is more frequently harmed by the adverse conditions associated with poverty than is men's. In turn, the cost of poor health can deplete the limited resources of the low-income poor.

LESS ACCESS TO HEALTH INSURANCE

Previous family and work patterns affect older women's access to adequate health care and health maintenance information. Specifically, the workplace determines such access through opportunities to enroll in group insurance plans. Most insurance systems exclude the occupation of homemaker, except as a dependent. As a result, older women who are never or sporadically employed generally have inadequate health insurance. In 1985, 4.5 million women age 45 to 65 lacked health insurance (Older Women's League, 1986). Low-income divorced or widowed women, unable to rely on their husbands' insurance, are especially disadvantaged. Divorced women are about twice as likely (14 percent) to lack health insurance as married women (7 percent), and are more likely to be uninsured than widows (9 percent) (Berk and Taylor, 1984). Some 40 percent of all divorced women and 27 percent of all widows not in the labor force have no private health insurance (Older Women's League, 1986). Some uninsured women gamble on staying healthy until qualifying for Medicare coverage at age 65. Since the incidence of chronic diseases is higher among older women than men, many women do not win this gamble. Yet they may not qualify for Medicaid. Tish Sommers, founder of the Older Women's League, represents this group of women. When she was diagnosed with cancer in her late fifties, she was too young to qualify for Medicare, too sick to obtain private insurance, and, as a divorcee, unable to turn to her former husband's insurance. Groups such as the Older Women's League have succeeded in advocating for conversion laws that require insurance companies to allow widowed and divorced women to remain in their spouse's group insurance for up to three years.

Even with adequate health insurance, older women spend 33 percent of their median annual income for out-of-pocket health care costs. It is estimated that, in 1986, Medicare paid for approximately 49 percent of the health care expenditures of older unmarried men, but only 33 percent of the expenditures of older single women (Older Women's League, 1987). (See Chapter 19 for a detailed discussion of the limitations of Medicare coverage that affect older women.)

Because of their lower socioeconomic status, older women are more likely than men to depend on Medicaid, forming over 60 percent of Medicaid recipients (Coalition on Women and the Budget, 1984). An insidious negative effect of this dependency is that health care providers, fearing financial losses, are often unwilling to accept Medicaid patients, making it difficult for older women to obtain adequate care. Male–female differences in longevity, marital status, and income are central in assessing the impact of recent increases in Medicaid co-payments and deductibles. Women outnumber men two to one among the frail elderly, for whom health care use and costs are greatest. This means that, as Medicaid costs are shifted to the patient, more low-income frail women will be unable to afford health care. Recent co-payment provisions in Medicaid may force some women to choose between prescriptions and groceries, or between clinic visits and the bus fare to get there.

HIGHER INCIDENCE OF CHRONIC HEALTH PROBLEMS

Limited insurance options and greater dependence on Medicaid are especially problematic because 85 percent of older women have some kind of chronic disease or disability. As discussed in Chapter 6, older women experience arthritis, hypertension, strokes, diabetes, most digestive and urinary problems (except ulcer and hernia), incontinence, most types of orthopedic problems, and visual impairments more frequently than do older men (Verbrugge, 1983). Women also face health problems specifically associated with their reproductive functions, such as breast, cervical, and uterine cancers—all of which have increased in recent years—as well as high-risk complications from hysterectomies. Tragically, women over age 60 who are most at risk of cancers of the reproductive system are least likely to have annual pap smears (Older Women's League, 1987). As noted in Chapter 6, although women suffer from more chronic health conditions, most of these are not life-threatening; they do, however, interfere with daily functioning and require frequent physician contacts. Although men tend to experience fewer daily aches and pains than women, when they do become ill, they are more likely to face life-threatening conditions and to require hospitalization. These differences in types of chronic health problems may be one reason why women live longer than men, even though they are less healthy (Kerzner, 1983). Male–female differences in death rates can also be attributed to immunity, environmental hazards, health habits and utilization of services, personality styles, and differences in reactions to and knowledge about disease and disability (Lewis, 1985).

Compared to their male counterparts, older women also experience more injuries and more days of restricted activity and bed disability. These measures are generally indicators of chronic disorders, such as high blood pressure and arthritis, although it may be that these variables reflect women's greater readiness to take curative action and spend more time in bed recuperating when they are ill. Among people aged 75 and over, sex differences in patterns of illness become even more striking, with three to four females for every male residing in skilled care facilities (U.S. Department of Health and Human Services, 1983). There are, of course, several factors besides health status that may account for this difference. As discussed in Chapter 10, older men are more likely to be married, with wives to care for them at home instead of being placed in a nursing home. Women over age 75, on the other hand, have few available resources for home-based care, and are often unable to afford home health services. In addition, it should be noted that men who survive to age 75 and older are the healthiest and hardiest of their cohort.

OSTEOPOROSIS

One particularly painful chronic condition disproportionately experienced by women is osteoporosis, or loss of bone mass. As noted in Chapter 6, women begin losing bone mass between 30 and 35 years of age, resulting in a 35 percent reduction in their bone mineral content by 65 or 70 years of age and a consequent increase in the risk of bone fracture. The higher incidence of hip fractures is one reason for the greater number of injuries and days of restricted activity among older women. It is also of concern because of the approximate 15 percent mortality rate within three months following a fracture. Most of these deaths result from post-operative complications, such as a pulmonary embolism, which has a higher incidence among older women (Lindsay, 1981; Nussbaum, 1981). The threat of hip fractures can create numerous fears among older women—of additional falls, further fractures, hospitalization, institutionalization, loss of independence, and death. As a result, an older woman's social world may become increasingly circumscribed, with accompanying feelings of isolation and loneliness. As for the expenses to society, the long-term care costs entailed by hip fractures are approximately $1.5 billion a year (Lindsay, 1985).

MENOPAUSE

The climacteric—the period of change between reproduction and nonreproduction—takes place in three phases: premenopause, menopause, and postmenopause. Premenopause is marked by a decline in ovarian function in which a woman's ovaries stop producing eggs and significantly decrease their monthly production of estrogen. The monthly menstrual flow becomes less frequent until it stops completely. The average age of menopause is 50 years, although it can begin as early as age 40 and as late as age 58. Menopause is complete when 12 consecutive months have passed without a menstrual period—usually about 2 years from its onset.

The major physical signs of menopause are irregular menstrual flow, hot flashes, and vaginal changes, such as a thinning and loss of elasticity of the vaginal walls. Hot flashes are caused by vasomotor instability, when the nerves over-respond to decreases in hormone levels. This affects the hypothalamus (the part of the brain that regulates body temperature), causing the blood vessels to dilate or constrict. When the blood vessels dilate, blood rushes to the skin surface, causing perspiration, flushing, and increased pulse rate and temperature. Hot flashes are characterized by a sudden sensation of heat in the upper body. Although 80 percent of women ages 45 through 55 experience some discomforts such as hot flashes and sweats during menopause, most find that these physiological changes do not interfere with their daily functioning nor cause psychological difficulties. Other symptoms reported by menopausal women, such as headaches, dizziness, palpitations, sleeplessness, depression, and weight increase, are not caused by menopause itself (Porcino, 1983).

Social attitudes can make menopause troublesome as well. Many of these discomforts are associated with society's tendency to view menopause as a disease, rather than as a normal biological process. Hence, many women anticipate that depression, loss of sexual desire and sexual attractiveness, and such signs of aging as wrinkled skin and weight gain are inevitable. Contrary to such expectations, menopause is not an illness or a deficiency. It can, however, be a major transition for many women. Menopausal symptoms thus provide another example of the interaction of normal physiological changes with psychosocial conditions and societal expectations.

The culturally prevalent model of menopause as a disease attributes changes to loss of estrogen. When thus defined as a "deficiency disease," a treatment implication is that estrogen must be replaced. Accordingly, the primary medical response to treating symptoms such as hot flashes has been estrogen replacement therapy. Estrogen does alleviate hot flashes and vaginal changes, including atrophy, dryness, itching, pain during intercourse, and frequent urination. (In addition, some studies suggest that women who use estrogen have far fewer hip and spine fractures due to osteoporosis.) However, estrogen merely postpones menopausal symptoms. When estrogen is stopped, even 20 years later, symptoms will recur. In addition, its use is controversial, because of the slight increase in the risk of endometrial cancer among women receiving estrogen for long periods. When there are no other solutions to major discomforts associated with menopause, women should be fully informed of the potential risks of estrogen, and treatment should be at low doses (often combined with progesterone), for short periods, and continuously monitored. Estrogen at any dose does not alter the aging process, depression, or insomnia (National Institute of Health, 1983).

When menopause is viewed as a normal life transition, however, lower estrogen levels among postmenopausal women can then be considered normal. Recently, many women have been using nonmedical approaches to minimize uncomfortable symptoms. These include hypnosis, biofeedback, relaxation techniques, exercise, support groups, herbal remedies, Vitamin E, and diets low in fats and preservatives.

Although the disease model of menopause links depression with the endocrine changes that occur, depresion among postmenopausal women appears to be more closely associated with psychosocial variables, particularly changes in women's roles and relationships, than with physiological factors. Menopausal women who experience depression tend to have invested heavily in childrearing responsibilities and to lack supportive social networks, other satisfying roles, and skills for effectively coping with their role changes (Bart, 1981; Neugarten, Wood, Kraines, and Loomis, 1968). Health care providers have often treated the symptoms of depression with drugs, or have assumed that middle-aged and older women were "too old" to benefit from therapeutic interventions. More recently, efforts have been made to provide women with ways of exerting control over their lives, such as assertiveness training, and to develop women's counseling and social support interventions as a means of combating depression. Such social support groups have been found to reduce women's feelings of isolation and to enhance their self-esteem and self-control.

Older Women's Social Status

Older women's physical and mental health problems are frequently intensified by the greater likelihood of their living alone. For example, older women who live alone are more likely to be diagnosed as malnourished. This is not surprising when the social functions of eating are considered. The older person living alone may derive no pleasure from eating and may skip meals, subsisting instead on such snacks as tea and cookies. The high poverty rates among older women who live alone, as we have seen earlier in this chapter, may also account for their poor eating habits. Even mild nutritional deficiencies may produce disorientation, confusion, depression, and reduced ability to respond to stress. One result is that a person with fewer immediate social supports may be less likely to resist infections and viral diseases. Their ability to live in the community may thus be sharply curtailed.

More than 40 percent of older women live alone for approximately one-third of their adult lives, primarily because of widowhood or divorce. In fact, only 33 percent of all women aged 65 and over live with their husbands, and only 20 percent live with other family members (Rix, 1984; U.S. Senate Special Committee on Aging, 1986). Among women aged 75 and over, the percentage living with their husbands drops to less than 25 percent, and the proportion living alone increases to nearly 50 percent (Rix, 1984).

WIDOWHOOD

As discussed in Chapter 10, the average age of widowhood for women is 56 years; therefore it is not surprising that 85 percent of all wives outlive their husbands. Because women generally marry men older than themselves, live longer than men, and, in their later years, seldom remarry after the deaths of their husbands, widowhood is a more common status for females than for males. Some 52 percent of women aged 65 and over are widowed, in contrast to 14 percent of men in this age group. This gap increases dramatically with age, with 73 percent of women over 80 years of age widowed. As noted above, the primary negative consequence of widowhood is low socioeconomic status; some 33 percent of older widows live alone and in poverty (Coalition on Women and the Budget, 1984). These economic conditions have numerous social implications; low-income women having fewer options to interact with others, fewer affordable and safe accommodations, and fewer resources to purchase in-home support services. The most negative consequence may be that older women's economic situation precludes continued independent living when health problems arise. For instance, a study of 300 older Detroit area residents found women living alone to be the highest risk group, and most at need for social and health services (Kahana and Kiyak, 1980). Despite these objective disadvantages of widowhood, recent studies are challenging the stereotype of the "lonely widow," and finding that widowhood does not necessarily produce the major, enduring negative emotional effects that typically have been reported (Hyman, 1983).

DIVORCE

Divorced women are even more vulnerable to social and economic problems. Compared to both their married and widowed peers, divorced women aged 65 and over have been found to have poorer health, higher mortality rates, and lower levels of life satisfaction (Hess and Waring, 1983). If divorced earlier in life, the disadvantages of having no financial support and often being employed in low-paying positions may have resulted in a lifetime of marginal economic security.

LIMITED OPPORTUNITIES TO REMARRY

Although remarriage may be viewed as a way to ensure economic security, older widowed and divorced women have fewer remarriage options than their male peers. The primary obstacles to remarriage are the disproportionate number of women to men age 65 and over, and the cultural stigma against women marrying younger men. At age 65 and over, remarriage rates are 2 per 1,000 for unmarried women compared to 17 per 1,000 for unmarried men. Some 77 percent of men 65 years and older are married, compared to 38 percent of women (U.S. Senate Special Committee on Aging, 1986). With the ratio of 80-year-old women to men being three to one, the chances for remarriage decline drastically with age (Hess and Waring, 1983). These differences lead to differential needs for support in the face of failing health (e.g., most older men are cared for by their wives, whereas most older women rely on their children for help). As discussed in Chapter 10, women comprise nearly 80 percent of the caregivers of elderly relatives (Brody, 1985). One half of these female caregivers are age 45 and over (Older Women's League, 1986). Increasingly, adult daughters who assist their widowed mothers are themselves in their sixties and seventies, and are faced with their own physical limitations. One consequence of this pattern is that older women may have to depend more on public support services. Older women are thus the primary informal providers of care, as well as the major users of public services (Rix, 1984). As invisible laborers, women's work is essential to the health care system and to their relatives' long-term care, but not supported by public policies.

In addition to having high rates of widowhood and increasing rates of divorce, the current cohort of older women had relatively high rates of remaining unmarried throughout their lives (approximately 8 percent for women now in their seventies and eighties), so that a cohort effect also may explain the large numbers of older women living without spouses. Another factor that increases the probability of being alone among this current cohort of older women is that approximately one in five has either been childless throughout her life or has survived her offspring (Hess and Waring, 1983).

It appears that widows without children tend to be more lonely and dissatisfied than widows who have grown children (Backman and Houser, 1982). The absence of children and spouse also increases the chance of being placed in a nursing home (Treas, 1977). This suggests that women are more likely to be institutionalized for social rather than medical reasons, and may be inappropriately placed in a nursing home, when alternative community supports might have permitted more independent lifestyles. As a result, women form 71 percent of nursing home residents, with the majority of them widowed or single, often dependent on Medicaid and lacking family members to assist them either socially or financially. After age 85, one in four women, especially never-married and widowed women, are in nursing homes (Hess and Waring, 1983).

In general, older women have fewer economic but more social resources than do older men (O'Rand, 1983). Older women tend to be skilled at forming and sustaining friendships with each other, which provide them with social support and intimacy. Even when their friends die, women generally establish new relationships, exchanging affection and material assistance outside their families (Powers and Bultena, 1980; Arling, 1980). Support groups for widows and family caregivers build on such reciprocal exchange relations among peers. With age, some women first become comfortable with being open about their lesbianism and their strong emotional bonds with other women, although they may face rejection from their adult children when they do so (Raphael and Robinson, 1980). One function of the affirmation of women's competencies by the women's movement has been to encourage them to support each other rather than depend on men, as evidenced by the growth of shared households, older women's support and advocacy groups, and intergenerational alliances.

Future Directions

Since women's low socioeconomic status compounds most of the problems they face in old age, fundamental changes are needed to remove inequities in the workplace, Social Security, and pension systems. Most such changes, however, will benefit future generations of older women, rather than the current cohort, which was socialized for work and family roles that no longer prevail. For example, recent efforts in some states to assure that women and men earn equal pay for jobs of comparable economic worth and to remove other salary inequities may mean that future generations of older women will have retirement benefits based on a lifetime of more adequate earnings. Some businesses and government agencies have initiated more flexible work arrangements with full benefits, which will allow men and women to share employment and family responsibilities more equitably. When such options exist, women may have fewer years of zero earnings to be calculated into their Social Security benefits, and will be more likely to hold jobs covered by private pensions.

Changes in Social Security that would benefit women workers have also been proposed by a number of federal studies and commissions. The current Social Security system is based on an outmoded model of lifelong marriage, in which one spouse is the paid worker, and the other is the homemaker. As the prior discussion of divorce and changing work patterns suggests, this model no longer accommodates the emerging diversity in employment and family roles. Nor for that matter has this model really represented the diversity of American families. The most commonly discussed remedy is earnings sharing, whereby each partner in marriage is entitled to a separate Social Security account, regardless of which spouse is employed in the paid labor force. Covered earnings would be divided between two spouses, with one-half credited to each spouse's account. Credits for

Women frequently provide emotional support within the multigenerational family.

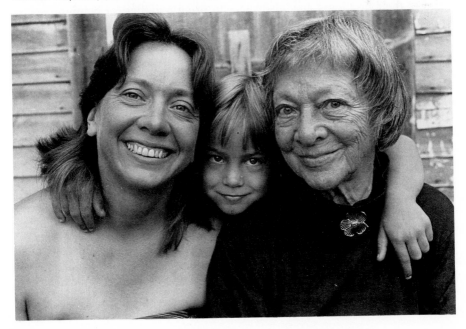

homemaking, benefits for widows under age 62, full benefits for widows after age 65, and the option of collecting benefits as both worker and wife have also been discussed by senior citizen advocacy groups and by some legislators. Given the large federal deficit and the concern with freezing Social Security benefits, the likelihood of any such changes being instituted in the next few years is small. Pension reforms have also been passed on the federal level that would increase by more than 20 percent the number of women covered by private pensions, by reducing the amount of time required for vesting. In the long run, changes are needed in society's view of work throughout the life cycle, so that men and women may share more equitably in caregiving and employment responsibilities. At the same time, employers must recognize that skills gained through home-making and voluntary activity are legitimate.

Such economic changes will ultimately enhance women's health and social well-being. An observable positive change in recent years is that more women of all ages are supporting one another, as illustrated by the intergenerational advocacy efforts of the Older Women's League and the National Action Forum for Women. Another promising change is the growth of social support groups among older women. Groups of older widows and women caregivers have been found to be effective in reducing women's isolation. They have encouraged group members to meet their own needs and have expanded women's awareness of public services to which they are entitled. This function of educating and politicizing older women has also helped many to see the societal causes of the difficulties that they have experienced as individuals. Awareness of external causes of their problems may also serve to bring together for common action women of diverse ages, ethnic backgrounds, socioeconomic classes, and sexual preference. As women unite to work for change, they can make further progress in reducing the disadvantages of their economic and social position.

Summary and Implications

Older women are the fastest growing segment of our population, making the aging society primarily female. In addition, the problems of aging are increasingly the problems of women. Threats to Social Security, inadequate health care, and insufficient pensions are issues for women of all ages. Increasingly, older women are not only the recipients of social and health services, but also are cared for by other women, whether as unpaid daughters and daughters-in-law, or as staff within public social services, nursing homes, and hospitals.

Women's family caregiving roles are interconnected with their economic, social, and health status. Women who devoted their lives attending to the needs of children, spouses, or older relatives often face years of living alone on low or poverty level incomes, with inadequate health care, in substandard housing, and with little chance for employment to supplement their limited resources. Older women face more problems in old age, not only because they live longer than their male peers, but also because, as unpaid or underpaid caregivers with discontinuous employment histories, they have not accrued adequate retirement or health care benefits. If they have depended on their husbands for economic security, divorce or widowhood increases their risks of poverty. As one of the poorest groups in our society, women account for nearly three-fourths of the elderly poor. The incidence of problems associated with poverty increases dramatically for older women living alone, for ethnic minority women, and for those age 75 and over. Frequently outliving their children and husbands, they have no one to care for them and are more likely than their male counterparts to be in nursing homes.

On the other hand, many women show remarkable resilience in the face of adversity. Fortunately, the number of exceptions to patterns of economic deprivation and social isolation is growing. With their lifelong experiences of caring for others, for example, women tend to be skilled at forming and sustaining friendships with each other, which provide them with social support and intimacy. Recently, increasing attention has been paid to older women's capacity for change and to their strengths, largely because of efforts of advocacy groups such as the Older Women's League. Current efforts to improve the employment and educational opportunities available to younger women will undoubtedly mean improved economic, social, and health status for future generations of women.

References

Arling, G. The elderly widow and her family, neighbors and friends. In M. Fuller and C. A. Martin (Eds.), *The older woman: Lavender rose or gray panther.* Springfield, Ill.: Charles C. Thomas, 1980.

Backman, L., and Houser, B. The consequences of childlessness on the social-psychological wellbeing of older women. *Journal of Gerontology,* 1982, *37,* 243–250.

Bart, P. Mental health issues: Is the end of the curse a blessing? *Health issues of older women.* Stony Brook: State University of New York, 1981.

Berk, M., and Taylor, A. Women and divorce: Health insurance coverage, utilization, and health care expenditures. *American Journal of Public Health,* 1984, *74,* 1276–1278.

Bernstein, M. C. Forecasting women's retirement income: Cloudy and colder and 25 percent chance of poverty. In M. Fuller and C. Martin (Eds.), *The older woman: Lavender rose or gray panther.* Springfield, Ill.: Charles C. Thomas, 1980.

Brody, E. Parent care as a normative family stress. *The Gerontologist,* 1985, *25,* 19–30.

Coalition on Women and the Budget. *Inequality of sacrifice: The impact of the Reagan budget on women.* Washington, D.C.: National Women's Law Center, 1984.

Estes, C. Older women and poverty. Presented at the annual meeting of the Western Gerontological Society, Denver, Colorado, March 1985.

Filner, B., and Williams, T. F. Health promotion for the elderly: Reducing functional dependency. *Healthy people: The Surgeon General's report on health promotion and disease prevention: Background papers.* Washington, D.C.: U.S. Government Printing Office, 1979.

Friends of the San Francisco Commission on the Status of Women. *Womennews,* December 1980, 1.

Helsing, K. J., and Szklo, M. Mortality after bereavement. *American Journal of Epidemiology,* 1981, *114,* 41–52.

Hess, B., and Waring, J. Family relationships of older women: A women's issue. In E. Markson (Ed.), *Older women.* Lexington, Mass.: Lexington Books, 1983.

Hyman, H. *Of time and widowhood: Nationwide studies of enduring effects.* Durham, N.C.: Duke University Press, 1983.

Kahana, E., and Kiyak, H. A. The older woman: Impact of widowhood and living arrangement on service needs. *Journal of Gerontological Social Work,* 1980, 3, 17–29.

Kerzner, L. Physical changes after menopause. In E. Markson (Ed.), *Older women.* Lexington, Mass.: Lexington Books, 1983.

Lesnoff-Caravaglia, G. (Ed.), *The world of the older woman.* New York: Human Sciences Press, 1984.

Lewis, M. Older women and health. *Women and Health,* 1985, *10*(2–3), 1–16.

Lindsay, R. Osteoporosis. *Health issues of older women.* Stony Brook: State University of New York, 1981.

Lindsay, R. The aging skeleton. In M. Haug, A. Ford, and M. Sheafor (Eds.), *The physical and mental health of aged women.* New York: Springer Publishing, 1985.

Markson, E. *Older women.* Lexington, Mass.: Lexington Books, 1983.

Minkler, M., and Stone, R. The feminization of poverty and older women. *The Gerontologist,* 1985, *25,* 351–357.

National Institutes of Health. *The menopause time of life.* U.S. Department of Health and Human Services, 1983.

Neugarten, B., Wood, V., Kraines, R., and Loomis, B. Women's attitudes toward the menopause. *Middle age and aging.* Chicago: University of Chicago Press, 1968.

Nussbaum, S. R. Management of osteoporosis. In A. H. Gorall, L. A. May, and A. G. Mulley (Eds.), *Primary care medicine.* Philadelphia: J. B. Lippincott, 1981.

Older Women's League. *OWL Observer,* Feb.–May, 1983.

Older Women's League. *Report on the status of midlife and older women in America.* Washington, D.C., 1986.

Older Women's League. *The picture of health for midlife and older women.* Washington, D.C., 1987.

O'Rand, A. M. Loss of work role and subjective health assessment in later life among men and unmarried women. In A. C. Kerckhoff (Ed.), *Research in sociology of education and socialization* (Volume 5). San Francisco: JAI Press, 1983.

O'Rand, A. M. Women. In E. Palmore (Ed.), *Handbook on the aged in the United States.* Westport, Conn.: Greenwood Press, 1984.

Porcino, J. *Growing older, getting better: A handbook for women in the second half of life.* Reading, Mass.: Addison-Wesley, 1983.

Powers, E., and Bultena, G. Sex differences in intimate friendships of old age. In M. Fuller and C. A. Martin (Eds.), *The older woman: Lavender rose or gray panther.* Springfield, Ill.: Charles C. Thomas, 1980.

Raphael, S., and Robinson, M. The older lesbian: Love relationships and friendship patterns. *Alternate Lifestyles,* 1980, 3 (2), 207–229.

Riley, M., and Riley, J. Longevity and social structure: The potential of the added years. In A. Pifer and L. Bronte (Eds.), *Our aging society: Paradox and promise.* New York: W. W. Norton, 1986.

Rix, S. *Older women: The economics of aging.* Washington, D.C.: Women's Research and Education Institute, 1984.

Scott, H. *Working your way to the bottom: The feminization of poverty.* London: Pandora Press, 1984.

Sommers, T. On growing old female: An interview with Tish Sommers. *Aging,* 1975, Nov.–Dec.

Treas, J. Family support systems for the aged: Some social and demographic considerations. *The Gerontologist,* 1977, *17,* 486–491.

U.S. Bureau of the Census. *Money income and poverty status of families and persons in the United States, 1985* (Advance Data from the March 1986 Current Population Survey). Washington, D.C.: U.S. Government Printing Office. Series P-60, No. 154, August 1986.

U.S. Bureau of the Census. Social and economic characteristics of the older population. *Current population reports: Special studies.* Washington, D.C.: U.S. Government Printing Office, Series P-25, No. 85, August 1979.

U.S. Bureau of the Census. A statistical portrait of women in the United States. *Current population reports: Special studies.* Washington, D.C.: U.S. Government Printing Office, Series P-23, No. 100, February 1980.

U.S. Department of Health and Human Services. *Women and national health insurance: Where do we go from here?* Report of the Secretary's Advisory Committee on the Rights and Responsibilities of Women. Washington, D.C.: U.S. Government Printing Office, 1983.

U.S. Senate Special Committee on Aging. *America in transition: An aging society.* Washington, D.C.: U.S. Government Printing Office, 1985.

U.S. Senate Special Committee on Aging. *Aging America: Trends and projections, 1985–1986 edition.* U.S. Department of Health and Human Services, 1986.

Verbrugge, L. Women and men: Mortality and health of older people. In M. W. Riley, B. B. Hess, and B. Bond (Eds.), *Aging in society.* Hillsdale, N.J.: Lawrence Erlbaum, 1983.

Verbrugge, L. An epidemiological profile of older women. In M. Haug, A. Ford, and M. Sheafor (Eds.), *The physical and mental health of aged women.* New York: Springer, 1985.

Von Mering, G., and O'Rand, A. M. Aging, illness and the organization of health care: A sociocultural perspective. In C. L. Fry (Ed.), *Dimensions: Aging, culture and health.* New York: Praeger, 1981.

Warlock, J. Aged women in poverty: A problem without a solution? In W. P. Browne and L. K. Olson (Eds.), *Aging and public policy.* Westport, Conn.: Greenwood Press, 1983.

Part V

The Societal Context of Aging

The final section of this book examines aging and the elderly from the broader context of society. The values and attitudes that policymakers and voters hold toward a particular group or topic are often the basis on which policies are made. To the extent that these policies also are grounded in knowledge, they can aid the status of that group. On the other hand, policies that are based solely on stereotypes or generalizations about a segment of society may be inadequate and even harmful.

Throughout this book we have reviewed the current state of knowledge about the physiological, psychological, and social aspects of aging. We have examined variations among older ethnic minority groups, between older men and women, and among other segments of the older population. The diversity in processes of aging has been emphasized. Differences in lifestyle, work patterns, and family and social experiences in earlier periods of life can have a significant impact on health and social functioning in old age. As a result, there are greater variations among the older population than among members of any other segment of society.

Despite these differences, stereotypes persist about "the typical older person." The focus of Chapter 17 is on the stereotypes and evaluations of older people held by younger persons and by the elderly themselves. How these attitudes are formed, and their implications for older people's self-concept and self-esteem, for the roles they are expected to fulfill, and for interactions with other age groups are examined in this chapter. The impact of attitudes on professionals' behavior toward older people and on decisions to work with older persons are also considered.

Attitudes toward older people also influence the social and health policies that are developed by federal, state, and local governments, as well as by employers regarding this population. As Chapter 18 points out, social policies and programs have evolved to address the special needs of some older people. Some age-based programs such as Medicare are directed toward all people who fulfill age criteria, whereas others such as Supplemental Security Income (SSI) and food stamps are based on financial need. The eligibility criteria and services provided through these programs and policies are often determined by the prevailing social values and by those of the political party and presidential administration in power. These values, in turn, reflect society's attitudes toward older people, their contributions and their responsibilities to society. For example, attitudes and values regarding older people's rights, whether chronological age is an appropriate basis for retirement laws, and whether care of the aging population is a societal or individual responsibility, all influence the development of social and health policies. The historical development of aging policy in the United States and changes in existing programs such as Social Security are also reviewed within the context of societal changes that influence values toward the older population. One societal change examined in this section is the growing economic security of a proportion of the elderly which, in turn, has fueled an attitude that the elderly are financially better off than other age groups. Such an attitude also stereotypes the elderly as being "all alike"; it overlooks both the economic diversity among older people and that younger and older generations engage in reciprocal exchanges throughout life.

Health policies toward the elderly also have evolved in response to society's values and expectations of responsibility and need. Chapter 19 describes these policies; the impact of demographic changes, especially the increased number of the old-old with multiple chronic illnesses; the growing need for long-term care for older persons; the rising costs of health care; and current attempts at cost containment and their impact on the quality of health services provided to the older population. Innovative community-based services, such as respite and adult day health programs, have emerged in response to the escalating costs of hospital and nursing home care, but public funding for these programs is limited. Health promotion programs are one way to reduce the impact of chronic illness and the need for costly medical care among older people. Such programs are an important element of a comprehensive health policy, and reflect the growing societal attitude of individual responsibility for one's own health. The goals and components of health promotion for this population are discussed in Chapter 19.

Finally, we examine in the Epilogue the implications of a changing older population upon future health and social policy and programming. As noted throughout this book, society is undergoing major transitions regarding the position of older people. Changes such as the termination of mandatory retirement, the growing numbers of older people returning to school, and the increased proportions of workers covered by employer pension plans suggest that the cohort entering old age in the next few decades will be far different from previous ones. These changes will have a dramatic impact on society as a whole, as described in the Epilogue. The following vignettes illustrate the impact of changing societal attitudes and policies regarding the elderly upon individuals who have been raised in different eras.

An Older Person Born at the Turn of the Century

Mr. O'Brien was born in 1900 in New York City. His parents had immigrated to the United States from Ireland ten years earlier, in search of better employment opportunities for themselves and a better life for their children. One of Mr. O'Brien's brothers died during a flu epidemic while still in Ireland; a sister and brother who were born in New York died of measles. Mr. O'Brien and his three surviving siblings worked from the age of 12 in their parents' small grocery store. He could not continue his education beyond high school because his father's death of tuberculosis at age 45 left him in charge of the family store. Mr. O'Brien thought of signing up for the newly created Social Security program in 1940, but he was confident that he would not need any help from the government in his old age. The family grocery was supporting him and his wife quite well; he planned to work until the day he died, and besides, his family had all died in their forties and fifties anyway. He has been a heavy smoker all his life, just as his father had been. As he approaches his seventy-fifth birthday, however, Mr. O'Brien has been having second thoughts about old age. His emphysema and arthritis make it difficult for him to manage the store. He has had two heart attacks in the past ten years, both of which could have been fatal if it had not been for the skills of the emergency medical team and their sophisticated equipment in his local hospital. Mr. O'Brien's savings, which had seemed substantial a few years ago, now are dwindling as he pays for his wife's care in a nursing home, and for his medications and doctor's care for his heart condition, emphysema, and arthritis. Despite these struggles, Mr. O'Brien is reluctant to seek assistance from the government or from his children and grandchildren. They, in turn, assume that Mr. O'Brien is financially independent because he still works part-time, and never seems to require help from anybody.

An Individual Born in the Post-War Baby Boom

Ms. Smith was born in 1946, soon after WWII ended and her father returned from his military duty. Her father took advantage of the GI bill to complete his college education and purchase a home in one of the newly emerging suburbs around Chicago. As Ms. Smith grew up, her parents gave her all the advantages they had missed as children of the Depression: regular medical and dental check-ups, education in a private school, a weekly allowance, and a college trust fund. She completed college, obtained a Master's degree in business, and now holds a middle-level management position in a bank. She has already begun planning a "second career" by starting work on a Master's degree in systems analysis. Recognizing the value of health promotion at all ages, she has been a member of a health club for several years, participating in aerobic exercise classes and jogging every day. She has also encouraged her parents, now in their late sixties, to participate in health promotion activities in their local senior center. Her parents both receive pensions, are enrolled in Medicare Parts A and B, and have planned for the possibility of catastrophic illness by enrolling in a supplemental health insurance program. Ms. Smith has encouraged her parents to get on the waiting list of an excellent retirement community nearby, which includes a life contract for residential and nursing home care, should they ever need it. She is also considering some long-term investments that will support her if she needs long-term care or costly medical care as she herself reaches old age. In this way, both Ms. Smith and her parents are planning for an independent and, to the extent they can control it through prevention, a healthy old age.

These vignettes illustrate the changing attitudes and expectations about aging held by younger cohorts. The influence of these attitudes on social and health policy, as well as on individuals' planning for their own aging, are discussed in the remainder of this book.

Chapter 17

Attitudes Toward Older People

The focus of this chapter is on attitudes toward aging and old age. Previous chapters have emphasized that aging is a natural process that all individuals experience; yet there are more mistaken beliefs and stereotypes about how aging occurs, about the causes and outcomes of age-related social, physical, and psychological changes, and about the well-being of older people than about any other period of life. These misconceptions are widespread; they are reinforced by messages on birthday cards, by books on "how to avoid aging," and by pills and creams to eliminate wrinkles and "age spots." The makers of such products, which represent reactions of society against the outcomes of aging, play on the general public's fears and lack of knowledge about aging.

Throughout this book, the variations in the experience of aging have been emphasized; differences across cultural and ethnic minority groups, between men and women, and among other subgroups of the older population have been discussed. Even among the population over age 65, there are notable differences in the health and social status of the young-old and the old-old. Nevertheless, misconceptions about the later years and about older people are generally based on the assumption that there are more similarities than differences in the over-65 population. Think how often you have heard someone say, "Older people are all alike," or "Old age is second childhood."

These misconceptions are problematic because they can have significant implications for social policy and for behavior toward older people. Negative evaluations and stereotypic beliefs about older people are part of the larger social context that may influence the behavior of younger people toward elderly persons (Green, 1981). These attitudes can also determine the types of health and social policies that are developed (Butler, 1969; Brubaker and Powers, 1976), and play a role in the older person's sense of self (Bennett and Eckman, 1973; Brubaker and Powers, 1976). Retirement laws, for example, were enacted on the basis of beliefs about the inefficiency and lost work time of older workers. Discrimination (i.e., a behavior that is based on socially held beliefs) against older workers has resulted from such mistaken beliefs. Fortunately, federal laws have been designed to protect employees experiencing age discrimination. At the same time, researchers have shown that older workers are just as efficient and less often absent than young employees. Despite such data and the elimination of most mandatory retirement laws, mistaken beliefs about older workers persist.

To the extent that a society reinforces misconceptions about a particular age or racial group, members of that group may feel that they are indeed different from others. These feelings may lead to self-deprecation and a sense of worthlessness. On the other hand, a society that values old age and views each older person as an individual with unique abilities to contribute to the well-being of the social system can benefit itself and its older members. We saw in Chapter 2 the more productive roles of many elderly in historical times, and in other cultures such as the Japanese, Black, and Native American. Compared to contemporary Western society, these cultures tend to value other people's contributions to the welfare of society, and to emphasize the reciprocal nature of older members' roles, although there have always been exceptions to this pattern.

It is important to understand the roots of stereotypes and negative values about aging and old age if we are to change these beliefs to benefit both society and older people. The tremendous increase in the population over age 65 makes it imperative that we develop an accurate understanding about older people and about the impact of negative attitudes on intergenerational contacts and on social policies affecting older people. The recent debates about whether policies and services aimed at the population over age 65 are discriminatory because they are age-based, or benefit the elderly at the expense of younger populations (Neugarten, 1982) are an indication of society's ambivalent attitudes toward this segment of the population. Other ways in which attitudes influence the development of social and health policies are discussed in Chapters 18 and 19.

Attitudes represent an organized set of beliefs, evaluations, or values held about a particular object or group of objects. Attitudes include several components: *cognitions* (described as beliefs or stereotypes), *evaluations* or affect, and *behavioral intentions* (Fishbein, 1967; 1975; Triandis, 1971). Each of these components may have a positive or negative *valence*. That is, we may hold positive stereotypes such as "The majority of older people are financially well-off," or negative stereotypes such as "Most elderly are poor." As we have seen, neither stereotype describes accurately the status of older people today. Unfortunately, negative attitudes often prevail regarding groups with which people have little or no familiarity. These attitudes may evolve from fears of the unknown, from feelings of potential threat or of competition for jobs or other scarce resources, or from anxieties about characteristics represented by the group that one may also possess. Thus, for example, Americans may hold negative attitudes about members of another nationality who are a very small minority of the American population; whites may have negative attitudes about ethnic minorities whose skills create competition for certain jobs. In the case of the older population, negative attitudes often evolve from anxieties about one's own aging, and from fears of becoming frail and dependent. With the rapid growth in the population of people over age 80, and their increased needs for health and social services, there is also a growing concern among younger generations about competition for scarce financial resources between the oldest and youngest segments of society. These concerns may lead to heightened negative feelings toward older people in the future, and have already resulted in a public "backlash" against the elderly, who are mistakenly viewed as taking away services from younger generations and contributing to the federal deficit, as will be discussed further in Chapters 18 and 19.

Myths and Stereotypes About Aging

Stereotypes are generalized and simplified *beliefs* about a group of people or objects, and they may be positive or negative. A positive stereotype is one that attributes favorable characteristics to all objects or persons in a particular category; for example, "All old people are wise." Conversely, a negative stereotype ascribes unfavorable characteristics to all objects or persons in a certain category; for example, "All older people are cognitively impaired."

By forming stereotypes, we simplify reality and attempt to increase the comprehensibility of the world. This may serve a useful function, particularly in an uncertain and unfamiliar environment, or with events that require a routine response. For example, an individual who is visiting a foreign country for the first time generally relies on his or her stereotypes of that country and its people. As he or she becomes more familiar with the country, these stereotypes often disappear. The danger of stereotyping, however, is that it leads to an oversimplification of reality, often causing us to ignore characteristics that do not fit into a particular stereotype and to minimize individual differences among members of certain groups. Thus, for example, the stereotype that "all elderly persons are lonely" does not take into account the numerous older persons who have active social networks. People who hold such a stereotype tend to view the socially active older person as "atypical," and thus fail to expand their views about the elderly beyond these "exceptions."

More importantly, stereotypes may influence the way a person interacts with the elderly, or even whether or not one chooses to have contact with them. Stereotypes held by voters and legislators often lead to ill-conceived and ineffective social policies. For example, stereotypes held by policy makers about cognitive disorders and mental functioning in old age led, until recently, to a proliferation of nursing homes that were no more than warehouses where older people waited to die. Only in the past two decades has there been a movement toward more humane, supportive institutional design and community programs, such as adult day health and senior centers intended to enhance older people's cognitive functioning. These shifts in social policy may be traced, in part, to changes in stereotypes about dementia and to the recognition that environmental factors can influence the behavior and well-being of older persons who have various cognitive disorders.

Another common stereotype is that older people are isolated from friends and family, and that intergenerational caring and sharing was more common in "the good old days." As we saw in Chapter 2, however, the myth of "the good old days" has very little empirical support. Most families who historically shared households and caretaking with grandparents and great-grandparents did so out of economic necessity, and such families were rare even a century ago. On the other hand, as we saw in Chapter 10, families today provide a significant proportion of social, emotional, and health care for their older members. Federal policies and cuts in services that place greater caregiving demands on families are based on stereotypes that long have been shown to be inaccurate.

Stereotypes held about a social group also may influence the self-concept and self-esteem of individuals in that group. As we saw in Chapter 8, one's self-concept is developed through interactions with the environment, and it represents one's cognitive definition of the self. Self-esteem, on the other hand, is an evaluation of the self that is influenced by external reinforcement of one's identity, and through the loss and gain of social roles. Thus, if older people receive messages from individuals around them and from the media that they are perceived to be confused, frail, unattractive, and helpless, they are likely to adopt some of these assumptions about aging into their own self-concepts, and to assume that such characteristics are inevitable. Such stereotypes can also lead to misperceptions about "appropriate role behaviors," such as how the grandparent role or the retired role must be expressed by older people. These definitions of one's identity that are often inconsistent with one's own needs can then lead to self-criticism and loss of self-esteem. One strategy for coping with these stereotypes, adopted by a significant number of elderly persons, is to deny one's own aging, and to define oneself as "middle-aged" or "young," even among people over age 70 (Bultena and Powers, 1978). Another strategy is to adopt the behaviors into one's repertoire, and to fulfill societal role expectations, even though the individual's personality or interests may be inconsistent with these stereotyped expectations (e.g., an older woman who feels she must fit the role of a nurturant grandmother, even if she has no interest in babysitting her grand-children).

Stereotypes may be exaggerated if the individuals who hold them have particular anxieties or fears about their own aging. For example, by defining older persons to be as different from themselves as possible, people may maintain the image that they will never be like "them," thereby denying their own aging.

Although the examples presented above suggest that unfavorable stereotypes can have negative consequences, positive stereotypes also can result in inappropriate policies or ineffective actions on the part of service providers. One example of such a mistaken generalization is the belief that most people age 65 and over receive private pensions, thereby depicting all older persons as being better off than they really are. As we saw in Chapter 12, although large organizations are now generally required by law to provide pensions for their retiring employees, most older retirees today, particularly those who worked in small or family businesses, and many widows of men who held such jobs, do not have any private pension coverage. Even though 65 percent of the current cohort of older Americans have no pensions, some policy makers assume that all older people have adequate income sources so that public support of older persons is unnecessary or, at best, is only supplemental income.

DEVELOPMENT OF STEREOTYPES

Stereotypes evolve through interactions with the world around us. To the extent that we have direct contact with many different older people, we are more likely to develop individually based opinions and less likely to form generalized stereotypes. If, however, our direct experience with the elderly is limited or nonexistent, we must rely on the information obtained from peers, family members, and the media. Many young people grow up with very little contact with older people. Their grandparents may live in a different part of the country; they may have few elderly neighbors; and they perhaps obtain all their knowledge about the elderly in school. If friends and family denigrate older people, they serve as role models for the child who has had little or no experience with this population. The opinions formed on this basis are often fragmentary and generalized to *all* or most members of that group (i.e., stereotyped). Fortunately, the opportunities for young people to interact with older people are increasing through inter-generational programming in schools, churches, and youth organizations.

There is some debate about the role of television in forming stereotypes. As with many other topics, it has been argued that television presents a distorted and negative view of older people, especially in advertisements (Bishop and Krause, 1984). Some researchers have suggested that people who watch several hours of TV each week will adopt negative attitudes toward older people (Kubey, 1980; Gerbner, Gross, Signorielli, and Morgan, 1980). However, a critical review of the literature in this area and a study of knowledge about and attitudes toward older

Children's attitudes about the elderly often are based on interactions with grandparents and great-grandparents.

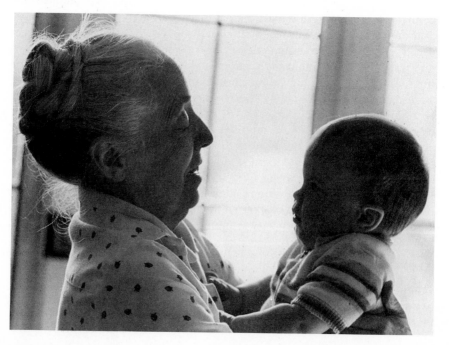

people among various age groups revealed that TV viewing has little impact on attitudes, and affects the knowledge of only some age groups (Passuth and Cook, 1985).

CHANGING STEREOTYPES

As stated above, stereotypic ideas about a given group often arise because of a lack of direct contact with that group. Generalizations may form on the basis of contact with a few of its members or from popular stereotypes communicated by the mass media, family members, peers, and society as a whole. The problem is not necessarily solved by increased contact, however. The "social contact hypothesis" suggests that contact with an "outgroup" may lead to more accurate perceptions of that group only under certain circumstances (Cook, 1969). Five factors are viewed as being critical to the reduction of stereotypes through social contact:

1. Equal status between ingroup and outgroup
2. A mutually interdependent relationship
3. A social climate favorable to egalitarianism
4. Outgroup participants who hold attributes that contradict stereotypes
5. A setting that promotes viewing the outgroup member as an individual, not as a member of a group

Although Cook tested this hypothesis with ethnic groups, one might expect his findings to apply to contacts between older and younger generations. Unfortunately, the conditions cited by Cook seldom exist between old and young in our society. Intergenerational contacts in Western countries generally are unequal, are not usually mutually interdependent (e.g., a young worker caring for an aged patient, or an older supervisor with a younger employee), and often occur in settings that promote stereotyping (e.g., in institutional settings). These conditions serve to reinforce stereotypes. In addition, such settings encourage stereotyping about the young by older persons. Even the relationship between grandparents and grandchildren may result in stereotypic views. On the one hand, those who remember loving grandparents who cared for them as children may develop idealized views of older people. On the other hand, those whose adult experiences include caring for a sick grandparent may generalize the stereotype of helplessness to all elderly. To the extent that intergenerational working or living situations can develop into egalitarian or interdependent arrangements, stereotypic beliefs will be reduced. Such mutually beneficial situations are possible through intergenerational homesharing and Foster Grandparents programs, through neighborhood efforts in which young and old work on community problems, as well as Phone Pals programs for latchkey children.

Increased contact with outgroups under the conditions recommended by Cook does not necessarily lead to greater liking for the outgroup. Both positive and negative characteristics of members of this outgroup are seen firsthand. As a result, perceptions become more *realistic*. Positive or negative stereotypes may persist, but it is more likely that these will be directed at individual group members, as one gets to know the diversity of the group. Thus, stereotypic responses to the group as a whole are diminished. The implications for ageist attitudes are clear. To the extent that younger persons interact with many different persons under egalitarian conditions and on an individual basis, the two groups can come to see each other as individuals with both good and bad traits, not as outsiders who are different from their peers merely because they differ in age. The latter perception is a form of prejudice, known as *ageism*, and will be described later in this chapter.

Another way to develop more accurate perceptions about the elderly is through coursework or other training in gerontology. Several researchers have reported a shift toward more realistic, less stereotypic perceptions among university students who took gerontology courses, and nurse aides who completed inservice training in geriatrics (Handschu, 1973; Beck et al., 1979; Kiyak et al., 1982). A review of research in this area, however, found that coursework may improve knowledge and create protective attitudes toward the elderly immediately following the course, but that it does not necessarily result in more realistic attitudes about the elderly in the long run (Coccaro and Miles 1984). It is also important to note that greater knowledge about older people does not result in more positive evaluations of this group (Holtzman and Beck, 1979; Michielutte and Diseker, 1985). Various courses that attempt to improve knowledge have been found to result in more positive, more negative, *and* more neutral evaluations of older people as a group (Kosberg, 1983). Although the number of elementary and secondary schools that teach gerontological topics has increased, more research is needed on the long-term effects of these programs on youth's evaluation of the elderly.

Unless the training program includes an opportunity to have contact with a variety of older persons, not only with the well elderly or with those in institutional settings, genuine attitudinal change is unlikely (Coccaro and Miles, 1984). It is also important to create a learning environment that encourages a view of the older population as a diverse group, and that avoids stereotyping by the nature of the material presented. Many textbooks and films, for example, depict older people in stereotypic roles. Instructors may also reinforce stereotypes by focusing course content on the diseases and losses associated with aging. It is important to portray the older population realistically, with its diverse elements.

The depiction of the elderly in the media also reflects society's attitudes about old age. There has been a growing effort by the media to draw attention to older persons who are successful and are continuing to make contributions in art, music, literature, science, and entertainment. Occasional news stories and documentaries about older people who have been exemplary in these areas can reinforce the fact that aging is not a disease or a lifestage to be feared, although ordinary older people who lead routine, satisfying lives, with whom most of us can identify, also need to be portrayed.

There also has been increased attention to the portrayal of older persons on television. Thanks to the vigorous efforts of the Gray Panthers and the National Council on the Aging, stereotypic and offensive portrayals of older persons are less common, while the presentation of older characters in more powerful and attractive roles has increased. As Atchley (1980) has noted, television portrayals of older persons are becoming more realistic and multifaceted. Older characters are shown in both a favorable and an unfavorable light, self-sufficient as well as dependent, and in positions of authority as well as lacking in power. For the first time in 1985, a television series portrayed the lives of four older women, all healthy, active, and intelligent. The success of this program surprised television producers and advertisers, and paved the way for other programs depicting older people in roles that did not suggest dependency or senility; this contrasted with earlier portrayals of nosy mothers-in-law, sickly grandfathers, and wizened old people who would be sought out only under extraordinary circumstances. Films portraying older people in independent, self-sufficient roles, such as *On Golden Pond* and *The Trip to Bountiful,* have also increased over the past several years.

Advertising can also serve to promote stereotypes or to present a more realistic view of aging. Unfortunately, advertisers have been slower than newspaper writers and television producers to integrate positive images of aging into their products. Aging continues to be associated with unattractiveness, a condition to be avoided, stopped, slowed, or ameliorated with products such as skin creams, make-up, vitamins, haircoloring, denture adhesives, and laxatives. To the extent that youth is idealized and old age is demeaned by these advertisers, negative attitudes toward this period in life, and toward this segment of the population, will be reinforced.

Nevertheless, societal attitudes toward aging and older people appear to have become more positive in recent years. Tibbitts (1979) attributes this positive change to the increasing visibility of older people in the media and in public roles, as well as to the growing positive self-evaluations of older people themselves. A positive shift has been found in college students' attitudes toward older people; in studies where they were asked to rank older people among various social minorities and disabled groups, they evaluated the elderly near the top (Nordby, 1985; Austin, 1985). It is difficult to assess whether older people are viewed more *accurately* today than they were 20 years ago, or if stereotypes have merely become more positive. Furthermore, it is difficult to determine if the public is more informed about the status of older people today, because comparative historical data on the factual knowledge held by the public are not available. Differences in measurement techniques over the years, as we will see later in this chapter, may account for these apparent changes toward more positive attitudes.

MEASURING STEREOTYPES

Stereotypes are measured in several ways. One of the earliest studies of attitudes toward aging and the aged (Tuckman and Lorge, 1953) involved a series of statements with which respondents were asked to agree or disagree. These statements were based on general knowledge and misconceptions; the responses could then be interpreted as to the level of accuracy or stereotypic thinking held by the respondent. It is important to reiterate that the respondent may be misinformed without feeling either negative toward or rejecting older persons; that is, both positive and negative stereotypes may be gleaned from responses to these statements.

A more recent and frequently used measure of beliefs about old age and elderly persons is the "Facts on Aging Quiz," developed by Palmore (1977). Using information derived from large national studies and from census data, Palmore prepared 25 statements describing the psychological, physiological, and demographic characteristics of persons age 65 and over. Slightly more than one-half of these items are factually true; the remainder are false. In a review of the research using this scale, Lutsky (1980) points out the consistency with which some items are missed by diverse respondent groups. It appears that many respondents are misinformed about the percentage of older persons in the general population and in long-term care settings as well as the extent of poverty and religiosity among the elderly; there is a tendency to overestimate the total number of elderly and those in institutions, as well as the number who are at or below the poverty level. As a result, respondents who, for example, do not know the percentage of older people in nursing homes are assumed to be stereotyping the elderly when, in fact, they do not *know* if the figures given in a statement are an overestimate or an underestimate. It is important to note that the "facts" in this quiz are based on studies conducted more than ten years ago; some of the information needs to be updated.

Other methods of measuring stereotypes include open-ended questions (e.g., the respondent is asked to describe characteristics of older people in his or her own words), word association techniques, adjective pairs, and projective techniques such as interpreting the meaning that a picture of a stimulus object has for the respondent (e.g., a picture of an older person engaged in "atypical" behavior). Since none of these methods has been tested widely in the area of attitudes toward the elderly, it is difficult to compare their relative merits.

Feelings Held Toward Older People

Affect is the evaluative dimension of attitudes that demonstrates liking or disliking, acceptance or rejection of a target group. Some gerontologists have suggested that societal values about aging have resulted in social stigmas, and therefore negative affect against elderly persons (Atchley, 1977; Butler, 1975). Research on

Interactions with a few older persons may result in positive affect toward those with whom one has contact, but not toward all elderly.

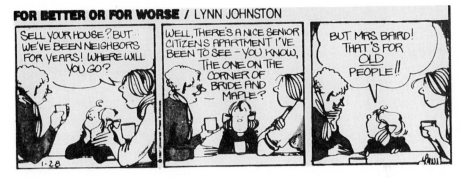

children's affect toward the elderly has shown that they respond positively to photos of older persons. At the same time, however, children associate old age with poor health and helplessness (Seefeldt et al., 1977; Hickey and Kalish, 1968; Thomas and Yamamoto, 1975). A review of studies in this area found negative expressions about older persons by young respondents (McTavish, 1971).

National surveys such as the one conducted by Louis Harris and Associates for the National Council on the Aging (1975) reveal that most people respond in a neutral manner in describing older persons. Thus, for example, in the Harris survey, only 8 percent rated older persons as not at all useful, 23 percent rated them as very useful, and the majority gave neutral evaluations. On the adjective pairs "friendly–unfriendly," and "wise–foolish," most respondents rated the older population on the positive ends of these scales.

The results of the Harris survey reveal that affect toward and stereotypes about older people may be inconsistent. That is, neutral evaluations in this study were often accompanied by stereotypes that the elderly are much worse off than they really are; 60 percent of the respondents believed that older people are lonely, 62 percent assumed that poverty was widespread, and 54 percent thought that older people felt useless, all of which are contrary to the facts about aging, as discussed in previous chapters. These beliefs, however, were not associated either with positive or negative evaluations of older people.

Many educators have bemoaned the lack of widespread interest among students in geriatric medicine, nursing, and dentistry, as well as the low priority given to treatment of older patients by psychiatrists, clinical psychologists, and social workers. These problems have often been attributed to the existence of negative attitudes toward older persons by the young. Despite these hypothesized associations between attitudes and behavior, few studies have been undertaken to test these relationships.

Most researchers have focused only on health care providers' *attitudes* (Chandler, Rachel, Kazelskis, 1986; Smith, Jepson, and Perloff, 1982; Green, 1981;

Taylor and Harned, 1978). Although differences in evaluations of older people have been reported among various health professionals, most groups hold neutral to positive perceptions. Knowledge about the elderly appears to vary more than does affect among different types and levels of health providers. In general, level of education has been found to be associated with knowledge about older people, but to have no impact on affect or evaluations of the elderly. A study of nurses revealed that respondents who had *less* experience with older people held more positive evaluations than those with more experience, although all respondents scored in the positive to neutral range (Taylor and Harned, 1978). However, a review of other studies of health professionals and the general public found that the *quality* of one's previous experiences with older people affects one's subsequent perceptions; to the extent that one's prior experiences have been positive, more favorable evaluations will be described by most respondents (Green, 1981). Such findings have relevance to the types of experiences that should be included in clinical training programs for health care providers. Students should have opportunities to interact with elderly in diverse settings—community clinics, senior centers, nursing homes, hospitals—and to view them in diverse roles, such as worker, volunteer, patient, and parent.

Studies of elderly persons' evaluations of their peers are rare. Somewhat surprisingly, respondents in their seventies are more likely than younger respondents to agree with stereotypic statements about the elderly (Ward, 1977). Studies that seek to determine respondents' preferences for people of various age groups have found that older respondents express greater preference for middle-aged persons than for older persons (Cameron and Cromer, 1974; Kogan, 1979). Such attitudes can be a significant barrier to recruiting older persons to age-based activities such as senior centers.

MEASURING AFFECT

One problem with research on evaluations of older people is the use of generalized stimuli such as "old people" or "young people" rather than a specific hypothetical person. Such general stimuli force the respondent to evaluate a whole class of people with no opportunity to indicate perceived variations among people within that group. Researchers who have asked respondents to rate *specific* older and younger stimulus persons have found equally positive evaluations of both age groups (Lawrence, 1974; Thomas and Yamamoto, 1975), or even more positive assessments of older stimulus persons (O'Connor et al., 1978). A study of attitudes of staff in facilities serving aged clients showed differences in evaluations of the stimuli "older persons in general," "my older clients," and "my own aging" (Kahana and Kiyak, 1982).

The most widely used measure of the affect dimension of attitudes is the semantic differential technique, using a series of adjective pairs (e.g., "good–bad," "friendly–unfriendly") within 5 to 7 points between them. A scale has been designed specifically to measure affect toward the elderly, and has been administered to diverse groups of adults and children (Rosencranz and McNevin, 1969). These scales may focus on specific stimulus persons, although, in the majority of studies, the stimulus is the general class of all elderly or young.

Preconceived Notions of Behavior Toward Older People

A third dimension of attitudes which has not been explored widely in gerontology is *behavioral intentions*. This term refers to the individual's preconceived notion of what he or she would do in certain situations with older persons. Knowledge about such behavioral intentions is helpful in developing educational and community programs for younger people who will be interacting with older people.

One method of measuring behavioral intentions is through the use of social distance scales, in which respondents are asked to indicate how comfortable they would feel with a stimulus person in various interpersonal situations (e.g., working with, eating with, living with that person or group of persons). A social distance scale has been designed specifically to ascertain how respondents would feel with persons of different ages in situations of increasing intimacy (e.g., "would sit next to the person on a bus" represents low intimacy; "would consider as a close friend" indicates high intimacy) (Kidwell and Booth, 1977). Increased age differences between the respondent and the stimulus person were found to lead to greater social distance, indicating less desirability of interacting with older persons. Older respondents expressed greater social distance from their age peers when compared with younger respondents.

Another method of measuring behavioral intentions is to ask respondents to rate their preference for working with the elderly. Studies of students in the health professions have revealed a generally low desire to work with older persons (Gale and Livesley, 1974; Geiger, 1978), even though evaluations of older persons may be just as positive as respondents' ratings of younger stimulus persons. This raises the issue of potential inconsistency among the three dimensions of attitudes. As we have already noted, positive affect toward older persons is not correlated with fewer stereotypes and a desire to interact with people in this age group (Gale and Livesley, 1974; Kahana and Kiyak, 1982). Furthermore, actual behavior toward older persons may be less related to any of the attitude dimensions than to social values or to the demands of a particular situation (Kahana and Kiyak, 1984). For example, a staff person in a nursing home with an institutional philosophy that older people should be encouraged to be independent may demonstrate such independence-oriented behavior in an effort to fit in with the organization's values, even though he or she believes that elderly in nursing homes are dependent.

Few studies have examined the relationship between attitudes and behavior toward older persons. This may be due to the difficulties of conducting the necessary longitudinal research, or of identifying behaviors that may be linked to specific attitudes. In the study by Kahana and Kiyak (1984), described earlier, staff in facilities for the elderly were found to display affect and behaviors that encouraged both dependency and independence. This study provided an opportunity to observe staff interacting with elderly clients within a few weeks after they completed questionnaires describing their stereotypes, affect, and behavioral intentions toward older persons. There was very little association between the staff person's self-reported affect and stereotypes and their observed behavior. In fact, the majority of behaviors were neutral, with few overtly positive or negative behaviors toward older clients. Behavioral intentions were most closely related to actual behaviors. That is, staff members who believed that older persons should be encouraged to take care of themselves were more likely to encourage independence-inducing behaviors than were staff who had endorsed behavioral intentions of encouraging dependency.

Ageism

Prejudice or rejection and labeling of a particular group of people develops because the individual attributes negative traits to all persons in that group. The societal impact of racial prejudice is widely recognized. But what is the effect of ageism, or prejudice against people merely on the basis of their age? Robert Butler (1969) coined the word *ageism* to describe the feelings of prejudice that result from misconceptions and myths about older people. This prejudice generally evolves from beliefs that aging makes people senile, unattractive, asexual, weak, and useless. Social discrimination on the basis of age may be a direct result of ageism, just as racism in the United States has reinforced social and political discrimination against ethnic minorities. The very existence of mandatory retirement has been a form of societal discrimination on the basis of age alone. Discrimination may be expressed in other ways. For example, older workers generally experience more difficulty finding new jobs, or reentering the job market. This is in part due to the prejudices held by employers regarding older people's abilities to learn new tasks or to keep up with the pace, and in part due to the large pool of new job candidates who are willing to work for lower salaries. Even with the passage of legislation that prohibits discrimination on the basis of age, older job applicants still frequently face signs of ageism when they meet many potential employers. Public agencies may also practice subtle forms of age discrimination by excluding older persons from their target populations or by underserving them.

It should be noted, however, that age discrimination may be practiced against other age groups as well. For example, many chore, nutritional, and low-cost health programs are aimed at persons over age 60, and exclude younger persons with disabilities who may also need these services. Young people may be rejected for a job because they "appear too young," and thus are assumed to be irresponsible. Policy debates regarding the potential discriminatory nature of age-based legislation are relevant in this discussion of age discrimination (Neugarten, 1982). However, the development of age-based programs may be a necessary consequence of society's attempt to meet the social and health needs of many older people.

Ageism on a societal level has also resulted in policies that serve to reduce the older person's independence and decision-making options. Until recently, frail elderly who could no longer maintain their own homes had no choice but to enter congregate living or institutional arrangements. Now, however, government funding of home-based services, such as hot meals, chore services, and health care through the Older Americans Act, has enhanced some options for living independently, while at the same time reducing the cost of health care for vulnerable elderly. These policy changes have taken place to some extent because of a shift in society's beliefs about the capabilities and needs of older persons (i.e., a reduction in ageism on a societal level).

It has also been suggested that some advocates of the elderly, in their zeal to improve the status of the more disadvantaged, have emphasized the need to do more *for* older people (Kalish, 1979). This form of ageism has been labeled "the new ageism." It is characterized by focusing on the least able elderly, who are viewed as powerless, dependent, and victimized, and by encouraging the development of services that do not enhance older people's independence. This "new ageism" may be just as detrimental to the self-esteem of older people as is the more typical form of ageism. It may also result in the expectation on the part of some older people that they must overcompensate for this perceived helplessness by remaining active in old age, even when they would prefer to become disengaged from social responsibilities. It is therefore important that advocates of the elderly, service providers, and older people themselves recognize the diversity in this population, and work toward maintaining the independence of the many elderly who are self-sufficient, while assisting those who need help.

The increased number of social and health services for older clients has produced unexpected problems in some cases. The staff of these services are often young, in many cases decades younger than the older client. This may result in interpersonal tension because the young staff person does not have the empathy to understand the special needs and concerns of older clients (Kahana and Kiyak, 1984; Behn and Stewart, 1982). Indeed, some aging advocates have suggested that programs funded through the Older Americans Act should hire only people age 60 and over.

Summary and Implications

Old age and the aging process are surrounded by more misconceptions than any other period of life. These mistaken beliefs grow out of people's fears about their own aging, and are reinforced by messages in the media and in advertising that emphasize the adverse effects of aging. Widely held beliefs about a particular group can have a significant impact on social interactions with members of that group, on social policies that influence the group, and on the self-concept of group members. In the case of older people, retirement and employment policies have been based on widely held beliefs—many of which have since been shown to be invalid—about how aging affects job performance. Surveys of public attitudes about aging have revealed that even the older population themselves endorse many negative descriptions of aging and old people.

Stereotypes are not unusual before we become acquainted with a particular group, but they must be replaced by accurate information as our familiarity with the group increases. Both positive and negative stereotypes may have unfortunate consequences for older people, because society may expect too much or too little from the aging person. Stereotypes can be reduced by gaining more knowledge about aging, and by increasing our contact with older people in an egalitarian or mutually interdependent setting. It is also important to interact with different types of older people in order to understand variations in the aging experience. The powerful impact of the media—television, newspapers, and magazines—can be used to dispel myths about aging as well as to create such myths. With increasing pressure from organizations concerned about older people, there has been a significant improvement in the portrayal of old age on television, and to a lesser extent in TV and print advertising.

Researchers have developed numerous measures of stereotypes about aging and old age. Most measures ask the respondent to agree or disagree with a series of statements that describe the "typical" older person. These methods often rely on factual information; thus it is difficult to distinguish stereotyped responses from simply not knowing the information precisely. Other methods, which rely less on factual knowledge but suffer from difficulties in interpreting the meaning of the information, are open-ended questions and word-association tests.

The evaluative or affective component of attitudes has been assessed by asking respondents to rate older people on a series of adjective pairs such as "friendly–hostile," "good–bad." Most studies have revealed neutral affect toward older persons, with college students expressing fewer positive responses than children or middle-aged adults.

Behavioral intentions toward older people have not been tested widely. Researchers using social distance scales have found preference for less social intimacy with older stimulus persons described in these scales, and less desire to work in settings with older people. But such intentions are generally not correlated with actual behavior toward older persons. Ageism is the tendency to label and judge an individual on the basis of age alone. Although age discrimination has been outlawed in employment, it is widespread in informal social situations, in organizations with older members, even in organizations that serve older people. Indeed, ageism may result in social policies that are intended to help older people, but actually may reinforce stereotyped beliefs and behaviors by younger people. As with stereotypes about aging in general, ageist attitudes can be detrimental for the psychological well-being of older people.

Further research is needed to determine the impact of social attitudes on behavior toward older persons, on policies aimed at this population, and on the development of older persons' self-esteem. Both cross-sectional and longitudinal studies are necessary. In particular, it is important to assess the effect of interventions aimed at changing attitudes. For example, what is the long-term influence of intergenerational programs that aim to develop more positive attitudes about the elderly in young children? How can the reduction of stereotypes influence a professional person's desire or willingness to work with older clients? These and other attitude-behavior associations must be examined if we are to gain a deeper understanding of the effect of attitudes on the lives of older persons, and on their social interactions with the young.

References

Atchley, R. C. *The social forces in later life* (2d ed.). Belmont, Calif.: Wadsworth, 1977.

Atchley, R. C. *The social forces in later life* (3rd ed.). Belmont, Calif.: Wadsworth, 1980.

Austin, D. R. Attitudes toward old age: A hierarchical study. *The Gerontologist*, 1985, *25*, 431–434.

Beck, J.D., Ettinger, R. L., Glenn, R. E., Paule, C. L., and Holtzman, J. M. Oral health status: Impact on dental student attitudes toward the aged. *The Gerontologist*, 1979, *19*, 580–584.

Behn, J. D., and Stewart, B. J. A behavioral study of the service provision encounter. Paper presented at meetings of the Gerontological Society of America. Boston, 1982.

Bennett, R., and Eckman, J. Attitudes toward aging: A critical examination of recent literature and implications for future research. In C. Eisdorfer and M. P. Lawton (Eds.), *The psychology of adult development and aging.* Washington, D.C.: American Psychological Association, 1973.

Bishop, J. M., and Krause, D. R. Depictions of aging and old age on Saturday morning television. *The Gerontologist*, 1984, *24*, 91–94.

Brubaker, T. H., and Powers, E. A. The stereotype of "old": A review and alternative approach. *Journal of Gerontology*, 1976, *31*, 441–447.

Bultena, G. L., and Powers, E. A. Denial of aging: Age identification and reference group orientations. *Journal of Gerontology*, 1978, *33*, 748–754.

Butler, R. N. Ageism: Another form of bigotry. *The Gerontologist*, 1969, *9*, 243–246.

Butler, R. N. *Why survive? Being old in America.* New York: Harper, 1975.

Cameron, P., and Cromer, A. Generational homophyly. *Journal of Gerontology*, 1974, *29*, 232–236.

Chandler, J. T., Rachel, J. R., and Kazelskis, R. Attitudes of long-term care nursing personnel toward the elderly. *The Gerontologist*, 1986, *26*, 551–555.

Coccaro, E. F., and Miles, A. M. The attitudinal impact of training in gerontology-geriatrics in medical school. *Journal of the American Geriatrics Society*, 1984, *32*, 762–768.

Cook, S. W. Motives in a conceptual analysis of attitude-related behavior. In W. J. Arnold and D. Levine (Eds.), *Nebraska symposium on motivation.* Lincoln: University of Nebraska Press, 1969.

Fishbein, M. (Ed.). *Readings in attitude theory and measurement.* New York: John Wiley and Sons, 1967.

Fishbein, M. *Belief, attitude, intention and behavior.* Reading, Mass.: Addison-Wesley, 1975.

Gale, J., and Livesley, B. Attitudes toward geriatrics: A report of the King's survey. *Age and Aging*, 1974, *3*, 49–53.

Geiger, D. L. How future professionals view the elderly: A comparative analysis of social work, law, and medical students' perceptions. *The Gerontologist*, 1978, *18*, 591–594.

Gerbner, G., Gross, L., Signorielli, N., and Morgan, M. Aging with television: Images in TV drama and conceptions of social reality. *Journal of Communication*, 1980, *30*, 37–47.

Grad, S. Incomes of the aged and nonaged: 1950–1982. *Social Security Bulletin*, 1984, *47*, 3–17.

Green, S. K. Attitudes and perceptions about the elderly: Current and future perspectives. *International Journal of Aging and Human Development*, 1981, *13*, 99–119.

Handschu, S. Profile of the nurses' aide: Expanding her role as psycho-social companion to the nursing home resident. *The Gerontologist*, 1973, *13*, 315–377.

Harris, L. and Associates. *The myth and reality of aging in America.* Washington, D.C.: National Council on Aging, 1975.

Hickey, T., and Kalish, R. A. Young people's perceptions of adults. *Journal of Gerontology*, 1968, *23*, 215–219.

Holtzman, J. M., and Beck, J. D. Palmore's "Facts on Aging Quiz": A reappraisal. *The Gerontologist*, 1979, *19*, 116–120.

Kahana, E. F., and Kiyak, H. A. *Attitudes toward the elderly: antecedents, content and outcome.* Final report submitted to the National Institute on Aging, 1982.

Kahana, E. F., and Kiyak, H. A. Attitudes and behavior of staff in facilities for the aged. *Research on Aging*, 1984, *6*, 395–416.

Kalish, R. A. The new ageism and the failure models: A polemic. *The Gerontologist*, 1979, *19*, 398–402.

Kidwell, I. J., and Booth, A. Social distance and intergenerational relations. *The Gerontologist*, 1977, *17*, 412–420.

Kiyak, H. A., Milgrom, P., Ratener, P., and Conrad, D. Dentists' attitudes toward and knowledge of the elderly. *Journal of Dental Education*, 1982, *46*, 266–273.

Kogan, N. A. A study of age categorization. *Journal of Gerontology*, 1979, *34*, 358–367.

Kosberg, J. J. The importance of attitudes on the interaction between health care providers and geriatric populations. *Interdisciplinary Topics in Gerontology*, 1983, *17*, 132–143.

Kubey, R. W. Television and aging: Past, present, and future. *The Gerontologist*, 1980, *20*, 16–35.

Lawrence, J. H. The effect of perceived age on initial impressions and normative role expectations. *International Journal of Aging and Human Development*, 1974, *5*, 369–391.

Lutsky, N. S. Attitudes toward old age and elderly persons. In C. Eisdorfer (Ed.), *Annual review of gerontology and geriatrics* (Vol. 1). New York: Springer, 1980.

McTavish, D. G. Perceptions of old people: A review of research methodologies and findings. *The Gerontologist*, 1971, *11*, 90–101.

Michielutte, R., and Diseker, R. A. Health care providers' perceptions of the elderly and level of interest in geriatrics as a specialty. *Gerontology and Geriatrics Education*, 1985, *5*, 65–85.

Naus, P. J. Some correlates of attitudes toward old people. *International Journal of Aging and Human Development*, 1973, *4*, 229–242.

Neugarten, B. L. *Age or need? Public policies for older people.* Beverly Hills: Sage, 1982.

Nordby, N. A. Acceptance of selected disabilities by university graduate students. Unpublished manuscript. Bloomington: Indiana University. Cited in D. R. Austin, Attitudes toward old age: A hierarchical study. *The Gerontologist*, 1985, *25*, 431–434.

O'Connor, C., Walsh, P., Litzelman, D., and Alvarez, M. Evaluations of job applicants: The effects of age versus success. *Journal of Gerontology*, 1978, *33*, 246–252.

Palmore, E. Facts on Aging: A short quiz. *The Gerontologist*, 1977, *17*, 315–320.

Passuth, P. M., and Cook, F. L. Effects of television viewing on knowledge and attitudes about older adults: A critical re-examination. *The Gerontologist*, 1985, *25*, 69–77.

Rosencranz, M. A., and McNevin, T. E. A factor analysis of attitudes toward the aged. *The Gerontologist*, 1969, *9*, 55–59.

Seefeldt, C., Jantz, R. K., Galper, A., and Serock, K. Using pictures to explore children's attitudes toward the elderly. *The Gerontologist*, 1977, *17*, 506–512.

Smith, S. P., Jepson, V., and Perloff, E. Attitudes of nursing care providers toward elderly patients. *Nursing and Health Care*, 1982, *3*, 93–98.

Taylor, K. H., and Harned, T. L. Attitudes toward old people: A study of nurses who care for the elderly. *Journal of Gerontological Nursing*, 1978, *4*, 43–47.

Thomas, E. C., and Yamamoto, K. Attitudes toward age: An exploration in school-age children. *International Journal of Aging and Human Development*, 1975, *6*, 117–129.

Tibbitts, C. Can we invalidate negative stereotypes in aging? *The Gerontologist*, 1979, *19*, 10–20.

Triandis, H. C. *Attitudes and attitude change.* New York: John Wiley and Sons, 1971.

Tuckman, J., and Lorge, I. Attitudes toward old people. *Journal of Social Psychology*, 1953, *37*, 249–260.

Ward, R. A. The impact of subjective age and stigma on older persons. *Journal of Gerontology,* 1977, *32*, 227–232.

Weinberger, L. E., and Millham, J. A multi-dimensional, multiple method analysis of attitudes toward the elderly. *Journal of Gerontology,* 1975, *30*, 343–348.

Chapter 18

Social Policies to Address Social Problems

A wide range of policies have been established within the past 20 years in efforts to improve the social, physical, and economic environments of older people described throughout this book. Approximately 50 major programs are directed specifically toward older persons, with another 200 programs affecting them indirectly. Prior to the 1960s, however, the United States lagged behind most European countries in its development of policy for the aging. Accordingly, the percentage of the Gross National Product spent and the extent of tax support for programs for the older population are greater in Europe than in the United States. For example, Social Security benefits were not awarded in the United States until 1940, whereas alternative Social Security systems were instituted in the nineteenth century in most western European countries. The United States has slowly and cautiously accepted the concept of public responsibility for dependent persons.

Since the 1960s, however, federal spending for aging programs has rapidly expanded, resulting in what has been called the "graying of the federal budget." Medicare has increased nearly tenfold since its inception in 1965, while Old Age Survivors Insurance under Social Security tripled between 1970 and 1979 (Clark and Menfee, 1981). The growth in federal support for programs benefiting older persons is vividly shown through budgetary figures. In 1960, the value of benefits for the elderly under federal programs was approximately $17 billion and represented 13 percent of the federal budget. By 1985, age-specific spending approached $265 billion, forming approximately 29 percent of the budget for an age group representing 11.8 percent of the population (U.S. Senate Special Committee on Aging, 1986).

It is important to recognize, however, that when Social Security and Medicare are excluded from these allocations, only about 4 percent of the total federal budget is devoted to aging programs. The growing percentage of allocations also masks the fact that funded services are often fragmented, duplicated, and inadequate in reaching those with greatest need (Minkler and Estes, 1984; Fisher, 1980). Without an integrated and comprehensive social policy toward older persons, the United States, despite growing allocations to age-based programs, is increasingly faced with complex unresolved policy dilemmas. Former Secretary of the Department of Health and Human Services Joseph Califano stated this succinctly: "To confront the graying of America may demand more political courage than any other domestic issue of the 1980s" (1981).

This and the next chapter describe the social and health programs, processes, and consequences of the "graying of America." First, policy is defined, types of policies are differentiated, and factors that affect policy development are identified. The relatively slow development of policies for older persons prior to the 1960s is contrasted with the rapid expansion of programs in the 1970s and the federal budget cuts of the 1980s; the policy impacts of the White House Conferences on Aging and of public perceptions about the "deservingness" of older persons are then reviewed. The two major programs that comprise the bulk of federal expenditures and thus shape public policy on old age are discussed:

first, Social Security, which comprises nearly 15 percent of federal expenditures, and then in Chapter 19, Medicare and Medicaid, which constitute nearly 7 percent of federal spending (U.S. House Select Committee on Aging, 1985). The development and coordination of direct social services, comprising less than 1 percent of federal expenditures for older people, and housing programs are also described. Each chapter concludes with a discussion of policy dilemmas, which have numerous implications for future directions discussed in the Epilogue.

Variations Among Policies and Programs

Policy refers generally to the principles that govern action directed toward specific ends. It is within the purview of social policy not only to identify problems, but also to take action to ameliorate them. The development of policy thus implies change in both means and ends: changing situations, systems, practices, or behaviors (Abel-Smith and Titmuss, 1979). The procedures governments develop for making such changes encompass planned interventions, bureaucratic structures for implementing interventions, and regulations governing the distribution of public funds. Policy for the elderly reflects society's definition of what choices to make in meeting their needs and how to share such responsibilities between the public and private sectors. Each policy development serves to determine which older persons should receive what benefits, from which sources, and on what basis.

Social programs are the visible manifestations of social policies. The implementation of the 1965 Older Americans Act, for example, resulted in a wide range of programs, including multipurpose senior centers, nutrition sites, homemaker and home health services, and adult day care. Some programs are designed specifically for older people, whereas others benefit them indirectly. Programs can be differentiated from each other in many ways; these dimensions are presented in Table 18–1 and described below.

1. *Eligibility criteria*   For example, in some programs, eligibility for benefits depends on *age alone* (i.e., a person's age entitles him or her to benefits such as Medicare at age 65), whereas in other programs, eligibility depends on *financial need* (i.e., a person's financial need entitles him or her to program benefits, such as Medicaid, food stamps, and public housing). Although *age entitlement* programs are categorical and specifically for older persons, *need entitlement* programs affect all age populations who meet particular income criteria. Need entitlement programs include taxation practices that redistribute income among the population and means-tested programs for low-income older and disabled persons, such as Supplemental Security Income.

2. *Form of benefits*   Another variation is the form in which benefits are

TABLE 18–1 Dimensions Along Which Programs and Policies Vary

	Examples
Eligibility	
On basis of age	Medicare
On basis of financial need	Supplemental Security Income
Form of benefits	
Cash	
Direct cash transfers	Society Security
Indirect cash transfers	Income tax exemption
Cash substitute	
Direct cash substitutes	Vouchers
Indirect cash substitutes	Medicare payments to service providers
Method of financing	
Contributory	Social Security
Noncontributory	Supplemental Security Income
Universal or selective benefits	
Universal—for all persons who belong to a particular category	Older Americans Act
Selective—determined on an individual basis	Food stamps

given—either *directly* or *indirectly* through a *cash transfer* or a *cash substitute*. Social Security benefits are a direct cash transfer, whereas tax policies that affect selected groups (e.g., personal income tax exemptions for older persons) are indirect cash transfers of funds from one segment of the population to another. An example of a direct cash substitute is vouchers for the restricted purchase of goods, such as food stamps and rent supplements. Medicare payments to service providers, rather than directly to beneficiaries, are indirect cash substitutes.

3. *Method of financing*   Programs also vary in how they are financed. Social Security and Medicare are *contributory programs;* benefit entitlement is tied to a person's contributions to the system through his or her status as a paid worker. On the other hand, Supplemental Security Income (SSI) is a *noncontributory program* available to older persons who meet financial criteria, regardless of their contributions through payroll taxes.

4. *Universal or selective benefits*   Programs differ according to whether they benefit populations on a universal or selective basis. Benefits from universal programs are available on the basis of social right to all persons belonging to a designated group—generally a category of people who have common needs

unmet by existing institutional arrangements. Eligibility is established by virtue of belonging to that group (e.g., to the older population). Medicare, the Old Age Survivors Insurance of Social Security, and the Older Americans Act are *universal-class* programs for all other Americans. In contrast, *selective benefits* are determined individually. Selective benefits include Supplementary Security Income, Medicaid, food stamps, and housing subsidies, which use economic need as a criterion.

Factors Affecting the Development of Policies

Despite the orderliness of these dimensions, the policy development process is not necessarily rational. A major characteristic of our public policy process is its shortsightedness—its general inability, because of annual budgetary cycles and the frequency of national elections, to deal with long-term economic and social trends, or to anticipate future consequences of policies established to meet today's needs or political imperatives. In an aging society, shortsightedness in policy development is fraught with dangers.

The complexity of the process of public policy formation for the elderly is also magnified by the variety of societal factors influencing it. These factors include values and beliefs; economic, social, and governmental structures; the configuration of domestic and international problems; powerful interest groups; and even random events or the chance appearance of charismatic political figures.

Two different sets of values have been played out in American social policies. In one, individual welfare is held to be essentially the individual's responsibility within a free-market economy unfettered by government control. The second set of values assumes individual welfare to be the responsibility both of the individual and the community at large. Government intervention is necessary to compensate for the free market's failure to distribute goods and opportunities equitably. Since the New Deal of the 1930s, public policy has oscillated between these two value orientations as public mood and national administrations have shifted. The increasingly frequent debate about the nature and extent of public provisions versus the responsibility of individuals, families, and private philanthropy thus has moral overtones. Judgments about the relative worth of vulnerable populations that compete for a share of limited resources, and about the proper divisions between public and private responsibilities are ultimately based on values (or preferences) held by individuals or groups. A major policy issue thus revolves around the question of whose values shape policy.

American *cultural values* of productivity, independence, and youthfulness, *public attitudes* toward governmental programs and toward the elderly, and *public perceptions* of older people as "deserving" have converged to create universal categorical programs that are limited to older persons, but available to *all* elderly, regardless of their income. In contrast, policies that use income (e.g., means-testing) to determine whether a person is "deserving" of services reflect our cultural bias toward productivity and independence; means-tested policies, such as Supplemental Security Income, are used to determine the eligibility of low-income elderly for financial assistance.

The American public tends to view older people as more deserving of assistance than other welfare recipients. In fact, public support for programs for older people has been ahead of benefits for the disabled, schools, and the poor, and second only to national defense (Klemmack and Roff, 1981; National Council on the Aging, 1981). While Congress debates how much to reduce public assistance programs that benefit primarily younger people, Social Security and Medicare have generally been viewed as inviolate and not to be cut drastically. The passage of such otherwise unpopular programs as a national health insurance for older people (i.e., Medicare) and guaranteed income for the elderly (i.e., Supplemental Security Income) can be partially explained by the fact that older persons as a group arouse public support and a favorable response from politicians who often cater to their votes.

Society's technical and financial resources and current economic conditions (e.g., unemployment, inflation, recession) also significantly influence policy development. Medicare and the Older Americans Act, for example, were passed during the 1960s and early 1970s. This was a period of economic growth and optimism, with government resources expanding under the so-called War on Poverty on behalf of both the young poor and the elderly. Adverse economic conditions also can create a climate conducive to the passage of income maintenance policies. For instance, Social Security was enacted in part because the Great Depression dislodged the middle class from financial security and from their belief that older people who needed financial assistance were undeserving of aid. A strategy to increase the number of persons retiring at age 65 was also congruent with economic pressures to reduce widespread unemployment in the 1930s. With economic constraints, program cost factors were salient. For example, a public pension was assumed to cost less than relying on local poorhouses, as had been the practice prior to the 1920s. Thus, a variety of economic and resource factors converged to create the necessary public and legislative support for a system of social insurance in the 1930s.

The influence of both economic resources and cultural values is also evident in the current public emphasis on fiscal austerity, private responsibility for the care of older persons, program cost-effectiveness, and targeting services to those most in need. Periods of scarcity tend to produce limited and often punitive legislative responses, as in the 1980s. For example, with the current high budget deficits, conservative legislators have advocated reducing Medicare benefits, even though such a move angers many older Americans and their advocates. In such instances, financial considerations generally supersede public support for older people.

The Residual and Incremental Nature of Policies for the Elderly

These cultural values, economic conditions, and consequent resource capability underlie the fact that American policy for the elderly tends to be *categorical, residual,* and *incremental.* As noted above, eligibility for categorical programs is determined by belonging to a particular age group. Residual and incremental policies assume that when the family or market economy does not adequately meet individuals' needs, then social and health programs attend to emergency functions. In other words, programs are developed to respond incrementally to crisis conditions, not to prevent problems from arising nor to attack their underlying causes.

In her critique of this approach, Estes (1979; 1984) maintains that our conceptions of aging have socially constructed the major problems faced by the elderly and thereby have adversely influenced U.S. age-based policies. These conceptions, discussed as the political economy perspective in Chapter 3, are:

1. Older people, not economic or social structural conditions, are defined as a "social problem."

2. Older people are seen as special and different, requiring separate programs.

3. The problems of older people are individually generated, best treated through medical services to individuals.

4. The use of costly medical services is justified by characterizing old age as a period of inevitable physical decline.

5. There is a growing perception that problems of the elderly cannot be solved by national programs, but rather by initiatives of state and local governments, the private sector, or the individual.

According to Estes, these are actually misconceptions that have fostered an old age policy structure that assumes that treating individuals through services, not through guaranteed income, health care, or employment, can solve "the problem" of aging. Yet, our societal failure to develop a comprehensive, coordinated policy framework has served to reinforce older persons' marginality and to segregate them (Estes, 1984; 1979).

Whereas Estes contends that policies for older people are inadequate, others maintain that the elderly are "busting the budget" and that expenditures for older persons are a primary reason for current fiscal crises, especially the growing federal budget deficit (Samuelson, 1978; Lammers, 1983). In reality, however, the net contribution of Social Security and Medicare to the federal deficit has been the same since 1980. Tax cuts, military defense hikes, and spiraling interest costs, not programs for the elderly, have primarily contributed to the federal deficit (Storey, 1986; Estes, 1984). Within this context of the types of programs and factors affecting policy development, we turn now to the development of public policy for older persons in the United States.

The Development of Aging Policy

1930–1950

Compared to European countries with similar levels of socioeconomic development, the United States has more slowly implemented policies affecting the aging population. Factors such as the lower percentage of older persons in the population in the past, a strong belief in individual responsibility, and the free-market economy partially explain this slower pace. Table 18–2 traces the historical development of aging policy. The Social Security Act of 1935 was the first major policy enacted for older persons. Justified as a "pay as you go" system of financing, the act is based on an implicit guarantee that the succeeding generation will provide for its elderly through their Social Security contributions. The original provisions of the act were intended to be only the beginning of a universal program covering all "major hazards" in life. Tragically, the concept of

TABLE 18–2 Major Historical Developments of Aging Policy

1935	Social Security Act
1950	Amendments to assist states with health care costs
1959	Section 202 Direct Loan Program of the Housing Act
1960	Extension of Social Security benefits
	Advisory commissions on aging
1961	Senate Special Committee on Aging
1961	First White House Conference on Aging
1965	Medicare and Medicaid, Older Americans Act, Establishment of Administration on Aging
1971	Second White House Conference on Aging
1972 & 1977	Social Security Amendments
1974	Supplemental Security Income
1974	Title XX
1974	House Select Committee on Aging
1974	Change in mandatory retirement age
1974	Establishment of the National Institute on Aging
1980	Federal measures to control health care expenditures
1981	Third White House Conference on Aging
1981	Social Services Block Grant Program
1986	Elimination of mandatory retirement

the program in its entirety, including a nationwide program for preventing sickness and ensuring security for children, was never realized.

After Social Security's passage, national interest in policies to benefit older persons subsided. An exception was provided by President Truman's advocacy to expand Social Security benefits and to launch a national health insurance plan. His efforts for a national health insurance were opposed by organizations such as the American Medical Association. President Truman did succeed, however, in his push for an amendment to Social Security in 1950 to provide financial help to states that chose to pay partial health care costs for needy older persons. This amendment then became the basis for the establishment of Medicare in 1965. In the late 1950s, Social Security benefits were extended to farmers, self-employed persons, and some state and local government employees. In approximately half the states, advisory commissions on aging were formed; and in 1961, the Senate Special Committee on Aging was established.

PROGRAM EXPANSION IN THE 1960s AND 1970s

Since the 1960s, programs directed at the welfare of older people have rapidly evolved, including Medicare, Medicaid, the Older Americans Act, Supplemental Security Income (SSI), the Social Security Amendments of 1972 and 1977, Section 202 Housing, and Title XX social services legislation. The pervasiveness of "compassionate stereotypes," which assumed all elderly to be poor, frail, ill-housed, and unable to keep up with inflation, undoubtedly influenced this rapid development (Binstock, 1983). As discussed in Chapter 17, policy issues are frequently framed in terms of ageism, whereby the same characteristics and status are attributed to a group labeled "the aged" (Binstock, 1984). A negative consequence of "compassionate ageism," for example, was a tendency to develop programs that obscured individual and subgroup differences among the elderly (Minkler, 1984). On the other hand, such stereotypes served to create a "permissive consensus" for government action on age-based services in the 1960s and 1970s, as illustrated by the discussion of programs below (Hudson, 1978).

The first White House Conference on Aging in 1961 was significant in highlighting older people's needs. Four years later, Medicare, Medicaid, and the Older Americans Act were passed. Although the Older Americans Act established the Administration on Aging at the federal level, as well as statewide area agencies to provide aging services, funding to implement these provisions was low. Therefore, one of the primary objectives of the 1971 White House Conference on Aging was to strengthen the Older Americans Act. In 1972, Social Security benefits were expanded 20 percent, and the system of indexing benefits to take account of inflation ("cost of living adjustments" or COLA) was established. Additional funding was provided for the Older Americans Act in 1973. The 1970s witnessed more developments to maintain the elderly's income: the creation of the Supplemental Security Income (SSI) program, protection of private pensions, formation of the House Select Committee on Aging, increases in Social Security benefit levels and taxes, and the change in mandatory retirement from age 65 to age 70. (As noted in Chapter 12, mandatory retirement was later abolished for most jobs in 1986.) During this period of federal government expansion, more than 40 different national committees and subcommittees were involved in legislative efforts affecting older people (Binstock, 1983).

A large constituency—including those older people who are not poor, frail, or inadequately housed—has benefited from the policy consensus built upon the "compassionate stereotype." In fact, Estes contends that human services professionals, such as administrators, medical personnel, and social service staff, gained from this program development more than did the elderly population most in need of services (1979), thus creating a "service enterprise." Despite these improvements in the benefits offered to older persons, many people with the greatest needs, such as older women and ethnic minorities, continue to be inadequately served by these programs, as described in Chapters 15 and 16.

PROGRAM REDUCTIONS IN THE 1980s

The 1980s have been characterized by diverse and often contradictory tendencies in public perceptions and support for aging programs. Aging advocates have urged more funding and legislation, especially for social services and housing, and have watched closely that Social Security not be cut. Concern over the future of Social Security was fueled by the near-term deficit facing the Social Security trust fund. As a result, Social Security was amended in 1983 to address financing problems. As public scrutiny of the costs of Social Security, Medicare, and Medicaid has grown, cost-efficiency measures have been implemented, oftentimes at the expense of assuring that low-income groups are not further disadvantaged.

Some policy analysts have suggested that the "compassionate stereotype" has been replaced in the 1980s by a new stereotype of the elderly as relatively well-off and benefiting at the expense of younger groups, thereby scapegoating the elderly or "blaming the victim" (Binstock, 1983; Minkler and Estes, 1984). For example, the 1985 report of the President's Council of Economic Advisors maintains that older families have been better able to keep with inflation, due to Social Security cost-of-living increases, than have younger families. Likewise, a Harvard University study that compared average government expenditures for children and elderly from 1960 through 1979 concluded that the absolute gain for each older person was much higher than the gain for each child (Preston, 1984). Yet, a 1981 Harris survey found that the public perceives the elderly as needier than the elderly themselves think they are (National Council on the Aging, 1981). The perception of poverty as typical of the elderly has actually increased since the same question was asked in 1974, although the elderly's relative income increased during the intervening time period. What is unknown is the extent to which these perceptions will shift with increasing public awareness of federal expenditures for aging programs along with the growing federal deficit. The potential for intergenerational conflicts is further discussed in the concluding section of this chapter.

We next review the programs that account for the majority of federal expenditures: Social Security (OASI) and Supplemental Security Income (SSI); tax provisions and private pensions that provide indirect benefits; social services through Title XX Block Grants and the "Aging Network" of the Older Americans Act; housing policies and subsidies and, in Chapter 19, Medicare and Medicaid. Of these, Social Security and health care represent the greatest percentage of federal funds expended on behalf of older persons, as illustrated in Figure 18–1.

Income Security Programs: Social Security and Supplemental Security Income

SOCIAL SECURITY

As noted earlier, the primary objective of the 1935 Social Security Act was to establish a system of income maintenance for older persons through individual

FIGURE 18–1 Federal Outlays Benefiting the Elderly, Fiscal Year 1985

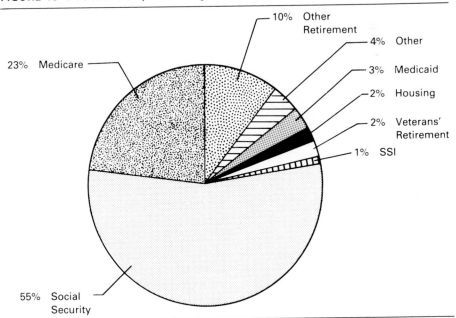

Source: Executive Office of the President, Office of Management and Budget, 1986.

insurance. A secondary purpose was to provide a basic level of protection for the most needy of the older population, initially through state plans for Old Age Insurance and, since 1974, through the federally funded Supplemental Security Income (SSI) program. A more recent objective has been to provide compensatory income to persons, regardless of age, who experience a sudden loss of income, such as widows, surviving children, and the disabled.

To meet these objectives, Social Security has four separate "trust funds": Old Age and Survivors Insurance (OASI); Disability Insurance (DI); Hospital Insurance (HI), which is funded through Medicare; and revenues for the supplemental insurance portion of Medicare. This discussion focuses on the combined OASDI fund, of which programs for the disabled are only 7 percent of the combined obligation. Funding for Medicare will be discussed in Chapter 19.

As described in Chapter 12, the Social Security system was based first on the concept of earned rights, rather than universal eligibility for all older persons. In fact, only 60 percent of the labor force was initially eligible to earn future benefits on the basis of the 1935 law. Coverage has since been expanded so that approximately 95 percent of the labor force is insured by Social Security (Kingson, Hirshorn, and Cornman, 1986). Social Security is thus distinguished by nearly universal coverage and wage-price indexing that protect recipients against economic changes over which they have no control. In 1981, the cost of Social Security benefits was $136.9 billion for all programs, with benefits for retired persons approximating $90 billion (Samuelson, 1983).

Contrary to public perceptions, Social Security was never intended to provide sole retirement income, but rather a minimum floor of protection. It was assumed that older people would have other pensions and individual savings. Nevertheless, a substantial percentage of the elderly rely on Social Security for most or all of their retirement income (providing about 35 percent of the total income going to all married older couples and about 45 percent to all unmarried older individuals) (Kingson, Hirshorn, and Cornman, 1986). In short, for most older households, Social Security provides the foundation for economic security.

Social Security is financed through separate trust funds, revenues raised equally from the taxing of employees and employers, and income based on current tax revenues. This method of financing partially underlies the fiscal crisis faced by the system in the early 1980s, when reserves were inadequate for projected benefits. That is, during times of economic recession, when high unemployment and low productivity result in less taxes collected from individuals and corporations, there is less money available for the Social Security funds. Because of this fiscal crisis, some critics of Social Security maintain that the elderly are bankrupting the economy, even though the immediate danger has been averted through remedial legislation passed in 1983. As noted in Chapter 12, Social Security trust funds are predicted to remain solvent for the next 75 years (U.S. Senate Special Committee on Aging, 1986). In fact, because of surpluses in its trust funds, Social Security actually contributes to reducing the federal deficit.

Yet media coverage that Social Security is going broke has fueled misunderstanding about the system's objectives and long-term stability.

Structural Factors Affecting Social Security   Rather than blame the elderly for the revenue shortage of the 1980s, we must recognize structural factors that underlie the threats of bankruptcy to Social Security. For example, unemployment played a major role by reducing revenues collected through taxes of employees paying into the system. For every 1 percent increase in unemployment, the loss of Social Security taxes was calculated to be $3 billion a year (Giwirtzman, 1982).

Other structural factors also affect the risk of revenue shortage. With increases in longevity and the number of retired workers in proportion to younger employees, fewer workers are paying into the Social Security system—the changing dependency ratio discussed in Chapter 12. The ratio of taxpayers to beneficiaries is projected to drop from 3.2 in the early 1980s to 2.2 by 2050—a decline of about one-third (Congressional Institute for the Future, 1984). With the change in the age of benefit eligibility from 65 to 62, more workers have retired early, thus draining an additional three years of benefits from the system. Since the 1972 and 1977 Social Security amendments, benefits have been indexed to changes in the Consumer Price Index during high inflation; this partially accounts for what younger people perceive to be the elderly's rapidly increasing monthly benefits.

Fundamental questions have been raised in the 1980s about the adequacy of benefits and the equity of costs between generations. Some future retirees fear that they will not receive a rate of return on their taxes comparable to that of many early recipients. The question of benefits for future retirees is made even more complicated by the "baby boom" generation's approaching retirement. In a 1985 Harris poll, 52 percent of those 25 years and over were not confident about Social Security's future viability (Yankelovich, Skelly, and White, 1985). This public misperception persists, despite long-range projections that the retirement benefits for today's younger worker will be considerably larger and over a longer time period (on average)—that is, they will have greater purchasing power—than those of today's retirees.*

Proposed Reforms of Social Security   Even though most people oppose reductions in benefits for current and future retirees (National Council on the Aging, 1981), private schemes are periodically proposed as alternatives to Social

---

*Social Security's actuaries project that a life-long worker, who earned average wages and retired at age 65 in 1985, would receive $548 a month; a similar worker retiring in 2000 would receive $659; and one retiring in 2015, $761. These figures are in inflation-adjusted dollars. The actual dollar amounts retired workers will receive in the future will be larger, of course (Kingson, Hirshorn, and Cornman, 1986).

Security, and ways to cut the costs of the existing system are frequently debated at the federal level. Nevertheless, the 1982 National Commission on Social Security Reform concluded that the nearly universal coverage and predictability of income provided by Social Security ensure that it will remain the cornerstone of the retirement income system (1983). Contrary to perceptions of intergenerational inequities, Social Security also benefits younger family members, by reducing their financial responsibility to their older relatives (Kingson, Hirshorn, and Cornman, 1986).

SUPPLEMENTAL SECURITY INCOME

Supplemental Security Income (SSI) is the central income transfer for the elderly living on the margin of poverty. SSI is financed fully by the federal government under the Social Security Administration, although states may supplement the federal payment. This has resulted in variability in benefits among states. California and New York, for example, tend to have substantial supplements for a larger number of recipients, whereas the majority of states either have few recipients receiving supplements or give token amounts to a larger number. The recent cutbacks in supplements by state governments have resulted in even more variability and inequities of SSI from state to state.

Although SSI is an important protective system for the least economically fortunate, it has not eliminated poverty among older persons, as evidenced by their 1984 poverty rate of 12.4 percent (U.S. Senate Special Committee on Aging, 1986). In fact, it has been estimated that at least half of low-income elderly who could benefit from SSI are not enrolled in the program. Some older people eligible for SSI resist applying because of the perceived stigma of dependency on the government. Even more elderly are unaware of SSI. Fortunately, some states have formed SSI outreach coalitions to promote awareness of the program. Another barrier is that older people who live with family members or who attempt to supplement their income by working may find their SSI payment reduced, thereby making it difficult for them to move out of their low-income conditions.

Private Pensions and Income Tax Provisions

PRIVATE PENSIONS

A smaller number of older persons receive a combination of government-supported public and/or private pensions in addition to their Social Security checks. As noted in Chapter 12, approximately 44 percent of the current labor force, primarily middle- and high-income workers, is covered by a private pension plan, which supplements Social Security. This translates into nearly 33 percent of the elderly receiving some income from public or private pensions. It is expected that fewer than 50 percent of retirees early in the next century will have private pension income, a small increase from the current situation (Clark, 1977).

The pension system tends to perpetuate systematic inequities by income, ethnic minority status, and sex, with lower income workers, often women and ethnic minorities, least likely to be in jobs that are covered by pensions and to have attained the vesting requirements (e.g., ten years on the same job). In many respects, private pensions exaggerate the division of the work force into an advantaged and disadvantaged sector (Crystal, 1982), favoring white males in technical, professional, or managerial positions. Retired civil service, military veterans, and railroad employees, for example, also receive cash benefits in addition to Social Security. This means that cash benefits from government-supported private savings plans and favorable tax policies accrue to those who are already relatively well-off.

INCOME TAX PROVISIONS

Pension plans are not the only "tax expenditures" related to aging. Some of the elderly also benefit from extra tax deductions, estimated to be worth over $2.5 billion annually (Crystal, 1982). Older people pay an average of 13 percent of their income in taxes, versus 23 percent for all ages (Nelson and Feldman, 1983). Many older people who file tax returns benefit from not paying a tax on Railroad Retirement and other government pensions. After these exclusions, however, less than 50 percent of the elderly receive benefits from the other tax-preferenced items because their incomes are below the taxable level (Kutza, 1981). Wealthy older persons also benefit from double income tax exemptions, property tax reductions, and preferential treatment of the sale of a home (e.g., exemption from capital gains taxation for sale of a principal residence after age 55). Tax provisions thus highlight the inequitable distribution of public benefits to older people. For example, 50 percent of the 1982 tax expenditures went to older individuals with incomes over $20,000, yet only 2 percent went to persons with incomes less than $5,000. Only this former group is able to deal with the economic hardships generally associated with old age by combining their private resources with these public tax expenditure items, Social Security, and Medicare (Nelson, 1982). As another illustration, the 1981 tax cuts benefited only about 36 percent of the elderly; the remainder had insufficient incomes to benefit from the special tax provisions (Select Committee on Aging, 1981). The outcome of these inequities is one standard of subsistence for the poor, defined by the public as "undeserving," a standard of social adequacy for the middle and downwardly mobile lower income elders, who are defined as the "deserving poor," and another standard for maintaining high-income elderly, or the "deserving nonpoor" (Nelson, 1982).

Tax benefits also illustrate how expenditures for one segment of the older population mean foregoing funds for another portion. In 1980, almost $26 billion went to expenditures for primarily high-income individuals, who form less than 6 percent of the elderly, compared to half that amount on welfare programs (e.g., SSI) for elderly poor, who, as we have seen in Chapter 12, form over 12 percent of the older population. Fundamental questions must be raised about the equity of using billions of tax dollars to maintain high-income lifestyles for a small percentage of older people when millions of others are in or near poverty at a time of intensified competition for federal resources (Nelson, 1983).

Not only are wealthier older people subsidized by tax benefits, but the federal government loses more income. Excluding Social Security and railroad retirement system benefits and veterans' pension income from taxation in the past has meant the loss of approximately $9.1 billion in federal taxes in 1981—another example of how the elderly can be perceived by others as draining the federal budget (Nelson, 1983; Samuelson, 1983).*

Housing Policy

Housing programs for older people have been secondary to income security and health care. A primary reason for this is that housing policy has been influenced by well-organized interest groups, such as builders and real estate developers, rather than by an aging constituency. As a result, only about 3 percent of older people have benefited from federally funded housing assistance programs (Pynoos, 1984). In addition, housing in the United States has generally received less public financial support than is the case in many other countries; for example, Great Britain provides publicly funded housing for one-third of its older population (Rubenstein, 1979). The cultural value placed on individual home ownership in the United States may partially explain this difference.

The major housing programs that have benefited older people involve subsidizing suppliers of housing to enable them to sell or rent housing for less than the prevailing market price. The Section 202 Direct Loan Program of the Housing Act of 1959 has provided housing for moderate-income older persons and for the handicapped whose incomes are too high to qualify for public housing, but too low to obtain housing in the private market. Under Section 202, low-interest loans are made to nonprofit corporations or to nonprofit consumer cooperatives.

Low-income older people are able to qualify for low-rent public housing. Although approximately 45 percent of such units are occupied by older people, only 2 percent of the aging population lives in public housing (Lammers, 1983).

---

*As of 1984, up to 50 percent of Social Security benefits have been treated as taxable for higher income beneficiaries, with the resultant revenue being transferred into the combined OASDI trust funds (approximately $4.1 billion in 1986) (Kingson, Hirshorn, and Cornman, 1986).

Section 236 housing programs provide private enterprise with additional means of developing quality rental and cooperative housing for low- and moderate-income persons, regardless of age, by lowering their housing costs through interest-reduction payments. Under rent supplement programs, landlords receive the difference from the federal government between the rental cost of a housing unit and 25 percent of the tenants' income available to pay for rent. Older people form an important segment of users of this rent supplement program (Kutza, 1981).

Other policies that indirectly affect older homeowners are property tax relief, energy assistance, and home equity conversion. Energy assistance for low-income homeowners to offset air conditioning and heating costs is provided under the federal government's allocation of block grant money to cities and states. Home equity conversions provide long-term homeowners with some discretionary income.

Most recent federal activity in the housing arena has been to maintain what exists, modifying programs only incrementally to serve larger numbers of older people. The policy focus has been to make better use of existing housing resources through homesharing, accessory apartments, and home equity conversions (see Chapter 11). Programs have not been geared to increasing the overall housing supply for the aging. Instead, concern over the growing budget deficit has resulted in reductions of the federally subsidized housing program. Another major need is for more congregate housing services, especially for low-income older persons. As indicated in Chapter 11, congregate housing is an important link in the long-term care continuum to enable older people to remain in the community. The best way to achieve this may be innovations that modify existing communities and neighborhoods to meet the elderly's housing needs rather than expensive housing supply programs (Newcomer, Lawton, and Byerts, 1986).

Social Services

A wide range of direct social service programs for older people have developed in response to needs unmet by income maintenance, health, and housing programs. Despite these developments, federal and state expenditures are primarily oriented toward income maintenance, health, and long-term care (U.S. House Select Committee on Aging, 1981; Newcomer, Estes, and Benjamin, 1983). Only 2 percent of the elderly's share of the federal budget is spent on social service programs (Senate Special Committee on Aging, 1986).

Funding for social services for older people derives from four federal sources: Medicare, Medicaid, amendments to the Social Security Act (Title XX), and the Older Americans Act of 1965. This section will focus on Title XX(of the Social

Services Block Grants) and the Older Americans Act as the primary basis of social service funding.

Title XX was established in 1974 to provide social services to all age groups; entitlements are means-tested (e.g., by financial need), with most Title XX services to older persons going to those who receive SSI. In terms of the program classification system discussed earlier, Title XX is a universal program aimed at redressing needs. Because income is an eligibility criterion, the elderly compete with a diverse group of Title XX recipients—primarily families with dependent children, the blind, and the disabled. An unfortunate consequence is that the poor and their allied service providers must thus compete for funds.

Title XX services are viewed as basic life-sustaining, self-care services to compensate for losses in health and the capacity for self-maintenance (Schram, 1982). Homemaker and chore services, home-delivered meals, adult protective services, adult day care, foster care, and institutional or residential care services financed by Title XX have generally assured a minimum of support for vulnerable older people, but have not improved their overall quality of life.

Under the federal Omnibus Budget Reconciliation Act of 1981, Title XX was converted to the Social Services Block Grant program at the same time that federal funds allocated to the states were reduced on the average by 20 percent. The Social Services Block Grant program was one of the initial decentralization efforts emerging from the new federalism of the 1980s. Block grant funding increased the states' discretion in determining clients' needs and allocating Title XX funds among the diverse eligible groups. For example, national income eligibility guidelines aimed at targeting programs to needy persons were eliminated. Accordingly, the competition for funds increased along with variability in services between and within states. As a result, most states have allocated a greater percentage of block grant funds to children than to older persons. Advocates for the elderly contend that the Social Services Block Grant program has discriminated against older persons and reinforced their economic and social marginality (Schram, 1982; Linemand and Pardini, 1983). In sum, limits to federal funding under decentralization along with fiscal crises in most cities and states have served to decrease revenues for social services under Title XX for the elderly at the same time that the demand for services has increased.

The Older Americans Act (OAA) seeks to alter state and local priorities to ensure that the elderly receive an appropriate share of social services allocations. Title III of the Older Americans Act is the single federal social service statute designed specifically for older people. Entitlements to services are universal, with the only eligibility criterion that one be over age 60. While the initial appropriation to the OAA in 1965 was only $7.5 million, its total 1983 budget was approximately $1 billion, and it served 3.2 million older persons (Newcomer, Estes, and Benjamin, 1983). The OAA was to create a national network for the comprehensive planning, coordination, and delivery of aging services. At the federal level, the Act charges the Administration on Aging (AOA), through the Commissioner on Aging, to oversee the activities of the Aging Network (i.e., the system of social services for the elderly), and to advocate for older persons nationally. The Federal Council on Aging is appointed by the president, and advises the Commissioner on Aging and the president.

The Older Americans Act also established State Units on Aging (SUAs). Each of these has a state advisory council to engage in statewide planning and advocacy on behalf of older persons' service needs. State Units on Aging designate local Area Agencies on Aging (AAAs) to develop and administer service plans within local areas. Approximately 700 Area Agencies on Aging operate at regional and local levels, and have advisory boards that include older persons. In addition to the federal, state, and local agencies responsible for planning and coordination, a fourth tier is composed of direct service providers in local communities. As described in Chapter 11, these include information and referral, transportation, outreach, homemaker services, day care, nutrition education and congregate meals (e.g., hot meals at senior centers and home-delivered meals), legal services, respite care, and senior centers. These services under OAA overlap with the goals and provisions of the Social Services Block Grants. Since 1984, the OAA has placed more emphasis on senior centers as coordinating points for services, particularly for congregate meals, for prevention of elder abuse, and for reaching low-income ethnic minority elderly.

The Older Americans Act, and the Aging Network which it created, although important, have been criticized for serving primarily nonpoor or newly poor older persons rather than those most in need. Critics maintain that OAA services improve or maintain the recently deprived elderly's past way of life and compensate for role losses by reintegrating them into society, but do not meet the poor's subsistence needs (Minkler and Estes, 1984). For example, senior centers tend to serve higher income and healthier older Caucasians who could otherwise afford to pay for such services. Programs that have relatively low per capita costs, but are also most likely to be used by middle-class elderly, such as special transportation services, mass health screening, and cultural and social activities, tend to be favored over adult day care, outreach, and homemaker services that could benefit the frail elderly.

Critics also contend that local and regional planning units have had limited influence on service agencies, have not advocated on behalf of older persons, and have not reduced rates of institutionalization (Minkler and Estes, 1984; Estes, 1979; Schram, 1982). They maintain that too much money has been spent on planning and coordinating services that are becoming even scarcer so that the actual services delivered have not been improved. Another criticism, as noted earlier, is that the Older Americans Act has benefited professional gerontologists, through jobs and research funds, more than the older people who are studied and served by professionals (Minkler and Estes, 1984; Estes, 1979).

Policy Dilemmas

AGE-BASED VERSUS NEEDS-BASED PROGRAMS

Ongoing debates about the need for *age-based programs* underlie most policy developments in the aging field. These debates highlight choices about whom to serve and how to restrict eligibility for program benefits. The major argument for age-based programs is that they are an efficient way to set a minimum floor of protection for beneficiaries, and are less stigmatizing than means-tested services. According to proponents of age-based programs, efficiency is enhanced by the fact that certain policies, such as Social Security and long-term care, exclusively or predominantly affect older people. Accordingly, it is argued that age-based programs involve fewer eligibility disputes and are less administratively intrusive into applicants' lives. Proponents maintain that programs based on age have greater chances to be funded, since older people, for the most part, are still perceived as a politically popular constituency.

Neugarten (1982; Neugarten and Neugarten, 1986), in particular, has argued strongly against age-based services. She maintains that age-based services reinforce the misperception of "the old" as a problem, thereby stigmatizing older people and adding to age segregation. The Older Americans Act, for example,

Maggie Kuhn is an outspoken advocate for intergenerational initiatives.

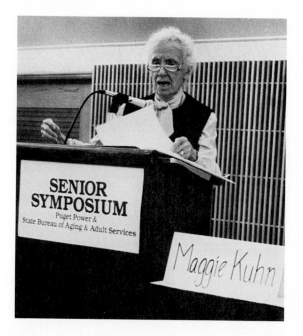

implicitly views anyone over age 60 as vulnerable and therefore needing services. Yet, as we have seen, there are many people over age 60 who are in good health, have an adequate income, and therefore do not need services. The use of age as a criterion for benefits assumes that older people are homogeneous and different from other age groups, but Neugarten maintains that old age in itself does not constitute a basis for treatment different from that of other ages. Age has become a poor predictor of the timing of life events, of people, health, income, and family status, and therefore of their interests and needs. Since age is not a useful indicator of changes within a person, it is an arbitrary criterion for service delivery. Instead, it is argued that economic and health needs, rather than age, should be the basis for selectively targeting services (Binstock, 1984). For example, the need for services increases after age 75, when an individual's health and income also tend to decline. Yet age-based programs have benefited the young-old who are relatively healthy and in the top third of the income distribution, and have even further disadvantaged low-income and frail elderly (Nelson, 1982).

With increasing fiscal restraints, the targeting of selected resources to the most needy has become more widely advocated. Although the average income of older people relative to that of the nonelderly has substantially improved, inequality among the elderly has actually increased (Crystal, 1986). As described in Chapters 15 and 16, most programs have not addressed the economic and social conditions of the most disadvantaged and vulnerable elderly: women, ethnic minorities, and those over age 75 (Estes, 1979). For example, 80 percent of Medicare benefits for older persons go to the nonpoor (Hudson, 1980). As noted earlier, upper-income retirees are helped the most by tax breaks (Nelson, 1983), and enjoy a disproportionate share of Social Security benefits relative to their past contributions. In 1983, only about 7 percent of all age-related federal costs went to programs specifically benefiting the elderly poor (Olson, 1984). In sum, social insurance and service strategies that attempt to meet the needs of both the poor and nonpoor elderly are now viewed by many as both costly and inefficient (Crystal, 1986).

Some advocates of targeting resources to the most needy favor a combination of categorical and group eligibility mechanisms. Under this model, a portion of Older Americans Act service monies, for example, could be restricted for allocation to SSI and older Medicaid recipients, thereby reaching individuals with the lowest incomes and presumably the most service needs (Kutza and Zweibel, 1982). Others advocate income maintenance policies that expand both SSI and Social Security benefits (Lammers, 1983).

INTERGENERATIONAL INEQUITY FRAMEWORK

A growing public argument that is closely related to the debate about aged-based programs is that the elderly are benefiting at the expense of younger age groups, who lack the political clout represented by senior organizations. This argument is being expounded in a growing number of newspaper and magazine editorials, and has resulted in the formation of groups such as Americans for Generational Equity (AGE) and the National Taxpayers Union. This backlash phenomenon has the potential to lead to destructive polarization between older and younger generations. The themes of the backlash argument are:

- America's elderly are now better off financially than the population as a whole.
- Programs for the elderly are a major cause of current budget deficits, economic problems, and increases in poverty among children.
- Children are the most impoverished age group.
- Young adults now have a harder time making ends meet and face a far stiffer tax burden than their parents did when they were the same age.
- Younger people will not receive fair returns for their Social Security and Medicare investments.

AGE maintains that the baby boom generation—the 78 million born between 1946 and 1964—will collectively face a disastrous retirement, and its children will, in turn, be much more heavily burdened with the support of its parents than any other generation in our nation's history. Underlying all these themes is that policies and programs for the elderly are "unfair" and result in intergenerational conflict. Policy questions then become framed in terms of competition and conflict between generations.

Admittedly, high inflation, lack of real wage growth, and runaway housing costs in the early 1980s have hurt young adults who are struggling to start jobs, families, and buy a home. Similarly, the growing divorce rate has thrown millions of children into one-parent households and poverty. (The poverty rate among children is over 20 percent [U.S. Bureau of the Census, 1985].) At the same time, the elderly are perceived as benefiting from Social Security, which thus far has been exempt from any budget-cutting measures. Another factor that feeds into the backlash is that old age benefits have only been cut by 3 percent in the 1980s, whereas human resources spending for all other groups has declined steadily by 7 percent (Storey, 1986).

It is true that the older population is financially better off than in the past. As noted in Chapter 12, 1 out of 3 elderly persons was poor in 1959, as compared to 1 out of 8 currently, an improvement that represents the effects of Medicaid and Medicare and the Older Americans Act (Uhlenberg and Salmon, 1986). Beneath the appearance of a dramatic decline in poverty among the older population is the reality that many of those who "moved out" of poverty have shifted from a few hundred dollars below the poverty line to a few hundred above it (Blaustein, 1982). In addition, the distribution of income among the elderly is extremely diverse and the level of inequality among them is extraordinarily high. As we have seen in earlier chapters, large pockets of poverty and near poverty persist among the elderly; about 23 percent of all elderly Hispanics, 36 percent of all elderly Blacks, 24 percent of older unmarried white women, 46 percent of older unmarried Hispanic women, and 63 percent of older unmarried Black women had below-poverty incomes in 1983. Many elderly only eke out an existence, with 6.2 million older people relying on Social Security checks that amount to $300 or $400 a month for 90 percent of their income (U.S. Senate Special Committee on Aging, 1986).

As noted in Chapter 12, the elderly are also more likely than other age groups to be among the "near poor" and the "hidden poor" (Cook and Kramek, 1986). Although Social Security has not yet been adversely affected, federal budget cuts of means-tested programs (e.g., food stamps, subsidized housing, Medicaid) in the early 1980s have fallen primarily on the low-income elderly who depend on multiple public benefits (Storey, 1986). For low-income elderly, the tax cuts and lessened inflation in the mid-1980s did not improve their economic status. Recent research also suggests that the low-income elderly are less likely to use formal or informal sources of support (Cook and Kramek, 1986; Uehara, Geron, and Beeman, 1986). Finally, the safety net for low-income seniors is extremely weak. For example, the SSI benefit for a single person is current $340 a month ($4,080 annually), approximately 75 percent of the poverty line ($5,410) (Villers Foundation, 1987).

CRITIQUE OF THE INEQUITY FRAMEWORK

The intergenerational inequity framework that attempts to measure the relative hard times of one generation against the relative prosperity of another has been widely criticized by aging advocates, especially by the Gerontological Society of America and the Gray Panthers (Kingson et al., 1986). The major criticisms of this framework are as follows: Contrary to the pessimistic argument that society will not be able to provide for future generations of elderly, the economy of the future, barring unforeseen disasters, will be able to support a mix of programs for all age groups. There is little real evidence of significant intergenerational conflict; instead, younger and older generations appear to recognize their interdependence and to support benefits to each other across the lifespan. For example, the Children's Defense Fund argues that funding for programs for the young should be increased at the cost of military spending, not at the expense of programs for the elderly. The American Association of Retired Persons agrees, and argues that older people's well-being contributes to the welfare of all other generations. Similarly, the public tends to be supportive of benefits for older generations (Navarro, 1984). For instance, the majority of respondents of all ages in a 1985 survey were opposed to cutting Social Security and Medicare benefits to reduce federal deficits, whereas only 30 percent were against reductions in military spending for the same purpose (U.S. Senate Special Committee on Aging, 1986).

The definition of fairness put forth by groups such as Americans for Generational Equity is narrow and misleading. Thus, the current preoccupation with equity between generations "blinds us to inequities within age groups and throughout our society" (Binstock, 1985). When fairness is equated with numerical equality, this assumes that the relative needs of children and the elderly for public funds are identical, and that equal expenditures are the equivalent of social justice. Even if needs and expenditures for each group were equal, this would not result in equal outcomes or social justice. By framing policy issues in terms of competition and conflict between generations, the intergenerational inequity perspective implies that public benefits to the elderly are a one-way flow from young to old, and that reciprocity between generations does not exist. By pitting young against old for the division of scarce resources, the intergenerational inequity framework assumes a "fixed pie," which can only be cut from the elderly or the young, and overlooks other ways of increasing public resources through economic growth, increased tax revenues, or reduced defense spending.

THE INTERDEPENDENCE OF GENERATIONS FRAMEWORK

This framework, advocated especially by the Gerontological Society of America, assumes that public and private intergenerational transfers are central to social progress. A major way in which generations assist one another is through the family; for example, through care for children and dependent adults, financial support, and inheritances. Such transfers within the family were estimated to be equivalent to 30 percent of the gross national product in 1979 (Morgan, 1983). Intergenerational transfers are essential to meeting families' needs at various points over the life course and to transmitting legacies of the past (e.g., economic growth, culture, values, and knowledge). Transfers based on public policy (e.g., education, Social Security, and health care programs) also serve intergenerational goals. For example, Social Security benefits are distributed widely across all generations and protect against risks to families' economic well-being over the course of their lives. It is erroneous to think of Social Security as a one-way flow of resources from young to old. Instead, younger generations have at least two important stakes in Social Security: they will be served by it when they become old, and, as stated earlier, programs that support their older relatives' autonomy currently relieve them from financial responsibilities. Similarly, when the problem of health care for the elderly is conceptualized as belonging to each of us as we age, then younger generations ask, "What health care resources would I want for each stage of my life?" (Clark, 1985). Likewise, it is erroneous to think of education as a one-way flow from adults to children. Rather, the elderly, now and in the future, benefit directly and indirectly from education programs that help to increase the productivity of the work force. The Gerontological Society's report on the interdependence of generations concludes:

A sufficiently broad policy framework for responding to the challenge of an aging society must include a concern for the long-term welfare of all age groups, an appreciation of policies that support the family as an institution, and an understanding of the significance of public and private investments in the human resources that will define the possibilities for the future (Kingson et al., p. 28).

The essentials in future policy developments are intergenerational alliances aimed toward benefiting the most needy, regardless of age, as well as preventive and early interventive strategies to forestall social, economic, and health problems for all age groups.

Who Is Responsible?

Another policy debate revolves around the division of responsibility between federal and state governments. Until recently, Social Security benefits, Medicare, Medicaid, SSI, and services under the Older Americans Act settled the question of responsibility for the elderly: It was to be a collective responsibility of the entire population, exercised through the national government. It was to be protection to which every older citizen was entitled, simply by virtue of age.

A growing view held by public officials in the 1980s is that the problems of the elderly and other disadvantaged groups cannot be solved with federal government policies and programs alone. Instead, solutions must come from state and local governments and from private sector and individual initiatives, such as advocacy and self-help. Individuals are assumed to be responsible for their own problems, and federal government interventions are considered to be harmful to national economic well-being. Recent policy changes have aimed to enhance the role of states through block grants, on the assumption that the states can most efficiently and innovatively respond to local needs. A limitation of this decentralized approach, however, is that states, which have the fewest resources for supporting community services, are generally the least likely to respond to the needs of the most disadvantaged (Hudson, 1984). As noted above, with decentralization, there is little assurance of policy uniformity and of equity for powerless groups across different states (Estes, 1984). National initiatives that establish stable, uniformly administered federal policies are usually necessary to bring the states with the most limited expenditures up to a minimum standard.

Decentralization also makes it more difficult for the elderly to influence policy development, since they must address officials in hundreds of different state and local agencies. Block grants, for example, have few central directives, thus allowing the most well organized and informed groups to influence the distribution of funds. Powerful interest groups, such as insurance companies, hospitals, and physicians, tend to have more political influence at the state level, with the low-income elderly faring poorly under decentralization (Estes and Lee, 1981; Reagan and Sanzone, 1981). Decentralization has also placed the elderly in competition with child welfare advocates, thereby fueling perceptions of inter-generational conflict (Minkler and Estes, 1984). Although decentralization can increase program responsiveness to a given area, broad inequities tend to result.

Issues of who is responsible become highlighted in policy debates about who should provide retirement security—individuals, families, employers, or the government. Recently, the federal government has encouraged individuals to take responsibility for themselves in old age, by granting special tax incentives for personal savings. However, changes in tax laws have curtailed some of these incentives such as Individual Retirement Accounts (IRAs). Some political conservatives would like to see Social Security totally replaced by private pensions and individual savings. As we have seen, however, Social Security is unlikely to be eliminated in our lifetimes.

Reductions in Government Support

What is more important than federal–state relations, however, is the level of public spending. Although government spending has increased in terms of total dollars, it has declined when measured as a percentage of the gross national product or as government expenditures per capita, corrected for inflation. The economically disadvantaged elderly appear to have been hurt the most by the budget cuts that have already taken place in the 1980s. For example, approximately 60 percent of the cuts in federal expenditures in 1982 occurred in means-tested programs, such as SSI, that formed only 25 percent of the federal budget (Palmer and Sawhill, 1983). Likewise, of the approximately $31 billion cut from social programs in 1983, an estimated $11.8 billion was in programs serving the elderly (Minkler and Estes, 1984).

Public spending levels are being substantially reduced at the same time that private and local spheres are being expected to be more responsible for dependent elders. Policy makers often assume that public programs reduce family involvement and that families could do more for their older relatives. However, as discussed in Chapter 10, the family has consistently played a major role in supporting older relatives in the community. Family members may be providing all the support that they are able or willing to do, although such assistance is not necessarily financial. When resources become scarce, the family tends to be viewed as a cost-effective alternative to nursing home placement and to publicly funded social services. Few public programs support families' caregiving. Instead, allocations for homemaker, nutrition, chore services, adult day care, low-income energy assistance, respite, and volunteer programs such as Retired Senior Volunteer Programs have all diminished in the 1980s. Yet those who work closely with families and their older relatives are vividly aware of the costs of care on the family. Proponents of public supports for family caregivers advocate financial subsidies, increased respite options for families, and educational and support groups to enhance care-giving efforts.

Not only is the family unable to carry expanded responsibilities, but the private nonprofit service sector cannot fill the gaps created by federal cuts. In fact, the 1986 federal tax law may reduce incentives for corporate giving. In addition, private contributions traditionally have not been concentrated on social services, so that increased private giving would not automatically flow into areas most severely cut. Instead, both public and private funds are decreasing as the aging population and their need for services increase (Wood and Estes, 1983).

Summary and Implications

This chapter has reviewed federal programs that benefit older persons. Since 1960, age-specific spending has increased significantly, mostly through Medicare and Old Age Survivors Insurance. Such growth, however, has not necessarily benefited those elderly who are most in need, because many programs are based on age alone as an eligibility criterion. This has resulted in many older people with the greatest needs, such as older women and ethnic minorities, continuing to receive inadequate benefits.

Age entitlement programs are often based on cultural values and public attitudes of all older people as deserving, as opposed to need entitlement programs that are based on cultural values of productivity and independence. U.S. public policies toward older people have been criticized for being fragmented and responding to crises rather than preventing problems and attacking their underlying causes.

The United States has developed policies aimed at older populations more slowly than European countries. The Social Security Act of 1935 was the first major policy aimed at older people. Social Security was expanded slightly in 1950 to support partial health care costs through individual states. These changes led to the enactment of Medicare in 1965. Since then, there has been a significant growth in the number of programs aimed at improving the welfare of older people: the Older Americans Act, Supplemental Security Income, the Social Security Amendments of 1972 and 1977, Section 202 Housing, and Title XX social services legislation. These programs have been strengthened by national forums such as the 1961 and 1971 White House Conferences on Aging. During the 1980s, however, there has been a decline in these programs. These cost-efficiency measures are based on a new stereotype of the elderly as having greater financial security than younger age groups. The fiscal crisis faced by the Social Security system in the early 1980s fueled this stereotype by speculations that the growing number of older persons was primarily responsible for the crisis, and would drain the system before future generations could benefit from it. However, numerous structural factors were responsible for the problems; changes that have subsequently been made in this system assure its future viability.

The debate over age-based versus needs-based programs has also led to the emergence of organizations that have expounded arguments about older people benefiting at the expense of younger age groups. Yet, evidence for such inequity is weak; numerous other organizations such as the Children's Defense Fund and the Gerontological Society of America recognize generational interdependence and the importance of seeking increased public support for all ages through other sources. This framework, known as the *interdependence of generations*, assumes that support from young to old and old to young benefits all ages and supports the role of families across the lifespan.

In sum, the aging policy agenda for the remainder of the twentieth century is full and complex. The current federal emphasis on fiscal austerity underlies all policy debates about how much the government should be expected to provide and for whom. Increasing public perceptions of the elderly as well-off, combined with decreased governmental resources, will undoubtedly affect the types of future programs and policies developed to meet the elderly's income, housing, and social service needs. Countering public resistance to more governmental expenditures for older people will be the advocates, lobbyists, and organized senior groups pressuring government to respond adequately to the rapid and disproportionate growth of older people.

References

Abel-Smith, B., and Titmuss, K. *Social policy.* London: George Allen and Unwin, 1979.

Binstock, R. H. The aged as scapegoats. *The Gerontologist,* 1983, 23, 136–143.

Binstock, R. Reframing the agenda of policies on aging. In M. Minkler and C. Estes (Eds.), *Readings in the political economy of aging.* Farmingdale, N.Y.: Baywood, 1984.

Binstock, R. H. The oldest old: A fresh perspective on compassionate ageism revisited. *Milbank Memorial Fund Quarterly: Health and Society,* 1985, 63, 437–438.

Blaustein, A. I. (Ed.). *The American promise: Equal justice and economic opportunity.* New Brunswick, N.J.: Transaction Books, 1982.

Califano, J. A. *Governing America.* New York: Simon and Schuster, 1981.

Clark, P. The social allocation of health care resources: Ethical dilemmas in age-group competition. *The Gerontologist,* 1985, 25, 119–126.

Clark, R. The role of private pensions in maintaining living standards in retirement. National Planning Association Report, No. 154, Washington, D.C., 1977.

Clark, R., and Menefee, J. Federal expenditures for the elderly: Past and future. *The Gerontologist,* 1981, 21, 134.

Congressional Institute for the Future. *Tomorrow's Elderly*, 1984.

Cook, F. L., and Kramek, L. Measuring economic hardship among older Americans. *The Gerontologist*, 1986, *26*, 38–48.

Crystal, S. *America's old age crisis: Public policy and the two worlds of aging*. New York: Basic Books, 1982.

Crystal, S. Measuring income and inequality among the elderly. *The Gerontologist*, 1986, *26*, 56–59.

Crystal, S. Where does reality begin and myth end? *Connection*, American Society on Aging, May–June 1986, 5.

Estes, C. *The aging enterprise*. San Francisco: Jossey-Bass, 1979.

Estes, C. Fiscal austerity and aging. In C. Estes, R. Newcomer, and Associates (Eds.), *Fiscal austerity and aging*. Beverly Hills: Sage, 1983.

Estes, C. Austerity and aging: 1980 and beyond. In M. Minkler and C. Estes (Eds.), *Readings in the political economy of aging*. Farmingdale, N.Y.: Baywood, 1984, pp. 241–255.

Estes, C., and Lee, P. Policy shifts and their impact on health care for elderly persons. *Western Journal of Medicine*, 1981, *135*, 511–517.

Fisher, C. Differences by age groups in health care spending. *Health Care Financing Review*, Spring 1980, 65–90.

Giwirtzman, M. Remarks made on television by the chairman of the National Commission on Social Security, which were reported in the *Los Angeles Times* (December 6, 1982), pt. 1, p. 16.

Hudson, R. B. The 'graying' of the federal budget and its consequences for old age policy. *The Gerontologist*, 1978, *18*, 428–440.

Hudson, R. Old-age politics in a period of change. In E. Borgatta and N. McCluskey (Eds.), *Aging and society: Current research and policy perspectives*. Beverly Hills: Sage, 1980.

Hudson, R. The new politics of aging. *Generations*, 1984, *9*, 5–7.

Kingson, E., Hirshorn, B., and Cornman, J. *Ties that bind: The interdependence of generations*. Washington, D.C.: Seven Locks Press, 1986.

Kingson, E., Hirshorn, B., and Harootyon, L. *The common stake: The interdependence of generations*. Washington, D.C.: The Gerontological Society of America, 1986.

Klemmack, D. L., and Roff, L. L. Predicting general comparative support for governments providing benefits to older persons. *The Gerontologist*, 1981, *21*, 592–599.

Kutza, E. *The benefits of old age: Social welfare policy for the elderly*. Chicago: University Press, 1981.

Kutza, E., and Zweibel, N. Age as a criterion for focusing public programs. In B. Neugarten (Ed.), *Age or need? Public policies for older people*. Beverly Hills: Sage, 1982.

Lammers, W. *Public policy and the aging*. Washington, D.C.: Congressional Quarterly, Inc., 1983.

Linemand, D., and Pardini, A. Social services: The impact of fiscal austerity. In C. Estes, R. Newcomer, and Associates (Eds.), *Fiscal austerity and aging*. Beverly Hills: Sage, 1983, pp. 133–157.

Minkler, M. Introduction. In M. Minkler and C. Estes (Eds.), *Readings in the political economy of aging*. Farmingdale, N.Y.: Baywood, 1984.

Minkler, M., and Estes, C. (Eds.), *Readings in the political economy of aging*. Farmingdale, N.Y.: Baywood, 1984.

Morgan, J. M. The redistribution of income of families and institutions and emergency hospital patterns. In G. Duncan and J. Morgan (Eds.), *Two thousand families—patterns of economic progress*. Ann Arbor, Mich.: Institute for Social Research, 1983.

National Commission on Social Security Reform. *Report of the National Commission on Social Security Reform*. Washington, D.C.: U.S. Government Printing Office, 1983.

National Council on Aging. *Aging in the eighties: America in transition*. Report of a 1981 poll by Louis Harris & Associates. Washington, D.C.: NCOA, 1981.

Navarro, V. The political economy of government cuts for the elderly. In M. Minkler and C. Estes (Eds.), *Readings in the political economy of aging*. Farmingdale, N.Y.: Baywood, 1984.

Nelson, C. T., and Feldman, A. M. *Estimating after-tax money income distribution using data from the March Current Population Survey*. U.S. Bureau of the Census, Current Population Survey, Special Publication Series P-23, No. 126, August 1983.

Nelson, G. Social class and public policy for the elderly. *Social Science Review,* 1982, *56,* 85–102.

Nelson, G. Tax expenditures for the elderly. *The Gerontologist,* 1983, *23,* 471–478.

Neugarten, B. Policy in the 1980s: Age or need entitlement. In B. Neugarten (Ed.), *Age or need: Public policies for older people*. Beverly Hills: Sage, 1982.

Neugarten, B., and Neugarten, D. Changing meanings of age in the aging society. In A. Pifer and L. Bronte (Eds.), *Our aging society: Paradox and promise*. New York: W. W. Norton, 1986.

Newcomer, R. J., Estes, C., and Benjamin, E. The Older Americans Act. In C. Estes, R. Newcomer, and Associates (Eds.), *Fiscal austerity and aging*. Beverly Hills: Sage, 1983.

Newcomer, R. J., Lawton, M. P., and Byerts, T. O. *Housing an aging society*. New York: Van Nostrand Reinhold, 1986.

Olson, L. K. Aging policy: Who benefits? *Generations,* 1984, *9,* 10–14.

Palmer, J. L., and Sawhill, I. V. (Eds.), *The Reagan experiment*. Washington, D.C.: The Urban Institute, 1983.

Preston, S. Children and the elderly in the U.S. *Scientific American,* December 1984, *251,* 44–49.

Pynoos, J. Elderly housing politics and policy. *Generations,* 1984, *9,* 26–31.

Reagan, M. D., and Sanzone, J. G. *The new federalism*. New York: Oxford Press, 1981.

Rubenstein, J. Housing policy issues in three European countries. Paper delivered at the meetings of the Gerontological Society of America, Washington, D.C., 1979.

Samuelson, R. J. Busting the U.S. budget: The costs of an aging America. *National Journal,* 1983, *10,* 256–260.

Schram, S. Social services for older people. In B. Neugarten (Ed.), *Age or need: Public policies for older people.* Beverly Hills: Sage, 1982.

Storey, J. Policy changes affecting older Americans during the first Reagan administration. *The Gerontologist,* 1986, *25,* 27–31.

Uehara, E., Geron, S., and Beeman, S. The elderly poor in the Reagan era. *The Gerontologist,* 1986, *26,* 48–55.

Uhlenberg, P., and Salmon, M. G. Change in relative income of older women, 1960–80. *The Gerontologist,* 1986, *26,* 164–170.

U.S. Bureau of the Census. *Money income and poverty status of families and persons in the United States: 1984.* Advance Data from the March 1985 Current Population Survey. Current Population Report, Series P-60, No. 149, August 1985.

U.S. House Select Committee on Aging. *Analysis of the impact of the proposed fiscal 1982 budget cuts on the elderly.* Washington, D.C.: U.S. Government Printing Office, 1981.

U.S. House Select Committee on Aging. *Tomorrow's elderly: Issues for Congress.* Washington, D.C.: Congressional Institute for the Future, 1985.

U.S. Senate Special Committee on Aging. *Aging America: Trends and projections, 1985–86 edition.* U.S. Department of Health and Human Services, 1986.

Villers Foundation, *On the other side of Easy Street: Myths and facts about the economics of old age.* Washington, D.C., 1987.

Wood, J. B., and Estes, C. L. The private nonprofit sector and aging services. In C. Estes, R. J. Newcomer, and Associates, *Fiscal austerity and aging.* Beverly Hills: Sage, 1983.

Yankelovich, Skelly, and White, Inc. *A fifty-year report card on the Social Security System: The attitudes of the American public.* Washington, D.C.: American Association of Retired Persons, 1985.

Chapter **19**

Health Care Policy
and Programs

Throughout this book, we have examined the interplay of social, physical, and psychological factors in how older people relate to their changing environments. We have seen numerous instances of how health status affects this interaction. Given the importance of health issues in old age and the increasing numbers of older people, it is not surprising that health care of the elderly has become one of the most critical and controversial policy issues facing our nation. Several previous chapters have mentioned the rapidly increasing costs of providing health care for our aging population. This chapter describes current programs and proposed alternatives, with attention to the key factors that must be considered in future policy decisions.

It begins by reviewing the statistics on public and private expenditures, their causes and impact. Next, Medicare and Medicaid, the two public programs that account for the largest increases in health care expenditures for the elderly, are described. Factors that underlie these escalating costs are identified, as well as significant problems and proposed reforms. Many of these proposals address the need for long-term care in a variety of community-based settings, as opposed to the institutional care for catastrophic medical conditions that has long dominated the health care system. The need for, and barriers to, community-based alternatives to institutionalization along a continuum of care are briefly reviewed. The chapter concludes by examining some of the benefits and limitations of health promotion as a programmatic strategy to prevent chronic illness, reduce health care costs, and enhance the elderly's quality of life.

Health Care Expenditures

In recent years, policymakers and service providers, as well as the general public, are increasingly concerned about the "crisis in health care." In 1984, the United States spent $387 billion on health, or about 11 percent of the gross national product (GNP). Of particular concern are health services for the elderly, which accounted for 30 percent of total health expenditures in 1984, or $120 billion; expenditures are projected to increase to $200 billion by the year 2000 (Davis, 1986). The average expenditure for personal health services for persons age 65 and over was nearly $4,200 in 1986, compared with approximately $1,000 for those under age 65 (Brickfield, 1986–87). These higher expenses are largely attributable to older people's greater health needs and use of hospital and nursing home care compared to their younger counterparts. For instance, at least 25 percent of older people are expected to face catastrophic illness at some point. Accordingly, the majority (66 percent) of the 1984 expenditures was for institutional care in hospitals and nursing homes (Waldo and Lazenby, 1984). By 1990, nursing home costs alone are projected to increase from $25 billion to $75 billion, not including individual out-of-pocket expenses (Jacobs and Abbott, 1983). As costs continue to grow, the danger increases that adequate health services will be outside the financial reach of many individuals and of society's willingness to pay.

These figures are of growing public concern because a large portion of the health expenditures for the elderly are borne by federal, state, and local governments, primarily through Medicare and Medicaid, as illustrated in Figure 19–1. In fact, Medicare and Medicaid are the fastest growing programs in the federal budget (Iglehart, 1983), and have surpassed Social Security as a troublesome policy arena in the 1980s. For example, federal expenditures for Medicare have been projected to rise from $74 billion in 1985 to $120 billion in 1989, a 60 percent increase in only four years (Davis, 1986). Current tax revenues are not expected to meet these increased expenditures. In fact, the Medicare trustees predict that the hospital insurance trust fund of the Medicare program will be depleted by the late 1990s (Trustees, 1985). As a result, Medicare is viewed as more vulnerable to budget cuts than Social Security, although public support for the program is strong.

Despite growing federal allocations, the average annual out-of-pocket health expenses borne by the elderly reached $1,500 in 1984—more than three times the amount spent by other age groups. Approximately 55 percent of this amount goes to nursing homes, home health care, and community long-term care services such as adult day care (Brickfield, 1986–87). As mentioned previously in this text, older

FIGURE 19–1 Sources of Payment for Health Care Expenditure for the Elderly, 1981

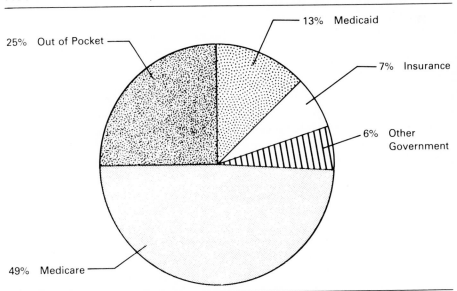

Source: Waldo and Lazenby, 1984, Health Care Financing Administration.

Americans now spend a higher proportion (and more in actual dollars) of their incomes on health care (15–16 percent) than they did before Medicare and Medicaid were established two decades ago (U.S. Senate Special Committee on Aging, 1985). These figures highlight the personal and public costs of extended life expectancy and the ability to manage chronic diseases among the elderly. This cost, although affordable to a growing and prosperous society, nevertheless presents major challenges for providing more economical and quality health care than at present.

FACTORS UNDERLYING GROWING COSTS

A number of structural factors underlie these escalating costs. First is the sucess of modern medical care. As noted in Chapter 6, these successes have assured an increase in the number of people who survive previously fatal illnesses in youth and middle-age, and have served to improve the physical well-being of the healthy young-old. However, they also have created more chronically ill old-old, who otherwise would have died, but who remain "one notch away from death," and who utilize a disproportionate amount of in-home and support services, especially in the last year of life (Avorn, 1986). This, in turn, has raised painful moral choices regarding what medical and legal steps should be taken in the care of dying elderly, given the general social and medical goal to preserve life at any cost.

A second related factor is the conflict between the curative goals of medicine and the long-term care needs of the elderly. As noted in Chapter 6, U.S. health services, based on a biomedical model, have focused on curing acute illnesses rather than caring for chronic diseases. As a result, greater weight in the financing and provision of services has been given to medical care, rather than health and social services for long-term support for the elderly. This situation has resulted in a growing demand for custodial services for the frail elderly, escalating long-term care costs, and increasing burdens on both the elderly and their families to provide such care—demands generally inadequately met by the medical profession or by publicly funded health programs. The reimbursement systems of Medicare and Medicaid, for example, are biased toward institutional medical services (e.g., hospitals and nursing homes). In both programs, enormous sums of public money are consumed by medical institutions serving a small percentage of older people in crisis. Long-term care services that do exist have resulted not from comprehensive planning, but rather from piecemeal reactions to pressing acute care needs in the health care system (Estes and Lee, 1985).

A third set of factors arise from the lack of coordination and unified funding in the United States health care system as a whole. No explicit, uniform mechanisms control the level of resources devoted to health care. Instead, most health services are provided privately, and are financed by a mix of public programs, private insurance, and direct patient payments. Patients are largely free to choose the physicians or health care providers they prefer; in turn, physicians may charge patients whatever they choose. There is neither effective market control nor governmental regulation of health expenditures. Whereas the health care of the elderly is, to a large extent, publicly funded (e.g., through Medicare and Medicaid), health services for the remainder of the population are financed primarily by private insurance. The separate public financing of health services for the elderly has meant that public pressure has focused on finding short-term ways to reduce such expenditures, without fostering a comprehensive policy that considers the health system as a whole.

We turn now to examining the two primary forms of public support for the elderly's health care: Medicare and Medicaid.

Medicare

The purpose of Medicare, or Title XVIII of the Social Security Act of 1965, is to provide older people with financial protection against the costs of hospital, nursing home, and physician care. A social value underlying Medicare is that the elderly are personally entitled to health care, and that society has an obligation to ensure their health. This assumption reflects a shifting of financial responsibility from the family to the state. Such a shift was assumed to benefit both the elderly and the young—who would be freed from shouldering the elderly's health care costs. Medicare's focus on the elderly also grew out of a compromise with the well-organized medical profession, which successfully opposed comprehensive health insurance for the general public. Support for a national health insurance for the elderly largely was garnered on pragmatic grounds that the greatest percentage of health care expenditures go to them.

The Medicare program has two basic components: Hospital Insurance (Part A) and Supplemental Medical Insurance (Part B), both oriented toward acute care. This focus has persisted, despite the growing need for long-term care for chronic illnesses. Part A, financed through the Social Security payroll tax, is available for all older persons who are eligible for Social Security. It pays for up to 90 days of hospital care and for a restricted amount of skilled nursing care and home health services. Recipients are responsible for their first day's hospital stay ($520 in 1987) and for copayments for hospital stays exceeding 60 days, costs which have escalated in the 1980s.

Part B supplemental medical insurance is financed through general tax revenues and has an additional monthly premium ($17.90 in 1987) paid by enrollees. Part B reimburses for some physician services, hospital outpatient services, home health care limited to certain types of health conditions and specific time periods, diagnostic laboratory and x-ray services, and a variety of miscellaneous services. Part A covers 99 percent of the older population, compared to 96 percent who are covered by Part B supplemental insurance.

Because of differences in health status among the elderly, particularly with the growing number of old-old, health expenditures within the older population are quite skewed. In 1981, 79 percent of the elderly had annual Medicare reimbursements of less than $1,000; 38 percent of these people received no Medicare payments. At the other extreme are the minority who require extensive care and treatment; 7.5 percent of the older population accounted for 66 percent of all Medicare payments, with an average payment of over $11,000 in 1981 (Davis, 1986).

Contrary to the assumption of many elderly that Medicare will cover their health care costs, Medicare only pays 80 percent of the *allowable* charges, not the actual amount charged by health providers. The patient must pay the difference between "allowable" and "actual" charges, unless the physician accepts "assignment" and agrees to charge only what Medicare pays. Individuals with both Part A and B must also pay an annual deductible for their medical expenses ($75 in 1986) and at least 20 percent of the remaining expenses.

For those who can afford more extensive coverage, private "medigap" insurance is available. In response to a growing concern with Medicare's limitations, 66 percent of the older population has purchased such insurance. However, the ability to afford private health insurance clearly varies widely by income. Of the poor or near-poor elderly, who suffer from more chronic illnesses than their higher income peers, only 47 percent have private insurance, compared with 78 percent of the high-income elderly (Davis, 1986). Even those who carry supplementary coverage can suffer burdensome medical expenses if they are seriously ill. Few "medigap" policies pick up physician charges in excess of Medicare's allowable fees, nor do they ordinarily cover prescriptions, dental care, or nursing home care. As a result, supplementary private insurance plans cover, on the average, only about 7 percent of the older population's health care bills (U.S. Senate Special Committee on Aging, 1985).

An additional problem is that Medicare has become so complicated that many older people do not understand how it works or to what it entitles them. Beneficiaries must deal with five different types of cost sharing and with seemingly arbitrary distinctions between covered and excluded services (Harvard Medicare Project, 1986).

Medicare's major limitation, however, is its focus on *acute care*, whereby it either excludes or gives little coverage to significant long-term care expenses, such as nursing homes, dental care and dentures, prescription costs, eye glasses and exams, hearing aids and exams, preventive health measures, and cosmetic surgery. In 1984, the average beneficiary paid an additional $550 for noninstitutional care not covered by Medicare, primarily for prescription drugs and deductibles (Davis, 1986). Medicare dollars are largely absorbed by acute care treatment of older people who are hospitalized for catastrophic illness at the terminal stage, as illustrated in Figure 19–2 (Waldo and Lazenby, 1984). Hospital payments in 1984 were slightly less than in 1981, when 75 percent of Medicare

FIGURE 19–2 Where the Medicare Dollar for the Elderly Goes, 1984

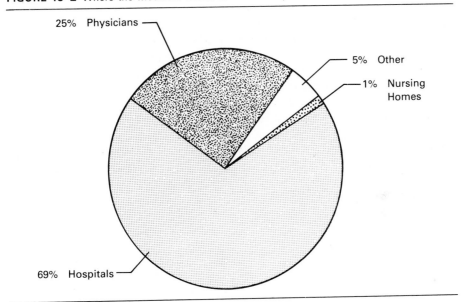

Source: Waldo and Lazenby, 1984.

expenditures covered hospital services (U.S. HCFA, 1982). In addition, approximately 25 percent of Medicare expenditures cover costs in the last year of life (Older Women's League, 1985). Another gap is that Medicare covers virtually none of the outpatient care provided by nonphysicians, including visiting nurses, home health services providers, and home health aides (Harvard Medicare Project, 1986). In 1981, for example, Medicare covered less than 1 percent of home health care costs (U.S. HCFA, 1982). An outcome of all these limitations is that Medicare covers only 45 percent of the health expenditures of the elderly (Davis, 1986). In turn, almost 75 percent of all noninstitutional care (e.g., home health care, homemaker services, adult day care) is privately financed by the elderly or their relatives (Liu, Manton, and Liu, 1986).

Many older people misunderstand the amount that Medicare and private insurance actually pay for extended periods of long-term care, a costly misunderstanding since custodial care constitutes about 25 percent of the elderly's health care expenses. When asked "Who will pay for long-term care?" the majority of members of the American Association of Retired Persons (AARP) said Medicare would be the primary payer, and private insurance and savings the secondary sources (Brickfield, 1986–87). The reality is, however, that the nursing home benefit through Medicare is available only for skilled care after a prior hospitalization; in addition, it is limited to a maximum of 100 days of care, yet most

---

Catastrophic Effects of Illness

Chronic health problems can be one of the fastest ways for the average person to deplete his or her resources. Addressing a Senate Subcommittee on Health and Long-Term Care, Mr. Howell, age 72, told how at age 58 he was strong and productive, shared $140,000 in savings with his wife, and was covered by four private health insurance policies. But then he had a stroke, his wife battled cancer for seven years before her death, and, after recovering from a near fatal bout of depression, Mr. Howell was involved last year in a serious automobile accident. He finds himself in the unfortunate situation of having spent nearly all of his life savings on health care and still worrying that the last few dollars will be gone soon.

---

older people end up needing about three times as many days of nonmedical custodial care as they do medical services. As a result, Medicare covers the expenses of less than 4 percent of the institutionalized elderly, which comprise only 2 percent of long-term care costs in nursing homes and in the home (Storey, 1983). Given the disparity between the elderly's perceptions of Medicare and what it actually covers, many older people only become aware of Medicare's limitations upon their first hospitalization or admission to a nursing home.

Medicare has also been criticized for providing disproportionate benefits to upper- and middle-income whites, compared to lower-income and ethnic minority elderly, even though, as described in Chapter 15, the latter face greater burdens of sickness and disability. As noted earlier in this chapter, upper- and middle-income older persons can better afford to supplement Medicare benefits with private health insurance and to meet increasing Medicare copayments and deductibles than can lower-income elderly (Estes, 1983; Minkler and Estes, 1984). These recent additional cost-sharing provisions may deter some of the elderly poor and near-poor from seeking health care.* Critics maintain that a two-tier system of health care delivery is developing: one level for those with private health insurance, Medicare, or the means to pay for expensive medical treatment; and another for those forced to rely on Medicaid or public charity, or to do without health care altogether (Torres-Gil, 1986). One aspect of this is that the proportion of income spent on health care declines as income rises. Those with incomes under $3,000 paid 10.2 percent of their earnings for health care in 1977, compared

---

*For example, the poor and near-poor elderly who have Medicare only average 4.2 physician visits per year, compared with 7 visits per year for those with both Medicare and Medicaid, and 6.5 visits for those with both Medicare and private health insurance. This lower utilization by the Medicare-only group cannot be attributed to better health status (Wilensky and Berk, 1983).

with 1.7 percent of income for those with incomes above $15,000 (Wilensky and Berk, 1983). People between ages 60 and 65, who are too "young" for Medicare and often no longer covered by job-related or other insurance, also often fall between the cracks. They are the most vulnerable to the loss of life savings for medical care.

THE IMPLICATIONS OF MEDICAL TECHNOLOGY

Medicare is popularly viewed as contributing to spiraling health care expenditures, primarily hospital costs. It is important to note, however, that the increase in Medicare expenditures has been due mainly to the rapid inflation in hospital costs and physicians' fees, not to the growth of the older population per se, nor to their increased utilization of services (Gibson, Waldo, and Levit, 1983; Estes, 1983). Health care payment mechanisms, including third-party payments based primarily on incurred costs and the fee-for-service reimbursement of physicians that is underwritten by government programs, offer little incentive for physicians or patients to reduce their use of costly medical technologies or out-patient care. Instead, there has been a built-in incentive for physicians to provide more hospital-based services. Hospital costs, for example, have increased an average of 16.2 percent per year from 1977 through 1984 (Waldo and Lazenby, 1984). Escalating hospital costs alone have diminished the intended purpose of Medicare to protect older people from the financial strain of needed medical care. Critics of the fee-for-service system for providers maintain that the primary beneficiaries of Medicare have been hospitals, physicians, insurance companies, and the medical supply and equipment firms, not older people with chronic care needs (Harvard Medicare Project, 1986; Estes, 1983; Minkler and Estes, 1984).

The Medicare payment system has other inequities. It is unfair to patients in that it allows physicians to accept or reject "assignment" (e.g., to decide whether to accept the fee set by Medicare as full compensation) on a case-by-case basis. In instances where the physician does not, the patient must pay the difference out-of-pocket or find a physician who will accept "assignment". An inequity for providers is that medical specialists and surgeons, as well as physicians in urban areas, tend to receive more compensation from Medicare than both general practitioners as a group and those in rural areas in particular.

There is growing agreement on the need for cost containment. What is less clear is how to do this while still ensuring quality medical care (Ball, 1985). One method used by the federal government has been to increase significantly the copayments and deductibles paid by the elderly. Although monthly premiums (which are required only for Part B) have only increased from $3 to about $15 during the past 20 years, copayments (e.g., costs shared by the older patient) have grown more than ten-fold. Copayments disproportionately burden the poor and the sick, since they are unrelated to income. For some low-income older people, the increased copayment may use up their money for transportation to doctors or for prescriptions (Coalition on Women and the Budget, 1983). Because co-payments are linked to service utilization, they are inherently unpredictable, which undermines the principle of insurance that Medicare was designed to promote (Harvard Medicare Project, 1986).

DIAGNOSTIC RELATED GROUPINGS (DRGs)

A system of prospective payment was instituted in 1983 to reverse the cost incentives for hospital decisions provided by the previous fee-for-service payment plan. Instead of reimbursing providers for each service for each patient, payment is determined by the diagnostic category in which each patient is placed. These categories, which are used to classify patients and thus set Medicare payments prior to the patient's admission, are called *diganostic related groupings,* or DRGs. Under the prior cost-based reimbursement system, hospitals were paid more if they provided more and longer services, resulting in higher subsequent costs. Now, a hospital that keeps patients longer than needed, orders unnecessary tests, or provides care inefficiently will be penalized financially. Hospitals that provide care at a cost below the established DRG fee can "pocket the difference." Although the DRG system has solved some problems, it has created others. From the point of view of the older population, a primary problem is that it applies only to Medicare patients, not to private-pay patients. Under pressure to hold down Medicare costs, the incentives can be great for hospitals to restrict Medicare patients' access to services and to discharge them too quickly (Nassif, 1986–87).

Another disadvantage of the DRG system is its failure to take account of the severity of the patient's illness within a given diagnostic category. Thus, for example, of two older persons hospitalized for hernia operations, one may take longer to recover than the other, because of poorer health status at admission. Such individual differences in prehospital health status are not considered by the DRG system. Preliminary studies of the impact of DRGs suggest an increased pressure on nursing homes, families, and home health care agencies to provide care for patients who are discharged from hospitals earlier, sicker, and thus in need of higher levels of post-hospital care than in the past. Since families and home health agencies often cannot provide these more complex levels of care, premature discharges have also resulted in a "revolving door" pattern of more patients in and out of hospitals (Jones, 1984; Bergthold and Estes, 1986). This has surfaced in numerous articles in the media about unnecessary deaths following such premature discharges of older people.

At the same time that hospital discharges to home health care have risen 37 percent since the passage of DRGs, the rate of growth in community-based home health services has slowed (U.S. Senate Special Committee on Aging, 1986). The search for cost-reduction carries the danger that providers may be encouraged to eliminate valuable services, substitute lower cost and less effective procedures, or deny needed care to older people. Even if the DRG system is successful in reducing the length of hospital stays, it will not lessen the growing numbers of elderly needing health care. In sum, Medicare cannot be saved by incremental "Medicare only" reforms. Cost-containment efforts must address all types of health services: hospitals, physicians, nursing homes, and all payees (individuals, Medicare, Blue Cross, commercial insurance, Medicaid, and third parties), and must be coupled with a commitment to quality care (Estes and Harrington, 1985).

REFORMING MEDICARE

Given the gaps, inequities, and spiraling costs of Medicare, a number of reforms have been proposed. Some proposals focus on how health care is provided. For example, increasing attention has been given to finding ways to reduce the disproportionately high costs of care in the last years of life; possibilities include rationing expensive health care interventions, such as organ transplants, artificial organs, and replacement joints, and questioning whether additional medical care is in the patient's best interest (Avorn, 1986). Our discussion in Chapter 14 about the right to die illustrates a slowly growing consensus that, in many instances, no good is served by prolonging the dying of an individual by days or weeks of intensive, expensive therapies (President's Commission, 1983). On the other hand, the question of when to provide what care is extremely complex, given our inability to predict accurately the future quality of life and to agree upon the basis for denying life-saving technologies. Who is to judge quality of life? For example, a recent study at the Palo Alto Medical Clinic found that the majority of their older patients who had died had nevertheless had a satisfactory quality of life in their last year, and thus were not clearly patients for whom life-sustaining technologies should have been terminated (Scitovsky, 1985).

Debates about rationing medical interventions are frequently framed in terms of intergenerational competition, with health care of the elderly viewed as consumption and that of the young as an investment. Callahan (1986), for example, argues that both young and old need to agree on a limit on the length of individual lives that a society can be expected to maintain at public cost. Critics of the current health care system maintain that a de facto rationing of medical care already exists, based on income and ability to pay (Avorn, 1986).

Other proposals involve changing Medicare procedures and regulations. These include generating new sources of revenue, removing the present prohibition against reimbursement for preventive care, combining Parts A and B into a single program, raising the age of initial Medicare eligibility to age 68 or 70, and shifting from an age- to a needs-based Medicare system (Ball, 1985; Callahan, 1986). A recent proposal to Congress is to make catastrophic health insurance for hospital care available to Medicare enrollees for an additional monthly premium; however, this overlooks the fact that most health catastrophes for the elderly generate expenses from nonhospital care (e.g., outpatient prescription drugs, dental and vision care, and nursing home care).

Comprehensive procedural revisions have been proposed to Congress by the Harvard Medical School. This plan has three goals: containment of Medicare expenditures; fairness to the elderly, to health care providers, and to other groups who are affected by the program; and simplicity. One of the most fundamental proposed changes in this plan is that Medicare should cover the cost of extended nursing home care, and provide more generous coverage of long-term care in outpatient settings, especially home health care and mental health services. The Harvard plan also proposes administrative simplification, decreased copayments and increased premiums adjusted according to ability to pay, and reforms in payments to physicians and hospitals. Rep. Claude Pepper has introduced legislation that would establish a new Part C under Medicare. This would provide comprehensive coverage of both acute and chronic health care needs. Although the proposed changes are unlikely to be passed in the near future because of the current political agenda of deficit reduction through cuts in domestic programs, they have served to move policy debates beyond merely cost containment (Harvard Medicare Project, 1986).

Although ours is the only major advanced industrial society that does not provide some form of publicly guaranteed, universally available health insurance, public support for a national health plan is growing. The Gray Panthers have been the strongest supporters of the elimination of Medicare and the creation of a National Health Plan. Even some members of the medical profession recognize the cost savings possible through a national system (Himmelstein and Wool-handler, 1986). It is argued that a national health plan would be less expensive than what is already spent through Medicare, Medicaid, private insurance, and out-of-pocket payments (Vladeck, 1983). Advocates of a national health service maintain that health care is a right to which all people, regardless of income or age, are entitled. They also contend that the health problems of the elderly cannot be solved effectively except as part of a broad-based program covering all age groups with universal accessibility, cost containment, and quality of care built into it. In 1986, this movement gained sufficient momentum to introduce a plan called "U.S. Health" in Congress that would replace Medicare, Medicaid, and most private insurance, and offer a complete health care benefit package. Although the legislation was not passed, it will probably lead to other efforts in this area. Rather than waiting for federal direction, the state of Massachusetts has taken the lead in this area by passing a Health Security Program, which has established universal access for all necessary medical services (Cockburn, 1986).

Medicaid

Medicaid was enacted in 1965. In contrast to Medicare, it is not a health insurance program for those age 65 and over, but rather a federal and state program of

The Older Women's League has pressed for changes in the health care system.

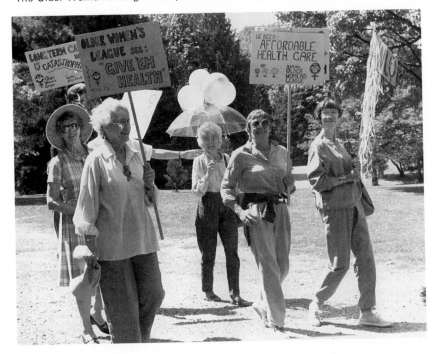

medical assistance for the needy, regardless of age. It covers older people as well as individuals eligible for assistance through Aid to Families with Dependent Children, and programs for the disabled and blind. Although more than half of the nation's poor do not meet the stringent eligibility requirements, Medicaid is the principal health care insurance provided for the poor. Approximately 16 percent of all older people are dependent on Medicaid, which covers 33 percent of older households living at or below the poverty line (Minkler and Estes, 1984).

Medicaid also differs from Medicare in that federal and state funds are administered through local welfare departments. Because Medicaid is tied to state welfare policy, it carries a stigma of welfare for some older people. This arrangement also results in variability among states in terms of eligibility requirements and the scope of health benefits provided. The states that have "generous" eligibility standards and benefits must pay for it in large part themselves, since there is no national policy uniform for all low-income elderly (Estes, 1984).

Federal regulations require that state Medicaid programs provide hospital inpatient care, physician services, skilled nursing facility care, laboratory and x-ray services, home health services, hospital outpatient care, family planning, rural health clinics, and early and periodic screening. In addition, many states provide up to 32 other optional services, including intermediate care, prescription drugs outside the hospital, some dental services, and eyeglasses (Muse and Sawyer, 1982). Unfortunately, however, these services are most vulnerable to state fiscal crises, so that in times of decreased revenues, Medicaid becomes a target for cutting costs. Since states have discretion to limit Medicaid coverage selectively, both in terms of services offered and program eligibility, the result is wide variations across states.

As with Medicare, Medicaid public expenditures have grown more rapidly than inflation. This is not because of an increase in the number of Medicaid recipients and the utilization rate of services, however (Gibson, Waldo, and Levit, 1983). Instead, price increases by health providers are the key factor in expenditure increases, whereas population growth and improvements in quality or complexity of care are negligible causes. Currently, Medicaid forms a growing proportion of many state budgets and is outrunning their capacities to raise the necessary revenues (Estes and Lee, 1981). Furthermore, many states have had to cut other programs in order to offset Medicaid increases at a time when overall state revenues have declined. With growing fiscal constraints at state and local levels, eligibility and scope of services have been reduced in most states. These benefit reductions, however, have not addressed the source of rising hospital and nursing home costs.

Older persons constitute a minority (15 to 17 percent) of the total users of Medicaid, yet they account for 40 percent of the total Medicaid expenditures (Davis, 1986). This disproportionate rate of expenditures is due to many of the same factors that underlie escalating Medicare costs. Another major cause is that Medicaid is the primary public source for funding nursing home care. In fact, approximately 55 percent of nursing home revenues come from Medicaid (Meiners and Gollub, 1984). Figure 19–3 illustrates how Medicaid funds are distributed, and shows that most of the Medicaid growth has resulted from nursing home costs. Such costs account for about 44 percent of the total Medicaid expenditures and 68 percent of the Medicaid funds spent specifically on older people (Waldo and Lazenby, 1984). Overall, nursing home expenditures, which are increasing at an average annual rate of 10 percent, form the fastest growing category of Medicaid expenses. Given the relatively small proportion of older people who are in nursing homes, this means that expenditures are concentrated on a small portion of elderly enrollees. For example, less than 34 percent of older Medicaid recipients account for more than 82 percent of the total Medicaid expenditures for nursing homes (U.S. HCFA, 1984).

Critics contend that Medicaid encourages unnecessary institutionalization, and benefits the major corporate enterprises that own an increasing percentage of nursing homes (Vladeck, 1980; Olson, 1984). Current estimates suggest that five to ten corporations will control 50 percent of all nursing home beds by 1990 (Harrington, 1984). The well-organized nursing home industry has often been able to promote regulations and other public policies favorable to its own

FIGURE 19–3 Where the Medicaid Dollar for the Elderly Goes, 1984

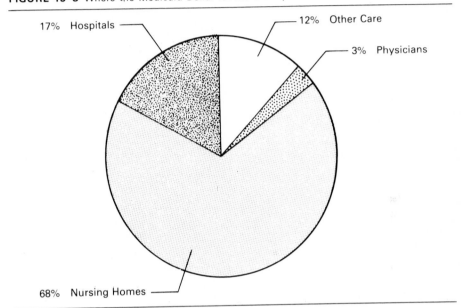

17% Hospitals

12% Other Care

3% Physicians

68% Nursing Homes

Source: Waldo and Lazenby, Health Care Financing, 1984.

interests. At the same time, future needs for skilled nursing home care are growing at a much faster rate than the state resources available through Medicaid.

Medicaid is also criticized for perpetuating class inequities, since some physicians refuse to take Medicaid patients because the fees allowed for reimbursement are generally below the prevailing cost levels. About 25 percent of physicians refuse to treat Medicaid patients, and most will accept them as no more than 20 percent of their load (Mitchell and Cromwell, 1983). Since the number of Medicaid beds in nursing homes is limited, Medicaid patients must often wait longer for placement than do private-pay patients (Crystal, 1982), and the proprietary homes available to them are frequently of lower quality.

One of the most controversial Medicaid requirements is that patients must first exhaust their own assets (excluding their house and car) on medical expenses until their remaining resources are below the levels set for eligibility. This "spend-down" qualification serves to impoverish even middle-class older patients and their spouses, especially wives. When the institutionalized spouse is a husband who has been the primary income earner during the marriage, any pension income in his name must be used to pay Medicaid. This leaves the wife with little or no income to support herself during his institutionalization or after his death. In response to this, the Older Women's League has proposed legislation that would permit states to shield one-half the marital property from the Medicaid

---

The Effects of the Medicaid Spend-Down Requirement

In order to secure needed care for her institutionalized, dying husband, and to avoid being left in poverty, Mrs. Hart filed for legal separation. Her husband's monthly retirement of $1,110 covered only half his nursing home charges. She had to use their stocks and securities to pay the bills. Within 18 months, half their life savings were gone and no end was in sight. The legal separation assigned their remaining assets to her and made him eligible for Medicaid. But Mrs. Hart feels guilty about the separation.

---

spend-down process. Some states have recently allowed the spouse needing nursing home care to transfer his or her assets to the less dependent spouse left in the family home. This serves to protect the spouse's income as well as the estate for heirs.

Since annual nursing home costs average $22,000, most private-pay patients soon deplete their assets. About 75 percent of nursing home patients receive at least partial Medicaid support, and the majority of patients end up on Medicaid within one to two years after admission (Crystal, 1982). In fact, 66 percent of single older people and 33 percent of married people who enter nursing homes face destitution within 13 weeks (U.S. House of Representatives, 1985). The spend-down requirement, coupled with nursing home restrictions against accepting patients who are already on Medicaid, means that Medicaid subsidies are available to the more middle-class elderly who have the financial resources to be admitted to a nursing home and eventually "spend-down"; ironically, they are less available to the "truly poor" who have to enter a nursing home initially as a Medicaid recipient.

Alternatives to Institutionalization

The words *long-term care* conjure up images of institutional facilities, of frailty, and of loss of independence. In actuality, however, long-term care includes ways to preserve an older person's independence. As noted in Chapter 12, it encompasses a range of services to meet the physical, social, and emotional needs of older persons with chronic illnesses or disabilities that interfere with their independence and ability to perform the activities of daily living. These services can be delivered in:

- the traditional *institutional facility* (e.g., nursing homes, hospitals, and outpatient clinics)

- *noninstitutional community settings* (e.g., nutrition programs, senior centers, adult day care, respite care, hospices, and transportation)
- a *person's home* (e.g., through skilled nursing care and occupational and physical therapy, social work services, chore services, home-delivered meals, emergency response systems, homemaker/home health aides, friendly visiting and telephone reassurance programs).

With over 20 percent of nursing home placements estimated to be incongruent with the older person's needs (Knight and Walker, 1985), community-based care is widely advocated as an alternative to inappropriate or premature institutionalization. Consumer surveys consistently show that older people prefer home care over hospitals or nursing homes (Jackson and Jensen, 1984; Brickfield, 1986–87). In addition, studies have found that patients recover from illnesses and accidents faster at home (U.S. General Accounting Office, 1982). Some innovative programs, such as New York state's Nursing Home without Walls, have demonstrated that nursing home candidates can be well cared for at home at a cost that is at least 25 percent below comparable nursing home care (Lombardi, 1986–87). Despite such evidence in support of in-home care alternatives, institutional care still dominates the long-term care system.

Ideally, a comprehensive system should include preventive health services, medical treatment, rehabilitation or therapy, and supportive health and social services. What exists is far from the ideal, however; there is no comprehensive long-term care system operating consistently around the country, nor is there a national policy on long-term care. Few incentives have existed to encourage the establishment of ongoing, cooperative arrangements among health and social service agencies.

A major obstacle to such a system is the method of financing health care for the elderly. As noted earlier, existing reimbursement mechanisms are not designed to provide community-based nonmedical services. Neither Medicaid nor Medicare adequately addresses noninstitutional components of the long-term care system, particularly services to enable older people to remain in the community, such as home health care, respite care, chore, and homemaker services. Less than 2 percent of Medicaid expenditures go to home health care services (e.g., skilled nurses, social workers, physical and occupational therapists). Even though Medicare is the largest single source of payment for home care, it only covers skilled nursing for the acute care needs of the homebound elderly for a limited time period. Once the patient's condition stabilizes and services are needed for health maintenance, coverage ceases, even when home care might prevent potential hospitalization or nursing home placement, which, as we have already seen, can be extremely costly for society and for patients themselves (Nassif, 1986–87).

Another major barrier is the current political climate that emphasizes cost containment, deficit reduction, and private initiatives. At the same time that

Medicare's prospective payment system (DRGs), described earlier in this chapter, is driving more patients prematurely into the community from the hospital, the federal government is imposing more restrictive interpretations on what Medicare reimburses for home care. This is resulting in reduced services to elderly patients, as well as financial losses to home care providers. Reimbursement per visit for each professional discipline is now being limited, which means that many home care agencies find it difficult to offer the more costly services, such as social work, speech pathology, and occupational therapy. Few private insurance programs include comprehensive home care coverage for long term custodial services (Nassif, 1986–87; Meiners, 1985).

HOME CARE

Despite these reimbursement barriers, home care has grown considerably in the past five years. Payment alternatives are being developed to enhance delivery of services. For example, one way to manage costs is for nonprofit community-based home care agencies, such as visiting nurse organizations, to operate on a "sliding scale" basis, adjusting fees according to a client's ability to pay. Such growth will undoubtedly continue, given the preference of most elderly to remain in their own homes, continued technological advances that will enable sophisticated medical care to be provided at home, the persistent shortage of nursing home beds, and the societal need for less expensive alternatives to institutional care (Holt, 1986–87).

The initiative to develop and expand noninstitutional community alternatives has been left primarily to states (Harrington, Newcomer, and Estes, 1985). Currently, states may apply to the federal Health Care Financing Administration for special exemptions (called *waivers*) from regulations that have restricted home care services. If the waivers can be presumed to prevent institutionalization, recipients in waivered states may receive services such as long-term nursing, case management, chore services, respite care, and even home repair (Nassif, 1986–87). Although such alternative programs have increased in the past 10 years, funds allocated to these programs have remained extremely small relative to total long-term care expenditures. No federal initiative has been taken to develop a comprehensive network of alternative services (Harrington, 1985).

OTHER FORMS OF COMMUNITY-BASED CARE

Respite care is an example of a community-based service widely recognized as desirable but implemented primarily through short-term demonstration projects. Respite care is provided in-home or out-of-home in adult day care centers or by temporary stays in nursing homes, geriatric units of rehabilitation centers, and Veterans Administration hospitals. The use of adult day care for respite purposes is limited, however; for example, only a small number of states cover adult day care on a statewide basis (U.S. Commerce Clearing House, 1984). Likewise, states vary considerably in the availability of nursing home respite beds, primarily because of the lack of coverage by Medicare or private insurance. Whether respite care significantly reduces the cost of institutional long-term care has yet to be documented. Some advocates argue, however, that even if respite does not reduce this risk, it is essential for the family caregiver's well-being. The Older Women's League, for example, has provided national leadership in proposing model respite legislation, components of which have been adopted as demonstration projects by some states. In this model, respite includes in-home, inpatient, and emergency care, and is integrated as part of a system of family support functions linked to case management and other coordinating mechanisms (Older Women's League, 1985). As is true of other community-based alternatives to nursing home placement, the greatest barrier to respite care is the limited funding options.

S/HMOS

Another demonstration effort being cautiously explored by the federal government is the Social Health Maintenance Organization or S/HMO. The S/HMO provides comprehensive social and home health services, including custodial care, within a preset budget, even for long-term chronic conditions. Medicare beneficiaries pay slightly higher premiums than exist elsewhere; Medicaid recipients pay nothing. The S/HMO demonstration will help test whether comprehensive health services, including long-term care, can be provided at a cost that does not exceed the public costs of Medicare and Medicaid (Nassif, 1986).

DISCHARGE PLANNING AND CASE MANAGEMENT

With the greater likelihood of Medicare patients being released from hospitals sicker and earlier because of cost incentives, discharge planning has grown in importance. Rather than simply arranging a nursing home placement, discharge planners need to confront the complex, time-consuming task of arranging for a package of care at home. Another service component that is being offered by a growing number of state and local programs is case management. Case management was first tested in a series of over 15 federally sponsored demonstrations from 1973–85. Under approved waivers or exemptions from Medicaid regulations, the federal government currently reimburses for case management services in over 40 states (Applebaum, 1986). Case management aims to increase service accessibility and to coordinate services offered by several agencies in a given locality. Case management staff, in both public and private agencies, perform outreach, eligibility screening, assessments, care planning, service arrangement, ongoing monitoring to assure appropriate delivery of services, and reassessment to adjust care plans to changing needs. The latter two functions distinguish case management from other social service activities and are crucial to the well-being of frail elderly with complex and changing situations.

Other Government Health Care Programs

Other government programs that support health care for older Americans include the Veterans Administration (VA), the Indian Health Service, as well as state and local government hospitals. As noted in Chapter 1, the VA service is the largest of these, providing care in over 172 hospitals and 101 nursing homes. The VA also contracts with community nursing homes and state veterans homes for additional care for eligible veterans. Older veterans accounted for 12 percent of the patients treated in VA facilities in 1982. With the rise in the number and average age of veterans over the next 20 years, it is expected that the group over age 65 will represent 37 percent of all veterans in the year 2000. The costs of health care to veterans will increase for the same reasons as the escalating health care costs for all elderly. In 1982, older veterans accounted for 27 percent of all hospital discharges and 32 percent of discharges from medical and surgical beds, even though they represented only 12 percent of the veteran population (Congressional Budget Office, 1984).

The Indian Health Service operates hospitals and community clinics for native Americans and Alaskan natives of all ages. Some state and local governments operate hospital care for their indigent population, many of whom are elderly. Health block grants, grants for preventive health care and health promotion for older people, as well as primary care, have also served to fill the gaps left by Medicare and Medicaid.

Future Directions

At the same time that concern mounts about public health care costs, the private sector is becoming more competitive in marketing private health care services to the upper-income segment of the older population that has the resources to purchase them. Growing awareness of the elderly's purchasing power is reflected in the diversity of emerging health care plans, hospital-sponsored outpatient and long-term care services, and advertising of such services to recruit older patients.

Another area ripe for marketing is long-term care insurance. Private insurers have recently begun to offer, albeit cautiously, long-term care insurance. These programs are not a panacea to the problems described above, however. Most policies still require that the older person pay a per diem toward the cost of nursing home care; they are usually unavailable to those over age 79, pay for only a limited period (generally up to three years), and do not cover Alzheimer's disease, which is one of the most common reasons for nursing home placements. A major restriction is that most policies do not cover custodial or personal in-home care services, primarily because insurance companies fear that the elderly would overutilize home care services rather than turn to family and friends (Brickfield, 1986–87; Leonard, 1986; Meiners, 1985). Although the development of private long-term care insurance has been praised by age-based organizations, it represents a major shift in both cost and values. Instead of having the general population meet a substantial part of long-term care costs through Medicaid, this shift proposes that the elderly should pool their own resources and spread the financial risks by assuming a higher proportion of long-term care costs through private insurance. Financing of long-term care via the private sector departs significantly from the assumptions of societal responsibility that underlie Medicare and Medicaid.

Although private long-term care insurance may be an option for middle- and upper-income Americans, the need is growing for federal and state programs to protect the elderly who cannot afford to pay for health care. A national long-term care policy is needed that would:

- be comprehensive, including preventive and restorative care, treatment and illness management services in both community and institutional settings.
- give incentives to providers to keep costs reasonable, to prevent unnecessary utilization, and to promote the use of appropriate services.
- have a financing system that provides protection from impoverishment.
- ensure access for those needing services regardless of financial resources, age, or disability, thereby providing age-integrated services (Estes and Harrington, 1985; Harrington, 1985; Crystal, 1982).

Policy debates need to move beyond juxtapositions of institutional versus home care, and consider other types of intermediate supportive living arrangements as well as the needs of caregiving families. Financing a full range of quality services along the long-term care continuum while controlling costs and meeting demand is a major challenge for our society.

Health Promotion with the Elderly

As noted in Chapter 6, health promotion programs are another recent policy response to the growing demand for both acute and long-term care. In an aging society with escalating health care costs, the question of prevention and early intervention assumes more importance than in the past. There is increasing concern on both a societal and personal level with health promotion as a way to forestall the onset of disability rather than with effecting a cure (Avorn, 1986). As

Dychtwald (1983), one of the leading proponents of health promotion for the elderly has noted, "If we are to survive the aging of America, we must first find ways to make our older citizens well" (p. 5).

As stated succinctly by the 1979 Surgeon General's Report, *Healthy People,* prevention not only improves the quality of life, but also can save dollars in the long run. Growing awareness of these benefits is not reflected in the allocation of health dollars, however. As discussed above, Medicare and most private health insurance plans do not pay for preventive services. Most health promotion efforts have been funded through short-term publicly funded demonstration projects or by private foundations. An encouraging sign, however, is the number of hospitals, health care clinics, and work sites that are beginning to offer health promotion services.

Although health promotion for the elderly is generally regarded as a positive direction, some limitations nevertheless exist. Most efforts have focused on the well elderly, not on the severely impaired who are the major users of health services. Health promotion programs have also been criticized for their emphasis on individual responsibility for change, thereby minimizing the societal factors that underlie individual health practices and use of services, such as access to affordable health care (Minkler, 1984; Crawford, 1978; Garfield, 1979). Likewise, some educational efforts ignore the roles of policymakers, health care providers, food manufacturers, and the mass media in creating social and economic environments that may counter health promotion interventions. In addition to educating individuals to adopt healthy habits, the broader social environment must be changed, for example, through training older people in advocacy and political action (Minkler and Fullerton, 1980). Another limitation is that, although the value of health promotion efforts is widely publicized, individuals often do not act on this information. Think about the number of people who continue to smoke, despite the empirical evidence linking smoking to lung cancer, or the small proportion of women over age 45 who have a Pap smear test and breast exam on a regular basis, even though such tests are important in detecting cancer (Thornsberry, Wilson, and Golden, 1986). As we are all aware, people do not always engage in healthy behaviors, even when they know that they should! The gap between health knowledge and health practices can be large.

To the extent that interventions focus primarily on individual change, their relevance is questionable for low-income and ethnic minority populations, whose health problems often stem from situational factors such as poverty over which individuals have little control. Accordingly, low-income populations, preoccupied with meeting basic needs, may view exercise and healthy foods as luxuries. To date, few health promotion efforts have been effectively implemented with low-income or ethnic minority groups (Minkler and Fullerton, 1980).

Even when individual behavioral change is a legitimate goal, sustaining health practices over time is difficult in the face of years of habit. In fact, little is known about the long-term changes resulting from many health promotion interventions, because most evaluations have been conducted soon after program completion, with no long-term follow-up. Health promotion programs that have been demonstration efforts have not been long-lasting nor widely replicated. Longitudinal research is needed to assess the long-range consequences of health promotion interventions for individuals and for health care costs, especially since programs to modify health-related behaviors may initially be very costly before they achieve long-run savings. Nevertheless, health promotion is clearly a growing area for the 1980s, and raises numerous opportunities for policy and program development and research.

Summary and Implications

With the growing health care expenditures by both the federal and state governments and older people themselves, spending for health care has become a source of concern for most Americans. The increasing proportion of the older population along with escalating hospital and physician costs have placed enormous pressure on the Medicare program—the financing mechanisms through which almost half of the funds for the elderly's care flow. The government's primary response to these Medicare costs has been cost-containment, particularly through the diagnostic related groupings (DRGs) which provide incentives for shortening the hospital stays of Medicare patients. Yet, this system of payment has placed growing pressures on families, home-care agencies, and nursing homes to care for sicker patients requiring higher levels of care. Recently, more proposals have been made for reforming the Medicare system, not just implementing incremental cost-cutting measures.

The other primary source of public funding for the elderly—Medicaid—has also been subject to cost-cutting measures. At the same time, copayments for health care services have increased, a cost that is disproportionately borne by low-income elderly. Medicaid is the primary source of funding nursing homes for the elderly. Unfortunately, in order to qualify for Medicaid, older people must first exhaust their resources, a requirement that has served to impoverish many older people and their spouses (although some states are modifying this requirement). Another major disadvantage of this method of financing nursing home care is that most nursing homes have a limited number of beds for Medicaid-paying patients and give first priority to placing private-pay patients. Given the gaps and problems with Medicare and Medicaid funding for nursing home care, a growing number of private companies are offering costly long-term care insurance options. Many of these, however, provide only limited institutional coverage and do not include home care benefits.

Long-term care does not just refer to nursing home care, but encompasses a range of other community-based options developed to support older people's independence, including home care, respite care, and case management. Unfortunately, most of these community-based services are not routinely covered by either Medicare or Medicaid, although some states have been able to obtain Medicaid waivers in order to offer more in-home services. Even though the number of community alternatives to nursing home placement is growing, many services remain fragmented and uncoordinated. There is growing consensus that a national long-term care policy is needed.

Health care services for the elderly have tended to focus primarily on acute care, and secondarily on long-term care or maintenance. With the growing public and professional awareness of the importance of lifestyle health behaviors in preventing illness and reducing health costs, however, health promotion programs have been implemented with older populations. More efforts are needed to develop health promotion interventions aimed at low-income and ethnic minority elderly as well as the old-old, and to evaluate their long-term consequences. Given the growing recognition of multiple causes of disease—biological, sociocultural, and environmental, as well as behavioral—a balanced health policy for the 1980s should include cost-containment efforts for primary, secondary, and long-term care, as well as efforts to expand programs in health promotion and disease prevention, a revamping of reimbursement systems, and a social support component.

References

Applebaum, R. *A guide to the evaluation of long-term care case management programs.* Seattle: University of Washington, Institute on Aging, 1986.

Avorn, J. Medicine: The life and death of Oliver Shay. In A. Pifer and L. Bronte (Eds.), *Our aging society: Paradox and promise.* New York: W. W. Norton, 1986.

Ball, R. Medicare: A strategy for protecting and improving it. *Generations,* 1985, *14,* 9–12.

Bergthold, C., and Estes, E. More or less? The impact of Medicare policy on home health care. Presented at meetings of the Gerontological Society of America, Chicago, November 1986.

Brickfield, C. Who will pay? *Generations,* 1986–87, *11,* 12–14.

Brown, E. R. Medicare and Medicaid: The process, values and limits of health care reforms. In M. Minkler and C. Estes (Eds.), *Readings in the political economy of aging.* Farmingdale, N.Y.: Baywood, 1984.

Callahan, D. Health care in the aging society: A moral dilemma. In A. Pifer and L. Bronte (Eds.), *Our aging society: Paradox and promise.* New York: W. W. Norton, 1986, pp. 319–339.

Coalition on Women and the Budget. *Inequality of sacrifice: The impact of the Reagan budget on women.* Washington, D.C.: National Women's Law Center, 1983.

Cockburn, A. Health care: Sowing the seeds of revolution. *Gray Panther Network,* Spring 1986, 3–5.

Congressional Budget Office. *Veterans Administration health care: Planning for future years.* Washington, D.C., 1984.

Crawford, R. You are dangerous to your health. *Social Policy,* Jan./Feb. 1978, 11–20.

Crystal, S. *America's old age crisis: Public policy and the two worlds of aging.* New York: Basic Books, 1982.

Davis, K. Paying the health-care bills of an aging population. In A. Pifer and L. Bronte (Eds.), *Our aging society: Paradox and promise.* New York: W. W. Norton, 1986.

Dychtwald, K. Overview: Health promotion and disease prevention for elders. *Generation,* 1983, *7,* 5–7.

Estes, C. Fiscal austerity and aging. In C. Estes, R. Newcomer, and Associates (Eds.), *Fiscal austerity and aging.* Beverly Hills: Sage, 1983.

Estes, C. Austerity and aging: 1980 and beyond. In M. Minkler and C. Estes (Eds.), *Readings in the political economy of aging.* Farmingdale, N.Y.: Baywood, 1984.

Estes, C., and Harrington, C. Fiscal crisis, deinstitutionalization, and the aged. *American Behavioral Scientist,* 1981, *24,* 811–826.

Estes, C., and Harrington, C. Future directions in long-term care. In C. Harrington, R. Newcomer, C. Estes, and Associates (Eds.), *Long-term care for the elderly: Public policy issues.* Beverly Hills: Sage, 1985.

Estes, C., and Lee, P. Policy shifts and their impact on health care for elderly persons. *Western Journal of Medicine,* 1981, *135,* 511–517.

Estes, C., and Lee, P. Social, political and economic background of long-term care policy. In C. Harrington, R. Newcomer, C. Estes, and Associates (Eds.), *Long-term care of the elderly: Public policy issues.* Beverly Hills: Sage, 1985.

Federal Council on Aging. *The need for long-term care: Information and issues.* A chartbook of the Federal Council on Aging. Prepared by Long Term Care Committee, Federal Council on Aging, DHHS Pub. No. (OHDS), 81-20704. Washington, D.C., 1981.

Garfield, J. Social stress and medical ideology. In C. Garfield (Ed.), *Stress and survival: The emotional realities of life threatening illness.* St. Louis: C. V. Mosby, 1979.

Gibson, R. M., Waldo, D. R., and Levit, K. R. National health expenditures, 1982. *Health Care Financing Review,* 1983, *5,* 1–31.

Harrington, C. Public policy and the nursing home industry. In M. Minkler and C. Estes (Eds.), *Readings in the political economy of aging.* Farmingdale, N.Y.: Baywood, 1984.

Harrington, C. Alternatives to nursing home care. *Generations,* 1985, *9,* 43–46.

Harrington, C., Newcomer, R. J., and Estes, C. *Long term care of the elderly: Public policy issues.* Beverly Hills: Sage, 1985.

Harris, R. Fitness and exercise. *Generations,* 1983, *7,* 23–26.

Harvard Medicare Project. Special report: The future of Medicare. *New England Journal of Medicine,* 1986, *314,* 722–728.

Himmelstein, D., and Woolhandler, S. Cost without benefit: Administrative waste in U.S. health care. *New England Journal of Medicine,* 1986, *314,* 441–445.

Holt, S. The role of home care in long-term care. *Generations,* 1986–87, *11* (2), 9–11.

Iglehart, J. K. Medicare begins payment of hospitals. *New England Journal of Medicare,* 1983, *308* (23), 1428–1432.

Jackson, B., and Jensen, J. Home care tops consumers' list. *Modern Health Care,* 1984, 88–90.

Jacobs, B., and Abbott, S. Planning for wellness: A community-based approach. *Generations,* 1983, *7,* 57–59.

Jones, A. Prospective payment: Curbing Medicare costs at patient's expense? *Generations,* 1984, *9,* 19–21.

Knight, B., and Walker, D. L. Toward a definition of alternatives to institutionalization for the frail and elderly. *The Gerontologist,* 1985, *25,* 358–363.

Leonard, F. The legal observer. *The OWL Observer,* 1986, *5,* 219.

Liu, K., Manton, K., and Liu, B. M. Home care expenses for the disabled, *Health Care Financing Review,* 1986, *7,* 33–49.

Lombardi, T. Nursing home without walls. *Generations,* 1986–87, *11,* 21–23.

Meiners, M. Long-term care insurance. *Generations,* 1985, *9,* 39–41.

Meiners, M., and Gollub, J. Long term care insurance: The edge of an emerging market. *Healthcare Financial Management,* 1984, *38,* 58–62.

Minkler, M. Blaming the aged victim: The politics of retrenchment in times of fiscal conservatism. In M. Minkler and C. Estes (Eds.), *Readings in the political economy of aging.* Farmingdale, N.Y.: Baywood, 1984.

Minkler, M., and Estes, C. *Readings in the political economy of aging.* Farmingdale, N.Y.: Baywood, 1984.

Minkler, M., and Fullerton, J. *Health promotion, health maintenance and disease prevention for the elderly.* Background paper for the 1981 White House Conference on Aging prepared for the Office of Health Information, Health Promotion, Physical Fitness and Sports Medicine, Department of Health and Human Services, USPHS, Washington, D.C., 1980. (Unpublished.)

Mitchell, J., and Cromwell, J. Access to private physicians for public patients: Participation in Medicaid and Medicare. *Securing access to health care.* President's Commission for the Study of Ethical Problems in Medicine and Biomedical and Behavioral Research, U.S. Government Printing Office, 1983.

Muse, D. N., and Sawyer, W. *The Medicare and Medicaid data book, 1981.* Washington, D.C.: U.S. Health Care Financing Administration, 1982.

Nassif, J. Z. The Social Health Maintenance Organization. *Caring,* 1986, *5,* 34–36.

Nassif, J. There's still no place like home. *Generations,* 1986–87, *11,* 5–8.

Older Women's League. *Respite services bill.* Washington, D.C., 1985.

Olson, L. K. Aging policy: Who benefits? *Generations,* 1984, *10,* 10–14.

Pifer, A., and Bronte, L. *Our aging society: Paradox and promise.* New York: W. W. Norton, 1986.

President's Commission for the Study of Ethnical Problems in Medicine and Biomedical and Behavioral Research. *Deciding to forego life-sustaining treatment.* Washington, D.C.: USGPA, 1983.

Samuelson, R. J. Busting the U.S. budget: The costs of an aging America. *National Journal,* 1978, *10,* 256–260.

Scitovsky, A. Medical costs in the last year of life. *Generations,* 1985, *9,* 27–29.

Storey, J. R. *Older Americans in the Reagan era: Impacts of federal policy changes.* Washington, D.C.: The Urban Institute Press, 1983.

Syme, S. L., and Berkman, L. F. Social class, susceptibility and sickness. *American Journal of Epidemiology,* 1976, *104,* 1–8.

Thornsberry, O., Wilson, R., and Golden, P. Health promotion and disease prevention: Professional data from the National Health Interview Survey, United States, January–June 1985. *NCHS Advance Data,* 119(5/14), 1986.

Torres-Gil, F. Hispanics: A special challenge. In A. Pifer and L. Bronte (Eds.), *Our aging society: Paradox and promise.* New York: W. W. Norton, 1986, pp. 219–243.

Trustees of the Federal Hospital Insurance Trust Fund and Trustees of the Federal Supplementary Medical Insurance Trust Fund. *1985 Annual Report.* Washington, D.C.: Department of Health and Human Services, 1985.

U.S. Commerce Clearing House. *Topical law reports, Medicare and Medicaid guide.* Volume 3-A. Chicago: State charts, 1984.

U.S. Department of Health, Education, and Welfare. *Healthy people. The Surgeon General's Report on health promotion and disease prevention.* Public Health Service, Office of the Assistant Secretary for Health and Surgeon General, Washington, D.C., 1979.

U.S. General Accounting Office. *The elderly should benefit from expanded home health care, but increasing these services will not insure cost reductions.* Washington, D.C.: GAO/IPE, 83–1, 1982.

U.S. Health Care Financing Administration (HC7A). *Medicare and Medicaid expenditures statistics.* Unpublished data. Baltimore, Md.: U.S. Department of Health and Human Services, 1982.

U.S. Health Care Financing Administration (HC7A). *National medical statistics: Fiscal years 1975 to 1982.* State 2082 Tables data tape. Baltimore, Md.: U.S. Department of Health and Human Services, 1984.

U.S. House of Representatives Committee on Ways and Means. *Background material on programs under the jurisdiction of the committee on ways and means.* Washington, D.C.: U.S. Government Printing Office, 1983.

U.S. House of Representatives Special Committee on Aging. Report on long-term care for Blue Cross and Blue Shield of Massachusetts, 1985.

U.S. Office of Management and Budget. *The budget of the United States government: Fiscal year 1981.* Washington, D.C.: U.S. Government Printing Office, 1980.

U.S. Senate Special Committee on Aging. *Developments on aging: 1981,* Part I. Washington, D.C.: U.S. Government Printing Office, 1982.

U.S. Senate Special Committee on Aging. *The proposed fiscal year 1983 budget: What it means for older Americans.* Washington, D.C.: U.S. Government Printing Office, 1982.

U.S. Senate Special Committee on Aging. *America in transition: An aging society.* Washington, D.C.: U.S. Government Printing Office, 1985.

U.S. Senate Special Committee on Aging. *Aging reports,* Spring 1985.

U.S. Senate Special Committee on Aging. *Aging America: Trends and projections, 1985–86 edition.* U.S. Department of Health and Human Services, 1986.

Vladeck, B. *Unloving care: The nursing home tragedy.* New York: Basic Books, 1980.

Vladeck, B. Long-term care: What have we learned? Paper presented at the Western Gerontological Society Meeting on Health and Aging. San Francisco, November 1983.

Waldo, D., and Lazenby, H. Demographic characteristics and health care use and expenditures by the aged in the U.S., 1977–1984. *Health Care Financing Review,* 1984, 6, 1–29.

Wilensky, G., and Berk, M. Medicare and the elderly poor. *Hearing on the future of Medicare.* U.S. Senate Special Committee on Aging, April 13, 1983.

Epilogue

In Chapter 1 we emphasized the importance of studying social gerontology. Reasons for this included the need to better understand our own aging and that of our parents and grandparents; the significant increase in the proportion of older people, especially the very old, in all countries; and historical developments that have dramatically changed the conditions of older people in society. Throughout the book, we have examined the physical and psychological status of people as they age, and how changes in these areas influence their social roles and behavior. In this final section, we turn briefly to the future of aging, to understand how future cohorts will differ from people who are currently aged 65 and older, and to anticipate how existing policies will influence the social well-being of the "future aged."

Trends That Affect Aging in the Future

The growth of the population over age 65, particularly those over age 75, provides a major challenge to society and to individuals themselves, as they anticipate living many more years after childrearing, education, and a career. The greatest increase in the aging population will occur early in the twenty-first century as the "baby boom generation" (i.e., those born between 1945 and 1960) reaches old age and creates the "senior boom." Since this population is already alive, we can predict with considerable accuracy that 17 percent of the U.S. population will be 65 and older in 2020, compared to 11.7 percent in 1985. People aged 55 to 65 will represent the largest subgroup of the population in 2020. In that same period, the proportion over age 75 will increase from 33 percent to 50 percent of all elderly (U.S. Senate Special Committee on Aging, 1986). Currently 2.5 million people in the United States are age 85 or older; it is estimated that these numbers will double by the year 2000. An even greater increase is expected in the population 100 years or older, from the current 25,000 to 100,000 by the turn of the century.

This future cohort of older people will differ from current cohorts in ways other than living longer. The era in which they were born and raised, their opportunities for education, their life expectancy, their health care and personal development were vastly different from those who were born between 1890 and 1920. In the United States and most other countries emerging from World War II and the Korean War, economic growth in the 1950s and 1960s appeared endless. Home ownership increased, especially in the newly developing suburbs and planned communities. Enrollment expanded in universities and colleges as the baby boomers reached college age. Advances in medicine and medical technology led to improvements in health care and reduced significantly the risks of mortality from major surgery and diseases, such as heart disease and cancer, that previously were assumed always to be fatal. With public resources seeming to be abundant, the federal government began to assume greater responsibility for the welfare of its citizens; programs to assist low-income families with children emerged in the

1960s (e.g., Aid to Families with Dependent Children and Head Start, low-interest loans to college students) along with services to help older people maintain their health and social well-being [discussed in Chapters 18 and 19]). More recently, with a less expansive economy, the trend has been toward a reduced role for government and an increased emphasis on individual responsibility and the private sector to provide services. Although it is clear that our country will not return to the levels of public spending characteristic of the 1960s, what is unclear is what the mix of public and private responsibility will be in the twenty-first century. We can predict, however, that the increasing rectangularization of the age pyramid will mean that older people will have to be more self-sufficient, and that proportionately fewer young persons will be available to care for the frail elderly.

Since the 1950s, the status of women and ethnic minorities has improved in the United States, although, as discussed in Chapters 15 and 16, older members of these populations have not necessarily benefited from improvements enjoyed by younger women and minorities. The passage of Civil Rights legislation, the women's movement, and increased demands from these segments of the population who were previously denied access to jobs and educational opportunities have resulted in more women and ethnic minorities completing college and obtaining professional degrees, entering the work force, and moving into higher level positions. On the other hand, these gains have not necessarily been widely distributed. Women, for example, still are paid only about 60 cents for every dollar earned by their male counterparts, and they remain concentrated in secondary sector industries and traditionally female-oriented, lower-paying occupations. The rapidly growing number of low-income women as heads of single-parent households, commonly referred to as the *feminization of poverty*, suggests that a large segment of women may reach old age without the support of a spouse and with few economic resources. Such women may, however, try out different types of household arrangements, such as home sharing and intergenerational group living, in an effort to reduce housing costs and meet emotional needs.

Implications for the Future

What do these changes mean for the future of aging? What will life be like for the baby boomers when they become the senior boomers? Unfortunately, we do not have a crystal ball to predict the future with certainty. Some factors are well beyond the control of social gerontologists, including economic conditions, international conflicts, fatal diseases such as AIDs, and natural disasters. We do know enough about the baby boom generation to begin to speculate about the future, however.

More of the future elderly will be members of four- and five-generation families, although probably not living together. Smaller family size may reduce the number of adult children and siblings available to provide support in times of illness or disability. These relationships will be further complicated by the growing number of divorces, step-families, gay and lesbian partners, and single parents. To what extent will younger members of "blended" families and those unrelated by blood but joined by years of sharing familial responsibilities assume the role of caregivers? Who will be responsible for the increasing numbers of never-married persons when they reach advanced old age if they can no longer care for themselves?

Future elderly will be better educated than current and previous cohorts. In 1960, less than 20 percent of the population over age 65 had finished high school. By 1982, approximately 45 percent of this age group had completed high school. The median education level among those under age 65 today is 12.5 years, and almost 13 years among the population under age 25 (U.S. Bureau of the Census, 1982). This means that the majority of older people in the future will be high-school graduates; many will have completed college (Congressional Institute for the Future, 1984). Because of the association between education, occupation, and income, these people are likely to earn more during their lifetimes. More individuals will have private pensions because of legislation during the past 20 years that requires some employers to institute pension programs. Furthermore, the increased number of women and ethnic minorities in jobs with pension plans may make it easier for many people in these groups to enjoy their old age rather than experience it as a time of destitution and despair. A countering force, however, is that more women than men are in part-time jobs and in small businesses, which are not covered by pensions, so that it is unclear at this point to what extent the proportions of women covered by pensions will increase. More people over age 70 may choose to continue working, given the elimination of mandatory retirement, although the pattern of early retirement will probably persist. Most older people will undoubtedly be healthier, having had the advantages of medical technology, preventive medicine, and widely available knowledge about ways of maintaining health. In the remainder of this chapter, we examine some of the trends in family patterns, work and retirement, living arrangements, and health care that have significant implications for the future.

CHANGING FAMILY RELATIONSHIPS

The added years due to increased life expectancy serve to prolong a person's relationships to others—spouse, parents, offspring, friends—whose lives are also extended. For example, more than half of the children born in 1910 and who survived to age 50 had experienced the death of a parent or sibling by their early teens (Uhlenberg, 1980). In contrast, today the loss of parents is not expected until the second half of adulthood, and the death of a child is no longer an anticipated part of family life. For current generations of young women, the death of the mother may occur close to the daughter's retirement age (Winsborough, 1978). These changes mean that a growing proportion of parents and children will share such critical adulthood experiences as work, parenthood, and even retirement and widowhood. Similarly, grandparents may survive to experience many years of their grandchildren's adulthood.

Extending the number of years we can expect to live has also meant that more adult children are involved in caring for frail parents and grandparents, to the point that parent care is now a normative experience for adult children (Brody, 1985). The irony of the myth that families used to care better for their older relatives is that nowadays more adult children provide greater care at more difficult levels and over much longer time periods than they did in the so-called "good old days." Increased life expectancy has combined with reduced fertility, so that for the first time, women can expect to spend more years caring for an aged parent than for a dependent child (*Family Ties*, 1986). Similarly, the average married couple has more living parents than children for the first time in history (Preston, 1984). These trends are likely to persist, given current patterns of reduced fertility, particularly the number of couples who are choosing not to have children.

The increase in longevity has also significantly changed grandparent–grandchildren roles. For example, we now anticipate that our grandparents will not die until our early adulthood, but until quite recently most grandparents did not live long enough to know their grandchildren well (Haraven, 1977). Now, as more women have their first children when they are teenagers, and more have their first child after age 35, first-time grandparenthood occurs for persons ranging in age from 35 to 75. Grandchildren encompass both infants and retirees, and grandparents include active middle-aged adults as well as frail, very old persons. Additional complicating factors are that grandparents and grandchildren are often separated by geographic distance and by divorce and remarriage of the grandchildren's parents; this results in the two generations at the extremes rarely seeing each other. Given such diversity, what are grandparents' rights and obligations? Without historical precedence, there are few clear culturally shared expectations about grandparent–grandchildren relationships.

As members of a person's social network survive longer, there is an increase in the complexity and the vertical links that cross generational lines of the networks. The growth of four- and five-generation families, combined with reduced fertility, have led to more vertical, intergenerational ties, but a decreasing number of horizontal relationships within generations (e.g., siblings, cousins), compared to families of the past. Individuals in a multigenerational family line interact in a much more complex set of family identities than is the case in a lineage with only two generations, those of parent and child. For example, who is responsible for a great-grandparent who falls and needs daily care: the grandparents who may themselves be frail, the parents who may both be employed, or grandchildren who are often still in school? Demarcations between generations are also becoming clearer. For example, active involvement in the daily demands of childrearing is now likely to be completed by the time women are grand-mothers. However, two social trends that blur such demarcations are the growing number of single adolescent mothers and the high rates of divorce. In these instances, grandparents often assume many of the tasks of parenting (Hagestad, 1986).

Two other demographic trends, in addition to the increase in longevity, have profoundly affected families. One is the decline in average family size, and the other is the smaller age difference common between a typical family's oldest and youngest child. Around the turn of the century, on the average, mothers bore 3.9 children, with as much as 15 years between the youngest and oldest child. The current estimate is about 1.8 children (Hagestad and Neugarten, 1985). As more and more women postpone marriage and childbearing into their late thirties and early forties, these trends toward smaller families and toward childbearing compressed into fewer years of a woman's life will continue. These changes suggest an increasing uniformity in childhood experiences and in parent–child relationships, factors that may affect future cohorts' caregiving experiences. For example, siblings who are closer in age and think of themselves as peers may be more likely to share caregiving tasks than to expect the oldest child or the unmarried daughter to be the primary caregiver—a pattern more common in large families in the past. On the other hand, with declining family size, the pool of potential caregivers is smaller, and this trend is likely to continue.

Another change with reduced fertility rates is that there are fewer individuals within each generation in which to invest emotionally. As a result, intergenera-tional relationships are not only more extensive, but also more emotionally intensive (Hagestad, 1986; Uhlenberg, 1980). As we saw in Chapter 10, parents remain invested in offspring for as long as they live. Adult children have a sense of obligation to their parents, and the family remains the major social support to older relatives. These family patterns, consistent for the past 20 years, will persist and perhaps even grow as the number of younger generations within a family increase, thereby distributing the responsibility across generations.

The widened gap between the mortality rates of men and women, which has produced a seven-year difference in the current life expectancy, is a third major demographic change that influences family relationships. As we saw in Chapters 10 and 16, the world of the very old is a world of women, both in society and within families. Some five-generation families may include three generations of widows. Most older women are widows living alone; most older men live with their wives. Such differences in widowhood and remarriage mean that men are more likely to maintain significant horizontal, intragenerational ties, primarily through their wives, until the end of their lives. In contrast, women turn more to intergenerational relationships for help and support throughout their lives, especially in old age (Hagestad and Neugarten, 1985). Even though more women are entering the marketplace traditionally dominated by men, they continue to place greater emphasis on interpersonal relationships. This, combined with the value placed by the women's movement on friendships and social support, suggests that women will continue to build diverse and extensive social networks to which they can turn in old age. For example, more older women in the future may choose to live with other women than today's elderly cohort. Another factor that may contribute to this trend is the growing number of women who choose not to marry; for these women, friends often represent a stronger social bond than relatives.

A social trend that interacts with these demographic changes is the increasing divorce rate. This increase may be inevitable in aging societies, because modern longevity makes marriage a greater long-term commitment than in the past. At the end of the nineteenth century, the average length of marriage until the time when one spouse died was about 28 years. In the late 1970s, it was over 43 years (Furstenberg et al., 1983). The chance of couples who married in the 1930s and 1940s reaching their golden wedding anniversary is less than 5 percent. In spite of increased life expectancy, no more couples reach this 50-year marker nowadays than did a century ago. But before 1974, most marriages ended with death; after 1974, more marriages ended with divorce than death. Nearly half of today's marriages are predicted to end in divorce (Glick, 1980; Goldman and Lord, 1983).

Trends in divorce and remarriage are shaping the life course and social networks of young and old. For women, divorce reduces their standard of living and creates an uncertain financial future. The more resources (e.g., education and income) that a divorced woman has available, the less likely she is to remarry, whereas this is reversed for men (National Center for Health Statistics, 1983). Therefore, men and women who have divorced but not remarried will differ from today's population. Among women divorcing in the 1980s will be a number of resourceful individuals who will already have lived for many decades on their own as they face old age at the turn of the century (Hagestad, 1986). These women may be innovative and adept at coping with the changes that aging brings (Riley and Riley, 1986).

For men, the primary consequence of divorce is disruption of family networks. Most common is reduced contact with children, which also generally means less interaction between paternal grandparents and grandchildren. Children have always faced family disruptions, but now divorce is the more common cause of disruption than is death (Spanier and Glick, 1980). It is estimated that more than 30 percent of all children under age 16 will experience the divorce of their parents. By the time children born in 1980 turn age 17, more than 80 percent of them will have spent some time living with only one parent, generally with the mother. Furthermore, among children whose parents remarry, nearly 40 percent will experience a second divorce (Furstenberg et al., 1983). A growing number of children, parents, and grandparents will thus devote substantial effort toward building reconstituted families and step-relationships, only to find them eventually dissolved. Recent trends in divorce and remarriage raise complex questions. How will children of divorce, remarriage, and redivorce approach relationships during their own adult years? What patterns of support will exist between aging parents and children in families disrupted by divorce?

As noted above, women tend to develop larger and more diverse inter-generational networks, often with other women, than do men. Recent trends in marital disruption may further weaken men's involvement across generations, as suggested by the dramatic decline in number of years that men were involved with their children between 1960 and 1980, and the growing numbers of women who had primary childrearing responsibilities (Antonucci, 1985). Social values toward sexual equality have increased in recent years, but demographic and social changes have created very different family worlds for men and women. An increasing proportion of men have only tenuous vertical ties along generational lines, yet women have retained strong links to both younger and older generations. What will be the relationships between aging fathers and children with whom they have had only sporadic contact for many years? What sort of responsibility will adult children feel toward an aging father who never paid child support? Will the mother–daughter relationship become even more important as the mainstay of family cohesion? And how will these changes affect the development of social policies regarding the care of frail elders?

At the same time that more women, both as single parents and as adult caregivers for parents and grandparents, are assuming more intergenerational responsibilities, their employment demands are expanding. The expectation and necessity for women to enter the paid workplace has grown, without any significant diminution in women's family responsibilities, as evidenced by the fact that women devote as much time to household tasks as they did 50 years ago. Similarly, employment tends to reduce caregiving responsibilities for sons to their aged parents, but not for daughters (Stroller, 1983; Brody, 1985). Such overload has been referred to as the "superwoman squeeze" (Friedan, 1981), or the "woman in the middle" (Brody, 1985). As increasing numbers of women enter the paid work force, traditional expectations about family caregiving can become an unbearable burden for women. Although such sex-based roles are slowly changing in terms of child care, the fact that women still assume primary care for children tempers any unrealistic expectations that men will soon become the primary caregivers of the elderly. Yet women who attempt to combine employ-ment and care of dependents often become physically and emotionally exhausted. A growing number of women are recognizing that they cannot "do it all," and are cutting back on employment responsibilities or turning to community agencies and other family members for assistance. At the same time that family caregivers are requesting more support, the current federal administration is expecting families to provide even more care as a cost-effective alternative to publicly supported services. Who will provide what care for elderly dependents remains a critical policy issue currently and for the future.

NEW DEFINITIONS OF WORK AND PRODUCTIVITY

An imbalance has existed between a population of increasingly long-lived people and decreasing opportunities for them to participate in society (Riley and Riley, 1986). Perhaps the most striking area in which social and cultural structures lag behind demographic changes is in employment. Since 1900, the labor force participation of the elderly has been eroding, and the competence of older workers for productive performance has been consistently underrated. As work opportunities for the older population have declined, pressures have mounted for socially rewarding roles in retirement. Today, people find that they are spending approximately 20 percent of their adult lives in retirement, compared with only 3 percent in 1900 (U.S. Senate Special Committee on Aging, 1986). The trend toward early retirement, combined with increased longevity, means that retirement as a life stage will become even more protracted. As people begin to comprehend how much of the adult lifetime is spent in retirement, there is growing awareness that formal retirement does not end the need for involvement in the larger society. Likewise, as members of successive cohorts retire at younger ages, are better educated, and perhaps healthier than their predecessors, it seems predictable that pressures from older people and from the public at large will modify existing work and retirement roles. Modifications in the workplace are already underway to offset the lag between changes in social structures and the recognition of older people's skills and productivity (Riley and Riley, 1986).

These workplace modifications include both incentives to maintain the older workers' productivity in the workforce as well as ways to ease the transition to retirement. Efforts to retain older workers in the labor force longer include redesigning jobs (e.g., job sharing, flexible and part-time schedules, conducting work at home) in order to accommodate older workers' needs and skills; providing retraining in the new technologies such as computers and robotics, counseling and other support services for new careers; and offering additional forms of compensation such as health benefits or tax credits. Some companies, such as Travelers Insurance, have set up data banks of retiree skills for temporary employment and job sharing. Local and federal government agencies have developed programs to make use of retirees' skills in voluntary and paid employment. For example, the Small Business Administration's SCORE program (Senior Corps of Retired Executives) makes use of retired business executives as counselors for new businesses.

In addition, changing social values about the "appropriate age" for schooling, employment, and retirement demand a reexamination of employment policies. The traditional compartments of education for the young, employment for the middle-aged, and retirement for the old are already undergoing major changes as more middle-aged and older persons enter college for the first time, or begin their studies for a graduate or professional degree. For example, since the *University of*

California Regents v. *Bakke* decision in 1978, more and more persons over age 35 have entered medical, dental, and law schools. From a developmental perspective, temporary "retirement" may be a more viable option for the young worker just starting a family, employment may be desirable for the teenager who is bored with school, and education attractive to the older person who can integrate his or her life experiences with academic content. Instead of the straight career trajectory traditionally followed in our society, movement in and out of the workforce, schooling, and family care may all need to be defined as legitimate options at various stages in the life cycle.

Women have moved in and out of the workforce for years, largely because of assuming family responsibilities, but they have often been penalized for their discontinuous work patterns through lower salaries and retirement benefits. However, with increasing numbers of career-oriented women who are committed to an ideology of shared family responsibilities, and with growing awareness of the possibility of two or three careers over the life course, movement in and out of the workforce may come to be viewed as a legitimate alternative for both men and women. This may also encourage individuals to integrate better their work and family lives.

The recognition of increased longevity has already led to the development of job retraining programs and adult education courses for older workers. In addition, more and more people in their forties and fifties are electing to move into second and even third careers. More organizations are allowing their employees opportunities for growth in their jobs by providing sabbaticals, extended vacations and leaves, retraining programs, and career development alternatives. Such strategies benefit employees by allowing them to explore new careers and volunteer and leisure interests; this, in turn, can serve to prevent job burnout or boredom, so that early retirement is not perceived as the only viable option. These programs also benefit employers in organizations that are undergoing rapid technological changes, such as automobile manufacturing companies that are adopting robotics and computerized assembly lines. By retraining their more experienced workers, such organizations can retain employees who have proven capable in the past.

There is disagreement, however, on the economy's ability to create such work alternatives. In the past decade, the U.S. economy has been characterized by lower growth in productivity, sharper competition from markets abroad, high inflation, and high unemployment. Few economists predict a return to the high growth rates of the 1950s and 1960s, when a rapidly expanding economy and low inflation provided jobs for almost all who wanted them, and improved retirement benefits for those who wanted to retire. There are also uncertainties about the potential impact of technological advances on job opportunities—whether these will produce new jobs or result in net job losses. However, some economists are predicting expansion for the economy toward the end of this century. If so, the older, more experienced workers who have taken advantage of job retraining programs could be leading the boom!

Other workplace options focus on easing the transition to retirement through retirement preparation programs. Retirement needs to be viewed not as a single and irreversible event, but as a process involving successive decisions. For example, IBM has a Retirement Education Assistance plan that provides tuition to employees and their spouses three years prior to retirement eligibility and ends two years after retirement; the plan aims to enable employees to develop new interests and prepare for new careers. Another model, common in some European countries and in Japan, is a "gliding out" plan of phased retirement that permits a gradual shift to a part-time schedule. Jobs can also be restructured, gradually allowing longer vacations, shorter work days, and more opportunities for community involvement during the pre-retirement working years. Volunteer opportunities that draw upon retirees' competence as well as provide them with chances to learn new skills can also blur the line between paid employment and retirement.

Such structural changes are a necessary first step, but our societal attitudes toward the productivity of the elderly must also be altered. As noted in Chapter 12, the meaning of productivity must be redefined to include more than employment. A more humanizing approach is to ask how we can develop and use our human potential in old age as part of a productive society. The vitality of the older population must be recognized out of a need to involve their skills and wisdom, through both paid and unpaid positions, in enriching our society (Butler and Gleason, 1985). Such fundamental redefinitions of old age and aging would move us beyond the artificially framed policy debates about young and old competing for scarce resources. They would also help to counteract the "new ageism" noted by Kalish (1979), and would serve, in the long run, to reduce the dependency, both real and perceived, of older persons. As suggested in Chapter 18, the interdependence of generations across the life span, when made explicit, can provide a future framework for policy and program development. Likewise, intergenerational programs in schools, community centers, nursing homes, retirement facilities, and adult day centers are growing. Such programs serve to utilize the elderly's skills, as well as provide children and youth with opportunities to interact with diverse older people; in other words, to build on the reciprocity that exists between generations. These cooperative, cross-age efforts may have the long run effect of reducing ageism and competition among age groups, so that young and old work together to benefit the most needy in our society, regardless of age. Perhaps in the future it will be unnecessary to develop age-based social and health policies, but rather to establish programs that address special needs.

In addition, future generations of elderly who need public assistance will be more likely to apply for it than previous cohorts. Because they will have grown up with much greater exposure to public assistance programs than current cohorts of elderly, future cohorts may be more adept at dealing with the system, and may feel less stigma from accepting such assistance. Some may even view this as a right, because of their previous contributions to society in the form of income taxes and Social Security taxes. At the same time, however, if trends toward reduced federal domestic spending and cost containment continue, there will be fewer public assistance programs on which older people can rely in the future.

LEISURE IN OLD AGE

As noted in Chapter 13, the concept of leisure is difficult to define; some gerontologists equate it with retirement or describe it as absence of work. Others have defined it as unobligated discretionary time (Kabanoff, 1980), or free time for pleasurable passive *or* active pursuits (Gordon, Gaitz, and Scott, 1976). Still others differentiate leisure from recreation in that the former is unstructured but the latter is planned free time (Atchley, 1971). Traditionally, leisure pursuits and the leisure role have been relegated to the retirement years, so that the traditional life trajectory consisted of education, employment, and childrearing, followed by leisure during retirement. According to this model of the life course, leisure opportunities are considered to be a reward for a lifetime of hard work and therefore are greater for affluent individuals and in societies with longer life expectancy and earlier retirement (Osgood, 1982; Robinson, Coberly, and Paul, 1985). Accordingly, a leisure industry has developed, particularly in retirement communities, to meet the recreational needs of the more affluent and healthy elderly. Think of the variety of social activities and recreational sports that are offered in many planned retirement communities.

Modifications in work patterns and organizational opportunities for career development, described in the previous section, suggest that definitions of leisure are also undergoing major changes. Work and leisure are becoming less compartmentalized and more evenly distributed across the life span through modified work schedules, sabbaticals, job sharing, lifelong education, phased retirement, as well as the increasing number of retirees who work part-time and engage in volunteer activities. This "blurring" of work and leisure is reinforced by increased organizational awareness of employee needs, such as on-the-job exercise and fitness programs, child care, staff training, and psychological counseling. To some extent, these factors are an outgrowth of the shift from the traditional work ethic to a more balanced view of work and leisure in this society (Robinson et al., 1985). Therefore, it is not unrealistic to expect that future cohorts of elderly will view leisure in retirement merely as a continuation of their leisure activities during their younger years, and will not regard it as a new stage in life. Given that many people choose to retire earlier than in the past, and that life expectancy beyond age 65 continues to increase, future elderly will benefit from the opportunity to adopt leisure activities into their preretirement years that can then be carried into the later years. Such integration of leisure throughout the life span will undoubtedly mean a smoother transition to retirement for many older people.

CHANGES IN LIVING ARRANGEMENTS

The movement away from farms and city centers to the suburbs has also resulted in the graying of the suburbs, with many people who had moved to these areas after World War II reaching retirement. A survey of 2,300 suburbs across the United States found that 11.8% of all residents were age 65 and older, with a far greater proportion in suburbs that were first developed in the 1940s (Logan, 1983). Elderly in older suburbs also have lower average incomes and lower home values than those in newer communities.

These trends will continue as the children of these migrants to the suburbs, who in turn built their homes in the suburbs and worked in nearby satellite communities, themselves age. Up until now, most health and social services, such as clinics, hospitals, senior centers, and nutrition sites, have been built near city centers with high concentrations of older people. Future cohorts will expect these services to be located closer to their homes in the suburbs, just as shopping centers, banks, and jobs have been moved outward from urban centers to these areas to accommodate the needs of this population. Think of the growing number of hospitals, nursing homes, and retirement communities that are being built in suburbs where 20 years ago family housing, shopping centers, and schools were the most prevalent type of construction, and 10 years ago, where "business parks" and office buildings were being constructed.

The growth of the suburbs was a natural outcome of the increased automobile ownership among Americans after World War II. The dependence on private automobiles made it unnecessary for many suburban communities to provide mass transportation, even after the oil crisis of 1973. This reliance on a private car may be implicit in middle-age and early old age. But what happens as the older person lives beyond age 75 and 80 in the suburbs, and experiences increased problems with vision, hearing, and reaction time, to the point where he or she must give up driving? Unfortunately, the assumption that people will be willing and able to drive long distances in advanced old age prevails, even among developers of retirement communities. It is not unusual for such communities to be built in physically beautiful locations, but far from places served by mass transportation, and without provisions for vans or other group transport options.

These problems may be alleviated in the future, with the growth of community-based, private and public programs that bring services to the older person's home (e.g., Meals on Wheels, chore workers, home health care, described in Chapter 11), as well as the increasing number of retirement communities that are self-contained. That is, some of these provide health and recreational services; even banking and shopping are nearby. With the trends toward computerized home-based banking and shopping services, future cohorts may not need to leave their homes to obtain services. As more people strive to remain in their homes, the market for home-based services will expand. Furthermore, the emergence of such programs as Emergency Medical Services (911), the Life Safety System or Lifeline Security Systems in retirement complexes, as well as Neighborhood Watch and programs by local utilities to watch over frail elderly living alone have offered a sense of safety for older people who choose to continue living in their own homes. These alternatives will continue to receive attention from future elderly as technological advances make home-based care and security systems available to more older people. For example, robotics is a field that has significantly altered the workplace, and is beginning to be applied in the homes of physically and sensory-impaired persons. The National Association of Home Builders is developing "Smart Houses," where computers and appliances can command each other and exchange feedback through advances in wiring.

Voice-activated computer systems that are being used widely by physically disabled individuals can also serve to enhance the independence of older people with chronic diseases. For example, these new systems can help older persons suffering from severe arthritis to correspond with family and friends, or to "write" their life history. It may be possible to compensate for impaired vision by using audible information instead of visual displays. An example of the use of audible announcements for people with visual or memory impairments is an electric range that can announce: "The front right burner is on high heat" or "The oven temperature is 350 degrees." Computer programs have also been developed to describe potential side effects of various medications and interactions among them. Although these programs are aimed at physicians, pharmacists, and other health professionals, it may be possible in the near future to buy such a program written in layman's language, type in the names and doses of medications one is taking, and then obtain a printout of potential side effects and special precautions. This would be particularly useful to the many elderly who are using numerous prescriptions and over-the-counter medications. Although too costly to implement at present, it is technically possible to conduct remote monitoring between a patient's home and a local health care facility for such things as a blood pressure and heart rate.

Technology also can be used to enhance options for recreation and enrichment for older people. For example, computers will increasingly be used for leisure, such as games linked by telecommunication channels or books read on microchips. Interactive television and videodiscs, special TV programming for the elderly, and open university via television can greatly expand the social worlds of homebound elderly. Technological advances will also benefit younger family members concerned with the financial costs and emotional burdens of caregiving. As robotics and computer systems become more cost-effective and user-friendly, they will be used by frail older people who would otherwise need to rely on family or paid caregivers, or move to a nursing home. These developments will be easier

Future cohorts of elderly persons will use computers to perform many of their daily tasks.

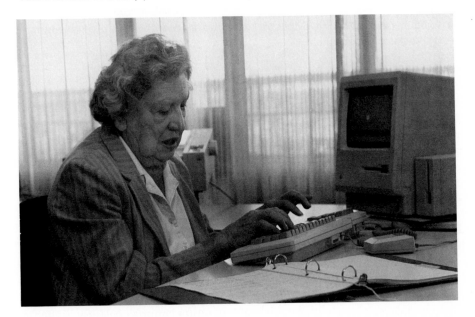

for future generations of elderly to adopt, because they will have grown up with computers and rapid technological advances in their work and leisure.

The cost of maintaining their homes has represented another major deterrent for many older people who wish to remain independent. In response, numerous banks and mortgage companies have begun to offer reverse mortgage plans, described in Chapter 11. In effect, these programs buy the older person's home at current market values, while allowing the individual to remain in it and to have additional financial resources. Some banks offer low-interest home improvement loans to older people, thereby making the home easier to maintain and more attractive to future buyers.

Shared housing is another means of helping older people remain in their own homes, as discussed in Chapter 11. Community programs that match older home-owners with other elderly, or with college students and younger working people who need housing, serve a useful function in making the cost of housing affordable to a wider cross-section of persons. These programs also provide security for frail older people who need occasional assistance from their healthier peers or younger people, but who do not require the constant care of nursing homes. Future cohorts of elderly may also continue the trends of their younger years by sharing housing with an unmarried companion. As society has become more accepting of unmarried couples and gay and lesbian partners living together, the advantages of such arrangements for older couples have become more evident. Thus, for example, sharing a home without marrying can reduce an older couple's expenses while maintaining their separate incomes from pensions and social security benefits. Most importantly, shared housing provides much-needed social companionship.

LONGEVITY IN HEALTH OR DISEASE?

Future cohorts of older people may be healthier and more independent well into their eighties and nineties. A strong argument has been put forth to this effect by Fries (1980), who has suggested that more people will achieve the maximum life span in future years because of healthier lifestyles and better health care during their youth and middle years. Furthermore, Fries argues that future cohorts will have fewer debilitating illnesses and will, in fact, experience "compressed morbidity" (i.e., only a few years of major illness in very old age). These elderly of the future may therefore expect to die a "natural death," or death due to the natural wearing out of all organ systems by approximately age 100. If this process does occur, it will have a significant impact on the type of health services needed by future generations of elderly, and on their demands for employment and leisure activities. Long-term care needs may be reduced, with more short-stay convalescent centers and short-term home health services being required.

A contrasting perspective on the health of future cohorts of elderly is offered by Verbrugge (1984). Based on her analysis of responses to the National Health Interview Survey from 1958 through 1980, Verbrugge notes that cohorts of middle-aged and older persons in each successive survey reported *more* short-term disability and days of restricted activity (i.e., morbidity rates) than did previous cohorts. Morbidity rates increased during this 22-year period for major life-threatening diseases (e.g., heart disease, cancer, diabetes, hypertension), as well as for nonlife threatening diseases (e.g., arthritis), but mortality rates did not. Earlier diagnosis and better health care for these conditions may be responsible for this trend toward survival from major illnesses. Thus, Verbrugge concludes that, although medical advances have prevented death from many acute conditions, older people experience more chronic conditions than did previous cohorts. As noted in Chapter 6, chronic conditions cannot be cured, but rather require long-term care. Verbrugge points out, however, that her findings may not be sensitive to the gradual changes in the health of Americans as a result of improved health habits (e.g., less smoking, less consumption of alcohol and saturated fats, increased exercise) being adopted by many people. A longer period of healthier lifestyles among people currently in their twenties and thirties may result in fewer chronic health problems when they reach old age.

Others have suggested that the average period of diminished vigor will increase because of the growing number of very old people who are most likely to have multiple chronic illnesses, and because some diseases are more likely to begin in old age (Schneider and Brody, 1983). Another perspective suggests that both phenomena will occur simultaneously (Rice and Feldman, 1983). That is, there will be an increasing number of people reaching advanced old age in very good health, while another segment of equally old people will experience prolonged morbidity.

HEALTH CARE DELIVERY IN THE FUTURE

One possibility that offers some promise is that future cohorts of elderly may cope with a longer lifetime of chronic diseases in different ways than previous generations. The increasingly high costs of hospitalization and nursing homes have already resulted in the growth of various options in health care.

A major area of expansion is home health care, provided by hospitals, private and nonprofit agencies, and local governments. These programs, described in detail in Chapter 19, allow older people to remain as self-sufficient as possible in their homes—values that future generations may be more likely to hold because of their greater opportunities for choice. Adult day centers and adult day health programs also provide family members with respite from full-time caregiving for a chronically ill or demented elderly person. But, as noted in Chapter 19, funding for such options is currently limited. What is unknown is the extent to which Medicare and Medicaid will be modified to cover more home health and community-based programs in the future. Certainly, legislation such as that introduced by Rep. Claude Pepper in 1987 point in that direction.

The growth in the number of hospitals over the past 20 years has led to increased competition for older patients. Many have developed special geriatric units, for both acute and chronic care. Some have established satellite clinics and provide health screening and foot care in senior centers and senior housing; others offer health education and health promotion activities for older persons and for family members of frail elderly in hospital and in community settings. Still others provide emergency response systems, home health care, information and referral, and free transportation to the hospital for older patients. The number of hospitals with long-term care beds, or planning to establish such beds or to convert acute care to long-term care beds has also increased significantly (Read and O'Brien, 1986).

A growing number of hospitals sponsor membership programs that provide a package of special services such as health screening, annual exams at reduced costs, telephone reassurance, and help with complex insurance forms. Such "health clubs" as Eldermed, Goldencare Plus, and Health Wise have sprung up around the country. Most are aimed at the financially better off portion of the elderly who have Medicare Parts A and B, *and* with supplementary "medigap" insurance. They do not address the needs of uninsured elderly, nor do they generally reduce the cost of outpatient medical care or hospitalization. Many of these programs do, however, offer discounts on eyeglasses and medication. As competition among hospitals increases, these clubs may eventually lead to lower health care costs for older people.

Other developments in the health care industry may also reduce costs for future generations. Health maintenance organizations (HMOs), for example, have attracted many older persons as members by providing comprehensive health care at lower average costs than private hospitals and physicians. These hospitals are also leading the way in preventive medicine and health promotion. Some existing private hospitals are converting to HMOs. Similarly, the increased number of alternative health care providers such as geriatric nurse practitioners offer older persons quality health services for chronic conditions without the high costs of traditional physician-based care. The growth of geriatric education in colleges of medicine, nursing, dentistry, social work, pharmacy, and in other areas such as nutrition and physical therapy suggest that a well-trained cadre of health care providers will become increasingly available to future elderly. These developments in hospital and community-based health services, combined with the increased number of health specialists training in geriatrics, offer hope for cost containment beyond what can be achieved by DRGs and incremental reforms in Medicare and Medicaid. They will also assure improved quality of medical care for older people.

LONG-TERM CARE IN THE FUTURE

Advances in long-term care for the chronically ill also offer future elderly the promise of greater options if they should ever need such care. As noted in Chapter 19, long-term care includes the array of community services that are needed on a continuing basis to enable people with chronic disabilities to maintain their physical, social, and psychological functioning, but these conditions do not generally require constant medical monitoring. Traditionally, such services have been provided by nursing homes, an alternative that has drained the resources of most older residents and their families. Currently, the possibility of long-term care for a chronic illness or functional limitation poses the greatest single threat to the economic security of all but the wealthiest of older Americans. Because of the limited help available in either our public programs or through the private sector to pay for potentially expensive long-term care, the need for a comprehensive, national long-term care policy, as well as for private long-term care insurance options, is likely to grow in the future.

Current expectations that families should assume more responsibility for long-term care are unrealistic, because of cost, and demographic and social trends that were discussed earlier. As noted, women, traditionally caregivers of the elderly, are now more likely to be employed than were previous generations; a typical life course of school, work, marriage, and caregiving no longer exists for most women. Yet few of our current or proposed programs adequately address the critical policy issue of the multiple demands on family caregivers. Geographic and occupational mobility may further reduce the family's ability to provide care, even though they may want to help their older relatives as much as possible. The problem of caring for elders with chronic illnesses is compounded by the increasing proportion of veterans living into advanced old age. This group has traditionally received federal funding for health services as a means of recognizing their contributions to society. Already, the Veterans Administration has raised the eligibility criteria for many health services as a means of cutting costs, thereby expecting families and the private sector to fill the gap. In sum, a major policy dilemma for the twenty-first century is: How much should long-term care services for the elderly cost, and who should pay for which services? What should be the role of government, the private sector, and the family in meeting the elderly's long-term care needs? These policy issues inevitably raise ethical dilemmas about the distribution of resources among various segments of society.

ETHICAL DILEMMAS

At the forefront of ethical dilemmas in an aging society is the issue of the prolongation of life. As a society, we have valued finding cures for dread diseases and forestalling death as long as possible. Medical technology has made it possible to extend life expectancy, but not necessarily *active* life expectancy, whereby a person is able to function fairly independently into advanced old age. We are far from achieving the goal of "squaring the life expectancy course," where a healthy life is followed by a quick illness and death (Black and Levy, 1981; Fries, 1980). Many elderly are now saved, often at great cost, from diseases that previously would have killed them, only to be guaranteed death from still another, at equally high or even higher costs. Life-support systems, organ transplants, and other advances in medical technology have made it possible to prolong the life of the chronically and terminally ill, and have blurred definitions of when life ends. For example, technology now allows the transplantation of various human tissues, and life can be prolonged by machines that keep the body functioning even if the conscious mind has died. But these advances have not necessarily ensured "quality of life."

The timing, place, and conditions of death are increasingly under medical control. The President's Commission for the Study of Ethical Problems in Medicine and Biomedical and Behavioral Research (1983) concluded that these new developments have made death more a matter of deliberate decision. For almost any life-threatening condition, some interventions can now delay the moment of death, but not its inevitability. Doctors and nurses have always dealt with dying, but not until the present technical advances have they had so much power and responsibility to control how long life lasts. As a result, these new medical capabilities demand a new set of ethics and practices (Older Women's League, 1986). At the core of these ethical issues is the question of who decides what for whom.

Decisions about whether and how to intervene can be excruciating for doctors, nurses, family members, and older patients. Where do you set the limits? At what point do you stop prolonging life, when the alternative is so final? How much suffering is "worth it" to stay alive? Which is more important: *quality* or *quantity* of life? And how do we measure or determine quality of life? Under what conditions and for which decisions should the wishes of the patient supercede those of his or her family members? What institutional mechanisms should be employed to resolve ethical conflicts? These decisions become even more complex when the older person is mentally incompetent, such as with an Alzheimer's patient. Medical professionals have been taught to spare no effort in keeping a patient alive. But increasingly, professionals and laypersons are questioning whether dying should be prolonged indefinitely when there is no possibility of recovery. Two powerful professions, medicine and law, are faced with clarifying both the definition of death and the rights, duties, and obligations of all those involved in the decision-making process.

Ethical considerations cannot be completely divorced from economic issues, however, given that 25 percent of Medicare expenditures cover costs in the last year of life (OWL, 1986). With pressures mounting to reduce medical bills paid with public funds, interventions to extend life are increasingly questioned. Does the quality of life gained justify the enormous expenditures often entailed by such interventions? When public resources are scarce, questions become framed in terms of how benefits should be distributed among various groups in society. As we have seen, the intergenerational inequity perspective maintains that economic imbalances caused by the provision of health care for the elderly potentially threaten the welfare of younger generations and of society as a whole (Callahan, 1986). Surrounding all such matters are issues of who should decide, in the aggregate and in individual instances, who receives what types of care.

Given our present social values for aggressive treatment, what options are available to control costs that do not significantly reduce adequate health care to the elderly? For example, under the DRG system, described in Chapter 19, the economic incentive can shift from keeping a person alive to allowing the patient to die, or, at least, to removing the patient from hospital care. As a result of policy shifts, there is the risk that, for economic reasons, life-sustaining treatment will be withheld from patients. In fact, opponents of "right to die" legislation fear that economic considerations may override compassionate concerns, with governments eventually requiring removal of life supports from the elderly as a way to control health care costs. They also argue that family members who are eager for their older relative's inheritance may put undue pressure on them to forego any life-sustaining technologies. When the former Governor of Colorado suggested the removal of life supports from terminally ill older patients as a way to reduce costs, there was a tremendous outcry from aging advocates.

Although the economic rationale for such decisions is generally condemned, there is growing public support for individual determination regarding life-sustaining treatment; as noted in Chapter 14, state legislatures are responding to this sentiment by passing "right to die" or "death with dignity" legislation. Hospital ethics committees continue to multiply throughout the country. And courts, albeit slowly, are upholding the right of individuals to make their own medical decisions. But court decisions have been conflicting, and definitions of *death* and *terminal condition* continue to be challenged, suggesting that the legal, medical, and ethical issues are far from settled. The question of who should control decisions about life and death will continue to be argued among doctors, families, and often lawyers. Conflicting pressures for change will likely give way to the creation of new norms, whereby more people will support the removal of life supports for the terminally ill and will want to have control over their own death. Countering these developments, however, will be a strong societal presumption about the value of aggressive treatment (Callahan, 1986).

Another closely related concern is *who* should receive life-saving techniques, such as organ transplants and kidney dialysis. Critics argue that with nearly 33 million people under age 65 without health care insurance and many more who cannot afford high-tech care, our health care system should first address such basic needs, rather than spending disproportionate resources for expensive procedures for only a few. Debates about an equitable provision of services versus targeting life-saving interventions for a few will intensify in the future. These debates will also be framed in terms of allocating scarce health care resources to the young, defined as an investment, versus the old. However, we have no accurate way of comparing the benefits of physical mobility allowed an older person by an expensive hip-and-joint replacement with those of an improved secondary education for a teenager, for example (Callahan, 1986).

Ultimately, these decisions come down to how much our society values the elderly. Our society's medical success story is that the conquest of infectious disease reduced the health care needs of the young while at the same time prolonging longevity. But with the accompanying persistence of chronic diseases, the elderly's health needs are now grossly disproportionate to their numbers. If high and ever-escalating health care costs are inherent in an aging and developed society, then we will have to face severe moral questions about the desirability of medical innovation, about the value we place on preserving and improving the elderly's health, and about the comparative rights of different generations to the necessary resources of life (Callahan, 1986). Just how much do we owe the elderly and why? What is our obligation to the elderly in the face of health care needs and prerogatives of other age groups? Finally, how many and what kinds of economic burdens should society be prepared to bear to ensure adequate health care for the older population? These larger ethical questions will translate into daily practice dilemmas for those who are faced with the reality of caring for chronically ill and dying elderly, as well as for children with acute medical needs in an era of diminishing resources for social and health services.

As the older population continues to increase, the decisions regarding the allocation and withholding of health care to individuals will assume greater importance. These decisions must be made by an informed and humanistic society; they cannot be left to policymakers, physicians, and attorneys only. What many today consider medical or geriatric issues will increasingly influence the lives of most Americans, young and middle-aged, not just the old (Avorn, 1986). For these reasons, it is important to understand the processes of aging, as well as the policies and services that affect the older population and how these policies are made, so that society as a whole can make informed choices. In the following section, we will review some of the many opportunities for careers in gerontology. Whether or not gerontology is chosen as a career, however, it is important for all of us to become informed about this field so that we can become better consumers, citizens, advocates, and caregivers to frail elderly within our families and in our communities.

CAREERS IN GERONTOLOGY

One reason for studying social gerontology is to determine the types of career opportunities in this field. It should be clear by now that gerontology holds great promise for practitioners, researchers, and teachers in diverse aspects of the field. As we have seen throughout this book, specialists in geriatric health care will assume a greater role in helping the growing population of older people to maintain their quality of life, both in terms of treating chronic diseases and in preventing health problems. The increasing number of geriatric training programs in schools of medicine, nursing, dentistry, pharmacy, social work, and public health attest to the importance of this field. Specialists in geriatric nutrition and physical and occupational therapy will be in greater demand in the future as options expand in housing and long-term care. Attorneys with special training in medical ethics and aging will become critical members of the gerontological team. The increased interest in leisure activities in old age will call for more recreation specialists. Architects and planners will be called upon to design housing that is sensitive to the needs of older people. Social workers and psychologists will be needed to work with older people and their families as counselors, advocates, support group facilitators, discharge planners, and case managers who coordinate services. Program planners, developers, and managers will have opportunities in a myriad of areas such as retirement housing for elderly, senior centers, adult day health programs, chore services, home health care, and respite care. There will even be opportunities for computer programmers and designers, as well as specialists in electronic communication, to design new products to help maintain older people's independence for as long as possible.

As noted throughout this book, more research is needed on the normal and pathological aspects of aging, and how age-related changes influence older people's social functioning. Researchers trained in sociology, psychology, economics, and political science must work with biologists, geneticists, nutritionists, and others in the basic and clinical sciences to examine these important issues in aging.

In many ways, the field of gerontology is limited only by one's imagination.

For those of you motivated and concerned about improving the quality of life for current and future generations of older people, we hope that the issues raised in this book will encourage you to join this exciting and challenging field.

References

Antonucci, T. Personal characteristics, social support and social behavior. In R. Binstock and E. Shanas (Eds.), *Handbook of aging and the social sciences* (2d ed.). New York: Van Nostrand and Reinhold, 1985.

Atchley, R. C. Retirement and leisure participation: Continuity or crisis? *The Gerontologist*, 1971, 2, 13–17.

Avorn, J., Medicine: The life and death of Oliver Shay. In A. Pifer and L. Bronte (Eds.), *Our aging society: Paradox and promise.* New York: W. W. Norton, 1986.

Black, P., and Levy, E. Aging, natural death and the compression of morbidity: Another view. *New England Journal of Medicine*, 1981, 304, 854–56.

Brody, E. Parent care as a normative family stress. *The Gerontologist*, 1985, 25, 19–30.

Butler, R., and Gleason, H. *Productive aging: Enhancing vitality in later life.* New York: Springer, 1985.

Callahan, D., Health care in the aging society: A moral dilemma. In A. Pifer and L. Bronte (Eds.), *Our aging society: Paradox and promise.* New York: W. W. Norton, 1986.

Congressional Institute for the Future. *Tomorrow's elderly.* 1984.

Family ties. *American Demographics*, 1986, 8(4), 11–12.

Friedan, B. *The second stage.* New York: Summit Books, 1981.

Fries, J. F. Aging, natural death, and the compression of morbidity. *The New England Journal of Medicine*, 1980, 303, 130–135.

Furstenberg, F., Nord, C. W., Peterson, J. L., and Zill, N. The life course of children of divorce: Marital disruption and parental contact. *American Sociological Review*, 1983, 48, 656–668.

Glick, P. Remarriage: Some recent changes and variations. *Journal of Family Issues*, 1980, 1, 455–478.

Goldman, N., and Lord, G. Sex differences in life cycle measures of widowhood. *Demography*, 1983, 20, 177–195.

Gordon, C., Gaitz, C. M., and Scott, J. Leisure and lives: Personal expressivity across the life span. In R. H. Binstock and E. Shanas (Eds.), *Handbook of aging and the social sciences* (1st ed.). New York: Van Nostrand Reinhold, 1976.

Hagestad, G. The family: Women and grandparents as kin-keepers. In A. Pifer and L. Bronte (Eds.), *Our aging society: Paradox and promise.* New York: W. W. Norton, 1986.

Hagestad, G., and Neugarten, B. Age and the life course. In E. Shanas and R. Binstock (Eds.), *Handbook of aging and the social sciences* (2d ed.). New York: Van Nostrand and Reinhold, 1985.

Haraven, T. Family time and historical time. *Daedelus*, Spring 1977, 57–70.

Kabanoff, B. Work and nonwork: A review of models. *Psychological Bulletin* 1980, *88*, 60–77.

Kalish, R. The new ageism and the failure models: A polemic. *The Gerontologist,* 1979, *19*, 398–402.

Logan, J. R. The graying of the suburbs. *Aging,* 1983, *345*, 4–8.

National Center for Health Statistics. *Monthly Vital Statistics Report,* Vol. 32, No. 4. Hyattsville, Md.: Public Health Service, 1983.

Older Women's League. *Death and dying: Staying in control to the end of our lives.* Washington, D.C., 1986.

Osgood, N. J. Work: Past, present and future. In N. J. Osgood (Ed.), *Life after work: Retirement, leisure, recreation, and the elderly.* New York: Praeger, 1982.

President's Commission for the Study of Ethical Problems in Medicine and Biomedical and Behavioral Research. *Deciding to forego life sustaining treatment.* Washington, D.C.: U.S. Government Printing Office, 1983.

Preston, S. Children and the elderly in the U.S. *Scientific American,* 1984, 59–85.

Read, W. A., and O'Brien, J. L. New trends in hospital-based services for the elderly. *Trustee,* Sept. 1986, 20–22.

Rice, D. P., and Feldman, J. J. Living longer in the United States: Demographic changes and health needs of the elderly. *Milbank Fund Memorial Quarterly/Health and Society,* 1983, *61*, 362–396.

Riley, M. W., and Riley, J. Longevity and social structure: The potential of the added years. In A. Pifer and L. Bronte (Eds.), *Our aging society: Paradox and promise.* New York: W. W. Norton, 1986.

Robinson, P. K., Coberly, S., and Paul, C. E. Work and retirement. In R. H. Binstock and E. Shanas (Eds.), *Handbook of aging and the social sciences* (2d ed.). New York: Van Nostrand Reinhold, 1985.

Schneider, E. L., and Brody, J. A. Aging, natural death, and the compression of morbidity: Another view. *New England Journal of Medicine,* 1983, *309*, 854–856.

Spanier, G., and Glick, P. Paths to remarriage. *Journal of Divorce,* 1980, 283–298.

Stroller, E. Parental caregiving by adult children. *Journal of Marriage and the Family,* November 1983, 851–858.

Uhlenberg, P. Changing configurations of the life course. In T. Harevan (Ed.), *Transitions: The family and the life course in historical perspectives.* New York: Academic Press, 1978.

Uhlenberg, P. Death and the family. *Journal of Family History,* Fall 1980, 313–324.

U.S. Bureau of the Census. *Current Population Survey,* March 1982, unpublished.

U.S. Senate Special Committee on Aging. *Aging America: Trends and projections, 1985–86 edition.* U.S. Department of Health and Human Services, 1986.

Verbrugge, L. Longer life but worsening health? Trends in health and mortality of middle-aged and older persons. *Milbank Memorial Fund Quarterly,* 1984, *62*, 475–519.

Winsborough, H. A demographic approach to the life cycle. In K. W. Back (Ed.), *Life course: Integrative theories and examplary populations.* Boulder, Col.: Westview Press, 1978.

Index